ORTHOPEDIC
INTERVENTIONS
FOR THE PHYSICAL THERAPIST ASSISTANT

ORTHOPEDIC INTERVENTIONS

FOR THE PHYSICAL THERAPIST ASSISTANT

Maureen Raffensperger, PT, DPT

Board Certified Clinical Specialist in Orthopaedic Physical Therapy
Professor/Director, PTA Program
Missouri Western State University

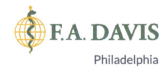

F.A. DAVIS

Philadelphia

F. A. Davis Company
1915 Arch Street
Philadelphia, PA 19103
www.fadavis.com

Copyright © 2020 by F. A. Davis Company

Printed in the United States of America

Last digit indicates print number: 10 9 8 7 6 5 4 3 2 1

Publisher: Margaret A. Biblis
Director of Content Development: George Lang
Senior Acquisitions Editor: Melissa A. Duffield
Senior Sponsoring Editor: Jennifer A. Pine
Content Project Manager II: Elizabeth Stepchin
Art and Design Manager: Carolyn O'Brien

As new scientific information becomes available through basic and clinical research, recommended treatments and drug therapies undergo changes. The author(s) and publisher have done everything possible to make this book accurate, up to date, and in accord with accepted standards at the time of publication. The author(s), editors, and publisher are not responsible for errors or omissions or for consequences from application of the book, and make no warranty, expressed or implied, in regard to the contents of the book. Any practice described in this book should be applied by the reader in accordance with professional standards of care used in regard to the unique circumstances that may apply in each situation. The reader is advised always to check product information (package inserts) for changes and new information regarding dose and contraindications before administering any drug. Caution is especially urged when using new or infrequently ordered drugs.

Library of Congress Cataloging-in-Publication Data

Names: Raffensperger, Maureen, author.
Title: Orthopedic interventions for the physical therapist assistant /
  Maureen Raffensperger.
Description: Philadelphia : F.A. Davis Company, [2019] | Includes bibliographical
  references and index.
Identifiers: LCCN 2018058582 (print) | LCCN 2018059083 (ebook) | ISBN
  9780803658950 | ISBN 9780803643710 (alk. paper)
Subjects: | MESH: Manipulation, Orthopedic—methods | Physical Therapist Assistants
Classification: LCC RM724 (ebook) | LCC RM724 (print) | NLM WB 535 | DDC
  615.8/2—dc23
LC record available at https://lccn.loc.gov/2018058582

Preface

After working with PTAs and teaching PTA students for well over 35 years, I am hopeful that this text is a testament to the respect I have for PTAs, and my optimism for the role of the PTA in the future of our profession.

As an orthopedic practitioner, it is important that the PTA understand the PT/PTA team, the use of evidence to inform practice, how tissues heal, and the effect of interventions on tissue healing. These basic principles are discussed in the first four chapters.

The remainder of the book is laid out by region. In each chapter, I have given a brief overview of the relevant anatomy and kinematics of the region. Common pathologies are then presented. The organization of pathologies is according to a description, contributing factors or causes, signs and symptoms, special tests, common interventions, prevention, and surgical interventions. A summary box of the pathology is presented after each discussion.

In this text, I have tried to focus on what PTAs do: data collection and intervention. I have provided the greatest detail on special tests and interventions. In addition to goniometry, manual muscle testing, and functional mobility testing, orthopedic physical therapy has many tests that are used by the PT to inform the diagnosis, and by the PT and PTA to inform patient progress. These tests become a keystone in the PTA's communication with the PT.

I have attempted throughout this book to provide information on common orthopedic pathologies and interventions that have been shown through research to be effective. Nevertheless, it is important to practice within the established plan of care (POC). Variance between the POC and suggested interventions in the text may provide the PTA with a deeper appreciation for the clinical reasoning that accompanies the PT evaluation.

Reviewers

Dianne Abels, M.S.P.T.
Associate Professor, Academic Coordinator of Clinical
    Education
Physical Therapist Assistant Program
Black Hawk College
Moline, IL

Morton Joseph Aime, PT, DPT, OCS, GCS
Assistant Professor
Arts, Sciences and Health Professions
Our Lady of the Lake College
Baton Rouge, LA

Jo Ann Beine, PTA, MLS
Faculty, Physical Therapist Assistant Program
PTA Department
Arapahoe Community College
Littleton, CO

Patricia Brady, PT, DSCPT
Instructional Specialist
PTA Department
Anne Arundel Community College
Arnold, MD

Nijah Chinn-Gonsalves, PT, MHA, DHS
Physical Therapist Assistant Program Director
Physical Therapist Assistant Program
ECPI University
Richmond, VA

Matthew Connell, MPT
Program Director
Physical Therapist Assistant Program
State College of Florida
Bradenton, FL

Sam M. Coppoletti, PT, DPT, CSCS
Program Coordinator/Educator
Department of Science and Health
University of Cincinnati Clermont College
Batavia, OH

Laura-Beth Falter, Registered Physiotherapist (Ontario),
BSc.PT, MSc.
(Rehabilitation Science)
Instructor
Faculty of Healthcare
triOS College
London, Ontario, Canada

Lisa Finnegan, PTA, ACCE
Instructor and Academic Coordinator of Clinical
    Education
Physical Therapist Assistant Program
College of Southern Nevada
Las Vegas, NV

Zachary D. Frank, DPT, MS (HCA)
Associate Professor
Allied Health
Washburn University
Topeka, KS

Michael B. Fritz, MS, ATC, PTA
Professor
Physical Therapist Assistant Program
North Shore Community College
Danvers, MA

Judith Gawron, MSPT, DPT
Professor
AHS (PTA) Department
Berkshire Community College
Pittsfield, MA

Ann Marie Herbert, MPT, OCS
Part-time Instructor, PTA program
Physical Therapy
Rehabilitation Health Center, Washtenaw Community
    College
Ann Arbor, MI

Kelly N. Jackson, PTA
Instructor
Physical Therapist Assistant Department
Clarkson College
Omaha, NE

Julianne Klepfer, BS PT/MASS
Assistant Professor
Physical Therapist Assistant Program
SUNY Broome Community College
Binghamton, NY

Heather MacKrell, PT, PhD
Program Director
Department of Health Science
Calhoun Community College
Tanner, AL

Jose Milan, PTA, M.Ed.
Dept. Chair/Associate Professor
PTA Department
Austin Community College
Austin, TX

Marisa C. Miller, PT
Assistant Professor
Health Programs
Walters State Community College
Morristown, TN

Deborah S. Molnar, PT, DPT, MSEd
PTA Program Director
Physical Therapist Assistant Program
State University of New York College of Technology at
    Canton
Canton, NY

Jeremy Oldham, MEd, BS, PTA
Academic Clinical Coordinator of Education
Physical Therapist Assistant Program
Allegany College of Maryland
Cumberland, MD

Jean E. Sanchez, PTA, BHS, MHS
Assistant Professor
Bachelors of Health Services Administration
Washburn University
Topeka, KS

Jacqueline Shakar, DPT, MS OCS LAT
PTA Department Chair
PTA Department
Mount Wachusett Community College
Gardner, MA

Lori Slettehaugh, MPT
Associate Professor
Physical Therapist Assistant Program
Kansas City Kansas Community College
Kansas City, KS

Roschella Stephens, PT, MS, CSCS
Faculty
Physical Therapist Assistant Program
Central Piedmont Community College
Charlotte, NC

Debbie Van Dover, PT, M.Ed.
Program Director, MHCC PTA Program
Health Professions
Mt. Hood Community College
Gresham, OR

Lisa J. Weaver, BS, PTA, LMT, NCTMB
Physical Therapist Assistant/Therapeutic Massage
    Instructor
Department of Health Science
Northeast Wisconsin Technical College
Green Bay, WI

Heather Brianne Wells, PT, DPT
Program Director
Physical Therapist Assistant Program
Wallace Community College
Dothan, AL

Rhonda Wesson, PTA
Full Time Faculty/Instructor
Physical Therapist Assistant Program
El Paso Community College
El Paso, TX

Krista M. Wolfe, DPT, ATC
Dean of Applied Sciences
Allied Health
Central Penn College
Carlisle, PA

Martha Yoder Zimmerman, PT, MA Ed
PTA Program Director/ACCE
Health Science Department
Caldwell Community College and Technical Institute
Hudson, NC

Acknowledgments

A project of this undertaking requires the support of many people. Foremost, I would like to thank my children, my sister, and my friends for their support, encouragement, and patience over the last several years, allowing me to prioritize the book.

I'd like to thank the staff of F.A. Davis, especially Melissa Duffield, Acquisitions Editor, and Jennifer Pine, Senior Sponsoring Editor. You are not just a publishing staff, but friends.

I'd like to thank my institution, Missouri Western State University, and my faculty colleagues for allowing me time to see this project through to completion.

I would like to express my appreciation to my physical therapy colleagues and my patients over the years. I've learned so much from you. Finally, I would like to thank my students for keeping the journey fresh.

Maureen Raffensperger

Contents

Chapter 9

Orthopedic Interventions for the Thoracic and Lumbosacral Spine 207

PART I

Physical Therapist Assistant and Orthopedic Management

Chapter 1

The Role of the Physical Therapist Assistant in Orthopedic Physical Therapy

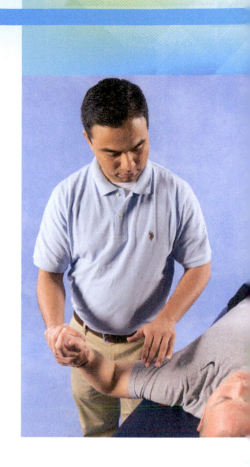

Patient Examination and Evaluation
>   **Medical History**
>   **Physical Examination**
>   **Medical Alert Flags**

The Role of the PTA
>   **Providing Interventions**
>   **Collecting Data**
>   **Communicating**
>   **Tying Them All Together With Critical Thinking**

Guiding Principles of Orthopedic Physical Therapy

Summary

LEARNING OUTCOMES

After reading this chapter, the student will:

1.1 Explain the importance of the plan of care in guiding the data collection and interventions to be utilized in treatment of the orthopedic patient.

1.2 Identify five significant findings in the patient history and explain their impact on orthopedic treatments.

1.3 Identify five significant findings in the patient physical examination and explain their impact on orthopedic treatments.

1.4 Discuss the use of special tests in the physical examination, and the importance of correctly reproducing and interpreting the tests used as a measure of patient progress.

1.5 Name five components of the physical therapist assistant's role in treating orthopedic pathologies using the problem-solving algorithm.

KEY WORDS

Cluster of tests	Red, yellow, orange, blue, and black flags	Plan of care
		Special tests

Introduction

The importance of physical therapy in treatment of orthopedic pathology is well accepted, and the physical therapist assistant (PTA) is a valuable extender of the physical therapist (PT) for this patient population. The PTA must have a thorough understanding of common orthopedic pathologies, their causes or contributing factors, associated symptoms, clinical signs, common interventions, and preventive measures. In addition to providing excellent patient care, the PTA must:

- Be particularly attentive to changes in the status of the patient
- Communicate effectively with the supervising PT
- Methodically collect data, including results of specific tests
- Provide evidence-based treatment interventions that are within the PT-prescribed **plan of care** (POC) for the patient
- Educate the patient

Patient Examination and Evaluation

The physical therapist performs the initial examination and evaluation of the patient. This includes taking a medical history and performing a basic physical exam followed by a more specific physical exam, all of which lead to establishing a POC for the patient. To provide appropriate care, the PTA must have a thorough understanding of the plan of care, including any contraindications or precautions, prior to treating the patient.

Medical History

When taking the patient's medical history and mindfully listening to the patient's description of his or her symptoms or complaints, the evaluating PT begins to discern the patient's problem and narrow the focus of the physical examination.

Common elements in the patient history include:

- A description of the patient's complaint
- Information regarding possible precipitating factors
- Time since onset
- Irritability
- Aggravating and relieving factors
- Diagnostic tests that have been performed (Table 1-1)
- Previous treatments or surgery
- Premorbid conditions including medical diseases or illnesses
- Current medications (Table 1-2)
- Occupational and/or daily activities
- Living situation
- Prior level of function

Physical Examination

The basic physical examination follows the history. In this basic physical examination, the PT conducts a systems review on the patient, screening each system: musculoskeletal, neuromuscular, integumentary, cardiovascular-pulmonary, gastrointestinal, and genitourinary. The physical therapist gathers information on the patient's present symptoms, assessing vital signs, range of motion, strength, sensation/proprioception, swelling, balance, coordination, reflexes, posture, tenderness to palpation, and functional mobility. After the basic examination, the PT should have one or more working hypotheses regarding the patient's condition.

A more specific physical examination follows, with the goal of supporting or refuting the hypotheses. The specific examination includes an assessment of the patient's response to joint mobilization, positions, movements, and **special tests**. There are hundreds of special tests in orthopedic physical therapy. These tests vary in diagnostic value. The PT often uses several tests to rule in or rule out a diagnosis. Some special tests increase in sensitivity or specificity when performed as part of a **cluster of tests**. If the literature supports using a cluster of special tests, this will be presented in the text.

The PTA must be familiar with the data collection techniques and special tests used by the PT so that he or she can fully interpret the findings of the examination, understand the POC, and adequately communicate changes in the patient's status to the PT. Throughout this text, the commonly collected data for each pathology is presented. Data which is assessed by the PT and PTA, with normal values, measurement scales, and parameters is presented in Table 1-3.

Medical Alert Flags

As the PT performs the physical examination, he or she makes note of medical "**red flags**" that may indicate more severe pathology. Red flag findings usually indicate the need to refer the patient to another medical professional for further testing. Some common red flags that the PT must be aware of are listed in Table 1-4.

Because PT is a doctoring profession, practitioners of physical therapy have become increasingly aware of red flags over the past two decades. More recently, the profession adopted the terminology of yellow, orange, blue, and black flags to indicate other factors that affect patient care and treatment. Categorizing findings in this way helps the PTA recognize the biopsychosocial factors that can impact patient symptoms and response to treatment.

Yellow flags are psychosocial factors, including beliefs the patient has about his or her physical problems. **Orange flags** are findings of psychiatric illness. **Blue flags** are

Table 1-1   Diagnostic Tests

Diagnostic Tests Provide Useful Information in the Evaluation and Treatment of Orthopedic Pathologies.

Test	Purpose
X-ray	To diagnose fracture, dislocation, arthritis, osteonecrosis, bone tumors.
Computed tomography (CT) scan	To diagnose tumor or fracture that does not show on x-rays, as well as pathology of the chest, abdomen, and pelvis. Superior to MRI for pneumonia, cancer, bone pathology, and bleeding in the brain.
MRI	To diagnose soft tissue pathology of muscle, ligament sprain, cartilage, and disc. Superior to CT for brain tumor and pathology of the spinal cord.
Bone scan	To diagnose stress fractures, arthritis, bone infection, and cancer.
Doppler ultrasound	To diagnose blood clots.
Angiogram	To visualize the blood flow through an artery or vein, to diagnose artery disease and aneurysm.
Myelogram	To diagnose herniated disc, spinal stenosis. Dye is injected into the subarachnoid space, followed by x-ray or CT.
Arthrogram	To diagnose pathology of joint ligaments, cartilage, tendons, and capsule.
Discogram	Determines the health of the intervertebral disc. Dye is injected into the disc followed by a CT scan.
Dual-energy x-ray absorptiometry (DEXA)	Measures bone density to diagnose osteopenia and osteoporosis.
Electromyography (EMG)	Determines and evaluates nerve and muscle function, to diagnose neuropathy, radiculopathy, and CNS pathology that affects muscle.
Nerve conduction velocity (NCV) study	Often done with an EMG to evaluate nerve function. Used to diagnose nerve entrapment.

Table 1-2   Common Medications Used to Treat Orthopedic Pathologies

Medication Class	Drug Names Generic (Brand)	Effects	Precautions	Common Side Effects (>1%)
Non-steroidal anti-inflammatory drug (NSAID)	naproxen (Aleve, Naprosyn) aspirin celecoxib (Celebrex) ibuprofen (Motrin, Advil) meloxicam (Mobic)	Reduce inflammation, reduce fever, relieve pain	Contraindicated with aspirin allergy Increases liver enzymes Increases blood pressure Increases risk of heart attack and stroke	Nausea, vomiting, upset stomach, bleeding
Non-narcotic pain reliever	acetaminophen (Tylenol)	Reduce fever, relieve pain	None	No major side effects
Narcotic pain reliever	dextropoxyphene (Darvocet, Darvon) meperidine (Demerol) hydrocodone (Lortab, Lorcet, Vicodin) morphine (MS Contin) oxycodone (Percodan) tramadol (Ultram)	Decrease pain	Risk of addiction	Constipation, drowsiness, fatigue, nausea, vomiting, confusion, dry mouth, itchy skin, sweating

Continued

Table 1-2 Common Medications Used to Treat Orthopedic Pathologies—cont'd				
Medication Class	Drug Names Generic (Brand)	Effects	Precautions	Common Side Effects (>1%)
Skeletal muscle relaxant	cyclobenzaprine (Flexeril) orphenadrine (Norflex) methocarbamol (Robaxin, Robaxisal) metaxalone (Skelaxin) carisoprodol (Soma)	Decrease muscle spasm	Should not be taken by patients with cardiovascular disease or heart failure, glaucoma, liver disease, and hyperthyroidism; increases risk of seizure	Altered taste (metallic), blurred vision, dry mouth, drowsiness, fatigue, dizziness, headache, constipation
Steroidal anti-inflammatory	hydrocortisone prednisone dexamethasone (Decadron)	Decrease inflammation, decrease pain	Suppresses the immune system Increases blood sugar Increases blood pressure Decreases bone density Increases risk of psychiatric reactions	Fluid retention, insomnia, mood swings, heartburn, upset stomach

Table 1-3   Data Collected in Orthopedic Pathology Assessment

Vital Signs

Heart rate:
Age predicted maximum: use either traditional formula of 220 − age or Tanaka formula of 208 − (0.7 × age).
Exercise at 60%–80% of age predicted max or use Karvonen formula of $(0.7 \times HR_{reserve}) + HR_{rest}$, where $HR_{reserve} = HR_{max} - HR_{rest}$.

Blood pressure:
Prehypertension >120 systolic or >80 diastolic.
Hypertension >140 systolic or >90 diastolic.
   Patient should not exercise if systolic is >210 or diastolic is >110.

Respiratory rate:
Normal respiratory rate for an adult is 12–16 breaths per minute.
   Patient should not exercise if respiratory rate is >45/minute.

Oxygen saturation (O$_2$ sat):
Normal is 95%–99%.
   Generally be cautious if O$_2$ sat drops below 90, and patient should not exercise if O$_2$ sat drops below 85.

Temperature:
Normal body temperature is 97.8°F–99°F.
   Patients should not exercise with a fever.

Balance

Graded using balance tools such as the Timed Up and Go (TUG), four-position standing test, Berg Balance Test, etc.
Generally may be graded on a 0–4 scale as follows:
0 – unable to assume or maintain a position without maximal support.
1 – able to assume the position with help, such as arm support or caregiver support. Cannot maintain position without support.
2 – able to assume the position, but cannot maintain against resistance.
3 – able to maintain balance against moderate resistance.
4 – able to maintain balance against maximal resistance.

Range of Motion (ROM)

May measure selected joints and record in degrees or assess functionally.

Deep Tendon Reflexes (DTRs)

0 – absent
1+ – diminished
2+ – normal
3+ – minimally hyperactive
4+ – very hyperactive

Table 1-3   Data Collected in Orthopedic Pathology Assessment—cont'd

Strength

May assess by manual muscle test (MMT), dynamometer, or functionally. Grades of MMT are:

5 – able to complete the motion against gravity and hold against maximal resistance. Normal.

4 – able to complete the motion against gravity and hold against moderate resistance. Good.

3 – able to complete the motion against gravity but cannot hold against additional pressure. Fair.

2 – able to complete the motion with effect of gravity minimized. Poor.

1 – palpable muscle contraction with attempts to perform movement; no visible movement. Trace.

0 – no muscle contraction evident. Zero.

Posture

Sagittal plane: plumb line falls through external auditory meatus, through acromion process, posterior to the hip axis of rotation, anterior to the knee axis of rotation, and through the lateral malleolus.

Frontal plane: head midline, shoulders level, scapula 2 inches from the spinous processes, iliac crest level, popliteal crease level, feet neutral.

Transverse plane: head neutral, shoulders and pelvis perpendicular to feet, feet slightly externally rotated and equal bilaterally. Feet not pronated or supinated.

Edema

1+ normal. When finger is pressed to skin, a barely detectable impression is left.

2+ slight edema. When a finger is pressed to the skin, an indentation remains for up to 15 seconds.

3+ moderate edema. When a finger is pressed to the skin, an indentation remains for 15–30 seconds.

4+ significant edema. When a finger is pressed to the skin, an indentation remains for >30 seconds.

Functional Mobility

Grade assistance and quality of movement in supine to sit, sit to stand, transfers, standing, gait.

Independent – able to perform without assistance, devices, or extra time.

Modified independent – able to perform independently with modifications to the environment such as devices or extra time.

Set-up – able to perform independently after having the environment set up to facilitate the task.

Supervision – able to perform but needs distant supervision and/or verbal/visual cues with or without an assistive device.

Standby assist (SBA) – able to perform but needs close supervision and/or verbal/visual cues with or without an assistive device.

Contact guard assist (CGA) – able to perform but needs close supervision and tactile cues and/or verbal/visual cues with or without an assistive device.

Minimal assist – able to perform with only minimal assistance (about <25%) from a caregiver. Patient does about 75% of the task.

Moderate assist – able to perform with moderate assistance (about 50%) from a caregiver. Patient does about 50% of the task.

Maximum assist – able to perform with maximal assistance (about 75%) from a caregiver. Patient performs about 25% of the task.

Dependent – unable to perform.

Continued

Table 1-3   Data Collected in Orthopedic Pathology Assessment—cont'd

Pain

Graded on numeric scale of 0–10, visual analog scale, pain questionnaire, or Wong-Baker faces scale.

Muscle Tone

Graded on numeric scale of 0–5 using Modified Ashworth scale.

0 – no increase in muscle tone.

1 – slight increase in muscle tone, manifested by a catch and release, or by minimal resistance at the end of the ROM.

2 – slight increase in muscle tone, manifested by a catch, followed by minimal resistance throughout the remainder (less than half) of the range.

3 – more marked increase in muscle tone through most of the ROM, but affected part moves easily.

4 – considerable increase in muscle tone, passive movement is difficult.

5 – affected part rigid in movement.

Cognition

Alert and oriented × 4 scale:

Person, place, time, and situation

Other tools:

St. Louis University Mental Status Exam (SLUMS)

Mini-Cog

Table 1-4   Examples of Red Flags[1]

System	Sign/Symptom
Cardiovascular	• Chest pain, shoulder pain, neck pain, or temporomandibular joint (TMJ) pain occurring in the presence of coronary artery disease, especially if relieved by nitroglycerin • Upper quadrant pain that is reproduced by lower extremity activity (i.e., biking, walking, or stair climbing) • Fatigue that lasts beyond the expected duration during or after exercise • Fainting (syncope) without any warning signs prior to the event • Posterior leg or calf pain
Pulmonary	• Persistent cough, dyspnea • Shoulder pain that is aggravated by lying supine
Gastrointestinal	• Shoulder, back, pelvic, or sacral pain that is affected by food, milk, antacids
Integumentary	• Presence of recently discovered lumps or nodules or changes in previously present lumps or nodules • Recent changes in moles • Presence of enlarged, painless, rubbery lymph nodes
Neuromusculoskeletal	• Muscle weakness with decreased deep tendon reflexes • Bone pain, aggravated by weight bearing, which is worse at night • Pain that is not related to activity • Progressive neurologic deficits such as weakness, sensory loss, reflex changes, bowel or bladder dysfunction • Painless weakness • Unexplained weight loss • Pain that is not relieved by positional change or rest and is present at night • Chest, back, hip, or shoulder pain without history of trauma

[1]Adapted from Goodman, C. C, & Snyder, T. K. (2012). *Differential diagnosis for physical therapists: Screening for referral* (5th ed.). St. Louis, MO: Saunders.

Table 1-5	Examples of Biopsychosocial Medical Alert Flags
Flag	**Examples**
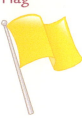	Yellow Flag: Catastrophizing, or thinking the worst about health problems. Having an excessive fear of movement, reinjury, or return to work. Being preoccupied with health. Having poor coping strategies.
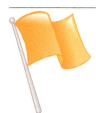	Orange Flag: Psychiatric illness including personality disorder, clinical depression.
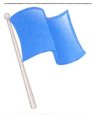	Blue Flag: Poor job satisfaction, poor relationship with coworkers or supervisor, unsupportive workplace, or belief that workplace that is not accommodating to altering job duties to facilitate return to work.
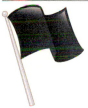	Black Flag: Policies or laws that do not facilitate return to work, conflict with insurance over claims, litigation, occupational hazards that are part of job.

perceived work-related factors that impact recovery. **Black flags** are similar to blue flags, but involve policies or rules involving the employee's return to work that impact recovery. Table 1-5 provides examples of yellow, orange, blue, and black flags.

The Role of the PTA

The role of the PTA on the PT-PTA team is dynamic. Patients often show significant changes from one treatment session to the next, making the practice of orthopedic physical therapy challenging and energizing. The PTA is responsible for providing procedural interventions, collecting pertinent data, and communicating with the supervising PT and others involved in the care of the patient.

Providing Interventions

After examining and evaluating the patient, the PT establishes the diagnosis, prognosis, plan of care, and goals for treatment of the patient. Several factors must be considered to determine whether the interventions are to be delegated to a PTA.[2]

- Are selected interventions within the scope of the PTA?
- Is the patient's condition sufficiently stable to delegate the intervention to a PTA?
- Are the intervention outcomes sufficiently predictable to delegate to a PTA?
- Does the PTA have the knowledge, skills, and abilities to provide the selected interventions?
- Have any risks and liabilities associated with the intervention been identified and managed?
- Have all payer requirements related to provision of PT services by a PTA been managed?

If the above considerations are met, the PT may direct the PTA to provide selected interventions. Using individual knowledge and experience, the PTA then chooses interventions that are within the plan of care established by the PT. The PTA may also modify interventions within the plan of care. Although the plan of care serves as a guide for treatment, choosing and modifying interventions requires that the PTA be knowledgeable about suitable and appropriate options.

Using the Problem-Solving Algorithm to Guide Interventions

The PTA constantly utilizes problem-solving processes in providing interventions. These processes include deciding when and how to provide selected interventions, when to modify the interventions, and how to ensure patient safety and comfort. The Departments of Education, Accreditation, and Practice of the American Physical Therapy Association collaborated to create the Problem-Solving Algorithm Utilized by PTAs in Patient/Client Intervention, which outlines these processes (Fig. 1.1). This algorithm is a very useful tool for PTA students and new graduates.

Collecting Data

Data collection occurs throughout the course of a patient's treatment to determine whether the patient is progressing. The PTA observes, questions, and assesses the patient to collect data (see Table 1-3). The PTA will subsequently reassess much of the data originally collected by the PT. The PTA may collect data regarding patient vital signs, cognition, range of motion, strength, end feel, edema, pain, balance, coordination, deep tendon reflexes, muscle tone, posture, functional mobility including gait, and/or special tests to determine whether the patient is progressing toward identified goals. The PTA reports data findings to the PT if the patient's progress is slow, if unexpected signs or symptoms are noted, and if the established goals are met.

Communicating

Of the three major components of patient care that the PTA provides, communication is the most crucial.

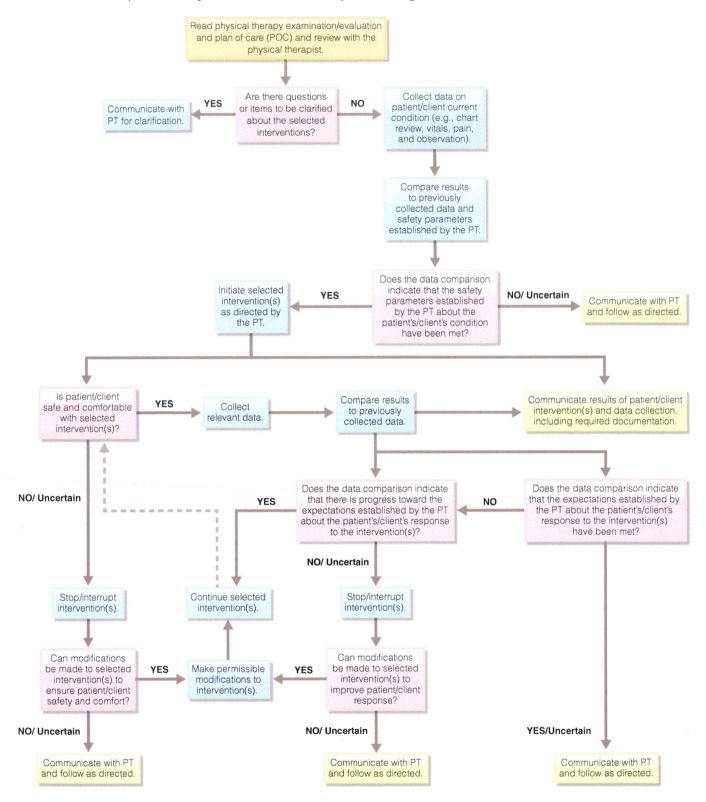

Figure 1.1 Problem-solving algorithm developed by the American Physical Therapy Association Departments of Education, Accreditation, and Practice. This algorithm outlines the problem-solving process used by PTAs when providing interventions.[3] *(American Physical Therapy Association. Problem-solving algorithm utilized by PTAs in patient/client intervention. In: A Normative Model of Physical Therapist Assistant Education: Version 2007. Alexandria, VA: American Physical Therapy Association, 84–85.)*

Box 1-1	**Examples of Active Listening Techniques of Restatement, Reflection, and Clarification**	
	Patient Says:	Example of PTA Response:
Restatement	"I hope I get better so that I can play with my grandkids."	"So, a goal of yours would be to be able to play with your grandkids?"
Reflection	"I hope my back gets better, so that I don't need surgery."	"It sounds like you are worried about the possibility of needing back surgery. I'm sure that would be difficult with your demanding job."
Clarification	"I'm not sure if therapy will help me since it didn't help the last time, and this time the problem is worse. I also have to consider that my daughter has to take time off work to bring me to therapy. I don't want to feel like a burden."	"So, are you most concerned about the likelihood that therapy will help the problem?"

Adapted from *Patient practitioner interaction: An experiential manual for developing the art of health care.*[4]

The PTA communicates verbally and nonverbally with the patient, the patient's family, the PT, health-care delivery personnel, and others. Due to the dynamic nature of orthopedic physical therapy and the relatively few number of patient visits, communication with the physical therapist is frequent.

Communicating With the Patient and Family

Patients want to know what is causing their symptoms, what the PT and PTA are doing about it, what they can do to get better, how long it will take to recover, how they can prevent recurrences, and the long-term expected outcome. The PT will have discussed these issues with the patient initially, and it is important for the PTA to be on the same page as the PT. Part of patient communication includes educating patients about their medical condition, but using confusing or complex medical terms that frighten the patients may have an adverse effect on their recovery. It's a good idea for the PTA to ask the PT about patient-specific considerations in communicating with the patient.

Listening to the patient is as important as talking. Active listening techniques include restatement, reflection, and clarification.[4] Box 1-1 gives examples of each of these forms of active listening.

Communicating With the PT

Effective communication between the PT and the PTA is paramount for successful patient care. Communication between the PT and the PTA should be open and honest, with information flowing in both directions. To avoid misunderstanding, the PTA clarifies any questions that he or she has about the examination findings and the proposed plan of care. The PT, in turn, needs to be informed of any unexpected responses, results of data collection, and progress toward goals. The PTA may suggest modifications to the plan of care to the PT, but any modification to the plan of care must be done by the PT. Six instances where communication with the supervising PT is essential are shown in the Problem-Solving Algorithm.

Communicating With Others

In addition to communication with the patient and the PT, the PTA communicates with other health-care providers and payers, often through written documentation. All documentation must accurately reflect the treatment provided in its entirety, not omitting anything that was done. Communication and documentation should be complete enough to allow another physical therapy provider to treat the patient in the absence of the original PTA. All documentation should be legible, accurate, timely, and concise.

Tying Them All Together With Critical Thinking

Critical thinking is fundamental to the practice of physical therapy. Data collected, interventions administered, and patient education presented are determined through critical thinking. Data collection informs intervention, which in turn leads to re-collection of data. Appropriate patient education is determined by data collection and includes information about interventions. Ultimately, communication with the PT and other health-care providers is necessary to share information. This is represented in Figure 1-2.

Guiding Principles of Orthopedic Physical Therapy

The following principles may be used to guide the PTA in treating patients with orthopedic pathologies:

1. Keep the patient as the primary concern.
2. Continually observe, think, listen, question. Remain curious.
3. Treat the patient holistically.

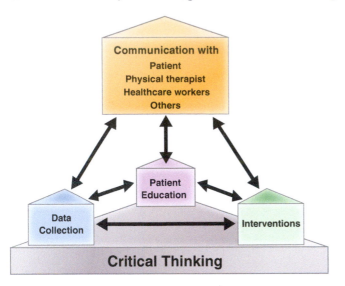

Figure 1.2 Critical thinking forms the foundation of physical therapy practice. The PTA collects data, provides interventions, and educates the patient and family. These components of care are what the PTA communicates to the PT and other health-care providers. Communication with other providers informs data collection, intervention, and patient education. All of these components are documented by the PTA.

4. Be mindful of tissue healing. Stress healing tissues as indicated in the plan of care.
5. Educate the patient but avoid using terminology that is frightening or worrisome.
6. Maintain communication with the supervising PT.
7. Follow the plan of care, using evidence to guide interventions.

SUMMARY

In the presence of an orthopedic pathology, physical therapy plays an important role in ensuring that the patient recovers as quickly and fully as possible. The PTA must have an understanding of the goals of orthopedic physical therapy, a knowledge of tissue healing, and an awareness of evidence-based interventions to assist the physical therapist in providing the highest standard of care. In the next three chapters, we'll be discussing each of these considerations.

REVIEW QUESTIONS

1. Discuss with your lab partner the impact on your treatment when you note each of the following in the patient history:
   a. Patient has a history of long-term use of prednisone (>7 years) for chronic COPD.
   b. Patient lives on the second floor of an apartment without an elevator.
   c. Patient complains of pain which began 2 years ago.
   d. Patient has a past medical history of spinal cord injury and paraplegia.
   e. Patient's job involves lifting over 50 lb several times a day.
   f. Patient rates pain 9/10 after getting out of bed, showering, and dressing.

2. Discuss with your lab partner the impact on your treatment when you note each of the following medical alerts on the initial evaluation:
   a. Patient has a history of depression and two suicide attempts.
   b. Patient's present complaint is due to a recent motor vehicle accident in which spouse died.
   c. Patient was hurt at work and states a deep dissatisfaction with his/her job.
   d. Patient states that the current problem is the worst thing that could happen, that it will never get better, and that pain is always a 10/10.

3. Read the following initial evaluation. Discuss with your lab partner the significant findings in the evaluation and plan of care. Describe at least six types of data that you would collect when providing care to this patient.

   The patient was seen for initial evaluation at home, on day 4 after elective total knee arthroplasty on the right. Vital signs: heart rate 75, blood pressure 138/74, respirations 14/min, O₂ saturation 98, temperature 98.4 degrees.

   The patient is a 65-year-old male who lives alone in a home with 3 steps to enter. There is a railing on the steps on both sides. The patient's niece is staying with him to help for the next week. He has a past medical history of chronic low back pain, unrepaired carpal tunnel syndrome bilaterally, and hypertension. He is employed at a local food plant, as a forklift driver. The patient states that he is eager to return to work, as he only has 2 weeks of paid time off. Prior level of function: the patient ambulated without a device independently, with complaint of pain in his knee. He was working full-time. Enjoys fixing old cars as a hobby.

   Objective findings: ROM is normal in upper extremities except right shoulder, which is limited to 140 degrees flexion and 120 abduction with complaint of pain (4/10). ROM in his left lower extremity, right hip, and right ankle is normal. R knee PROM measures 15–100, AROM measures 25–95. Strength in upper extremities is 5/5, with the exception of R shoulder strength in abduction which is 4/5 with pain (5/10). Pain in R knee is rated as 2/10 at best and 7/10 at worst.

   The patient is able to go sit to stand with CGA from a kitchen chair with arms. He requires min assist from a recliner. He ambulates with a wheeled walker with CGA/SBA, 40 feet, WBAT on the right. The patient goes supine to sit, and sit to supine, with min assist for his right leg. The patient ambulates up and down 3 steps with bilateral rails with CGA and verbal cueing.

The patient states that he has a home exercise program, and he demonstrates the exercises accurately. He uses ice at home for pain and swelling. The patient's wound is covered with a sterile dressing. Staples in place, with minimal yellow drainage noted.

4. You are the PTA assigned to the patient described in the previous question. You have been treating the patient for a week, and the patient is not showing any progress in gait. Applying the Problem-Solving Algorithm, discuss the options that you have. How would the plan of care affect your options?

REFERENCES

1. Goodman, C. C., & Snyder, T. K. (2012). *Differential diagnosis for physical therapists: Screening for referral* (5th ed.). St. Louis, MO: Saunders.
2. Crosier, J. (2010). PTA direction and supervision algorithms. PT in motion. Retrieved from http://www.apta.org/PTinMotion/2010/9/PTADirectionAlgorithmChart/ (accessed Nov 27, 2016).
3. American Physical Therapy Association (2007). Problem-solving algorithm utilized by PTAs in patient/client intervention. In *A normative model of physical therapist assistant education: Version 2007* (pp. 84–85). Alexandria, VA: American Physical Therapy Association.
4. Davis C. M. (2011). *Patient practitioner interaction: An experiential manual for developing the art of health care* (5th ed.). Philadelphia, PA: F.A. Davis.

Chapter 2

Evidence-Based Physical Therapy Practice

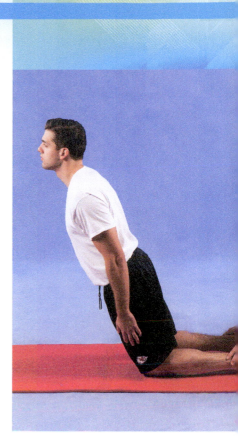

LEARNING OUTCOMES

At the end of this chapter, the student will:

2.1 Explain the concept of tiers of evidence, give an example of evidence in each tier, and explain how evidence in each tier impacts physical therapy practice.

2.2 Name the factors that led to the use of evidence to guide clinical decision making in the physical therapy profession.

2.3 Explain the role of the physical therapist assistant in applying evidence to practice.

2.4 Describe the role of the physical therapist assistant in contributing to the body of evidence in physical therapy practice.

2.5 Name and briefly describe the major sections of a research article.

2.6 Compare type I and type II errors.

2.7 Explain reliability, validity, sensitivity, and specificity.

2.8 Explain the relevance of minimal clinically important difference (MCID) in interpreting results of physical therapy interventions.

2.9 Explain how clinical practice guidelines (CPGs) contribute to best practice.

Introduction

The profession of physical therapy is on the cusp of arguably the most dynamic time in its history. In this environment, it is mandatory that practitioners of physical therapy use evidence to guide physical therapy practice and inform patient outcomes. Therefore, the interventions presented for the pathologies in this book are based on evidence of effectiveness. To put this evidence into perspective, however, the physical therapist assistant (PTA) must first understand what constitutes evidence, how the strength of the evidence is prioritized, and how the PTA integrates evidence into practice.

The application of evidence delivers vibrancy to the practice of physical therapy. Research can inform best practices, and be a source of variety and support in intervention choices. However, a significant component of evidence comes from the clinical expertise of the supervising physical therapist. As PTAs begin their practice they will themselves accumulate information about intervention effectiveness that will become a source of evidence for their future patients.

Why All This Talk About Evidence-Based Practice?

The concept of evidence-based medicine was first espoused by a team led by Gordon Guyatt, MD, in 1992.[1] In 1999, the American Physical Therapy Association (APTA) House of Delegates wrote a position statement in support of "development and utilization of **evidence-based practice** that includes the integration of best available research, clinical expertise, and patient values and circumstances related to patient/client management, practice management, and health policy decision making."[2] Since that time, there has been a huge increase in the amount of physical therapy research.[3] In a nutshell, the last two decades have seen an increase in the desire, the ability, and the need to base physical therapy practice on

evidence. **Evidence-based practice (EBP)** is now a guiding principle for the physical therapy profession. Several factors have driven the decision to apply evidence to practice:

- The improved ability to communicate and consume information directly resulting from the advances in technology and from the rise of the Internet.
- Increased patient awareness about their treatment options, in large part due to their use of the Internet to gain information.
- Improved ability to disseminate information to the physical therapy community.
- Requirements from third-party payers that PT practitioners demonstrate efficacy in their interventions, in response to rising health-care costs.
- Physical therapists and physical therapist assistants applying evidence to practice for the single purpose of improving outcomes for their patients.

Tiers of Evidence

So, what is *evidence*? Certainly, evidence includes research, but evidence includes clinical expertise as well. Evidence comes in many forms, and is typically ranked, in tiers, by the rigor of the process that produced it.[4] Evidence that ranks higher on the scale is considered more applicable, having greater **validity** and dependability. The lower the tier, the less dependable or credible the evidence. An example of how evidence may be ranked into six tiers is shown in Figure 2.1.

Tier 6: Expert Opinions, Anecdotal Data, and Experience

On the evidence hierarchy, anecdotal clinical experience and expert opinion rank as the lowest tier of

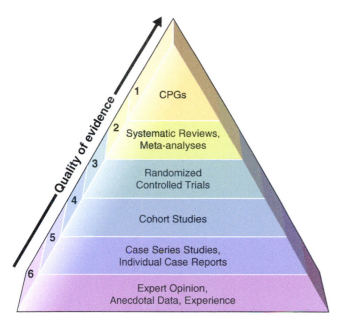

Figure 2.1 Six major tiers of evidence. Evidence is ranked according to strength. Lowest-strength evidence includes expert opinions and experience. Highest-tier evidence comes from systematic reviews, meta-analyses, and Clinical Practice Guidelines.

evidence—Tier 6. At this level of evidence, no study of the intervention has been performed.

Tier 5: Case Series Studies, Individual Case Reports

Moving up the hierarchy, the next level of evidence includes individual case reports, case series studies, and case-control studies. Each of these is also known as a **retrospective study,** that is, the study is performed by examining outcomes after treatment is completed. An individual **case study** involves exploring in retrospect one patient's condition and the effectiveness of interventions. An example of a case study is a report of a patient who sustained a patellar tendon rupture after a patellar fracture, titled *"Patellar tendon rupture following a patellar fracture."*[5]

A **case series study** analyzes an intervention effect on a small number of people who are similar in their medical conditions or their outcomes. Such studies are simply studying the effect of the intervention in general. An example of a case series study is an analysis of the effect of neuromuscular electrical stimulation (NMES) on quadriceps strength in three patients after a total knee arthroplasty titled *"Neuromuscular electrical stimulation for quadriceps muscle strengthening after bilateral total knee arthroplasty: a case series."*[6]

In a **case-control study,** subjects with a condition (case subjects) are compared with subjects who appear similar except for the absence of the condition (control subjects). This type of study design is used to identify factors that may contribute to a condition, but it allows for very limited conclusions due to a lack of **randomization** of the subjects. An example of a case-control study done by Barton et al. compared the amount of foot pronation in people with a specific knee pathology versus people without this knee pathology. This study, titled *"Foot and ankle characteristics in patellofemoral pain syndrome: a case control and reliability study"* sought to determine whether foot pronation is a contributing factor in developing this knee pathology.[7]

Tier 4: Cohort Studies

Cohort studies are in the next higher tier of evidence because they provide stronger evidence for a **hypothesis.** In a **cohort study,** subjects are grouped according to similar characteristics, such as age or gender. The study compares how the groups respond to an intervention. Because the subjects are followed over time, a cohort study is a **prospective study** (also called **longitudinal study**). Wideman et al. did a cohort study examining recovery from depression in patients with work-related injuries titled *"Recovery from depressive symptoms over the course of physical therapy: a prospective cohort study of individuals with work-related orthopaedic injuries and symptoms of depression."*[8]

Tier 3: Randomized Controlled Trials

A **randomized controlled trial** (RCT) is the next higher tier of evidence. An RCT is a study in which subjects are randomly assigned to the **experimental group** or the **control group.** The experimental group receives the treatment or intervention that is being studied; the control group does not. A comparison of the outcomes of the two groups is conducted prospectively. An example of an RCT is a comparison study done by Crossley et al. on the effectiveness of physical therapy in reducing patellofemoral pain. The study is titled *"Physical therapy for patellofemoral pain: a randomized, double-blinded, placebo-controlled trial."*[9]

The important distinction between an RCT and a case-control design is the randomization of a subject's assignment to a group in the RCT design. This method provides us with the expectation that the two groups are comparable and strengthens the evidence. To further strengthen the study, often the subjects are **blind** to the intervention they are receiving. This means that the subjects do not know to which group or intervention they are assigned. Better yet, the study may be a **double-blind** study, in which case both the subjects and the investigators collecting results are prevented from knowing the group to which the subject has been assigned.

Tier 2: Systematic Review, Meta-analysis

Near the top of the hierarchy, offering very powerful evidence, are **systematic review** and **meta-analysis.** A systematic review rigorously looks at research findings that address a specific question and discusses them in terms of outcomes. An example of a systematic review is a study of the efficacy of joint mobilization as a treatment for lateral ankle sprains by looking at the outcomes of multiple studies titled *"The efficacy of manual joint mobilisation/manipulation in treatment of lateral ankle sprains: a systematic review."*[10]

Meta-analyses similarly consider multiple studies by employing a method of statistical analysis that quantitatively combines the results. Meta-analysis is often done with a systematic **literature review**. An example of a meta-analysis was done by Brudvig et al. that explored the literature regarding treatment of shoulder dysfunction called *"The effect of therapeutic exercise and mobilization on patients with shoulder dysfunction : a systematic review with meta-analysis."*[11] By statistically combining the results found on multiple studies, the analysis gains **power**.

Tier 1: Clinical Practice Guidelines

A relatively recent result of the increase in evidence in the physical therapy profession is the development of **clinical practice guidelines** (**CPGs**). These guidelines of recommended interventions are developed by teams of physical therapists after a systematic review of the literature with adequate quantity and quality of studies. An example of a CPG was published on the management of plantar fasciitis by McPoil in 2008.[12] CPGs have been developed for many common orthopedic pathologies and are used to inform common interventions. The Orthopaedic Section of the APTA is committed to developing CPGs for physical therapy management of patients with musculoskeletal impairments. The most up-to-date CPGs can be found online at https://www.orthopt.org/content/practice/clinical-practice-guidelines. Practitioners and students of physical therapy should use the CPG to guide treatment whenever possible. Because of the strength of the evidence for these select pathologies, this text designates the availability of a CPG by this icon: **CPG**

The Role of the Physical Therapist Assistant in Evidence-Based Practice

Although a knowledge of research findings can be used by the PT in examining the patient and establishing the plan of care, the PTA can also employ a knowledge of EBP to deepen understanding of the evaluation findings and interventions employed. Using EBP leads the PTA to choose interventions within the plan of care that are supported by research. PTAs who are aware of research findings can address patient concerns more clearly and confidently. PTA knowledge of the evidence improves the effectiveness of the PT-PTA team.

In addition to using EBP to influence intervention choices, the PTA can take a more active role by producing

clinical research. It starts with curiosity and a desire to improve patient outcomes. PTAs who are interested in clinical research can expand their knowledge in a variety of ways:

- Alert colleagues about their interest in clinical research.
- Read the physical therapy journals each month.
- Become familiar with PubMed, the National Library of Medicine's electronic database (http://www.ncbi.nlm.nih.gov/pubmed).
- Take advantage of the APTA's resources for members, including PTNow ArticleSearch, the Portal to Evidence-based Practice (http://www.ptnow.org/ArticleSearch).
- Collect data on interventions that can be published.
- Publish findings to disseminate research results.

How to Read a Research Article

Scholarly research articles are written with a predictable sequence of sections: Abstract, Introduction, Methods, Results, Discussion, and Conclusion. Each of these sections contains distinct information. The following descriptions tell you what to expect to find in each section.

The Abstract

The **abstract** is found at the beginning of the article and serves as a brief summary of the purpose, question, method, results, and significance of the research. The abstract is the fastest way to determine whether the study addresses one's interests.

The Introduction

The **introduction** provides background information to the reader, summarizes previous research on the topic, and ends with a statement of purpose and possibly a hypothesis, which states the anticipated findings of the study. The summary of existing related research, called a literature review, clarifies the significance of and need for the study. Within the Introduction, the authors may state either the **purpose** of the study or put forth a hypothesis about what they hope to discover.

The Methods Section

The **methods** section lists and describes the steps and procedures used in the study, including information on research design (for example, whether it was a cohort study, RCT, or case study), subject selection, materials used, and details of the intervention and data collection. The information provided here is meant to be sufficiently detailed that the study could be replicated by other researchers.

The Results Section

The **results** section presents the findings of the study. This section typically includes the raw data and a statistical analysis of the data but does not include a subjective interpretation of the study results. Statistical considerations discussed below are helpful in interpreting this section.

The Discussion and the Conclusion

In the **discussion** section, the authors interpret their findings. This section often includes the clinical relevance of the findings, study limitations, and suggestions for further research on the topic. In the **conclusion,** the authors summarize the purpose and findings of the study.

Statistical Considerations

Type I and Type II Errors

The purposes for conducting research are to discover the causes of a given pathology, the value of the investigators' diagnostic tests, the trustworthiness of the investigators' equipment, the reproducibility of the investigators' data collection, and the effect of the investigators' interventions. In the process, the investigators hope that the data collected indicates true relationships. In other words, that the findings are without error. As discussed above, by establishing a control group, using large numbers of subjects, randomizing the subjects to the experimental or control group, and using a method that "blinds" subjects and investigators, the investigators increase the likelihood that their results are true.

However, it is impossible to be completely certain that the results obtained *are* true, that they are not due to chance. Two types of errors can be made while performing research. They are known as type I and type II errors. A **type I error** occurs when the investigator concludes that a relationship exists when in fact it does not. In other words, the results have led to a false-positive result. We are left to believe a falsehood. A **type II error** occurs when the investigators conclude that no relationship exists when in fact it does. In other words, the results have led to a false-negative result. We are left failing to believe a truth. Figure 2.2 depicts these two types of errors.

Probability

When analyzing data, the investigators report on the strength of the findings in terms of the probability of committing a type I error. It is generally accepted that this probability should be no more than 5%. This is called the ***p*-value,** and is usually denoted as an italicized p. If the results report a $p < 0.05$, there is less than a 5% probability of a false positive; if $p < 0.01$, there is less than a 1% probability of a false positive.

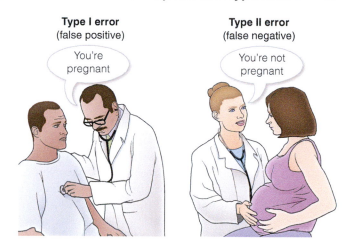

Figure 2.2 Conclusions drawn from research may be made in error. Type I errors result in believing an untruth and type II errors result in not believing a truth.

Sensitivity and Specificity

Type I or type II errors may be due to the results of our testing. The likelihood that we will believe something that is not true, as depicted in Figure 2.2A, has to do with test **specificity.** Specificity is a measurement of a test's ability to correctly rule out non-cases. In this example, if a pregnancy test has come back positive (falsely), we could say that the test was not very specific, that it didn't rule out this non-case. Test specificity is reported in terms of percentage. A test that led to a false-positive conclusion 30% of the time would have a specificity of 100% − 30%, or 70%.

The likelihood that we will reject something that is true, as depicted in Figure 2.2B, depends on test **sensitivity.** Sensitivity is a measurement of a test's ability to correctly detect a case. In this example, if a pregnancy test has come back negative (falsely), we could say that the test was not very sensitive, that it didn't identify this case. The sensitivity is similarly given in terms of percentage. A test that led to a false-negative conclusion 40% of the time would have a sensitivity of 60% (100% − 40%).

To remember the difference between specificity and sensitivity, it may be helpful to use the mnemonics SPin and SNout. SPecificity is a measure of a Positive test correctly ruling *in* a truth (a disease, condition, or effective intervention). SeNsitivity is a measure of a Negative test correctly ruling *out* a non-truth (a disease, condition, or effectiveness of an intervention).

Physical therapy practitioners have studied the sensitivity and specificity of many of the special tests that are used in orthopedic physical therapy. An understanding of these numbers leads to understanding why the physical therapist initially may have performed several tests and why a given test may be preferred over others.

Reliability

In conducting research, researchers may use instruments to collect data. PTAs often rely on instruments and tools to assess their patients. In both instances, the **reliability** of the instrument used is paramount. Reliability is determined by the accuracy and the consistency of the measurements provided. Instruments are measured by studying **intra-tester reliability** and **inter-tester reliability**.

Intra-tester (or intra-rater) reliability is a measurement of the reproducibility of an instrument when one investigator uses it over several trials. For example, if a PTA repeatedly used a goniometer to measure Q-angle and obtained the same measurement, that goniometer would be found to have good intra-tester reliability.[13]

Inter-tester (or inter-rater) reliability is a measurement of the reproducibility of an instrument when used by multiple investigators in one trial. Using the above example, if the PTA measured Q-angle and then had several colleagues repeat the process, the goniometer would be found to have good inter-tester reliability if the measurements each investigator obtained were the same.

Validity

Validity is the measurement that reflects the degree to which the instrument is measuring what it is supposed to measure. An instrument must be reliable to be considered valid. Beyond that, it must yield results that reflect what it claims to measure. In an example of validity, researchers have compared results obtained in measuring shoulder range of motion using an inclinometer with those obtained using a goniometer.[14] This study was intended to validate the use of the inclinometer.

Minimal Clinically Important Difference

Since Jaeschke and coworkers[15] first wrote of the concept of **minimal clinically important difference (MCID)**, investigators have been attempting to quantify the true benefit of physical therapy interventions from the patient perspective. MCID is defined as the smallest change that is perceived as a benefit by the patient. The importance of MCID lies in the fact that although studies may show a statistically significant difference between interventions, the patients may not perceive a difference. Statistical significance is not the same as clinical significance. Recent studies have looked at the MCID of various scales that are used to assess pain, balance, function, gait speed, and disability to determine the amount of improvement needed on each assessment instrument in order for the patient to notice a benefit.[16–20]

SUMMARY

Physical therapy practitioners must appreciate the importance of applying evidence to therapy interventions to substantiate their treatment choices. Such evidence comes from many sources with varying degrees of strength. Randomized controlled trials, systematic reviews, meta-analyses, and CPGs provide the strongest evidence. The role of the PTA in using evidence is to clarify the established plan of care, to supplement treatment options within the plan of care, and to provide a foundation of discussion between the PTA and the supervising physical therapist. The PTA may also contribute to the body of evidence by conducting research.

REVIEW QUESTIONS

1. Using the hierarchy of evidence chart, rank the following studies in terms of their power.
   a. The effect of stretching of the Achilles' tendon on ankle sprain recurrence: a randomized controlled trial.
   b. Ankle dorsiflexion range of motion in a patient with recurrent ankle sprain: a case study.
   c. Clinical practice guidelines for ankle sprain.
   d. Is limited ankle dorsiflexion range of motion a factor in ankle sprain? A longitudinal cohort study.

2. Name and briefly describe the sections of a research article.

3. Are the following possible examples of type I or type II errors?
   a. A research article that concludes that patient education cannot decrease the risk of knee injury.
   b. A research article that concludes that the strength of the biceps brachii is a factor in knee injuries.

4. A PTA is testing a new device that measures proprioceptive sense. When the device is used by two examiners, the results are identical. Is this an example of intra-tester reliability, inter-tester reliability, or validity?

5. A PTA is testing a new device that measures muscle strength. When compared to an existing dynamometer, this device gets results which are similar. Is this an example of intra-tester reliability, inter-tester reliability, or validity?

6. What is the significance of MCID to you as a PTA?

7. In what ways can you, as a PTA, be involved in EBP?

REFERENCES

1. Evidence-Based Medicine Working Group. (1992). Evidence-based medicine. A new approach to teaching the practice of medicine, *JAMA, 268*, 2420–2425.
2. HOD statement on evidence.

3. Herbert, R., Jamtvedt, G., Hagen, K. B., Mead, J. M., & Chalmers, I. (2011). *Practical evidence-based physiotherapy*.

4. West, S., King, V., Carey, T. S., Lohr, K. N., McKoy, N., Sutton, S. F., & Lux, L. (2002). Systems to rate the strength of scientific evidence: Summary. *Evidence Report/Technology Assessment: Number 47*. AHRQ Publication No. 02-E015, March 2002. Agency for Healthcare Research and Quality, Rockville, MD. https://www.ncbi.nlm.nih.gov/books/NBK11930/

5. Jackson, S. M. (2012). Patellar tendon rupture following a patellar fracture. *Journal of Orthopaedic and Sports Physical Therapy, 42*, 969–969.

6. Stevens, J. E., Mizner, R. L., & Snyder-Mackler, L. (2004). Neuromuscular electrical stimulation for quadriceps muscle strengthening after bilateral total knee arthroplasty: A case series. *Journal of Orthopaedic and Sports Physical Therapy, 34*, 21–29.

7. Barton, C. J., Bonanno, D., Levinger, P., & Menz, H. B. (2010). Foot and ankle characteristics in patellofemoral pain syndrome: A case control and reliability study. *Journal of Orthopaedic and Sports Physical Therapy, 40*, 286–296.

8. Wideman, T. H., Scott, W., Martel, M. O., & Sullivan, M. J. L. (2012). Recovery from depressive symptoms over the course of physical therapy: A prospective cohort study of individuals with work-related orthopaedic injuries and symptoms of depression. *Journal of Orthopaedic and Sports Physical Therapy, 42*, 957–967.

9. Crossley, K., Bennell, K., Green, S., Cowan, S., & McConnell, J. (2002). Physical therapy for patellofemoral pain: A randomized, double-blinded, placebo-controlled trial. *American Journal of Sports Medicine, 30*, 857–865.

10. Loudon, J. K., Reiman, M. P., & Sylvain, J. (2014). The efficacy of manual joint mobilisation/manipulation in treatment of lateral ankle sprains: A systematic review. *British Journal of Sports Medicine, 48*, 365–370.

11. Brudvig, T. J., Kulkarni, H., & Shah, S. (2011). The effect of therapeutic exercise and mobilization on patients with shoulder dysfunction: A systematic review with meta-analysis. *Journal of Orthopaedic and Sports Physical Therapy, 41*, 734–748.

12. McPoil, T. G., et al. (2008). Heel pain—plantar fasciitis: Clinical practice guidelines linked to the international classification of function, disability, and health from the orthopaedic section of the American Physical Therapy Association. *Journal of Orthopaedic and Sports Physical Therapy, 38*, A1–A18.

13. Weiss, L., DeForest, B., Hammond, K., Schilling, B., & Ferreira, L. (2013). Reliability of goniometry-based Q-angle. *Physical Medicine and Rehabilitation, 5*, 763–768.

14. Kolber, M. J., & Hanney, W. J. (2012). The reliability and concurrent validity of shoulder mobility measurements using a digital inclinometer and goniometer: A technical report. *International Journal of Sports Physical Therapy, 7*, 306–313.

15. Jaeschke, R., Singer, J., & Guyatt, G. H. (1989). Measurement of health status: Ascertaining the minimal clinically important difference. *Controlled Clinical Trials, 10*, 407–415.

16. Clement, N. D., Macdonald, D., & Simpson, A. H. R. W. (2013). The minimal clinically important difference in the Oxford knee score and Short Form 12 score after total knee arthroplasty. *Knee Surgery, Sports Traumatology, Arthroscopy*. doi: 10.1007/s00167-013-2776-5.

17. Ebert, J. R., Smith, A., Wood, D. J., & Ackland, T. R. (2013). A comparison of the responsiveness of 4 commonly used patient-reported outcome instruments at 5 years after matrix-induced autologous chondrocyte implantation. *American Journal of Sports Medicine, 41*, 2791–2799.

18. Franchignoni, F., Vercelli, S., Giordano, A., Sartorio, F., Bravini, E., & Ferriero, G. (2014). Minimal clinically important difference of the disabilities of the arm, shoulder and hand outcome measure (DASH) and its shortened version (QuickDASH). *Journal of Orthopaedic and Sports Physical Therapy, 44*, 30–39.

19. Kukkonen, J., Kauko, T., Vahlberg, T., Joukainen, A., & Aärimaa, V. (2013). Investigating minimal clinically important difference for Constant score in patients undergoing rotator cuff surgery. *Journal of Shoulder and Elbow Surgery, 22*, 1650–1655.

20. Kwok, B. C., Pua, Y. H., Mamun, K., & Wong, W. P. (2013). The minimal clinically important difference of six-minute walk in Asian older adults. *BMC Geriatrics, 13*, 23.

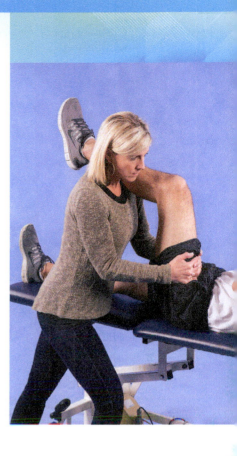

Chapter **3**

The Goals of Orthopedic Physical Therapy

LEARNING OUTCOMES

After reading this chapter, the student will:

3.1   Identify the primary goals of physical therapy.
3.2   Describe the stages of tissue inflammation and healing and discuss physical therapy interventions appropriate for each stage.
3.3   Compare and contrast the gate control and neuromatrix theories of pain.
3.4   Explain central sensitization and discuss its implications in physical therapy intervention.
3.5   Compare how contractile and noncontractile tissues stretch and describe the implications for physical therapy intervention.
3.6   Describe the concave-convex rule and the importance of this understanding when performing joint mobilization.

3.7 Explain the rationale for neural mobilization.
3.8 Name and briefly explain the four principles of muscle performance.
3.9 Discuss considerations in concentric, eccentric, isometric, and plyometric muscle performance exercises.
3.10 Discuss the importance of proprioceptive, balance, and neuromuscular retraining in physical therapy interventions.
3.11 Discuss the major components of an aerobic exercise program that is based on the FITT model.

KEY WORDS

Accessory movement	Multiple angle isometrics	Repetition maximum
Central sensitization	Muscle spindle	Reticulin fibers
Collagen fibers	Neuromatrix	Sarcomere
Elastic response	Neuromatrix theory of pain control	Sliders
Elastin fibers	Neuropathic pain	Strain
Gate theory of pain control	Neuroplasticity	Stress
Golgi tendon organ	Neurotag	Tensile strength
Ground substance	Nociceptive pain	Tensioners
In-parallel addition	Nociplastic pain	Therapeutic neuroscience education
In-series addition	Perturbation	Tissue necking
Irritability	Physiological movement	
Microtearing	Plastic response	

Introduction

The vision of physical therapy is to "optimize movement to improve the human experience" (http://www.apta.org/Vision/). This may be accomplished by a wide variety of goals and methods. To optimize movement for example, the physical therapist assistant (PTA) may address tissue healing, pain modulation, tissue mobility, muscle performance, neuromotor control, cardiovascular fitness, functional movement, postural correction, and education. This chapter reviews each of these goals and provides intervention strategies.

Tissue Healing

The goal of tissue healing is to restore tissue to its pre-injury state in order to decrease pain, improve function, and minimize risk of reinjury. This is done by understanding normal tissue healing, observing the patient's signs and symptoms, and providing appropriate interventions at the appropriate time.

Tissue healing after injury occurs in a predictable fashion in three overlapping stages. These are the inflammatory stage, proliferative or repair stage, and maturation or remodeling stage. There are distinct clinical signs, cellular changes, and appropriate physical therapy interventions for each stage.

Stage I: Inflammation

The inflammation stage begins at the onset of tissue injury and generally lasts 3 to 6 days. It is characterized by the cardinal signs of inflammation: warmth, swelling, redness, pain, and loss of function. Pain occurs even at rest in this stage. Cellular changes that are occurring include an initial vasoconstriction followed by vasodilation, which causes the localized warmth and redness. The arteries in the affected area become more permeable, allowing fluid to accumulate in the tissue, resulting in swelling. Macrophages arrive to clean up dead cells, bacteria, and debris. As the macrophages finish clearing up the area and begin to die, their cell death summons fibroblasts to the area. The cellular change from macrophages to fibroblasts indicates the onset of stage II healing.

Although the inflammatory stage is a necessary part of the tissue healing process, during stage I it is important to control the effects of inflammation and to avoid prolonging the insult to the tissues. Interventions appropriate for this stage are support, protection, rest, ice, compression, and elevation. These interventions are collectively referred to by the acronym PRICE. Therapy should focus on minimizing the loss of motion, strength, and function by employing passive range of motion, assistive devices, and tissue mobilization.

Stage II: Proliferation and Repair

The proliferative stage usually begins as early as day 3 and ends by day 21. In this stage, the signs of inflammation cease. Pain is no longer experienced at rest but does occur when the tissue is stretched. The fibroblasts are busy in stage II, manufacturing and depositing collagen fibers. In this stage the collagen is immature, thin, and not well organized. It is bound together by weak hydrogen bonds that are easily formed and broken.

In stage II healing, it is important to stretch the tissue while the collagen bonds are easily altered. Stretch in this phase will align the collagen fibers and promote normal range of motion. Gentle strengthening exercises may also be initiated.

Table 3-1	Treatment Guidelines for Each Stage of Tissue Healing
Stage of Tissue Healing	Treatment Guidelines for Inflammation
Stage I	Protection, rest, ice, compression, elevation, support, PROM, use of assistive devices, minimize loss of motion and strength
Stage II	Stretch to align collagen fibers and promote normal range of motion, gentle strengthening exercises
Stage III	Progressive resistive exercises, eccentric strengthening, plyometric exercises, sport- or occupation-specific activities

Stage III: Maturation and Remodeling

In stage III, after the collagen is deposited in the area during the rebuilding period, it gradually matures, thickens, and bonds permanently through covalent bonding. Signs of inflammation are gone, and the clinical findings at this point may be limited range of motion, weakness, and pain with stretch beyond the point of tissue resistance. The maturation and remodeling stage begins at approximately 3 weeks and can last up to 1 year.

During this stage of healing, physical therapy interventions include progressive resistive exercises, eccentric strengthening, plyometric exercises, and sport- or occupation-specific activities.

Table 3-1 provides treatment guidelines for the three stages of tissue healing.

In summary, the three stages of healing can be understood using the analogy of building a house (Fig. 3.1). In stage I, the area is cleared of debris so that the rebuilding may occur (top left). In stage II, the collagen fibers have been deposited in the area, but do not resemble the tissue being replaced because they are haphazardly arranged. But the fibers are "on site" and ready to be built into tissue (bottom left). In stage III, the collagen

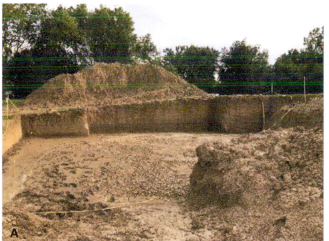

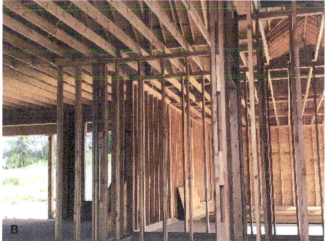

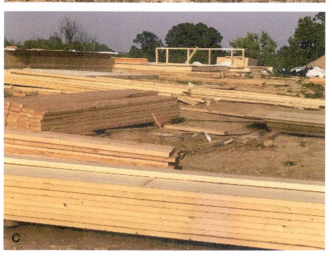

Figure 3.1 The three stages of healing can be likened to building a house. In stage I (A), the area is cleared; in stage II (B), the materials needed for rebuilding arrive on site; in stage III (C), the materials organize into a recognizable structure.

organizes and the structure resembles the original tissue (top right).

Irritability

The concept of **irritability** may be applied to tissues as they heal.[1] Degree of irritability is largely related to stages of inflammation. A tissue with high irritability will have a very low tolerance for exercise. Examination of the patient may be abbreviated due to irritability, and the patient may have pain that lingers for several hours after movement. Patients will often report pain of 7 or higher on a 0 to 10 scale. Range of motion will be limited actively more than passively.

Moderately irritable tissues will become painful with movement, but less quickly. Symptoms subside more quickly. Patients will tolerate more activity. Patients will usually rate pain as 4 to 6 out of 10 and demonstrate range of motion that is similar actively as compared to passively.

A tissue with low irritability will tolerate exercise without a lingering increase in pain. Patients will generally rate their pain as 3 or less and will demonstrate equal active and passive range of motion.

Pain

Frequently, a goal in physical therapy is to minimize or relieve pain. Pain is a warning system that protects us from things that may be harmful or dangerous. It is an unpleasant experience, but it serves an important function. Pain has been discussed and researched for centuries, but two theories regarding pain control, the gate theory and the neuromatrix theory, are helpful in understanding how pain behaves and how it is best treated.

The Gate Theory of Pain Control

Melzack and Wall postulated the **gate theory of pain control** in 1965.[2] According to this theory, pain is carried as an input from peripheral pain receptors to the central nervous system (CNS) by small-diameter, unmyelinated nerve fibers called C-fibers. Larger-diameter A-fibers, which are faster conducting, myelinated fibers, carry input that is not painful. When a painful stimulus activates the C-fibers, an interventionary stimulation of the faster A-fibers will block the pain input from reaching the brain. In this way, the A-fibers are said to close the "gate" so that the C-fiber input is suppressed. According to this theory, when the brain is made aware of the pain, it may send a signal down to the spinal cord to further decrease input from the C-fibers. Figure 3.2 represents what is happening at the spinal cord according to this theory.

The gate theory improved our understanding of pain in several ways. It explained our observation that a nonpainful stimulus can be used to inhibit pain; for example, rubbing your head after bumping it. It also

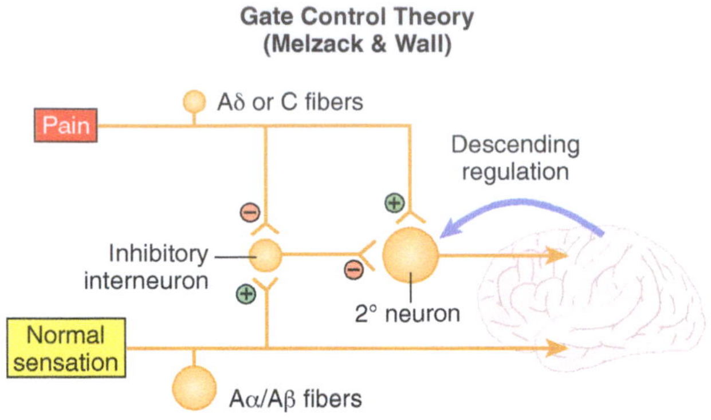

Figure 3.2 Depiction of the mechanism of the gate control theory of pain as described by Melzack and Wall. Painful stimuli are blocked in the spinal cord by stimulation of faster nerve fibers carrying nonpainful stimuli, closing a "gate" on pain.

provided an explanation for the influence of the brain and emotions on pain.

The Neuromatrix Theory of Pain

Limitations in the gate theory became apparent in instances such as phantom limb pain, where there is no possible input from the site of pain. By the late 1990s, Melzack began to describe a **neuromatrix**, or network of nerves in the brain that generate pain.[3,4] In describing the neuromatrix, he theorized that it is genetically determined but modified by sensory experiences, stress, and cognitive influences.

The **neuromatrix theory of pain control** differs from the gate theory in important ways. In particular, according to this theory, pain is not an input, but an output. Pain is produced by the brain. The nociceptive input that results from stimulation by something that may cause harm is carried by nerve fibers to the brain, but it is the brain that interprets this input and determines whether the experience is painful.

For the brain to interpret nociceptive stimuli, many areas of the brain become involved. These areas communicate with each other in patterns that are unique to each individual. Communication occurs among areas of the brain that store information such as memories, beliefs, knowledge, understanding, cultural expectations, emotions, fears, and social context. The places in the brain that are activated by nociceptive input make up what is known as the person's pain **neurotag** (Fig. 3.3). The input travels rapidly throughout the brain, lighting up the person's unique pain pathways, so the brain can judge whether the stimulus poses a threat or danger. If the brain determines that it does, the input results in pain.

Central Sensitization

The nervous system is constantly undergoing change, and these changes are evidence of **neuroplasticity**. An example of neuroplasticity is seen in the changes that

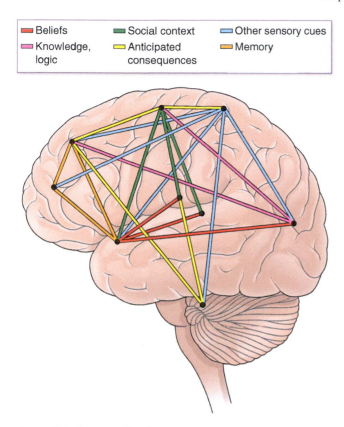

| ■ Beliefs | ■ Social context | ■ Other sensory cues |
| ■ Knowledge, logic | ■ Anticipated consequences | ■ Memory |

Figure 3.3 An example of a pain neurotag. When the brain perceives a dangerous stimulus, a personally unique pathway is activated that involves many areas of the brain.

occur if neuron A stimulates neuron B repeatedly. Changes occur in both neurons that make it easier and more likely for neuron A to stimulate B. Simply put, "nerves that fire together, wire together." The pathway becomes more efficient. Considering the pain neurotag, the more often the patient's brain uses these pathways, the easier it becomes to activate the pain neurotag again. The system becomes overly sensitive, in a phenomenon called **central sensitization**.[5]

Woolf defined central sensitization in 2011 as an amplification of neural signaling within the CNS that elicits pain hypersensitivity.[5] This phenomenon explains how pain becomes chronic and may exist without pathology. The pain neurotag has become so efficient, fueled by fear and catastrophizing, that the patient experiences prolonged pain that is out of proportion to the pathology.

Recent clarifications from the International Association for the Study of Pain (IASP) have described three types of pain.[6] **Neuropathic pain** is the result of disease or a lesion of the nervous system. Pain which is a result of actual or threatened damage to non-nervous tissue is referred to as **nociceptive pain**. **Nociplastic pain** is the descriptor used for pain in which changes (plasticity) in central nervous system sensitization appear to be contributing to the chronicity of the symptoms.

Treating patients with chronic pain is difficult, and it is extremely important for the PTA to be aware of this sensitivity. Patients with chronic pain benefit from education regarding the neuroscience of pain perception. This has been called **therapeutic neuroscience education.** Basic to this education is the understanding that pain is not an input to the brain, but an output from the brain. The patient must disassociate pain with harm and understand that pain with movement may still be safe. The PTA is instrumental in reducing the fear or sense of threat the patient feels, to calm the brain. The words we use to educate the patient must be carefully chosen. It has been shown that an understanding of pain provided in a single educational session may result in improvement in physical function and decreased brain activity.[7–13]

Tissue Mobility

Improving mobility to soft tissue is often a goal in orthopedic physical therapy to restore normal patterns of functional movement and to minimize the risk of reinjury. Limited mobility may be due to shortening of soft tissues including muscle, tendon, ligament, joint capsule, nerve, fascia, and skin. Rarely is only one structure involved. Stretching or release of the involved tissues has been shown to improve mobility. This may be due to an improved stretch tolerance in the tissues, an actual lengthening of the tissues, or both. An understanding of tissue response to stretching is important to provide a safe, effective, and targeted stretch.

Indications and Contraindications for Mobility Activities

The indications for mobility exercises include impaired soft tissue or joint mobility, the presence of contractures, decreased function due to limited motion, muscle weakness that unopposed may lead to shortening of the opposing muscles and subsequent deformity, and injury prevention.[14]

Contraindications to mobility exercises include the presence of a bony block, acute inflammation or infection, sharp pain with stretching, tissue trauma, hypermobility, or cases in which shortened structures provide stability/function.[14] An example where stretching is contraindicated in order to provide stability may be found after surgery for glenohumeral instability. The surgeon may restrict shoulder external rotation range of motion to improve the stability of the joint. An example of selective shortening to improve function can be found in treating patients with quadriplegia secondary to spinal cord injury. These patients may benefit from allowing their finger flexors to shorten to provide a functional tenodesis grasp.

Soft Tissue Response to Stretch

Soft tissues respond to stretch in two major ways: change in structure and change in function. Examples

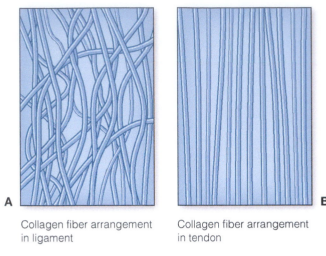

Collagen fiber arrangement in ligament

Collagen fiber arrangement in tendon

Figure 3.4 Type I collagen with randomly oriented fibers (A) and aligned fibers (B).

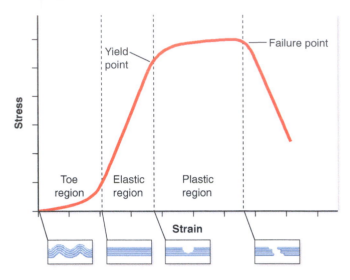

Figure 3.5 Stress-strain curve of noncontractile tissue. Collagen fibers straighten out in the toe region and begin to be stretched in the elastic region. However, irreversible changes occur only in the plastic region with microtears of the tissue. Tissue failure follows with continued tissue stress.

of change in structure are microtears and tissue lengthening. Functional changes that occur lead to increased tolerance of the tissue to stretch. Functional changes are discussed in further detail in the Neurophysiology section below.

The structural changes that result from stretch of non-contractile tissue, contractile tissue (muscles), and nerves are unique and will be discussed separately.

Noncontractile Tissue

Noncontractile soft tissue (tendons, ligaments, joint capsules, fascia, and skin) is made up of a **ground substance** containing fibers of **collagen, elastin, and reticulin.** Each of these fibers has different properties and serves different purposes. The tissue response to stretch is largely influenced by the concentration and arrangement of collagen and elastin.

The tissue's ability to withstand compression is largely influenced by the amount of proteoglycans in the **ground substance,** the gel-like substance that supports, nourishes, and hydrates the soft tissue fibers. Ground substance is composed primarily of water and proteins. The proteoglycans in the ground substance serve to resist compressive forces.

Collagen fibers provide the tissue with **tensile strength**—that is, the amount of resistance the tissue has to stretching and tearing. Tissues gain tensile strength with an increased proportion of collagen fibers and by the alignment of the fibers in the tissue. An alignment of fibers in a parallel, organized fashion provides more strength than that of a haphazard alignment (Fig. 3.4).

Elastin fibers, as their name implies, are stretchy and allow tissues to extend. Stretching of elastin fibers results in lengthening of the fibers with a return to prestretch length upon release. Reticulin fibers are a type of thin collagen. They add bulk to the tissue and support the collagen fibers.

When noncontractile tissue is stretched, the behavior of the tissue can be represented by a stress-strain curve, as depicted in Figure 3.5. An applied load, or **stress,** results in tissue elongation or deformation, which is called **strain.** It is important for the PTA to understand the association between the amount of stretch and the changes in soft tissue in order to stress the tissue adequately without causing tissue failure.

Progressive stress to a tissue leads initially to an **elastic response,** causing tissue lengthening which is temporary. If the stress is released at this time, the tissue will quickly revert back to the original length. With continued stress on the tissue, a **plastic (permanent) response** occurs due to tearing of the tissue. The four regions of the graph depict distinct responses of soft tissue to stress: the toe region, the linear region, the plastic region, and the tissue failure region.[15]

Toe Region

During this phase, there is a considerable amount of tissue elongation with very little load, as the wavy collagen fibers straighten. If the stress is removed, the tissue quickly recoils back to the original length, and the collagen fibers regain their crimp.

Elastic Region

During this phase, tissue elongation requires a greater load to be applied to the tissue, as collagen fibers have straightened and aligned along the line of stress. The relationship between tissue stress and elongation approaches a 1:1 ratio. Yet, stretching to the end of the elastic region causes no tissue damage, and elongation is completely reversible when the stress is removed—the fiber recoils to its original length with an elastic response.

Plastic Region

Lasting tissue changes occur in the plastic region, as the bonds between collagen fibers, and eventually the fibers themselves, are torn. **Microtearing** in the tissue is necessary to permanently elongate the tissue. Stretching to increase tissue length involves applying stress into the plastic region.

Late in the plastic region the tissue displays a large amount of deformation with little or no additional stress. This phenomenon is called **tissue necking** and immediately precedes complete tissue failure or rupture. The term *necking* reflects the observation that tissue becomes thinner and develops a "neck," much like stretched taffy immediately before it breaks apart. The PTA should be aware of the feel of tissue necking to avoid applying additional stress if this begins to occur.

Tissue Failure

This region refers to the macrofailure of the tissue, or complete rupture.

Contractile Tissue

Contractile tissue refers to the muscle fiber. Skeletal muscle is comprised of muscle fibers and noncontractile "wrappings"—the epimysium, perimysium, and endomysium. The noncontractile components of a muscle respond to stretch as described above. The response of muscle fibers to stretch, however, is unique.

Muscle fibers are the cellular unit of the muscle. These fibers are long, often running the entire length of the muscle. They are made up of smaller fibers, called myofibrils, which contain actin and myosin myofilaments. At the microscopic level of the myofilaments the anatomy of the **sarcomere** can be seen. The sarcomere is the contractile unit of a muscle, and describes a section of the myofibril between discs called Z-lines. The actin filaments attach onto the Z-lines. Thicker myosin filaments pull the actin filaments toward each other, shortening the sarcomere. This results in overall muscle shortening that occurs during a concentric contraction.

With increased tension or stretch of the muscle, the connective tissue bonds between actin and myosin filaments are stressed, which may lead to the sarcomere yielding to the stress. The PTA may feel a sudden increase in muscle length, in a phenomenon call "sarcomere give."[16]

With sustained stretch or upon frequent stretching, the muscle fibers add additional sarcomeres to increase resting length, as shown in Figure 3.6. Because the sarcomeres are added to the length of the muscle fibers, it is called an **in-series addition**.[17–21]

Two mechanoreceptors play a role in muscle response to stretch: the **muscle spindle** and **Golgi tendon organ** (**GTO**). The muscle spindle is located in the muscle belly

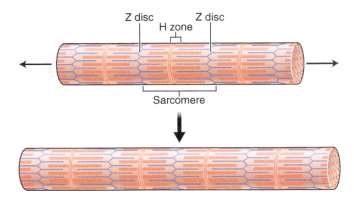

Figure 3.6 Stretch of a muscle results in additional sarcomeres being added to the length of the myofibril, termed an in-series addition. This results in a longer muscle or changes in the tension within the sarcomeres.

and senses the amount and velocity of stretch. Both end-range stretching and quick stretching increase the input from the muscle spindle to the brain. The response to muscle spindle firing is activation of the alpha motor neuron to the muscle, increasing muscle tension and resistance to stretch.

Golgi tendon organs, located at the musculotendinous junction of skeletal muscles, sense the amount of tension in the area. As the muscle stretches or contracts, the GTO is stimulated. This leads to inhibition of the muscle and decreased resistance to stretch. It is thought that the GTO plays a role in regulating muscle output in response to fatigue to prevent muscle injury.

Nervous Tissue

Nerves may impair movement as a result of either a structural or functional abnormality. Structurally, a mechanical limitation such as nerve tightness, compression from nearby structures, or decreased sliding between the nerve and the adjacent tissue may impair motion. Functionally, stretch hypersensitivity of the nerve may limit mobility. Pain, pressure, restricted movement, and stress may cause the nerve to become overly sensitive to these stimuli and fire more readily. In physical therapy, nerves are moved and manipulated to increase nerve length or tolerance to stretch and to decrease sensitivity of the nerve. This will be discussed further in Nervous System Mobilization.

Types of Stretch
Static Stretch

Static stretch is elongating the tissue to the point of a stretching sensation or slight discomfort and holding this position. Various studies have explored the optimal hold time for a static stretch, with conflicting evidence. A hold time of 30 to 60 seconds for three repetitions is common. Static stretching is used to increase range of motion.

Cyclic Stretch

A cyclic stretch is an intermittent, gradual stretch that is held briefly, released, and applied again. Typically, cyclic stretching involves stretch times of 5 to 15 seconds applied multiple times. Cyclic stretching is regarded as a more comfortable form of stretching that is still very effective.

Ballistic Stretch

Ballistic stretching refers to a technique that uses fast, bouncing movements to stretch tissues. Because of the high speed of stretching involved, ballistic stretching is linked to tissue injury. It is best used in athletic patients prior to participation in a sport or activity that calls for high-velocity end-of-range movements, such as basketball, football, or running.

Facilitative Stretch

The facilitative stretch techniques require the patient to actively contract muscles to facilitate or inhibit movements to increase the effectiveness of the stretch. Proprioceptive neuromuscular facilitation techniques such as contract-relax and hold-relax are examples of facilitative stretching. These techniques are effective in increasing range of motion.

Types of Mobilization

Soft Tissue Mobilization

Soft tissue mobilization (STM) includes transverse friction massage and myofascial release. STM may be performed using devices such as those pictured in Figure 3.7 to assist the PTA. This is referred to as instrument assisted soft tissue mobilization or IASTM. The goal of both STM and IASTM is to relax muscle and fascial tension, decrease pain, increase blood flow, and stretch soft tissue. If fascial restriction is determined to be the cause of pain or limited motion, the patient may benefit from soft tissue mobilization.

Joint Mobilization

Joint mobilization may be included in the plan of care to treat pain and limitation of motion arising from the joint capsule or ligaments. There are two types of motion when joints move: **physiological movement** and **accessory movement.** Physiological movement is a voluntary movement of one bone on another, such as flexion and abduction. Accessory movement, or joint play, is nonvoluntary movement that occurs at the same time between the joint surfaces, such as rolling and sliding. Accessory movement is necessary for full range of motion. One purpose of joint mobilization is to normalize the accessory movements of the joint, allowing for normal physiological movements.

The accessory movements are compression, distraction, rolling, spinning, and gliding. Compression is a movement of joint surfaces closer together, and distraction is a pulling of joint surfaces apart. To differentiate rolling, spinning, and gliding, consider the comparisons shown in Figure 3.8. When we perform joint mobilization, we use both gliding and joint distraction.

Concave-Convex Rule

The concave-convex rule describes the direction of the accessory glide that occurs during physiological movement. The direction depends on the shape of the moving bone.

If the moving bone has a convex surface relative to the surface of the stationary bone, the direction of the glide is *opposite* that of the movement of the bone. As an example, when performing shoulder abduction, the convex humeral head slides *down* on the concave glenoid as the arm is raised *up* (Fig. 3.9A).

If the moving bone has a concave surface relative to the surface of the stationary bone, the direction of the glide is in the *same* direction as that of the bone. As an example, when performing sitting knee extension, the concave surface of the tibia moves *up* as the lower leg is raised *up* (Fig. 3.9B).

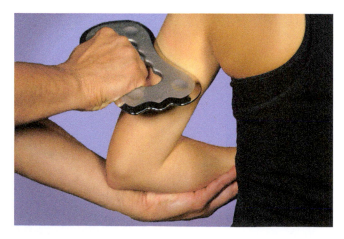

Figure 3.7 Tools such as these may be used for augmented soft tissue mobilization (ASTM).

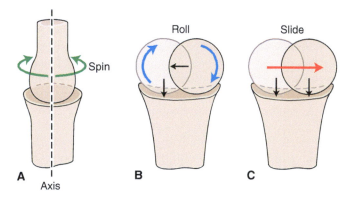

Figure 3.8 Examples of joint motions of spinning (A), rolling (B), and sliding or gliding (C). The movement of sliding is often used in joint mobilization.

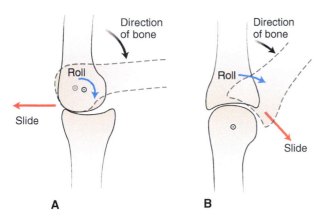

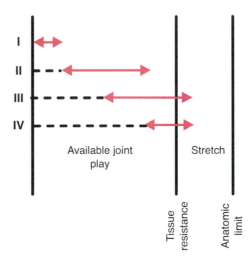

Figure 3.9 The concave-convex rule describes the direction of movement of the bone in relationship to the direction of the slide within the joint. When a convex surface of a bone moves on a concave surface, the movement of the bone is opposite that of the sliding in the joint (A). When a concave surface of a bone moves on a convex surface, the movement of the bone is the same as that of the sliding in the joint (B).

Figure 3.10 The relative amplitude of four grades of oscillatory joint mobilization.

Box 3-1 | **Grades of Oscillatory Mobilization**

- **Grade I:** Small-amplitude movement at the beginning of the accessory range of movement.
- **Grade II:** Large-amplitude movement from early in the range to about midrange.
- **Grade III:** Large-amplitude movement from midrange to the end of the available range of movement.
- **Grade IV:** Small-amplitude movement at the end of the available range of movement.

Box 3-2 | **Grades of Sustained Mobilization**

- **Grade I:** Small-amplitude movement that does not stress the capsule, but just distracts the joint enough to relieve muscle tension and neutralize the pressure in the joint. No separation of the joint is noticeable. A grade I sustained distraction is used prior to oscillatory mobilization.
- **Grade II:** Large-amplitude movement that takes up the slack in the joint to the point of tissue resistance. Grade II distraction separates the joint surfaces and significantly reduces joint play.
- **Grade III:** Larger large-amplitude movement that stretches the joint past the point of tissue resistance, stretching the capsule and surrounding tissues.

Open-Packed vs. Close-Packed Position

The open-packed position of the joint is usually the position in which the patient is placed for joint mobilization. It is the position of least joint congruency and least bone-to-bone contact. Additionally, in this position the ligaments and capsule are in a slackened position and the joint volume is maximized. This allows for the most joint play.

Conversely, the close-packed position of a joint is the position of most congruency. In this position, the joint surfaces have the most contact, capsule and ligaments are most taut, and joint volume is minimized. This position is not generally used for joint mobilization, but is often used to test ligament stability. The open-packed and close-packed positions for each joint are provided in the anatomy chapters.

Grades of Joint Mobilization

Joint mobilization may be performed as an oscillatory or sustained motion. As an oscillatory motion, there are four grades of joint mobilization, as described in Box 3-1. Grades I, II, and III are generally used to decrease pain, whereas grades III and IV are primarily used to

increase range. Oscillatory mobilizations are performed at a rate of about 1 to 3 per second, for up to 2 minutes. This sequence is repeated several times. Figure 3.10 depicts the relative amplitude of oscillatory mobilizations.

In using sustained mobilizations, there are three grades, as described in Box 3-2. Grade I is used to decrease pain, grade II is used to decrease pain and maintain range of motion, and grade III is used to increase range of motion. Sustained mobilizations are applied for 6 to 10 seconds, followed by a 3 to 4 second rest, for about two minutes. Figure 3.11 depicts the relative amplitude of sustained mobilizations.

Indications and Contraindications for Joint Mobilization

Joint mobilization may be used to improve joint motion and to decrease pain. It also may improve the flow of synovial fluid in the joint, improving nutrition to the articular and meniscal cartilage.

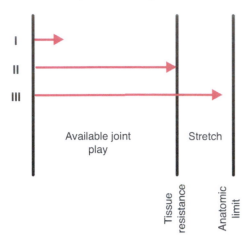

Figure 3.11 The relative amplitude of three grades of sustained joint mobilization.

Box 3-3   Treatment Guidelines for Joint Mobilization

1. Position the patient in a comfortable resting position, placing the joint to be mobilized near the edge of the table.
2. Position the joint in an open-packed position.
3. Determine the type of joint mobilization and grade to be performed based on the plan of care and purpose of joint mobilization.
4. Ensure your ability to maintain good body mechanics by changing table or stool height.
5. Stabilize one side of the joint, either manually or mechanically by using the treatment table, towels, etc.
6. Using one or both hands, slightly distract the joint surfaces (grade I sustained mobilization).
7. Adhering to the concave-convex rule, apply force to the other side of the joint.
8. Continuously assess patient.
9. Reassess patient's pain and joint mobility after joint mobilization.

Relative contraindications include osteoporosis, rheumatoid arthritis, fracture, joint hypermobility, cancer, and neurologic symptoms. Pregnancy is a relative contraindication: Pregnant or postpartum patients may have increased ligament laxity requiring extra caution, and prolonged supine positioning should be avoided during pregnancy after the fourth month. Treatment guidelines for joint mobilization can be found in Box 3-3.

Nervous System Mobilization

Treatment of the nervous system may involve exercises that tense (stretch) or slide the nerve. Nerve-tensioning exercises (**tensioners**) are done as an oscillatory stretch, because blood flow to the nerve is reduced as the

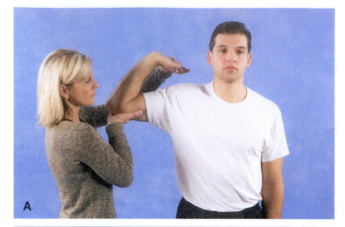

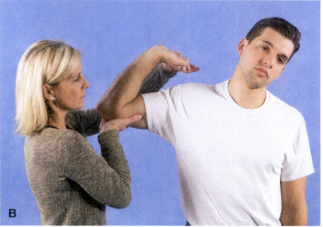

Figure 3.12 Nerve tensioning for the ulnar nerve. The nerve is initially stretched over the elbow and wrist (A). Maintaining this position while simultaneously side bending the head increases the tension on the nerve (B). An oscillatory stretch is applied by holding for 10–20 seconds and then releasing.

nerve is stretched. Because of this, static stretches of a peripheral nerve are not generally recommended. The goal of nerve tensioning is to increase the nerve's ability to tolerate stretch. Figure 3.12 depicts a nerve-tensioning exercise.

An alternative treatment for reduced range of motion in the nervous system is nerve **sliders** (also known as nerve flossing). These exercises lengthen the nerve over one joint while simultaneously shortening it over another joint. As a result, the nerve is moved within the nerve bed with very little stretch applied to the nerve. The goal of nerve gliding is to reduce sensitivity of the nerve and improve mobility between the nerve and the adjacent tissue.

Muscle Performance

Physical therapist assistants often provide interventions to increase muscle performance. These interventions often take the form of resistance exercises, which are used to increase strength, power, or endurance. Strength refers to the muscle's ability to generate force, power is a measure of force per unit of time, and endurance refers to a muscle's ability to perform contractions over a long period of time.

Principles of Muscle Performance

There are four principles that must be understood by the PTA to choose the optimal parameters for muscle performance interventions. These are the specific adaptation to imposed demands (SAID) principle, the transfer of training principle, the overload principle, and the reversibility principle.

Specific Adaptation to Imposed Demands (SAID) Principle

The SAID principle refers to the finding that the greatest benefit from exercise is specific to the demands of the exercise. In other words, if we exercise to strengthen a muscle eccentrically in a lengthened range, the muscle will gain the most strength *eccentrically in a lengthened range*. If we want to help someone become a better swimmer, the training should occur in a pool. If we want to enhance endurance, we will get the best result by endurance training.

Transfer of Training Principle

The transfer of training principle (or the overflow principle) seems to contradict the SAID principle at first glance. The transfer of training principle states that when enhancing muscle performance using a specific method or focus, gains occur in other areas as well.[22–24] For example, when patients exercise to increase power, they also gain strength. Strengthening concentrically increases strength eccentrically. Plyometric training transfers into sport-specific gains. Whereas the SAID principle tells us the very best muscle performance exercises, the transfer of training principle tells us that there is carryover between different modes of exercise.

It has been shown that there is a transfer of training effect from one side of the body to the other.[25–27] The effect seems to be an increase in strength of the same muscle on the untrained side as that of the side undergoing training. This effect has been found in upper and lower extremities. This principle can be employed when working with a patient with pain or immobilization that makes it difficult to exercise the involved extremity.

Overload Principle

The overload principle states that to improve muscle performance, the muscle must be challenged. Exercises must be progressed in intensity, repetitions, or sets as the muscle adapts to greater challenges. Generally, providing resistance equal to 30% to 50% of 1 **repetition maximum** (RM) for 25 to 35 repetitions will increase muscular endurance.[28] Resistance in the range of 70%

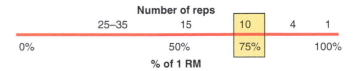

	Number of reps			
25–35	15	10	4	1
0%		50%	75%	100%
		% of 1 RM		

Figure 3.13 Muscle strength is increased by performing about 10 to 15 repetitions of an exercise at 70% to 90% of 1 RM. Endurance is increased by performing 25 to 35 repetitions of an exercise at 30% to 50% of 1 RM. Ability to perform 10 repetitions of an exercise before fatigue correlates with about 75% of 1 RM.

to 90% of 1 RM for 4 to 12 repetitions is recommended for strength training.

One repetition maximum is defined as the amount of weight the patient can lift only one time. On the second attempt to lift the load, fatigue or weakness makes it impossible to lift and maintain a steady contraction with good form. The patient's RM can be assessed by having the patient perform the movement with progressively heavier loads, until the load that can be lifted one time is determined. A good estimate of the RM may be made, however, with the understanding that if a patient can lift a load about 10 times, the resistance is approximately 75% of 1 RM (Fig. 3.13).[29]

Sedentary patients may be exercising in the range of 30% to 40% of 1 RM, whereas healthy patients are often exercising in a range from 40% to 80% of 1 RM. Athletes may be given resistance loads in the range of 80% to 90% of 1 RM. When choosing exercise intensity, it is important that the PTA understand the goals of the resistance exercises and be aware of any contraindications to muscle loading.

There are many protocols for progression of resistance exercises. More important than the specific protocol used, however, is adhering to the overload principle, which mandates continual reassessment of patient performance and progressive resistance in exercises.

Reversibility Principle

The reversibility principle refers to the loss of gains in muscle performance if training ceases. Detraining begins to occur within a week after the patient stops exercising. Patients need to be educated on the importance of maintaining the gains in strength through regular exercise.

Types of Muscle Contraction

Muscles can contract while shortening, lengthening, or remaining the same length. Each type of muscle contraction has advantages and disadvantages, but all are useful in rehabilitating orthopedic pathologies.

Concentric vs. Eccentric Contraction

Concentric muscle contraction generates less force and requires more energy compared with eccentric exercise. Eccentric exercise leads to greater hypertrophy of the

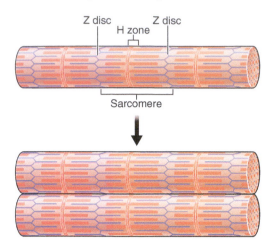

Figure 3.14 Hypertrophy of a muscle results from additional sarcomeres being added in parallel to existing sarcomeres, resulting in larger-diameter muscle fibers.

muscle. Both concentric and eccentric exercise lead to muscle growth, either by in-series addition of sarcomeres (Fig. 3.6) or by adding sarcomeres parallel to the muscle fiber, in what is termed an **in-parallel addition** (Fig. 3.14).[30–32]

Although research is inconclusive on the effects of exercise on connective tissues, eccentric exercise is often used to hypertrophy tendons in the area. However, eccentric exercise has been linked with more muscle soreness. The physical therapist may prescribe eccentric exercise later in the rehabilitation process for more athletic patients and for patients with tendon pathologies such as Achilles and patellar tendinopathy where tendon hypertrophy is desired.[33]

Often a patient will perform a concentric-eccentric exercise: concentric on the raising phase and eccentric on the lowering phase. It is possible to have the patient perform only the concentric or eccentric phase by assisting the patient to complete one phase of the exercise. Alternatively, the patient may shift the focus to one phase by more slowly performing that part of the exercise. For example, it is common to have the patient raise the extremity to a count of 3 and lower to a count of 6 to emphasize the eccentric component.

Isometric Contraction

Isometric exercise leads to strength gains if it is performed at an intensity of 60% of maximum or greater. Isometric contraction may be employed early in the rehabilitation process because it is gentle. It may also be the method chosen when joint movement is not possible or is contraindicated or when the goal is to promote joint stability.

Strength gains from isometric exercise occur only in that part of the range of motion where contraction occurs and up to 10° in either direction from the stop point. To strengthen through the entire range of motion, the patient must perform isometric contractions at least every

20° through the range. Isometric exercises done this way are called **multiple angle isometrics** (MAI).

Plyometric Exercise

Plyometric exercise is used to increase the power and agility of a muscle. Power refers to the muscle's ability to do work in a short amount of time. Plyometrics use stored energy to create an explosive, high-velocity response in muscle. A plyometric activity includes an eccentric lengthening of a muscle followed by a concentric contraction of the same muscle.

An example of plyometric exercise is jumping from a box to the floor and then springing off the floor. In jumping off a box, the quadriceps, gastrocnemius, and soleus are eccentrically lengthened upon landing and then quickly contracted concentrically in a vertical jump. The energy stored in the stretch phase of the exercise is released in the shortening phase. An indication of muscle power is seen in the patient's ability to reverse from the stretched to the shortened position quickly. Plyometric exercises are best used before a patient returns to sports or activities that involve rapid acceleration and deceleration.

Proprioceptive and Kinesthetic Awareness and Neuromuscular Control

The purpose of proprioceptive and kinesthetic retraining is to relearn kinesthetic and proprioceptive sense. Kinesthesia (sense of movement) and proprioception (sense of position) are provided by the muscle spindles, GTOs, and receptors in skin and in and around the joints. This information, along with vestibular system information from the inner ear, is processed in the brain, resulting in a sense of position and movement.

The ability to quickly process information from these receptors and generate an appropriate motor response is crucial to prevent injury and maximize function. The physical therapist is likely to include proprioceptive retraining when there has been muscle, tendon, ligament, or joint injury, or removal of ligament or cartilage, with a subsequent decrease in proprioceptors in the area. Proprioceptive and kinesthetic retraining involves exercising on an unstable surface. Exercise has been shown to be effective in retraining proprioceptive awareness.[34–36]

Recently this type of intervention has included visual and verbal feedback to help patients normalize movement patterns. Such training has been used, for example, to decrease the risk of knee ligament injury related to the pattern of landing from a jump. Whether working on an unstable surface to retrain and enhance the proprioceptive pathways in the brain, or working on neuromuscular control, the patient is learning to rapidly integrate proprioceptive input and respond appropriately.

Balance, Agility, and Coordination

Balance, agility, and coordination involve the ability to maintain one's center of gravity over one's base of support. Agility implies the ability to do this with speed and grace, and coordination implies the ability to do it smoothly and efficiently. Balance, agility, and coordination require input from the somatosensory, visual, and vestibular systems. Input is processed at the spinal cord and brain level, resulting in movements that maintain the desired body position.

With **perturbation** (efforts to disrupt balance), patients may attempt to maintain balance by using one of three strategies: an ankle, hip, or stepping strategy. For minor perturbation, the patient will initially use small ankle movements to maintain balance. With greater perturbation, the patient may additionally employ hip flexion or extension to restore balance. If the challenge to balance is great enough, the patient may step to keep the center of gravity over the base of support. While these strategies occur subconsciously in healthy people, patients may need to relearn these strategies.

Numerous studies have shown that physical therapy is effective in improving balance, agility, and coordination.[37–43] The basic tenet in balance, agility, and coordination activities is to provide a challenge while ensuring patient safety. Treatment guidelines for progressing balance activities are found in Box 3-4.

Interventions for patients with balance disorders must consider any factors that are affecting balance, such as limited motion, weakness, pain, and fear. Typically, agility and coordination activities are added to the orthopedic rehabilitation program after motion and strength are normalized and pain and inflammation are resolved. Agility training and sport-specific drills are established based on signs of patient readiness.

Aerobic Endurance

Aerobic fitness both affects and is affected by orthopedic pathology. For example, spinal discs are slower to heal in patients with low aerobic endurance. Pathologies that lead to pain and difficulty walking may lead to a loss of aerobic fitness.

The indicator of aerobic fitness is maximum oxygen consumption, or VO_{2max}, the maximum amount of oxygen that the body can take in and use per minute. VO_{2max} is measured in milliliters of oxygen per kilogram of body weight per minute. As fitness increases, VO_{2max} increases. The therapist can administer bicycle, treadmill, or walking tests to determine an approximate VO_{2max}.

In prescribing aerobic conditioning exercises, it is important to determine or estimate the patient's maximum heart rate (MHR) and target heart rate (THR). MHR is affected largely by age. An estimate of MHR can be determined by subtracting the patient's age (in years) from 220. For example, 220 – 80 (years) = 140, so an 80-year-old patient's MHR would be about 140 beats per minute (bpm). Tanaka[44] found that the formula 208 – (0.7 × age [years]) was a more accurate estimate of MHR. Using the previous example, the patient's MHR would be calculated as follows: 208 – (0.7 × 80) = 152 bpm.

Using MHR, the patient's THR can be determined. The THR is the heart rate that you want the patient to sustain during exercise. One way to calculate THR is to take 70% of the MHR. An alternative formula developed by Karvonen takes resting heart rate into account.[45] Resting heart rate is initially determined. From this, heart rate reserve is calculated by subtracting resting heart rate from MHR. Using this figure, the Karvonen formula for calculating THR is $HR_{rest} + (0.7 \times HR_{reserve})$.

When a patient's heart rate response may be blunted due to medication or cannot be assessed (while running on a treadmill, for example) a perceived exertion scale, such as the Borg Rate of Perceived Exertion (RPE) Scale, may be used. Using the Borg scale, the patient assigns a numerical value to how hard he or she is working, from 6 to 20, as shown in Table 3-2. The Borg rating has been shown to correlate to heart rate.[46,47]

When training to increase aerobic conditioning, the patient should be encouraged to exercise according to the FITT model:

- Frequency: 3 to 5 days per week
- Intensity: 60% to 90% of maximum heart rate (70% average in healthy person)
- Time: 20 to 45 minutes or more
- Type: rhythmic exercise of large muscle groups (for example, running and cycling)

Box 3-4	Treatment Guidelines for Progressing Balance Interventions

1. Move from a stable surface to an unstable surface (sitting on a chair to sitting on a swiss ball).
2. Move from a hard surface to a soft surface (standing on the floor to standing on foam).
3. Raise the center of gravity (short kneeling to tall kneeling).
4. Narrow the base of support (wide standing to narrow standing).
5. Progress from eyes open to eyes closed.
6. Add perturbation (toss a ball to the patient) in any position.
7. Move from static stability to dynamic stability (standing on, to walking on, a balance beam).
8. Add conflicting inputs (turn head side-to-side while walking straight).
9. Add cognitive distraction during movement (have patient talk while walking).

Table 3-2	Borg Rate of Perceived Exertion Scale[48]	
Rating	**Perceived Exertion**
6	No exertion
7	Extremely light
8	
9	Very light
10	
11	Light
12	
13	Somewhat hard
14	
15	Hard
16	
17	Very hard
18	
19	Extremely hard
20	Maximal exertion

From: Borg, G. *An introduction to Borg's RPE-scale*. (Ithaca, NY: Mouvement Publications, 1985).

Posture

Postural training is an important component in the treatment of some orthopedic pathologies. Posture may be affected by tight or weak muscles and by learned behaviors. Stretching and strengthening may be used to address postural impairments. In addition, the patient may require activities that increase kinesthetic awareness—using a mirror, wearing a device that provides feedback, or watching a demonstration by the PTA, for example. Proper posture will often feel abnormal and stiff to patients who have habitually assumed a poor posture. An effective teaching technique is to have the patient move into an overcorrected position and then relax to midway between their starting posture and the overcorrected position and attempt to hold this position as long as possible. Postural retraining should be done frequently throughout the day, up to every hour, so that eventually the patient naturally adopts the correct posture.

Functional Mobility

Physical therapist assistants incorporate functional mobility in orthopedic rehabilitation. Patients often require training in bed mobility, gait, and stair climbing. The patient may need to relearn how to perform functional tasks while adhering to restrictions or precautions. Having to use braces or splints may challenge traditional movement strategies. Therapy may include instruction in activating core muscles during functional movements to prevent reinjury. Gait training with assistive devices may be necessary to unload a limb while the patient is recovering.

SUMMARY

The therapist's plan of care in orthopedic rehabilitation often involves multiple goals, as discussed above. Interventions provided by the PTA will be varied to address all of the goals. It is not unusual in orthopedic physical therapy to be working on goals addressing tissue mobility, pain, strength, and functional mobility simultaneously.

In the next chapter, we will discuss in detail how tissues heal so that as we address the patient's goals, we can tailor interventions according to these healing timetables.

REVIEW QUESTIONS

1. Discuss the fundamental differences between the gate theory of pain control and the neuromatrix theory of pain control.

2. Compare and contrast the effects of stretch on contractile vs. noncontractile tissue.

3. Discuss the role central sensitization plays in chronic pain.

4. Explain the concave-convex rule to your lab partner. Discuss how an understanding of joint accessory movement and this rule are important in joint mobilization.

5. Explain the difference between neural tensioning exercises and sliding exercises. When would the therapist be likely to include each in the plan of care?

6. Explain the four principles of muscle performance: SAID, transfer of training, overload, and reversibility principles. Give an example of how each principle may affect your practice as a PTA.

7. Explain the role of concentric, eccentric, and isometric exercise in the plan of care.

REFERENCES

1. *Maitland's peripheral manipulation: Management of neuromusculoskeletal disorders* (5th ed.) Vol. 2: 9780702040672: Medicine & Health Science Books @ Amazon.com. Retrieved from: https://www.amazon.com/Maitlands-Peripheral-Manipulation-Management-Neuromusculoskeletal/dp/0702040673/ref=sr_1_1?s=books&ie=UTF8&qid=1499653361&sr=1-1&keywords=maitland%27s+peripheral+manipulation (accessed: July 10, 2017).
2. Melzack, R., & Wall, P. D. (1965). Pain mechanisms: A new theory, *Science, 150*, 971–979.

3. Melzack, R. (1999). Pain—an overview, *Acta Anaesthesiologica Scandinavica, 43,* 880–884.

4. Melzack, R. (2001). Pain and the neuromatrix in the brain, *Journal of Dental Education, 65,* 1378–1382.

5. Woolf, C. J. (2011). Central sensitization: Implications for the diagnosis and treatment of pain. *Pain, 152,* S2–15.

6. Kosek, E., et al. (2016). Do we need a third mechanistic descriptor for chronic pain states? *Pain, 157,* 1382–1386.

7. Louw, A., Butler, D. S., Diener, I., & Puentedura, E. J. (2013). Development of a preoperative neuroscience educational program for patients with lumbar radiculopathy. *American Journal of Physical Medicine and Rehabilitation, 92,* 446–452.

8. Louw, A., Diener, I., Butler, D. S., & Puentedura, E. J. (2011). The effect of neuroscience education on pain, disability, anxiety, and stress in chronic musculoskeletal pain. *Archives of Physical Medicine and Rehabilitation, 92,* 2041–2056.

9. Louw, A., Diener, I., Landers, M. R., & Puentedura, E. J. (2014). Preoperative pain neuroscience education for lumbar radiculopathy: A multicenter randomized controlled trial with 1-year follow-up. *Spine, 39,* 1449–1457.

10. Louw, A., Puentedura, E. L., & Mintken, P. (2012). Use of an abbreviated neuroscience education approach in the treatment of chronic low back pain: A case report. *Physiotherapy Theory and Practice, 28,* 50–62.

11. Moseley, G. L. (2003). A pain neuromatrix approach to patients with chronic pain. *Manual Therapy, 8,* 130–140.

12. Moseley, G. L. (2005). Widespread brain activity during an abdominal task markedly reduced after pain physiology education: fMRI evaluation of a single patient with chronic low back pain. *Australian Journal of Physiotherapy, 51,* 49–52.

13. Moseley, G. L., Nicholas, M. K., & Hodges, P. W. (2004). A randomized controlled trial of intensive neurophysiology education in chronic low back pain. *Clinical Journal of Pain, 20,* 324–330.

14. Kisner, C., & Colby, L. A. (2012). *Therapeutic exercise: Foundations and techniques.* Philadelphia, PA: F.A. Davis.

15. Hammer, W. I. (2007). *Functional soft-tissue examination and treatment by manual methods.* Burlington, MA: Jones & Bartlett Learning.

16. Bottinelli, R., Eastwood, J. C., & Flitney, F. W. (1989). Sarcomere 'give' during stretch of frog single muscle fibres with added series compliance. *Quarterly Journal of Experimental Physiology, 74,* 215–217.

17. De Deyne, P. G. (2001). Application of passive stretch and its implications for muscle fibers. *Physical Therapy, 81,* 819–827.

18. Lynn, R., & Morgan, D. L. (1994). Decline running produces more sarcomeres in rat vastus intermedius muscle fibers than does incline running. *Journal of Applied Physiology, Bethesda Maryland, 1985, 77,* 1439–1444.

19. Scott, A. B. (1994). Change of eye muscle sarcomeres according to eye position. *Journal of Pediatric Ophthalmology and Strabismus, 31,* 85–88.

20. Williams, P. E. (1990). Use of intermittent stretch in the prevention of serial sarcomere loss in immobilised muscle. *Annals of Rheumatic Disease, 49,* 316–317.

21. Williams, P., Watt, P., Bicik, V., & Goldspink, G. (1986). Effect of stretch combined with electrical stimulation on the type of sarcomeres produced at the ends of muscle fibers. *Experimental Neurology, 93,* 500–509.

22. Cormie, P., McGuigan, M. R., & Newton, R. U. (2010). Adaptations in athletic performance after ballistic power versus strength training. *Medicine and Science in Sports and Exercise, 42,* 1582–1598.

23. Young, W. B. (2006). Transfer of strength and power training to sports performance. *International Journal of Sports Physiology and Performance, 1,* 74–83.

24. Zaras, N., et al. (2013). Effects of strength vs. ballistic-power training on throwing performance. *Journal of Sports Science and Medicine, 12,* 130–137.

25. Latella, C., Kidgell, D. J., & Pearce, A. J. (2012). Reduction in corticospinal inhibition in the trained and untrained limb following unilateral leg strength training. *European Journal of Applied Physiology, 112,* 3097–3107.

26. Lee, M., & Carroll, T. J. (2007). Cross education: Possible mechanisms for the contralateral effects of unilateral resistance training. *Sports Medicine, Auckland, New Zealand, 37,* 1–14.

27. Pearce, A. J., Hendy, A., Bowen, W. A., & Kidgell, D. J. (2013). Corticospinal adaptations and strength maintenance in the immobilized arm following 3 weeks unilateral strength training. *Scandinavian Journal of Medicine and Science in Sports, 23,* 740–748.

28. Petty, N. J. (2011). *Principles of neuromusculoskeletal treatment and management: A handbook for therapists.* Elsevier Health Sciences: London, UK.

29. Reynolds, J. M., Gordon, T. J., & Robergs, R. A. (2006). Prediction of one repetition maximum strength from multiple repetition maximum testing and anthropometry. *Journal of Strength and Conditioning Research, 20,* 584–592.

30. Roig, M., O'Brien, K., Kirk, G., Murray, R., McKinnon, P., Shadgan, B., & Reid, W. D. (2009). The effects of eccentric versus concentric resistance training on muscle strength and mass in healthy adults: A systematic review with meta-analysis. *British Journal of Sports Medicine, 43,* 556–568.

31. de Souza-Teixeira, F. & de Paz, J. A. (2012). Eccentric resistance training and muscle hypertrophy. *Journal of Sports Medicine and Doping Studies, S1.* doi: 10.4172/2161-0673 .S1-004. Retrieved from: https://pdfs.semanticscholar.org/96d5/ 9d0785bdf61e39950c1d3b158f2e42b45e80.pdf?_ga=2 .191679215.458144152.1538958428-1303887332 .1538958428

32. Vikne, H., Refsnes, P. E., Ekmark, M., Medbø, J. I., Gundersen, V., & Gundersen, K. (2006). Muscular performance after concentric and eccentric exercise in trained men. *Medicine and Science in Sports and Exercise, 38,* 1770–1781.

33. Murtaugh, B., & Ihm, J. M. (2013). Eccentric training for the treatment of tendinopathies. *Current Sports Medicine. Reports, 12,* 175–182.

34. Hwang, J. A., Bae, S. H., Do Kim, G., & Kim, K. Y. (2013). The effects of sensorimotor training on anticipatory postural adjustment of the trunk in chronic low back pain patients. *Journal of Physical Therapy Science, 25,* 1189–1192.

35. Lephart, S. M., Pincivero, D. M., Giraldo, J. L., & Fu, F. H. (1997). The role of proprioception in the management and rehabilitation of athletic injuries. *American Journal of Sports Medicine, 25,* 130–137.

36. Lephart, S. M., Pincivero, D. M., & Rozzi, S. L. (1998) Proprioception of the ankle and knee. *Sports Medicine (Auckland, New Zealand), 25,* 149–155.

37. Burschka, J. M., Keune, P. M., Oy, U. H., Oschmann, P., & Kuhn, P. (2014). Mindfulness-based interventions in multiple sclerosis: Beneficial effects of Tai Chi on balance, coordination, fatigue and depression. *BMC Neurology, 14,* 165.

38. Chen, B., Mok, D., Lee, W. C. C., & Lam, W. K. (2014). High-intensity stepwise conditioning programme for improved exercise responses and agility performance of a badminton player with knee pain. *Physical Therapy in Sport: Official Journal of the Association of Chartered Physiotherapists in Sports Medicine* doi: 10.1016/j.ptsp.2014.06.005.

39. Hiroyuki, S., Uchiyama, Y., & Kakurai, S. (2003). Specific effects of balance and gait exercises on physical function among the frail elderly. *Clinical Rehabilitation, 17,* 472–479.

40. Karthikbabu, S., Nayak, A., Vijayakumar, K., Misri, Z., Suresh, B., Ganesan, S. & Joshua, A. M. (2011). Comparison of physio

ball and plinth trunk exercises regimens on trunk control and functional balance in patients with acute stroke: A pilot randomized controlled trial. *Clinical Rehabilitation, 25,* 709–719.

41. Lee, J., & Seo, K. (2014). The effects of stair walking training on the balance ability of chronic stroke patients. *Journal of Physical Therapy Science, 26,* 517–520.

42. Martínez-Amat, A., Hita-Contreras, F., Lomas-Vega, R., Caballero-Martínez, I., Alvarez, P. J., & Martínez-López, E. (2013). Effects of 12-week proprioception training program on postural stability, gait, and balance in older adults: A controlled clinical trial. *Journal of Strength and Conditioning Research, 27,* 2180–2188.

43. Seo, K., Kim, J., & Wi, G. (2014). The effects of stair gait exercise on static balance ability of stroke patients. *Journal of Physical Therapy Science, 26,* 1835–1838.

44. Tanaka, H., Monahan, K. D., & Seals, D. R. (2001). Age-predicted maximal heart rate revisited. *Journal of the American College of Cardiology, 37,* 153–156.

45. Karvonen, J., & Vuorimaa, T. (1988). Heart rate and exercise intensity during sports activities. Practical application. *Sports Medicine (Auckland, New Zealand), 5,* 303–311.

46. Alberton, C. L., Antunes, A. H., Pinto, S. S., Tartaruga, M. P., Silva, E. M., Cadore, E. L., & Martins Kruel, L. F. (2011). Correlation between rating of perceived exertion and physiological variables during the execution of stationary running in water at different cadences. *Journal of Strength and Conditioning Research, 25,* 155–162.

47. Chen, M. J., Fan, X., & Moe, S. T. (2002). Criterion-related validity of the Borg ratings of perceived exertion scale in healthy individuals: A meta-analysis. *Journal of Sports Science, 20,* 873–899.

48. Borg, G. (1985). *An introduction to Borg's RPE-scale.* Ithaca, NY: Mouvement Publications.

Chapter 4

Interventions to Promote Healing in Various Tissues

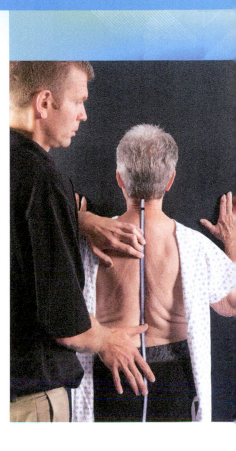

Ligament
> Ligament Pathology: Sprain
> Ligament Healing
> Physical Therapy Interventions During Ligament Healing

Tendon
> Tendon Pathology: Strain, Tendinopathy, and Tenosynopathy
> Tendon Healing
> Physical Therapy Interventions During Tendon Healing

Muscle
> Muscle Pathology: Strain
> Muscle Healing
> Physical Therapy Interventions During Muscle Healing

Cartilage: Articular Cartilage and Fibrocartilage
> Cartilage Pathology: Degeneration and Tear
> Cartilage Healing
> Physical Therapy Interventions During Cartilage Healing

Peripheral Nerves
> Peripheral Nerve Pathology: Neurapraxia, Axonotmesis, and Neurotmesis
> Peripheral Nerve Healing and Repair
> Physical Therapy Interventions During Nerve Healing

Bone
> Bone Pathology: Fracture
> Fracture Healing
> Fracture Management
> Physical Therapy Interventions During Bone Healing

Summary

LEARNING OUTCOMES

After reading this chapter, the student will:

4.1 Discuss the healing process in ligament, tendon, muscle, cartilage, nerve, and bone.

4.2 Describe the grades of ligament sprain, tendon strain, muscle strain, and nerve injury.

4.3 Identify common physical therapy interventions suitable for pathologies of ligament, tendon, muscle, cartilage, nerve, and bone.

KEY WORDS

Axonotmesis	Neurapraxia	Soft callus
Closed reduction	Neurotmesis	Synovial sheath
Coaptation	Open reduction, internal fixation	Tendinopathy
Compound fracture	(ORIF)	Tendinosis
Comminuted fracture	Osteoblast	Tendonitis
Denervated	Osteoclast	Tenosynopathy
External fixation	Paratenon	Tenosynovitis
Extraarticular ligaments	PRICE approach to treatment:	Wallerian degeneration
Fracture hematoma	Protection, Rest, Ice, Compression,	
Hard callus	Elevation	
Intraarticular ligaments	Simple fracture	

Introduction

All tissues respond to injury in a similar fashion: healing begins immediately after injury with an inflammatory response, followed by repair and remodeling. Although the basic processes are similar between tissue types, there are tissue-specific considerations: injured tissue must be replaced with healthy tissue of the same type, that is, bone is replaced by bone, cartilage by cartilage, et cetera.

Every body tissue responds to injury or stress by undergoing predictable changes. We say that "form follows function." In rehabilitation, we use this principle to stress the injured tissue to promote a return to pre-injury structure, or form. The challenge comes in stressing tissues to the optimum amount, at the optimum time, to promote healing. A deeper understanding of how tissues heal is necessary.

This chapter discusses specific considerations for each type of tissue healing. Factors such as the vascularity of the tissue, the patient's age and health, and the extent of the injury all affect the rate at which the tissue will heal.

Ligament

Ligaments are composed primarily of type I collagen and water. Type I collagen is strong and thick, and the collagen fibers run in bundles lengthwise down the ligament. Ligaments were once considered simple and inert structures, but we now understand that ligaments have a highly complex arrangement of fibers and that they vary in composition depending upon specific function. Proprioceptive receptors within ligaments play an important role in joint position sense.

Ligament Pathology: Sprain

A stretch or tear of the ligament is called a sprain. Ligament sprain is graded in severity as follows:

- Grade I ligament sprain: Stretching and microtearing of some fibers of the ligament; no detectable joint laxity.
- Grade II ligament sprain: Partial tearing of the ligament; some joint laxity usually results.

- Grade III ligament sprain: Complete tearing or rupture of the ligament; significant joint laxity is common.

Figure 4.1 depicts grades of ligament sprain.

Ligament Healing

Ligament healing occurs in three, overlapping stages. In stage I, the tissue becomes inflamed. Macrophages in the area are actively removing dead cells. In stage II, fibroblasts are producing collagen that will be used to rebuild. In stage III, the collagen aligns and matures to resemble the preinjury tissue. This process is described under inflammation in Chapter 3. However, the timetable for ligament healing may be prolonged due to the relatively limited blood supply that is typical of ligaments (see Box 4-1).

Initially after tearing of part or all of a ligament, the area forms a hematoma. Fibroblasts produce collagen that aligns along the length of the ligament. However, the remodeled "scarred" area will have a persistence of small-diameter collagen with weak bonds even months after injury. The end result is that the healed ligament may have only about 50% of the tensile strength of the preinjury ligament.[1,2]

While ligaments in general are subject to a slow timetable of healing, there are other factors that impact ligament healing. The location of the ligament is one factor. As an example, two ligaments that have been studied extensively are the medial collateral ligament (MCL) and the anterior cruciate ligament (ACL) of the knee. Of interest when comparing these two ligaments is that the MCL is likely to heal after rupture, whereas the ACL is not likely to heal after rupture. It has been generalized from this observation that **intraarticular**

Box 4-1	Approximate Timetable for Ligament Healing
Stage I (inflammatory)	0–14 days
Stage II (repair)	2 weeks–2 months
Stage III (remodeling)	2 months–1 year

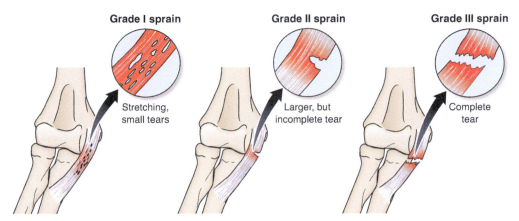

Grade I sprain   **Grade II sprain**   **Grade III sprain**

Stretching, small tears   Larger, but incomplete tear   Complete tear

Figure 4.1 Grades I–III of ligament sprain. Grade I involves microtearing of some ligament fibers. Grade II is a partial tear. Grade III is a complete tear.

ligaments don't heal as well as extraarticular ligaments. It has been suggested that synovial fluid in which intraarticular ligaments are immersed may interrupt the formation of a hematoma and thereby interrupt this essential stage in healing.

Some ligaments appear to have properties, other than location, that allow them to heal more readily than other ligaments. For example, injury to the ACL causes the ligament to release enzymes that destroy new tissue during the repair stage of healing. Injury to the MCL does not result in the same enzyme destruction.[3]

Physical Therapy Interventions During Ligament Healing

Ligament recovery appears to depend on a number of variables, including the amount of movement to which the ligament is subjected.[4–7] Controlled early motion is beneficial for ligament recovery. Exercise has been shown to increase the number and thickness of collagen fibers in the healing ligament and improve fiber alignment. An "exercised" ligament has been shown to withstand greater forces before failing than a nonexercised ligament. As soon as safely possible, the body part should be mobilized and weight-bearing should be progressed.

During the inflammatory stage of ligament healing, interventions should focus on controlling the inflammatory response. Use the **PRICE approach to treatment: P**rotection, **R**est, **I**ce, **C**ompression, **E**levation. Progressive weight-bearing, multiple-angle isometric exercise, and ligament protection are common interventions during this stage.

During the repair stage of healing, weight-bearing is progressed. Exercise should gently stress the ligament to orient the collagen fibers in parallel along the ligament.[4,6] However, the ligament should not be overstressed during this phase, to avoid harming the healing ligament.

In the remodeling phase, activities are advanced to include increased ligament stress, concentric and eccentric exercise, plyometric exercise, and proprioceptive retraining.

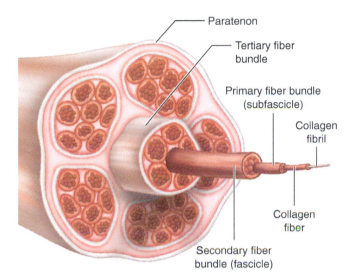

Paratenon

Tertiary fiber bundle

Primary fiber bundle (subfascicle)

Collagen fibril

Collagen fiber

Secondary fiber bundle (fascicle)

Figure 4.2 Tendons are arranged in bundles of collagen fibers. The outside is either a synovial sheath or a loose covering called a paratenon.

Tendon

Tendons are composed primarily of type I collagen and water. The collagen fibers are arranged in bundles (fascicles) and run lengthwise down the tendon. The tendon transmits forces from the muscle to the bone. Tendons are stronger than muscle and have a tensile strength equal to that of bone.

Tendons have two types of coverings: a **synovial sheath** or a **paratenon**. Synovial sheath coverings are lined with synovial cells, which lubricate the tendon. Synovial sheaths are often present where tendons have to glide over multiple joints, such as in the hand. Tendons without a synovial sheath have a paratenon instead, a loose covering consisting of connective tissue. Figure 4.2 depicts the structure of tendon.

Tendon Pathology: Strain, Tendinopathy, and Tenosynopathy

Tears of the tendon are called tendon strains. Similar to a ligament sprain, a tendon strain is graded on a scale from I to III as follows:

- Grade I: Microtearing of the tendon; little to no weakness or loss of function.
- Grade II: Partial tear of the tendon; moderate weakness and loss of function is common.
- Grade III: Complete rupture of the tendon; significant weakness and loss of function.

Chronic overuse and microtearing of the tendon may lead to degenerative changes in the tendon with or without inflammation. It was previously believed that inflammation was the cause of tendon pathology, but many recent studies demonstrate microscopic changes in the tendon without inflammation. These changes include tendon thickening, immature collagen formation, and formation of new blood vessels.[8-10]

Tendon pathology with inflammation is called **tendonitis**. Degenerative changes in the tendon without signs of inflammation are called **tendinosis**. An inclusive term used to describe pathologies of the tendon with or without inflammation is **tendinopathy**. Similarly, if the pathology involves the synovial sheath covering, it may be referred to as **tenosynovitis** or **tenosynopathy**.

Because the tendon is attached to contractile tissue, symptom reproduction with a tendon pathology may occur during contraction of the attached muscle. The area may also be painful to palpation and to stretch of the tissue. Pain on palpation, stretch, and contraction indicates a muscular or tendinous pathology. These maneuvers form the basis for many special tests of muscle and tendon pathologies.

Tendon Healing

Tendon healing follows the inflammation/repair/remodeling processes but with a longer timetable due to a relatively limited blood supply and compromised diffusion of nutrients. The inflammatory stage may last for up to 3 weeks after injury. Stage III may not begin until 6 to 8 weeks after injury. See Box 4-2 for an approximate timetable of tendon healing.

Two problems commonly develop after tendon injury. The first is adhesion to surrounding tissue. Tendon healing relies on fibroblasts from the paratenon and surrounding structures to produce collagen. Because of this, adhesions are common. Second, the tensile strength of tendon is commonly decreased for a year or more after injury and may reach only 40% to 60% of preinjury levels.[11]

Physical Therapy Interventions During Tendon Healing

Initially after tendon injury, interventions focus on controlling the inflammatory response. The plan of care will often include the PRICE approach to treatment.

Because of the risk of adhesive scarring, it is essential to glide the tendon early in the healing process. Most commonly this is accomplished by passive range of motion in the early stages of healing, to protect the tendon against the forces produced by muscle contraction. At approximately 2 months after injury, intervention may include active range of motion with gravity eliminated. By 3 to 4 months after injury, progressive resistance may be included in the plan of care, with maximum muscle contraction allowed after 4 months.

Because the healing process varies and depends on so many factors, initial stress on healing tendons should be minimal. Observe the patient for changes in symptoms as exercise is progressed. The PTA should seek a balance between tissue protection and early mobilization. When in doubt about how much to stress the tissue, the PTA should consult the supervising physical therapist for direction.

Muscle

Muscle is made up of contractile muscle fibers containing actin and myosin myofilaments, surrounded by noncontractile tissue that envelops the fibers and arranges them into bundles. The noncontractile tissues include the endomysium, perimysium, and epimysium. Satellite cells lie dormant on the outside of the muscle fiber. When muscle injury occurs, these satellite cells activate and play a major role in healing, as discussed below. Figure 4.3 depicts muscle anatomy.

Muscle Pathology: Strain

Muscle injury is called strain. It is graded in severity from I to III:

- Grade I muscle strain: Microscopic damage to the muscle with few fibers stretched or torn; although painful, muscle has normal strength and function.
- Grade II muscle strain: Many of the muscle fibers are torn; noticeable loss of strength.
- Grade III muscle strain: Complete tear of the muscle; complete loss of strength in the muscle; possibly noticeable change in the superficial contour of the muscle.

Because the muscle is contractile, symptoms of pathology are similar to those of tendon pathology. Pain on palpation, stretch, or contraction may indicate a muscular

Box 4-2	Approximate Timetable for Tendon Healing[16]	
Stage I (inflammatory)	0–21 days
Stage II (repair)	3–6 weeks
Stage III (remodeling)	6 weeks–1 year

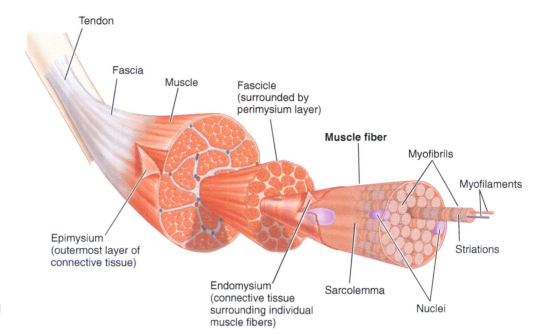

Figure 4.3 Anatomy of muscle. The muscle fiber is the cellular unit of muscle. It is wrapped with endomysium. Muscle fibers are bundled into fascicles, wrapped with perimysium. Within each fiber are myofibrils made of actin and myosin myofilaments.

Box 4-3	Approximate Timetable for Muscle Healing
Stage I (inflammatory; satellite cells)	**0–3 days**
Stage II (repair)	**3 days–8 weeks**
Stage III (remodeling)	**8 weeks–1 year**

pathology, and these maneuvers form the basis for the special tests for muscle pathologies.

Muscle Healing

When a muscle is strained repair occurs through the stages of healing as described previously. Although muscle is highly vascular, rebuilding after injury takes some time. During the inflammatory stage, bleeding stops and phagocytosis occurs. The satellite cells activate; the cells divide, travel to the injured area, and patch the original muscle fiber or form a new fiber (Fig. 4.4). If the muscle injury disrupts the endomysium, the satellite cells are unable to multiply and a connective tissue scar replaces the injured tissue. The rebuilding phase may take up to 8 weeks after injury. In stage III, the muscle is remodeled and the repaired or replaced fibers mature. See Box 4-3 for an approximate timetable for muscle healing.

Physical Therapy Interventions During Muscle Healing

Initially after muscle injury, interventions focus on controlling the inflammatory response. Use the PRICE approach to treatment.

During the repair stage, passive range of motion allows the muscle and tendon to move while protecting the muscle from the force of contraction. Around 2 months after injury, intervention may include active range of motion with gravity eliminated. By 3 to 4 months after injury, progressive resistance may be included in the plan of care, with maximum muscle contraction allowed after 4 months. Surgical repair after complete tear may progress more slowly.

Cartilage: Articular Cartilage and Fibrocartilage

There are three types of cartilage: articular (or hyaline) cartilage, fibrocartilage, and elastic cartilage. Articular and fibrocartilage are involved in the movement system and will be discussed further. The main components of most types of cartilage are collagen, elastin, and proteoglycans/glycosaminoglycans (GAGs) (see Table 4-1).

Articular cartilage lines the ends of bones. Articular cartilage is made up of water, type II collagen, chondrocytes, and proteoglycans/glycosaminoglycans (GAGs). Proteoglycans are protein compounds that make the cartilage capable of withstanding compression. Articular cartilage is avascular, which significantly compromises its ability to heal.

Fibrocartilage makes up the meniscus of the knee and labrum of the hip and shoulder. Fibrocartilage is composed primarily of water and type I collagen. It contains a small amount of elastin and proteoglycans. The collagen fibers in fibrocartilage run circumferentially to allow the tissue to absorb compressive forces and resist shear.

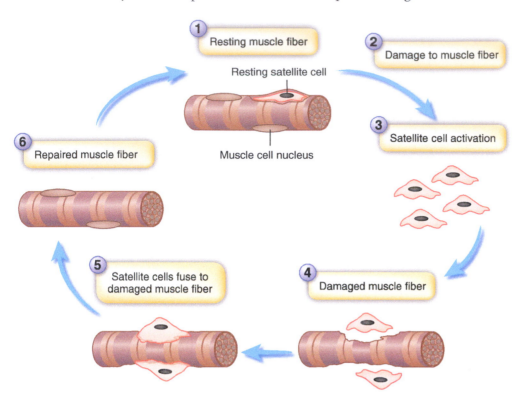

Figure 4.4 Healing process for muscle. Satellite cells on the muscle fiber form a patch to repair the injured tissue.

Table 4-1	Components of Cartilage
Type I collagen	Strong, thick, permanently bonded protein fiber. Found in mature scars, tendons, skin, and fibrocartilage.
Type II collagen	Protein fiber found in articular cartilage.
Type III collagen	Thin, temporarily bonded protein fiber found in second stage of healing.
Elastin	Very thin protein fiber that increases flexibility or elasticity of tissue.
Proteoglycan/ glycosaminoglycan	Molecules that increase compressive strength.

Cartilage Pathology: Degeneration and Tear

Pathology of the articular cartilage may arise from trauma, wear and tear, or joint immobilization. As articular cartilage wears, it becomes soft and may fray, crack, and deteriorate. The consistency of the cartilage changes from a firm, slippery substance to that of hard-boiled egg white. Areas where the cartilage is worn are called articular cartilage defects. If unrepaired, articular cartilage defects may lead to osteoarthritis of the joint.

Examples of fibrocartilage pathology are commonly seen in the knee, hip, and shoulder. Injury to the meniscal cartilage may be a result of trauma or wear-and-tear and manifests in the form of cartilage tears. The labrum of the hip and shoulder may tear or partially detach from the bony rim due to repetitive stress or trauma.

Cartilage Healing

In articular cartilage, the stages of healing described above generally result in a mechanically weak scar due to the lack of blood flow. However, recent advances in surgical repair of articular cartilage, including microfracture of the subchondral bone to stimulate blood flow to the area, autograft transplantation of articular cartilage from other areas of the joint, and chondrocyte harvesting and reimplantation, are proving to be successful treatments.

The outer third of the knee meniscus is vascular, but the middle and inner thirds are progressively less vascular. Meniscal cartilage tears in the outer one-third will heal if repaired. Repair or stitching of the meniscus ensures that the tear lies flat and relatively undisturbed while the tissue heals. If the tear is in the middle or inner third, however, that portion of the cartilage is generally removed, because healing is unlikely in those regions. Surgical removal of meniscal cartilage is called meniscectomy.

Physical Therapy Interventions During Cartilage Healing

Physical therapy interventions in the presence of cartilage injury depend on the location and extent of the injury. Decreasing the stresses on the cartilage may include

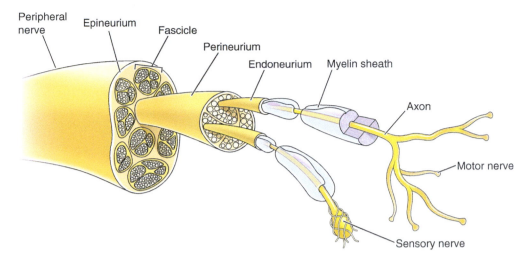

Figure 4.5 Anatomy of a peripheral nerve. Axons of sensory, motor, and autonomic neurons are bundled in the nerve fiber. Each axon is wrapped in an endoneurium and bundled into clusters by a perineurium. The epineurium surrounds the entire nerve.

avoiding certain movements, such as the end range of hip flexion or extension in the case of a hip labral tear. Weight-bearing may be restricted. Open-chain or isometric strengthening may be used to maintain strength.

Peripheral Nerves

Neurons (nerve cells) are composed of dendrites, a cell body, an axon, and axon terminals that synapse on the dendrites of other neurons. Peripheral nerves are a bundle of axons that may represent sensory neurons, motor neurons, and/or autonomic system neurons. Each neuron is supported by Schwann cells that form a fatty myelin sheath around the axon. The axon and Schwann cells are then covered by a thin, delicate membrane called the endoneurium. Bundles of axons are segregated into fascicles by a perineurium. Many clusters of fascicles, along with blood vessels, are surrounded by an epineurium, to form a peripheral nerve (Fig. 4.5).

Peripheral Nerve Pathology: Neurapraxia, Axonotmesis, and Neurotmesis

Pathology of peripheral nerves includes overstretch, laceration, or crushing injuries. Peripheral nerves are capable of repair if the perineurium and epineurium are left intact. Nerve injury was initially classified into three categories: neurapraxia, axonotmesis, and neurotmesis.[12] Further study led to five degrees of peripheral nerve injury (Fig. 4.6).[13]

- First degree (**neurapraxia**): Minor injury to the nerve that causes temporary weakness and loss of sensation. The endoneurium, perineurium, and epineurium are not disrupted. Recovery is full, and generally occurs within 6 to 8 weeks.
- Second degree (**axonotmesis**): Injury to some axons, but the endoneurium remains intact. Recovery is possible.

- Third degree: The endoneurium is partially disrupted. The perineurium and epineurium remain intact, and recovery is possible.
- Fourth degree (**neurotmesis**): Injury in which everything is disrupted except the epineurium. Recovery is not possible without surgical repair.
- Fifth degree: More severe form of neurotmesis; the nerve is completely severed, including the epineurium. Recovery is not possible without surgical repair.

Peripheral Nerve Healing and Repair

After peripheral nerve injury, signs of inflammation and healing occur very quickly. If the axon is disrupted, it dies from the point of injury distally, in a process called **Wallerian degeneration**. Schwann cells proliferate and travel into the area where the axon was, forming tubules that act as channels to direct new axon sprouts across the lesion and to the tissue that was originally innervated by the axon (Fig. 4.7). This tissue is known as the target tissue. Multiple small-diameter axon sprouts form in the area and grow through the channels at a rate of about 1 mm/day or 1 inch/month.

During the final stages of healing, axons that reach the target tissue increase in diameter as they mature. However, the thickness of the axon and myelin sheath is not usually restored to preinjury levels. Even with proper nerve healing, the axon may go astray and not successfully reach the target tissue. In this case, the target tissue remains **denervated**, lacking a nerve supply. Without innervation, the target tissue undergoes changes that include bone and muscle atrophy and capsule fibrosis.

In fourth- and fifth-degree (neurotmesis) injuries, fibroblasts in the endoneurium activate to rebuild the nerve. The fibroblast action results in thick scar tissue, which is difficult for axonal sprouts to penetrate. For this reason, surgical repair is necessary in these higher degrees of peripheral nerve injury.

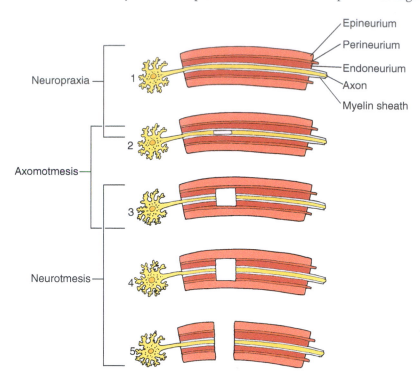

Neuropraxia

Axomotmesis

Neurotmesis

Epineurium
Perineurium
Endoneurium
Axon
Myelin sheath

Figure 4.6 Degrees of nerve injury.

Surgical repair may involve bringing the severed ends of the nerve together and stitching the nerve fascicles together (**coaptation**). If the nerve ends cannot be suitably aligned or approximated, a nerve autograft may be performed. Commonly, the patient's sural nerve is taken from the calf and grafted onto the injured tissue. Alternatively, synthetic collagen tubes to guide the nerve growth may be inserted so the patient is not subjected to further nerve damage.

Physical Therapy Interventions During Nerve Healing

Physical therapy interventions during nerve healing must ensure that nerve tension is applied carefully at first to avoid injuring the axon sprouts or the perineurium. A thorough understanding of the extent of injury, the nature of the repair if applicable, and the process of nerve healing should be applied to determine how to treat the regenerating peripheral nerve. Some stress of neural tissue helps to promote healing, but extreme tension applied early in recovery is harmful.[14] The plan of care in the early stages of recovery may include the use of modalities such as electrical stimulation or superficial heat. Mirror therapy may be used to rebuild the brain map for injured areas.[15,16]

Bone

Bone is made up of about 30% organic material, mostly collagen, and 70% mineral, mostly calcium and phosphate. The primary cell responsible for producing bone is the **osteoblast**. The cell responsible for absorbing bone

is the **osteoclast**. Bones are in a constant state of being formed or absorbed by these two cells.

Bone Pathology: Fracture

Common pathologies affecting bone include osteomalacia, osteoporosis, and tumors. This discussion, however, focuses on the process of healing after fracture.

Fracture is the most common injury or pathology of bone that the PTA encounters. Figure 4.8 depicts various types of fractures. From a clinical standpoint, fractures are described using the Salter classification, which includes the following information about the fracture:

- Site of the fracture. Describing the place on the bone that is injured; common terms are diaphyseal, epiphyseal, or intraarticular fracture.
- Extent of the fracture. Fractures may be complete (all the way across the bone) or incomplete. Incomplete fractures include hairline fractures or cracks. Greenstick fractures are a common incomplete fracture in children.
- Configuration of the fracture. The direction of a complete fracture including a classification of transverse, oblique, or spiral. The term **comminuted** is used to describe a fracture with more than two fragments.
- Relationship of the fracture fragments to each other. Fragments can be displaced or nondisplaced. Additional terms (rotated, impacted) may describe the displaced fragments.
- Open vs. closed fracture. A closed fracture (also called a **simple fracture**) is one in which the skin

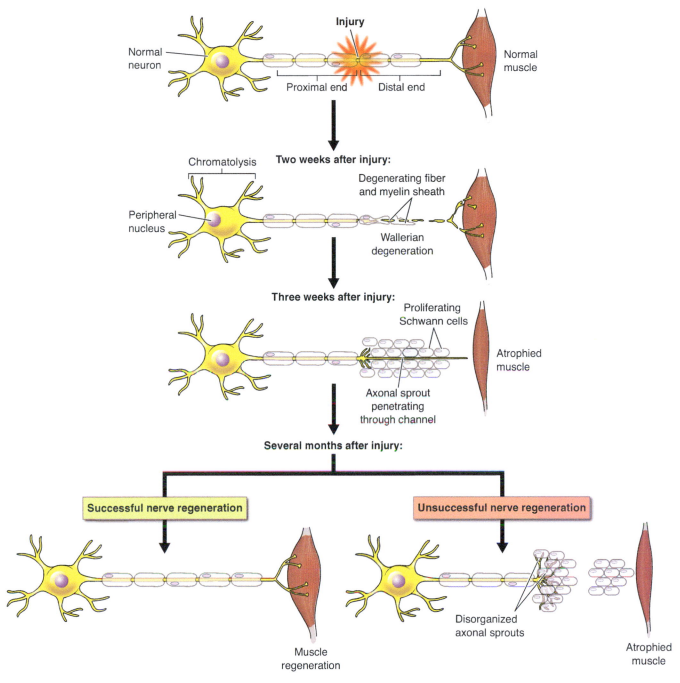

Figure 4.7 Repair after nerve injury. After axonal injury, the axon deteriorates distal to the injury. Nerve sprouts are guided by Schwann cells toward the denervated tissue, growing at a rate of about 1 inch/month. Likelihood of reinnervation of the target tissue is higher with less severe injury. Neurotmesis may lead to permanent loss of innervation.

over the fracture is intact. An open fracture (also called a **compound fracture**) is one in which the skin over the fracture is not intact.

- Complicated vs. uncomplicated. A complicated fracture refers to any local or systemic complication from the fracture or treatment of the fracture. Complications may include infection, vascular compromise, and delayed union or nonunion of the bone ends.[17]

Fracture Healing

There are two primary mechanisms by which the bone heals after fracture. If the bone ends are brought into close approximation, the bone will heal by primary repair. Primary repair requires the bone ends to be brought tightly together and stabilized. In this type of healing, osteoclasts travel through the fracture line and remove dead bone on either side of the fracture. Osteoblasts then fill in these areas with new bone cells.

More commonly, the ends of the fracture are not held so tightly together, and healing occurs through a secondary repair. A blood clot (**fracture hematoma**) forms in the area of the break. A small portion of the bone on the fracture ends dies. Phagocytes clean the area of debris, then fibroblasts and chondrocytes produce a fibrocartilage **soft callus** in the area, filling in the gap between the bone surfaces. During this phase of healing the fracture site may be referred to as "sticky." Soft callus is usually seen between 4 days and 3 weeks after fracture.

Osteoblasts begin to enter the area of the soft callus, producing bone cells and converting the soft callus to a **hard callus,** which is complete about 5 to 6 weeks after fracture. The hard callus shows up on an x-ray, and at this point the fracture is united. For several more months,

possibly up to a year, the hard callus will be remodeled by osteoclasts and osteoblasts until the preinjury diameter of the bone is restored (Fig. 4.9).

Bone fractures may be slow to heal (delayed union), or fail to heal (nonunion). Factors that have been shown to adversely affect bone healing include inadequate reduction of the bone ends, inadequate fracture stabilization, tobacco or nicotine use (smoking, chewing tobacco, and nicotine gum or patches), advanced age, severe injury, anemia, diabetes, poor nutrition including vitamin D deficiency, some medications, and infection.

Fracture Management

Initially after a fracture, the physician or surgeon determines whether the fracture requires intervention. If the fracture ends are in close approximation, with good alignment, and the fracture is stable, no intervention may be necessary.

If, however, the fracture is not stable, intervention may be necessary. Intervention may be any of the following:

- **Closed reduction:** The bone ends are approximated with or without the use of anesthesia. After closed reduction, traction or external fixation may be used to maintain the position of the bone ends.
- **Open reduction, internal fixation (ORIF):** Surgical realignment of the fracture ends. After alignment, fracture ends are held in position by plates, screws, nail, pins, rods, or wires. Bone grafting over the fracture site may be employed if the bone ends are not close to each other.
- **External fixation:** Casting, splinting, and/or external fixator hardware are employed to stabilize the bone fragments.
- **Traction:** Pins are inserted in the distal segment and weight or distraction is applied to the bone to maintain alignment. Traction is frequently employed for cervical spine fractures.

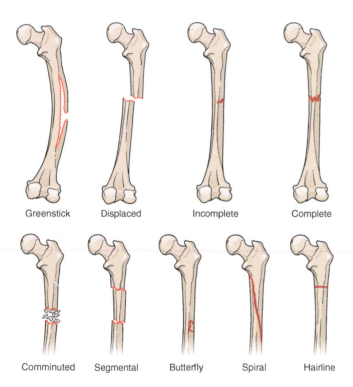

Greenstick   Displaced   Incomplete   Complete

Comminuted   Segmental   Butterfly   Spiral   Hairline

Figure 4.8 Types of bone fractures.

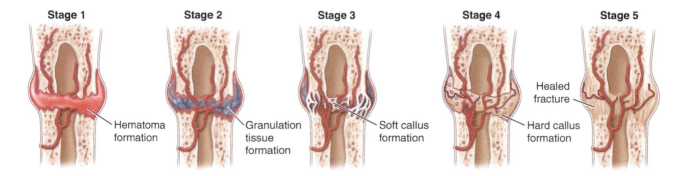

Stage 1   Stage 2   Stage 3   Stage 4   Stage 5

Hematoma formation   Granulation tissue formation   Soft callus formation   Healed fracture   Hard callus formation

Figure 4.9 Stages of bone healing. A hematoma forms in the area between the bone ends. Fibroblasts and chondrocytes form a soft callus by about 3 weeks. Osteoblasts change the soft callus to a hard callus by about 6 weeks. Bone remodeling lasts for several months after fracture.

Physical Therapy Interventions During Bone Healing

Immobilization of the fracture ends is imperative for bone healing to occur, but it often leads to weakness in surrounding muscles, shortened ligaments and tendons, and decreased density of the bone itself. Although these deleterious effects of immobilization are unavoidable to some extent, therapy in the immobilization stage is aimed at minimizing these changes. Body parts that are not immobilized should be kept moving and strong. Range-of-motion exercises to the joints proximal and distal to the immobilized segment are important to avoid unnecessary loss of motion. Aerobic exercise using the uninvolved extremities may be performed.

Strengthening the muscles that cross the immobilized area may be performed isometrically in a cast, splint, or fixator, if indicated. Strengthening the uninvolved extremities and core muscles is beneficial to maintain overall strength. In addition, because of the principle of overflow, strengthening the contralateral extremity may lead to strength gains in the immobilized extremity as well.

SUMMARY

Many variables influence tissue healing, including the type of tissue, the extent of the injury, and the patient's age and health. Physical therapist assistants play an important role in maximizing healing by understanding the healing process of distinct tissue types. Therapeutic exercise and modalities can be used to control inflammation, restore motion and strength, minimize pain, and promote normal function.

REVIEW QUESTIONS

1. Discuss the implications of using the terms to describe pathology ending in –itis vs. –osis vs. –opathy (for example, tendonitis/tendinosus/tendinopathy).

2. You are treating a patient with a fracture as well as soft tissue injury in the area. How does the treatment for the fracture affect the soft tissue injury? How might this affect your physical therapy treatment?

3. Describe neurapraxia, axonotmesis, and neurotmesis. What are the implications for recovery of nerve function in each level of injury?

4. Discuss the terms open reduction, closed reduction, internal fixation, and external fixation.

5. What are the factors that impact ligament healing? What is the effect of exercising a ligament?

6. Describe the three signs which indicate a contractile tissue (muscle or tendon) pathology.

REFERENCES

1. Frank, C. B. (2004). Ligament structure, physiology and function. *Journal of Musculoskeletal Neuronal Interaction, 4,* 199–201.
2. Thornton, G. M., Shrive, N. G., & Frank, C. B. (2003) Healing ligaments have decreased cyclic modulus compared to normal ligaments and immobilization further compromises healing ligament response to cyclic loading. *Journal of Orthopedic Research, Official Publication of the Orthopedic Research Society, 21,* 716–722.
3. Goodman, C. C., & Fuller, K. S. (2014). *Pathology: Implications for the physical therapist.* St. Louis, MO: Elsevier Health Sciences
4. Buckwalter, J. A. (1995). Activity vs. rest in the treatment of bone, soft tissue and joint injuries. *Iowa Orthopedic Journal, 15,* 29–42.
5. Thornton, G. M., Johnson, J. C., Maser, R. V., Marchuk, L. L., Shrive, N. G., & Frank, C. B. (2005). Strength of medial structures of the knee joint are decreased by isolated injury to the medial collateral ligament and subsequent joint immobilization. *Journal of. Orthopedic Research, Official Publication of the Orthopedic Research Society, 23,* 1191–1198.
6. Tipton, C. M., James, S. L., Mergner, W., & Tcheng, T. K. (1970). Influence of exercise on strength of medial collateral knee ligaments of dogs. *American Journal of Physiology, 218,* 894–902.
7. Vailas, A. C., Tipton, C. M., Matthes, R. D., & Gart, M. (1981). Physical activity and its influence on the repair process of medial collateral ligaments. *Connective Tissue Research, 9,* 25–31.
8. Ashe, M. C., McCauley, T., & Khan, K. M. (2004). Tendinopathies in the upper extremity: A paradigm shift. *Journal of Hand Therapy, Official Journal of the American Society of Hand Therapy, 17,* 329–334.
9. Fredberg, U., & Stengaard-Pedersen, K. (2008). Chronic tendinopathy tissue pathology, pain mechanisms, and etiology with a special focus on inflammation. *Scandinavian Journal of Medical Science Sports, 18,* 3–15.
10. Waugh, E. J. (2005). Lateral epicondylalgia or epicondylitis: What's in a name? *Journal of Orthopedic and Sports Physical Therapy, 35,* 200–202.
11. Hampson, K., Forsyth, N. R., El Haj, A., & Maffulli, N. (2008). "Tendon tissue engineering." In N. Ashammakhi, R. Reis, & F. Chiellini (Eds.), *Topics in tissue engineering* (Vol. 4, pp. 1–20). https://www.oulu.fi/spareparts/ebook_topics_in_t_e_vol4/abstracts/hampson.pdf. Accessed 4/15/2019.
12. Seddon, H. J. (1943). Three types of nerve injury. *Brain, 66,* 237–288.
13. Sunderland, S. (1951). A classification of peripheral nerve injuries producing loss of function. *Brain Journal of Neurology,74,* 491–516.
14. Topp, K. S., & Boyd, B. S. (2006). Structure and biomechanics of peripheral nerves: Nerve responses to physical stresses and implications for physical therapist practice. *Physical Therapy, 86,* 92–109.
15. Hoermann, S., Franz, E. A., & Regenbrecht, H. (2012). Referred sensations elicited by video-mediated mirroring of hands. *PloS One, 7,* e50942.
16. Selles, R. W., Schreuders, T. A. R., & Stam, H. J. (2008). Mirror therapy in patients with causalgia (complex regional pain syndrome type II) following peripheral nerve injury: Two cases. *Journal of Rehabilitation Medicine, 40,* 312–314.
17. Roy, S. H., Wolf, S. L., & Scalzitti, D. A. (2012). *The rehabilitation specialist's handbook.* Philadelphia, PA: F.A. Davis Company.

PART II

Upper Extremities

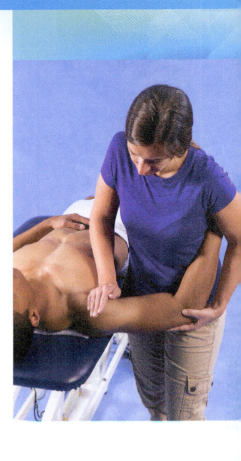

Chapter 5

Orthopedic Interventions for the Shoulder

Anatomy and Physiology

Common Pathologies

LEARNING OUTCOMES

At the end of this chapter, the student will:

5.1 Describe the anatomy of the shoulder complex.

5.2 Describe normal shoulder range of motion.

5.3 Explain normal kinematics of the shoulder joints, including scapulohumeral rhythm.

5.4 Describe anterior, posterior, inferior, and distraction mobilization techniques of the glenohumeral joint, and glide mobilization techniques of the acromioclavicular and sternoclavicular joints, and their purposes.

5.5 Discuss common shoulder pathologies and typical presentation.

5.6 Discuss contributing factors to various shoulder pathologies and, when relevant, preventive measures.

5.7 Describe the clinical tests that the physical therapist may have used to diagnose common shoulder pathologies and how to administer the tests.

5.8 Describe common treatment interventions for shoulder pathologies in the nonsurgical patient.

5.9 Discuss common treatment after surgical intervention including patients with rotator cuff repair, subacromial decompression, inferior capsular shift, Bankart repair, and conventional and reverse total shoulder arthroplasty.

5.10 Discuss the relationship between shoulder instability and subacromial impingement, and between subacromial impingement and rotator cuff tendinopathy.

5.11 Describe clinical alerts for shoulder pathologies.

KEY WORDS

Acromioplasty	Distal clavicle excision	Multidirectional instability
AMBRI	Dynamic stability	Osteophytes
Arthroplasty	Dyskinesia	Plane of the scapula
Bankart lesion	Force couples	Scaption
Capsular pattern	Glenoid labrum	Scapular stabilizers
Congenital hypermobility syndrome	Hemiarthroplasty	Scapulohumeral rhythm
Coracoacromial arch	Idiopathic	Sclerosis
Coracoacromial ligament resection	Instability	Static stability
Degenerative joint disease (DJD)	Irritability	Subluxation
Dislocation	Manipulation under anaesthetic (MUA)	TUBS

Anatomy and Physiology

The shoulder complex contains four joints with relatively sparse bony and ligamentous restraint. This anatomical arrangement gives the shoulder more mobility than any other joint while providing a large envelope of upper extremity movement around the body. Stability is provided primarily by the soft tissues and muscles in the area. In addition to the **static stability** of the ligaments, capsule, and glenoid labrum, we will discuss the **dynamic stability** provided by the muscles. This dynamic stability relies heavily on normal joint motion in four joints, normal muscle strength in three force couples, and precise timing of contractions.

Bone and Joint Anatomy and Physiology

The shoulder involves three bones and four joints acting in a complicated interplay of movements. The shoulder *girdle* involves the sternoclavicular joint (SC), the acromio-clavicular joint (AC), and the scapulothoracic articulation (ST). The shoulder *joint* refers to the articulation of the glenoid of the scapula with the humeral head (GH) (Fig. 5.1). It is essential that all four of the joints in the shoulder complex move and function normally to contribute to full movement of the shoulder.

Ultimately, the shoulder has three degrees of freedom, allowing for about a 240° arc of motion in flexion/extension and abduction/adduction and a 180° arc of motion in internal rotation/external rotation and horizontal abduction/horizontal adduction. For the purpose of this chapter, motions that involve raising the arm into shoulder flexion, abduction, or scaption will be called arm *elevation*. **Scaption** is elevation in the **plane of the scapula**, which lies about 30° to 45° toward the sagittal plane from the frontal plane.[1]

The bones and joints of the shoulder complex are summarized in Table 5-1.

Soft Tissue Anatomy and Physiology

The shoulder relies on soft tissues, including the labrum, capsule, and ligaments, to increase static stability of the joint. Other relevant soft tissues that are found in the shoulder include the nerves and bursae.

Glenoid Labrum

The glenoid fossa has a fibrocartilage tissue called the **glenoid labrum** that stands up off the rim of the glenoid by about a quarter of an inch. This increases the depth of the glenoid by up to 50% and helps to stabilize the humeral head.[2,3] The labrum serves as an attachment site for the glenohumeral ligaments and the tendon of the long head of the biceps (Fig. 5.2). The relationship of the labrum and biceps tendon becomes important in *SLAP lesions* (Box 5-3).

Joint Capsule

The glenohumeral joint capsule is a loose-fitting structure, particularly inferiorly. This allows the humeral head to drop down into the baggy folds of the inferior capsule during arm elevation (Fig. 5.3). A normally lax capsule will allow for about one-quarter inch movement of the humeral head anteriorly and posteriorly and about an inch of movement inferiorly.[4] The importance of this redundancy in the inferior capsule will be discussed in the pathology of *adhesive capsulitis*.

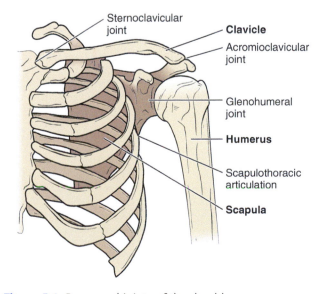

Figure 5.1 Bones and joints of the shoulder area.

Sternoclavicular joint
Clavicle
Acromioclavicular joint
Glenohumeral joint
Humerus
Scapulothoracic articulation
Scapula

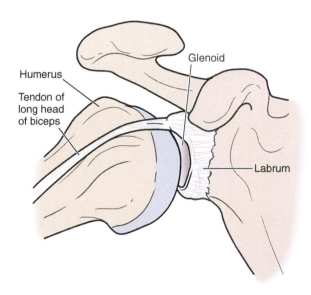

Figure 5.2 The glenoid labrum increases the stability of the humeral head.

Humerus
Tendon of long head of biceps
Glenoid
Labrum

Table 5-1 Bone and Joint Anatomy and Physiology Of the Shoulder

Joint	Anatomy	Normal ROM and Movements	Landmarks	Clinical Considerations
Glenohumeral	Ball-and-socket shape with 3 degrees of freedom. Convex humeral head articulates with concave glenoid of scapula. Glenoid faces anterior to frontal plane about 30° ("plane of the scapula").	Humerus: Flexion – 0°–180° Extension – 0°–60° Abduction – 0°–180° Adduction – 0°–60° Internal rotation* – 0°–70° External rotation*– 0°–90° * at 90° of shoulder abduction	Greater tubercle of humerus Lesser tubercle of humerus Bicipital groove Coracoid process of scapula Acromion process of scapula	Glenoid is shallow, pear-shaped. Much smaller than humeral head. Less than half of humeral head is in contact with glenoid at any one time, increasing mobility. Scapulohumeral rhythm – 2/3 of arm elevation comes from the GH joint. Close-packed position: full shoulder abduction with external rotation Loose-packed position: about 45° scaption Capsular pattern: greatest limitation in shoulder external rotation, then abduction, then internal rotation. Flexion is least limited.
Sternoclavicular	Saddle shape with 3 degrees of freedom.	Clavicle: movements include elevation/depression, protraction/retraction, and axial rotation. Elevation and posterior rotation in full arm abduction	Medial end of clavicle at suprasternal notch	Bony connection between axial and appendicular skeleton Close-packed position: full shoulder elevation and protraction Loose-packed position: arm at side
Acromioclavicular	Plane joint allows 3 degrees of freedom, but movement occurs primarily in two planes.	Minimal gliding and rotation at end range of arm elevation	Step-off at lateral end of clavicle	Link between acromion shape (flat, curved, hooked, or convex) and damage to structures below Close-packed position: 90° shoulder abduction Loose-packed position: arm at side
Scapulothoracic	Scapula lies on thorax between 2nd and 7th ribs. Medial border of scapula is 2 inches from the spinous processes.	Scapula: elevation, depression, protraction, retraction, upward rotation, downward rotation, tilt, internal rotation, external rotation. Scapula upwardly rotates on thorax 60°.	Spine of the scapula ending in acromion process Coracoid process on anterior scapula Supraspinous, infraspinous, and subscapular fossae Axillary border, medial border, inferior angle	Functional joint, not true joint (no joint capsule or bony articulation) Scapulohumeral rhythm – 1/3 of arm elevation comes from upward rotation of the scapula

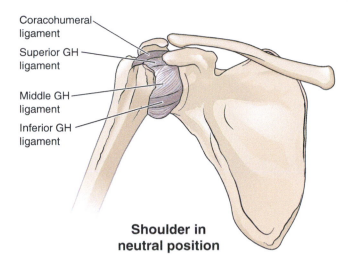

**Shoulder in
neutral position**

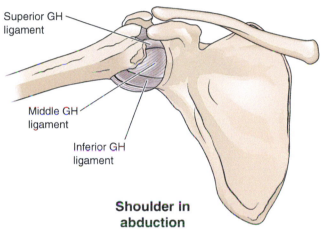

**Shoulder in
abduction**

Figure 5.3 The shoulder joint capsule hangs in loose folds inferiorly when the arm is adducted. In shoulder elevation, these folds allow the humeral head to slide inferiorly on the glenoid.

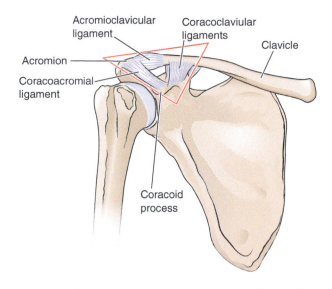

Figure 5.4 The acromioclavicular, coracoclavicular, and coracoacromial ligaments form a triangle of ligaments superior to the shoulder.

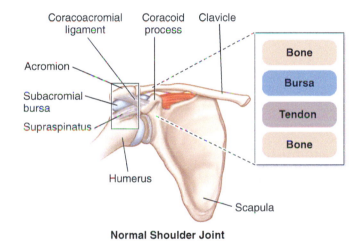

Normal Shoulder Joint

Figure 5.5 The coracoacromial arch is formed by the coracoid process, coracoacromial ligament, and acromion.

Shoulder Ligaments

There are three glenohumeral ligaments: superior, middle, and inferior. These ligaments are thickenings of the capsule and form the shape of a "Z" on the anterior and inferior shoulder to enhance the stability of the joint.

Many other ligaments stabilize the shoulder complex. The coracohumeral ligament runs from the coracoid process downward and laterally to attach to the superior humeral head. It helps counteract the force of gravity when the arm hangs by the side and also plays a role in assuring normal mechanics of the shoulder as the arm is elevated. Tightness of this ligament may restrict shoulder motion; laxity may cause shoulder instability.[5]

The sternoclavicular joint is stabilized by a joint capsule, several sternoclavicular ligaments, and muscles. However, the most important stabilizer of the SC joint is the costoclavicular ligament that connects the proximal clavicle to the first rib.

Superior to the glenohumeral joint lie three ligaments that form a triangle over the glenohumeral joint (Fig. 5.4). These three ligaments are the acromioclavicular ligament, coracoacromial ligament, and coracoclavicular ligament. Both the acromioclavicular ligament and the coracoclavicular ligaments stabilize the AC joint.

The coracoacromial ligament spans two processes on the same bone: the acromion and the coracoid of the scapula. In this way, it doesn't serve a function of holding two bones together, as most ligaments do. However, with its bony attachments, it forms the **coracoacromial arch** (Fig. 5.5). This curved complex creates a protective roof over the humeral head and helps to stabilize the humeral head against superior and inferior translation.[6] The supraspinatus muscle, tendon of the long head of the biceps, and subacromial bursa lie between this arch and the humeral head. This relationship of soft tissue sandwiched between two relatively unyielding structures (coracoacromial arch on top and humeral head on the bottom) has been implicated in *subacromial impingement syndrome*. This pathology will be discussed later in the chapter.

The shoulder capsule, ligaments, and labrum anatomy of the shoulder complex are summarized in Table 5-2.

Bursae

There are several bursae in the shoulder area to help cushion the many muscles that need to glide on each other. The two primary bursae of importance are the

Table 5-2 Connective Tissue Anatomy and Physiology
Of the Shoulder

Structure	Anatomy	Function	Clinical Considerations
Joint capsule	Loose-fitting structure, particularly inferiorly, to allow the humeral head to drop down during elevation.	Stabilizes the joint. Lined with synovium to produce synovial fluid.	Tightness in the inferior capsule can cause range-of-motion restrictions. Laxity in the capsule can lead to instability.
Glenohumeral ligament	Three glenohumeral ligaments: • superior glenohumeral ligament • middle glenohumeral ligament • inferior glenohumeral ligament Form the shape of a "Z" on the anterior and inferior shoulder.	Enhance the stability of the GH joint.	Laxity of these ligaments compromises the stability of the joint.
Coracohumeral ligament	Runs from the coracoid process downward and laterally to attach to the superior humeral head.	Counteracts the force of gravity when the arm hangs by the side. Offers additional stability for superior and anterior shoulder.	Tightness may restrict shoulder motion; laxity may cause shoulder instability.
Coracoacromial ligament	Runs across the top of the shoulder from coracoid process to the acromion.	With the coracoid process and acromion, forms a roof over the top of the shoulder, referred to as the coracoacromial arch.	The space between the humeral head and coracoacromial arch is very small. Muscles and bursae under the arch may swell if inflamed, resulting in pinching of the soft tissues.
Coracoclavicular ligament	This ligament runs from the coracoid process to the underside of the clavicle. Two parts: • conoid ligament • trapezoid ligament	Provides most of the stability of the clavicle relative to the acromion.	If AC ligament is stretched or torn, the coracoclavicular ligament can provide stability to the clavicle.
Acromioclavicular ligament (AC)	Cover the superior and inferior aspect of the joint.	Stabilizes the AC joint.	If the AC ligament is stretched or torn, the distal clavicle will elevate on the acromion.
Sternoclavicular ligaments (SC)	Several SC ligaments. Most important is the costoclavicular ligament.	Stabilizes the SC joint by connecting the clavicle to the first rib.	Movement at this joint is necessary to have full shoulder motion.
Glenoid labrum	Rim of fibrocartilage that stands up off the glenoid by about a quarter of an inch.	Increases the depth of the glenoid by up to 50% and helps to stabilize the humeral head.[2,3] Attachment site for the glenohumeral ligaments and the tendon of the long head of the biceps.	Tears in the labrum cause pain and shoulder instability.

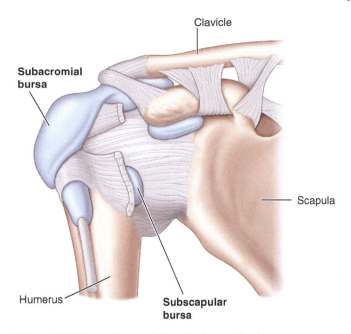

Figure 5.6 The subacromial and subscapular bursae.

subacromial (also called the subdeltoid) and the subscapular bursae.

The subacromial bursa lies under the deltoid muscle, acromion process, and coracoacromial arch. It forms a cushion between the deltoid and the rotator cuff muscles. This bursa may become inflamed in *shoulder impingement syndrome*. If the subacromial bursa becomes inflamed and swells, it can further reduce the space under the coracoacromial arch. The subscapular bursa lies under the tendon of subscapularis and on top of the anterior rim of the glenoid. It cushions the subscapularis tendon from the scapula. Figure 5.6 depicts these two bursae of the shoulder.

Nerves

The most significant neural structure in the shoulder region is the brachial plexus. This network of nerves is formed by the nerve roots of C5–T1. The roots join and split as they become peripheral nerves that often contain a representation of multiple nerve root levels (Fig. 5.7). The brachial plexus travels through the axilla, just anterior and inferior to the shoulder. It supplies nerves to most of the shoulder as well as the arm, forearm, and hand. A basic understanding of the nervous system anatomy in the shoulder is important when treating patients with plexus and peripheral nerve injuries.

Nerves that exit the plexus provide innervation to the muscles in the shoulder area. Special attention should be paid to the axillary and long thoracic nerves. The axillary nerve innervates the deltoid and the teres minor. This nerve is often damaged in brachial plexus injuries. The long thoracic nerve innervates the serratus anterior. This nerve is vulnerable as it runs very

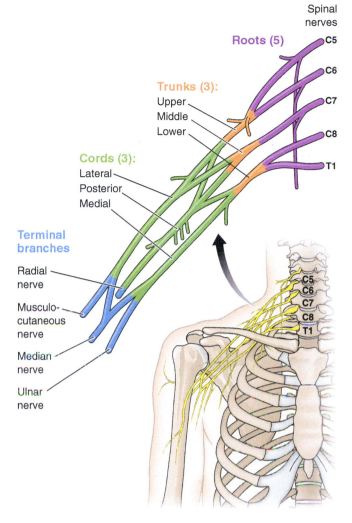

Figure 5.7 The brachial plexus. Nerve roots from C5–T1 merge and divide prior to becoming peripheral nerves.

superficially down the lateral chest wall. Stretch or tear injuries may result in medial *scapular winging* due to serratus anterior denervation (Box 5-1).

Muscular Anatomy and Kinesiology

The muscles that overlie the shoulder are essential to provide dynamic stability to the joint. Before understanding the kinematics of the shoulder complex, a thorough knowledge of kinesiology of the shoulder is needed. Table 5-3 contains a review of muscles with origin, insertion, innervation, action, and clinical relevance.

Several of the muscles in this region are collectively referred to as **scapular stabilizers**. These muscles include the serratus anterior, rhomboids, levator scapulae, and trapezius muscles. These muscles may be a focus for strengthening due to their common action of controlling the scapula.

Box 5-1 Scapular Winging

Winging of the scapula occurs due to muscle weakness, most commonly of the serratus anterior muscle. In this condition, the medial **border of the** scapula protrudes from the thorax, resembling a wing. The long thoracic nerve, which innervates the serratus anterior, may be the cause of winging. The nerve runs superficially along the anterolateral chest wall and is vulnerable to injury. The resulting serratus anterior weakness causes the scapula to move medially toward the spine due to the largely unopposed scapular adductors. Weakness of the serratus **anterior** impacts the effectiveness of the upward rotation force couple and may impact activities of daily living that involve arm elevation.

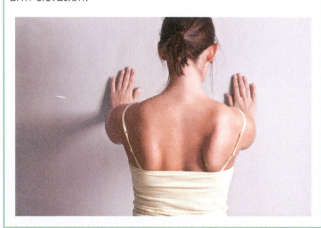

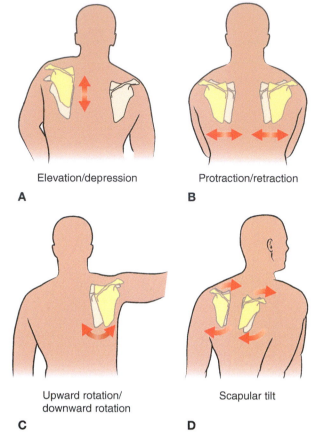

Figure 5.8 Scapular movements include elevation/depression (A), protraction/retraction (B), upward/downward rotation (C), and scapular tilt (D).

Kinematics

Scapulothoracic (ST) Joint

The scapula can slide on the thorax in movements that we call elevation and depression, protraction and retraction, and upward and downward rotation. When the scapula elevates, it tilts anteriorly to maintain contact with the ribcage. With depression, a posterior tilting occurs. Likewise, with protraction the scapula internally rotates in the transverse plane as it follows the curve of the ribcage. Internal rotation of the scapula causes the underside of the scapula to turn more inwardly and the scapula to lie more in the sagittal plane. With retraction, the scapula externally rotates and comes to lie more in the frontal plane. Figure 5.8 depicts the movements of the scapula.

Movements of the scapula increase both mobility and stability of the shoulder complex. Stability is increased as movements allow the scapula to maintain contact with the thorax and the humeral head to maintain a central position on the glenoid with various arm positions. Movements of the scapula also contribute to overall mobility of the arm. In arm elevation, the scapula upwardly rotates about 60°, contributing about one-third of the range to the overall motion. This will be discussed under "Scapulohumeral Rhythm," later.

Acromioclavicular (AC) Joint

Because of the connection between the acromion of the scapula and the distal clavicle, the movements of the scapula as discussed above are transmitted to the AC joint. The amount of movement of the AC joint has been debated through the years, but recent studies suggest that movement is minimal.[7] However, the movements of scapular tilting and internal/external rotation of the scapula do occur here.

Sternoclavicular (SC) Joint

With only minimal movement occurring at the AC joint, the motions of the shoulder girdle are, in large part, transmitted to the SC joint. With scapular upward rotation, the acromion elevates, elevating the distal clavicle. This occurs in the first 90° of shoulder abduction and accounts for up to 30° of distal clavicle elevation. With continued elevation, the coracoclavicular ligament becomes taut and pulls on the clavicle causing it to rotate posteriorly. The *S*-shaped clavicle spins, elevating the lateral end similar to a crank handle movement. At least half of

Table 5-3   Muscle Anatomy and Kinesiology
Of the Shoulder

Muscle	Origin	Insertion	Innervation	Primary Action	Clinical Considerations
Upper trapezius	Occipital protuberance and the cervical vertebrae upwardly rotate, elevate, and retract the scapula.	Distal clavicle	11th cranial nerve (spinal accessory)	Upward rotation, elevation, and retraction of the scapula	One of three muscles in the upward rotation force couple, weakness may lead to impingement syndrome.
Middle trapezius	Spinous processes of C7-T5	Acromion process	11th cranial nerve (spinal accessory)	Retraction of the scapula	
Lower Trapezius	Spinous processes of T6-T12	Superior aspect of the spine of the scapula	11th cranial nerve (spinal accessory)	Depression, upward rotation, and retraction of the scapula	One of three muscles in the upward rotation force couple, weakness may lead to impingement syndrome. Action of scapular depression is used to raise the body going sit-to-stand, or in walking with an assistive device.
Levator scapulae	Transverse processes of C1-4	Medial border of the scapula between the superior angle and the root of the scapular spine	Dorsal scapular nerve	Elevation and downward rotation of the scapula. In addition, it has weak retraction ability.	
Rhomboids (major and minor)	Spinous processes of C7-T5	Medial border of the scapula	Dorsal scapular nerve	Retraction, downward rotation, and elevation of the scapula	Injury to the dorsal scapular nerve results in lateral scapular winging.
Serratus anterior	Lateral side of ribs 1–9	Runs deep to the scapula and inserts on the medial border of the scapula	Long thoracic nerve	Upward rotation and protraction of the scapula Maintains medial border of scapula against thorax	One of three muscles in the upward rotation force couple, weakness may lead to impingement syndrome. Injury to the long thoracic nerve results in medial scapular winging.
Pectoralis minor	Anterior surface of the third, fourth, and fifth ribs	Coracoid process	Medial pectoral nerve	Depression, downward rotation, and anterior tilting of the scapula	Tightness leads to rounded shoulder posture. May contribute to thoracic outlet syndrome.

Continued

Table 5-3 Muscle Anatomy and Kinesiology—cont'd

Of the Shoulder

Muscle	Origin	Insertion	Innervation	Primary Action	Clinical Considerations
Supraspinatus	Supraspinous fossa of the scapula	Runs under the acromion and coracoacromial arch to insert on the greater tubercle of the humerus	Suprascapular nerve	Scaption of the humerus With the other rotator cuff muscles it pulls the humeral head down and in against the glenoid.	One of four rotator cuff muscles. Most commonly involved muscle in impingement syndrome.
Infraspinatus	Infraspinous fossa of the scapula	Greater tubercle of the humerus	Suprascapular nerve.	External rotation of the humerus With the other rotator cuff muscles, it pulls the humeral head down and in against the glenoid.	One of four rotator cuff muscles
Teres minor	Lateral border of the scapula, near the inferior angle	Greater tubercle of the humerus	Axillary nerve	External rotation of the humerus With the other rotator cuff muscles, it pulls the humeral head down and in against the glenoid.	One of four rotator cuff muscles
Subscapularis	Underside of the scapula in the subscapular fossa	Lesser tubercle of the humerus	Upper and lower subscapular nerves	Internal rotation of the humerus With the other rotator cuff muscles, it pulls the humeral head down and in against the glenoid.	One of four rotator cuff muscles
Latissimus dorsi (Lats)	Spinous processes of the lower thoracic and all of the lumbar vertebrae, the lower four ribs Often has additional origins from posterior iliac crest and the inferior angle of the scapula.	Anterior humerus at the intertubercular groove	Thoracodorsal nerve	Extension, adduction, and internal rotation of the humerus Depression of the scapula Extension of the lumbar spine	Action of scapular depression is used to raise the body going sit-to-stand, or in walking with an assistive device.
Teres major	Inferior angle of the scapula	Runs through the axillary area to the anterior shoulder, inserting on the lesser tubercle of the humerus	Lower subscapular nerve	Extension, adduction, and internal rotation of the humerus	Only scapulohumeral muscle that is not part of the rotator cuff

Table 5-3　Muscle Anatomy and Kinesiology—cont'd

Of the Shoulder

Muscle	Origin	Insertion	Innervation	Primary Action	Clinical Considerations
Pectoralis major	Two heads: • Sternal head originates from the sternum • Clavicular head originates from the proximal clavicle	Anterior humerus at the greater tubercle	Medial and lateral pectoral nerves	Horizontal adduction, internal rotation, and adduction of the humerus	
Anterior deltoid	Distal clavicle	Deltoid tuberosity	Axillary nerve	Flexion and horizontal adduction of the humerus	
Middle deltoid	Acromion process	Deltoid tuberosity	Axillary nerve	Abduction of the humerus	
Posterior deltoid	Scapular spine	Deltoid tuberosity	Axillary nerve	Extension and horizontal abduction of the humerus	
Coraco-brachialis	Coracoid process	Humerus, about midway down the shaft	Musculocutaneous nerve	Flexion of the humerus	
Biceps brachii	Long head: superior aspect of the glenoid fossa and the glenoid labrum Short head: coracoid process	Radial tuberosity on the proximal radius	Musculocutaneous nerve	Flexion of the shoulder, flexion of the elbow, supination of the forearm	Long head serves as a restraint to superior translation of the humeral head.
Triceps brachii, long head	Inferior aspect of the glenoid fossa	Olecranon process of the ulna	Radial nerve	Extension of the shoulder Extension of the elbow	This is the only head of the triceps that affects shoulder.

the elevation of the distal clavicle comes from posterior rotation at the SC joint.

The SC joint also allows for protraction and retraction, which accompanies protraction and retraction of the scapula on the thorax. About 15° to 30° of movement may occur in either direction.

Glenohumeral (GH) Joint

During arm elevation, the convex humeral head moves on the slightly concave glenoid. Rolling of the humeral head is accompanied by a slide in the opposite direction, in keeping with the concave-convex rule as discussed in Chapter 3. The oversized humeral head must glide inferiorly as the arm is elevated to take advantage of the small glenoid. In this way, the humeral head is kept from rolling off the glenoid.

This inferior glide also serves to keep the humeral head from migrating upwardly into the coracoacromial arch and pinching the soft tissues against the underside of the acromion. In addition to inferior glide, elevation of the arm must be accompanied by external rotation of the humerus to attain full shoulder range of motion (Fig. 5.9). External rotation decreases impingement of the soft tissues between the humeral head and the acromion,[8] particularly as arm elevation increases.[9] In shoulder abduction, full internal rotation of the humerus restricts range to 60°, and neutral rotation restricts motion to 90°. Limited shoulder external rotation range has implications on range of motion primarily into abduction and scaption.

Watch Out For...

Watch out for the rotation position of the shoulder when exercising patients into flexion, abduction, or scaption. Remember to keep the shoulder in neutral rotation or external rotation to avoid impingement. Likewise, avoid cardinal-plane abduction when working with patients who have a shoulder impingement syndrome. Move them in the scapular plane instead.

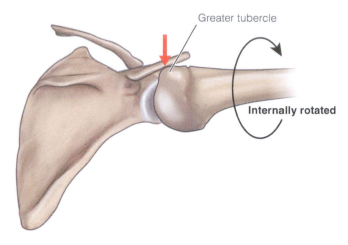

Greater tubercle

Internally rotated

A

Acromion

Greater tubercle

Externally rotated

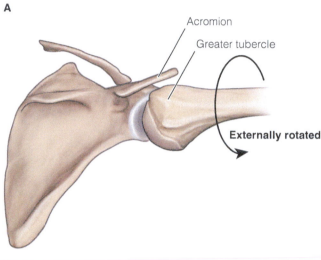

B

Figure 5.9 With the shoulder in internal rotation, as the arm is elevated the soft tissues are compressed between the greater tubercle of the humerus and acromion (A). External rotation of the humerus decreases this impingement under the coracoacromial arch (B).

Because of the relative size of the humeral head and the shallow depth of the glenoid, stability of the shoulder joint depends upon the labrum, capsule, ligaments, and muscles. The primary muscle stabilizers are the rotator cuff muscles, latissimus dorsi, teres major, and the biceps brachii long head. Muscles may perform as a stabilizer in several ways. They may move the joint into a position that tightens ligaments to create a passive barrier, they themselves may form a barrier by passive tension, and they may actively contract to pull the bone against the destabilizing force.

It has been shown that subscapularis is a barrier restraint to anterior displacement of the humeral head and that infraspinatus and teres minor form a posterior barrier (Fig. 5.10). The long head of biceps, latissimus dorsi, teres major, and subscapularis contract to stabilize against superior translation of the humeral head. Contraction of supraspinatus stabilizes against inferior translation.

Front of Shoulder

Anterior capsule

Subscapularis tendon

Glenoid

Humeral head

Infraspinatus tendon

Posterior capsule

Back of Shoulder

Figure 5.10 Superior view of the glenohumeral joint. Anterior and posterior rotator cuff muscles form a barrier to humeral head displacement.

An understanding of the role muscles play in joint stability is important in treatment, as we'll see in the pathology of *shoulder instability*.

The rotator cuff muscles act together to stabilize the GH joint. While each muscle of the rotator cuff is individually responsible for creating motion at the GH joint, acting together the cuff has the important function of pulling the humeral head down and in against the glenoid, stabilizing the joint. Aside from increasing the stability of the joint, this motion counteracts the pull of the deltoid in arm elevation, as we'll discuss in "Force Couples," later.

Scapulohumeral Rhythm

A large contributor to the overall motion of arm elevation is movement of the scapula on the thorax. Inman et al. investigated the scapular contribution to shoulder abduction in 1944.[10] They reported a scapular setting phase for the first 30° and then two degrees of humeral motion for every one degree of scapular motion. This 2:1 ratio has come to be termed **scapulohumeral rhythm** (Fig. 5.11).

Since the early report by Inman et al. this biomechanical relationship has been well studied. We now appreciate that there is significant variability in the amount and timing of scapular upward rotation during arm elevation. In spite of this variability, as a clinician you should consider the scapulothoracic movement to be essential to full arm elevation and to contribute roughly one-third, or 60°, to the total motion.

Because of the ligamentous connections between the acromion, clavicle, and sternum, the 60° of scapular movement occurs with slight movement at the AC joint and significant movement at the SC joint.

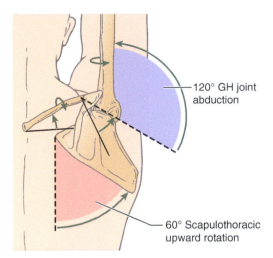

Figure 5.11 Scapulohumeral rhythm. The ratio of humerus to scapular motion is 2:1. Of the 180° of arm elevation, scapular upward rotation contributes 60°, and humeral abduction contributes 120°.

Watch Out For...

Watch out for excessive scapular motion as a result of restricted glenohumeral movement. Patients will compensate for the limitation of GH motion by increased scapular movements. As you work to increase shoulder ROM, target the joint that is restricted. You may need to stabilize the scapula to focus your exercises on the glenohumeral joint.

Force Couples

Movements throughout the body rely on muscles contracting synergistically to create a smooth pattern of motion. Nowhere is this more evident than in the shoulder complex. During the motion of arm elevation, the rotator cuff and deltoids work together to create the glenohumeral component of the motion. Simultaneously, three scapular upward rotators create the scapulothoracic component of the motion. Let's look at these two important **force couples**.

Scapular Upward Rotators

The three strongest scapular upward rotators are upper trapezius, lower trapezius, and serratus anterior. Serratus anterior is the strongest muscle of the three, but all must work at varying points in the range to ensure smooth upward rotation of the scapula. This upward rotation of the scapula contributes to the total movement of the arm and allows the glenohumeral muscles to maintain a favorable length-tension relationship throughout the range (Fig. 5.12).

In this force couple, upper trapezius is a very minor contributor. If a patient displays weakness in scapular upward rotation, the PTA should focus on lower trapezius and serratus anterior.

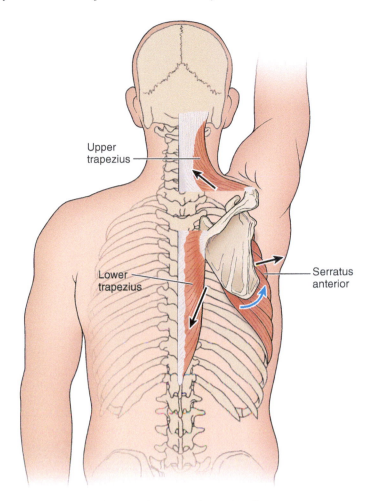

Figure 5.12 The scapular upward rotation force couple: upper trapezius, lower trapezius, and serratus anterior.

Rotator Cuff and Deltoid

At the glenohumeral joint, the rotator cuff has a perfect line of pull to bring the humeral head down and in against the glenoid, stabilizing it against the upward shear (sliding) force that is created by the deltoid muscles. This allows the deltoid to abduct the humerus rather than causing superior migration of the humeral head (Fig. 5.13). With a *rotator cuff tear*, an abnormal movement pattern is often seen involving elevation of the humerus against the acromion as the deltoid contracts unopposed by the rotator cuff.

In this force couple, the contribution of supraspinatus to depression of the humeral head is questionable. The line of pull of the other three rotator cuff muscles would indicate a more prominent role in depressing the humeral head.

Joint Mobilization

To reduce pain or increase range of motion, joint mobilization may be a useful intervention. According to the concave-convex rule, movement of the convex humeral head on the concave glenoid is accompanied by a slide

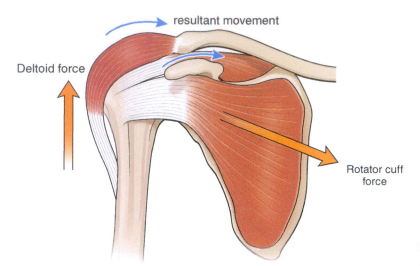

resultant movement

Deltoid force

Rotator cuff force

Figure 5.13 Arm elevation force couple: deltoid and rotator cuff.

Table 5-4	Direction of Slide Used to Increase Range of Motion
Limited Range	**Direction of Slide in Mobilization**
GH Flexion	GH inferior glide
GH Abduction	GH inferior glide
GH Internal rotation	GH anterior and posterior glides
GH External rotation	GH anterior and posterior glides
GH Horizontal abduction	GH anterior glide
GH Horizontal adduction	GH posterior glide
General shoulder motion	GH distraction
Scapular elevation	SC inferior glide
Scapular depression	SC superior glide
General scapular motion	Scapular distraction

of the humeral head in the opposite direction than the movement of the humeral shaft. The loose-packed position of the shoulder is in the plane of the scapula and elevated about 45°. It is important to remember that the glenoid lies in the scapular plane, so anterior and posterior glides will be applied perpendicular to this plane. Table 5-4 lists the movements of the shoulder and the associated glide mobilizations used to increase range of motion.

Watch Out For...

Watch out for correctly mobilizing the glenohumeral joint in the plane in which it lies. Remember the glenoid does not lie in the sagittal plane. Anterior mobilization should be done in an anteromedial direction. Posterior mobilization should be done in a posterolateral direction. Mobilizing in a straight plane will be uncomfortable for the patient and less effective.

Glenohumeral Joint

Anterior Glide

Anterior glide of the humerus on the glenoid is used to increase rotation and horizontal abduction. The patient may be positioned supine or prone. If positioned prone, a towel is placed under the clavicle to support the scapula. The examiner supports the patient's arm and applies a gliding force anteriorly and medially using the ulnar border of the hand, as shown in Figure 5.14.

Posterior Glide

Posterior glide of the humerus on the glenoid is used to increase rotation and horizontal adduction. The patient lies supine with a towel under the scapula. The examiner supports the patient's arm and applies a gliding force posteriorly and laterally using the ulnar border of the hand, as shown in Figure 5.15A.

As an alternate position, the patient is supine with the shoulder flexed to 90° and the elbow flexed. The examiner supports the scapula and applies a force at the elbow through the long axis of the humerus while stabilizing the scapula, as shown in Figure 5.15B.

Inferior Glide

Inferior glide of the humerus on the glenoid is used to increase shoulder abduction or flexion. The patient is positioned supine, with the shoulder in the loose-packed position. Stabilizing the scapula, the examiner glides the humeral head inferiorly. This technique may be applied in the sagittal plane to increase flexion and in the frontal plane to increase abduction, as shown in Figures 5.16 and 5.17.

Distraction

Distraction of the glenohumeral joint is used for general capsule tightness or pain. The patient is positioned supine, with the shoulder in about 40° of flexion. The examiner grasps the proximal humerus in the patient's axilla and

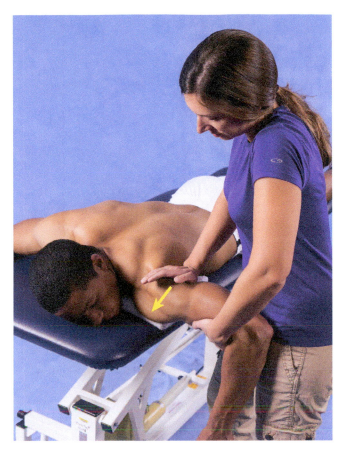

Figure 5.14 Anterior glide of the glenohumeral joint increases GH rotation.

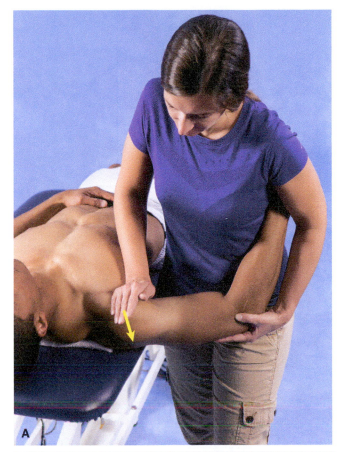

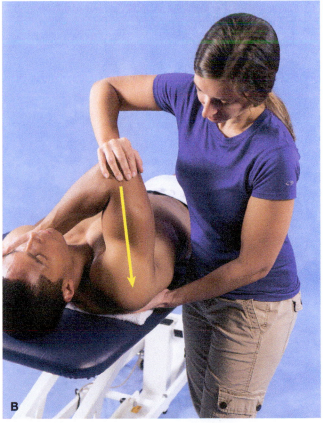

Figure 5.15 Posterior glide of the glenohumeral joint increases GH rotation. This can be performed with the patient's arm in slight abduction (A) or at 90° flexion (B).

pulls laterally to distract the joint surfaces, as shown in Figure 5.18.

Sternoclavicular Joint

Superior Glide

Superior glide of the clavicle on the sternum is used to increase scapular depression. The patient is positioned supine. The examiner's fingers are positioned under the proximal end of the clavicle. A superior glide is applied, as shown in Figure 5.19.

Inferior Glide

Inferior glide of the clavicle on the sternum is used to increase scapular elevation. The patient is positioned supine. The examiner's thumbs are positioned on the top of the proximal end of the clavicle. A downward glide is applied, as shown in Figure 5.20.

Acromioclavicular Joint

Posterior Glide

Posterior glide of the clavicle on the acromion is used to increase mobility of the AC joint. The patient is positioned sitting with the affected side toward the examiner. The examiner stabilizes the acromion posteriorly and with the heel of the hand applies a posteriorly directed force on the distal clavicle (Fig. 5.21).

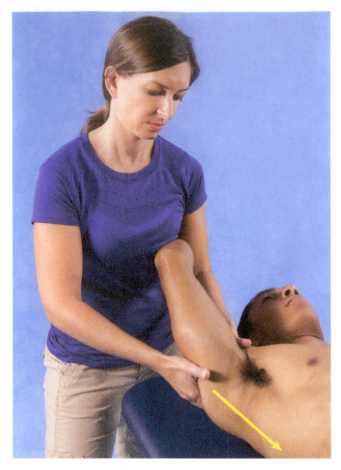

Figure 5.16 Inferior glide of the glenohumeral joint in flexion is used to increase GH flexion.

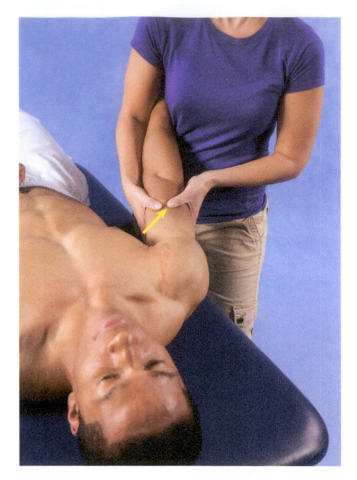

Figure 5.18 Distraction mobilization of the glenohumeral joint is used for general joint hypomobility and pain.

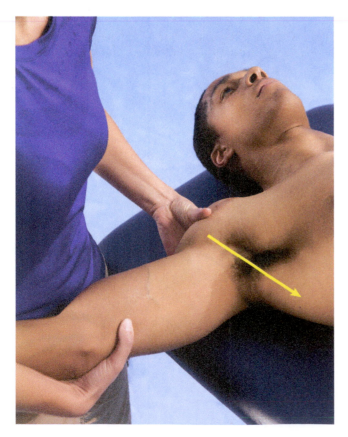

Figure 5.17 Inferior glide of the glenohumeral joint in abduction is used to increase GH abduction.

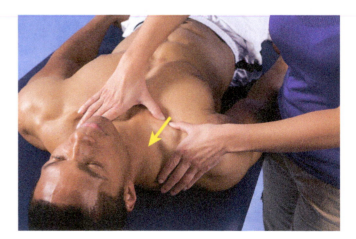

Figure 5.19 Superior glide of the sternoclavicular joint is used to increase scapular depression.

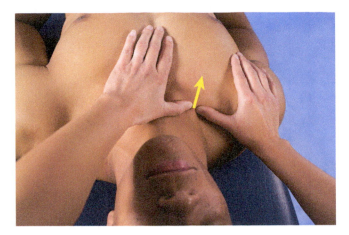

Figure 5.20 Inferior glide of the sternoclavicular joint is used to increase scapular elevation.

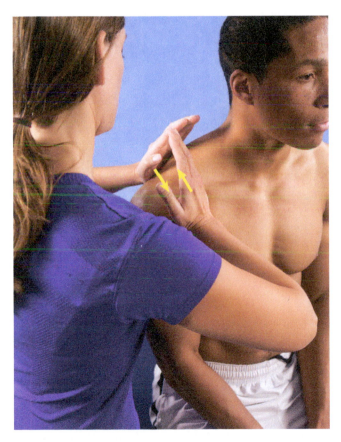

Figure 5.21 Posterior glide of the clavicle on the acromion is used to increase mobility of the AC joint.

Scapulothoracic Joint

Distraction

Distraction of the scapulothoracic joint is used to increase all scapular motions. The patient is positioned side-lying with the affected side up. The examiner supports the arm by draping it over his or her arm. Grasping the inferior angle and the acromion, the examiner gradually works under the scapula, loosening the soft tissue. The scapula can be moved in any direction (Fig. 5.22).

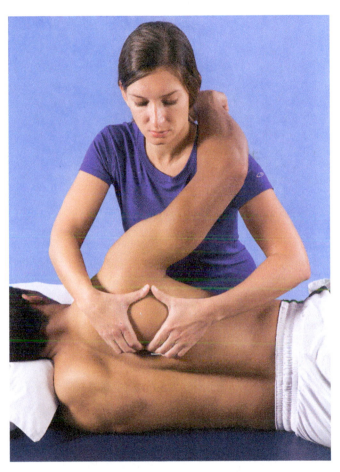

Figure 5.22 Distraction of the scapulothoracic joint is used to increase all scapular motions.

Common Pathologies

Adhesive Capsulitis
Shoulder Instability—Subluxation/Dislocation
Subacromial Impingement Syndrome
Rotator Cuff Tendinopathy/Tear
Posterior Internal Impingement
Bicipital Tendinopathy
Acromioclavicular Sprain/Separation

Thoracic Outlet Syndrome
Osteoarthritis of the Shoulder
Fractures
    Proximal humerus
    Clavicle
    Scapula

Slight abnormalities in shoulder biomechanics can lead to pathology of the soft tissues around the shoulder, including the rotator cuff, the glenohumeral capsule, and the neurovascular structures of the neck and shoulder. Pathologies of the shoulder frequently lead to other pathologies. For example, instability of the shoulder may contribute to rotator cuff tendinopathy, and tendinopathy may lead to rotator cuff tear. In this section, we'll explore common shoulder pathologies and treatment approaches.

Adhesive Capsulitis   CPG

Adhesive capsulitis is commonly referred to as "frozen shoulder". Under normal circumstances, the redundant folds of the inferior capsule allow for the humeral head to drop down as the arm is raised. In adhesive capsulitis, this excessive volume of capsule is reduced as the capsule becomes inflamed, thickens, and forms fibrous adhesions (Fig. 5.23).[11] This scar tissue significantly impairs movement.

Causes/Contributing Factors

Adhesive capsulitis may be primary or secondary. Primary adhesive capsulitis is **idiopathic,** without a known cause.

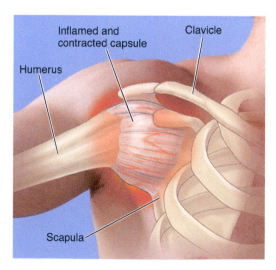

Figure 5.23 In adhesive capsulitis, the shoulder capsule becomes inflamed and forms adhesions.

Age seems to be a factor, as the majority of cases are seen in people between the ages of 40 to 65. It is more common in women; approximately 70% of people who develop adhesive capsulitis are women.

Secondary adhesive capsulitis has been linked to trauma or immobilization of the shoulder. It may be that a minor trauma sets off an exaggerated and prolonged inflammatory response, which causes the fibrosis of the capsule.[12]

Some medical conditions increase the risk. For example, adhesive capsulitis has been strongly linked to diabetes with an increased risk of up to 4 times that of nondiabetics. It is more common in people with thyroid disorders, cardiovascular disease, and Parkinson disease.[13] People who have had a previous episode of adhesive capsulitis are at higher risk.

Symptoms

The initial symptoms of frozen shoulder are pain and loss of motion. The pain will be diffusely felt in the shoulder area and may be referred down the arm as well. Patients often complain of increased pain with movement and at night. A loss of motion, both passively and actively, is evident in elevation and rotation. A **capsular pattern** of limitation may be seen, because the joint capsule is the limiting structure. In the shoulder, the capsular restriction causes external rotation and shoulder abduction to become the most limited movements. Limited shoulder external rotation range has implications on range of motion into abduction and scaption as well.

According to the CPG for adhesive capsulitis, diagnosis may be based on a loss of range of motion of more than 25% in two or more planes and a greater than 50% loss of passive external rotation when compared to the uninvolved side, or passive external rotation of less than 30°.[14]

The course of the disorder has been frequently described to occur in stages: a painful stage without loss of motion, a freezing stage, a frozen stage, and a thawing stage. The first stage lasts up to 3 months. During this time, the patient complains of sharp pain on end range of motion, ache at rest, and difficulty sleeping. The freezing stage typically lasts from months 3 to 9, with range of motion becoming more and more restricted. The frozen stage follows, in which the pain generally decreases but motion

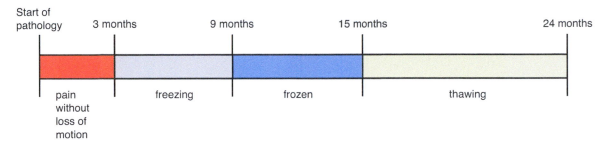

Figure 5.24 Time line for adhesive capsulitis.

remains significantly restricted. This stage typically is from months 9 to 15. At this point, the capsule has thickened and become adherent. In the final thawing stage, motion and strength gradually return. This stage typically lasts from months 15 to 24.[15–17] Mobility deficits will still persist after 2 years in nearly half of those affected.[18] Figure 5.24 depicts the typical time line for the stages of adhesive capsulitis.

Clinical Signs

There are no special tests for adhesive capsulitis. According to the Clinical Practice Guideline,[14] adhesive capsulitis should be considered if:

- The patient's age is between 40 and 65
- The patient reports a gradual onset and progressive worsening of pain and stiffness
- Pain and stiffness limit sleeping, grooming, dressing, and reaching activities
- Glenohumeral passive ROM is limited in multiple directions, with external rotation the most limited
- External rotation or internal rotation ROM decreases with increased abduction from 45° to 90°
- End-range passive movements of the shoulder reproduce the patient's complaint of pain, and
- Joint glides are restricted in all directions

Common Interventions

Patients with adhesive capsulitis may benefit from modalities, joint mobilization, and gentle stretching exercises. A home exercise program of stretching exercises will often be indicated. Patient education about the progression of the disorder is beneficial.

Prior to stretching or joint mobilization, the patient may benefit from electrical stimulation, short wave diathermy, or ultrasound to decrease pain and increase tissue extensibility.[19–22]

Therapeutic exercise is commonly part of the plan of care for patients with adhesive capsulitis. The most important consideration in choosing exercises is the **irritability** of the tissue. If the tissues are extremely irritable, gentle stretching in a pain-free range is recommended. Pendulum exercises to decrease pain and maintain or

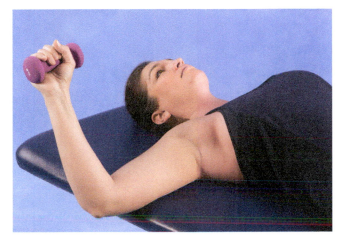

Figure 5.25 Low-load stretch into external rotation may be effective in increasing ROM in adhesive capsulitis.

increase range-of-motion are often included in the plan of care during this time. Prolonged, low-load stretch into external rotation using a small weight or can is very effective (Fig. 5.25). As the symptoms show less irritability, more aggressive stretching may be used.

Watch Out For...

Watch out for the degree of irritability of the shoulder capsule. Aggressive stretching may be detrimental during the inflammatory stage when the tissues are very irritable.[23]

Joint mobilization may be used to decrease pain and increase ROM in patients with adhesive capsulitis. Anterior glides and posterior glides have been shown to increase external rotation range of motion.[24] Inferior glides may be used to improve flexion and abduction ROM.

Surgical intervention for adhesive capsulitis is unusual but can be used for cases that do not respond to other, more conservative approaches. Surgical options include a **manipulation under anaesthetic (MUA)** and arthroscopic release of the capsule. Physical therapy after surgical intervention is similar to that for the nonsurgical patient.

The Bottom Line: for patients with adhesive capsulitis

Description and causes	Tight, scarred shoulder capsule more prevalent in females and people with diabetes and thyroid disorders
Test	None. Clinical signs of limitation of motion actively and passively, usually in a capsular pattern.
Stretch	Capsule, with focus on restoring ROM in all planes. Use low-load stretch, joint mobilizations.
Strengthen	NA
Train	NA
Avoid	Painful, aggressive stretching

Shoulder Instability— Subluxation/Dislocation

The glenohumeral joint has abundant mobility and is provided minimal stability by the capsule, ligaments, and labrum. If the humeral head moves partially off the glenoid, it is considered shoulder **subluxation**; if it loses contact with the glenoid, it is a **dislocation** (Fig. 5.26). Shoulder **instability** occurs in an anterior, posterior, or inferior direction. A patient may experience instability in more than one direction, in which case it is considered a **multidirectional instability.** Ninety-five percent of shoulder instability is in an anterior direction.

When a shoulder subluxation or dislocation occurs, there may be extensive soft tissue damage. The humeral head will often tear the labrum and glenohumeral ligaments on the side of the glenoid as it slides off and stretch the capsule on the opposite side. The risk of recurring episodes of dislocation is high, especially in younger patients where recurrence can approach 90%.[25–27]

Causes/Contributing Factors

There are two major causes of shoulder instability: trauma and joint capsule laxity. In other words, the person who sustains a traumatic dislocation is "torn loose," and the person who sustains an atraumatic dislocation may be "born loose."

Two acronyms are used to describe these classifications: **TUBS** and **AMBRI**. TUBS is the acronym for a dislocation that is Traumatic, Unidirectional, causing a **Bankart lesion,** and usually requiring Surgery to correct. A Bankart lesion is a detachment of the anterior labrum and inferior GH ligament that results from an anterior dislocation (Fig. 5.27). Surgery to repair the labrum and GH ligaments is often needed to prevent recurrence.

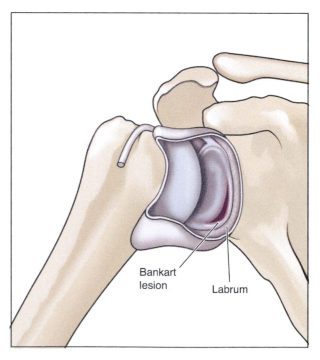

Figure 5.27 A tear of the anterior labrum called a Bankart lesion is often a result of a traumatic dislocation of the GH joint.

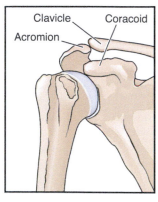
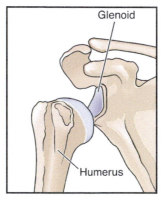

Normal anatomy   Dislocated shoulder

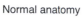

Figure 5.26 Normal relationship of the humeral head with the glenoid (A) and anterior-inferior shoulder dislocation (B).

AMBRI is the acronym for a dislocation that is **A**traumatic, **M**ultidirectional, frequently **B**ilateral, responding to **R**ehabilitation, and if therapy is not successful, requiring a surgical correction called an **I**nferior capsular shift (see surgical options below).

TUBS dislocation is most common in young male patients (80% to 90% are teenagers, 85% to 90% are males) due to motor vehicle accidents, sports injuries, or falls. Contrast this to the patient with AMBRI dislocation who may have a congenital hypermobility of many joints, may have had recurrent episodes of subluxation or dislocation, and probably has soft tissue laxity with or without bony changes in the glenoid that contribute to instability simply when raising the arm overhead. This patient will have a multidirectional instability, most commonly in an anterior and inferior direction. Expect this patient to have a good response to physical therapy that includes strengthening of the muscles around the joint to increase dynamic stability.

Contributing factors to AMBRI dislocation include a flattened glenoid, muscle weakness in the scapular and shoulder area, and **congenital hypermobility syndrome.**[28] Patients may be assessed for their degree of congenital hypermobility using the Beighton Score. A score of 4 or greater is considered to be hypermobile (Fig. 5.28).

Symptoms

Prior to subluxation or dislocation, the patient will often report a feeling of apprehension. With subluxation, the joint may feel as if it moves out of the socket and then slides back in place. With dislocation, the patient will feel a "giving way," which is usually painful. After dislocation, the patient may report a sensation of pain and weakness in the arm due to the momentary stretch of the brachial plexus. This is called "dead arm syndrome."

If the instability is in an anterior direction, the position of most risk to dislocate is in an abducted and externally rotated position. If the patient has posterior instability, the position at most risk is an abducted and internally rotated position. The patient needs to be instructed to use caution when performing activities in the position of risk.

Clinical Signs

After shoulder subluxation or dislocation, it is common to find increased movement of the humeral head on the glenoid when compared to normal subjects or to the unaffected side. The special tests for this pathology are used to assess the degree and direction of glenohumeral instability. There are numerous tests for instability, including those below.

Apprehension Test (Anterior Instability)

The apprehension test is done with the patient in sitting or supine. The patient's arm is positioned at 90° abduction with the elbow flexed. The shoulder is then slowly externally rotated. A positive test is indicated by a sense of apprehension with or without pain (Fig. 5.29).[29–31]

10-Point Beighton Score for Joint Hypermobility

1- point for extension of the 5th metacarpal past 90º on each hand

1- point for ability to bring the thumb down to the forearm on each side

1- point for elbow hyperextension on each arm

1- point for knee hyperextension on each leg

2- points for touching the floor with palms flat while keeping knees extended

TOTAL: 10 points

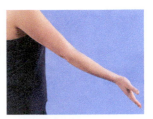
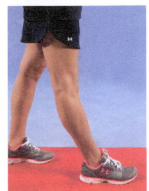
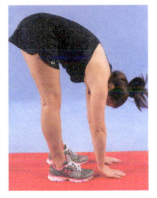
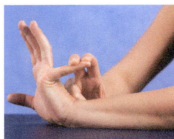
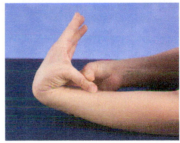

Figure 5.28 Beighton Score may be used to assess hypermobility

Some examiners apply an anteriorly directed force at the shoulder while taking the patient to end range of external rotation. Other examiners have found that if the patient is unstable, apprehension will be elicited without this force simply by increasing the amount of abduction and external rotation.

Surprise Test (Anterior Instability)

This test is also called the anterior release test. The patient is positioned supine. The examiner supports the arm in neutral rotation and at 90° abduction. In this position, the examiner applies a posterior gliding force to the humeral head with the other hand while taking the patient's arm into a position of end-range external rotation. At this point, the posterior force on the humeral head is released. A positive test is indicated by a sense of apprehension or reproduction of the patient's symptoms. See Figure 5.30.

Anterior Drawer Test (Anterior Instability)

The patient is positioned supine with the affected upper extremity supported by the examiner. The shoulder is

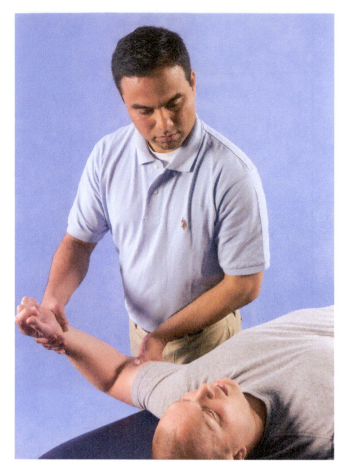

Figure 5.29 Apprehension test for anterior shoulder instability.

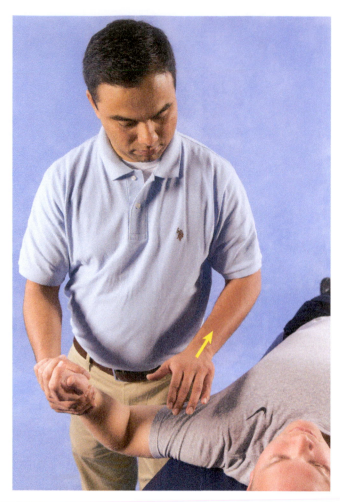

Figure 5.30 Surprise test for anterior shoulder instability. A posterior force is applied while the shoulder is externally rotated and then suddenly released.

abducted to about 90°, with slight flexion and external rotation. The examiner stabilizes the patient's scapula with one hand and with the other hand glides the humeral head forward and medially, bearing in mind the orientation of the glenoid, as shown in Figure 5.31.

The degree of anterior translation of the humeral head is compared to the unaffected side or graded using the modified Hawkins classification.[32] The grade of instability is determined by what the examiner palpates.[33] Box 5-2 describes the grades of shoulder instability.

Posterior Drawer Test (Posterior Instability)

The patient is positioned supine and the examiner supports the patient's upper extremity. The scapula is stabilized while the examiner glides the humeral head posteriorly and laterally, bearing in mind the orientation of the glenoid (Fig. 5.32). The modified Hawkins scale is used to grade the amount of translation of the humeral head.

Kim Test (Posterior or Posteroinferior Instability)

The patient is sitting with the arm supported at 90° of abduction. With one hand, the examiner applies an axial (or compressive) load while abducting the arm an additional 45°. With the other hand, the examiner

simultaneously glides the humerus posteroinferiorly. A positive test is indicated by pain or reproduction of the patient's symptoms. This test is also used to assess the integrity of the glenoid labrum for posterior/posteroinferior tear. See Figure 5.33.

Sulcus Sign (Inferior or Multidirectional Instability)

The patient is sitting with the arm at the side. The examiner grasps the patient's forearm below the elbow and provides a traction force inferiorly (Fig 5.34A). The test is positive with the finding of excessive translation of the humeral head and reproduction of the patient's symptoms (Fig. 5.34B). Greater than 1 cm between the anterior acromion process and the humeral head is considered to be excessive.[34] A positive test indicates inferior laxity, multidirectional instability, and/or a superior labral tear.

Rowe's Test (Multidirectional Instability)

The patient stands forward flexed with the arm relaxed. The examiner applies forces to assess anterior, posterior,

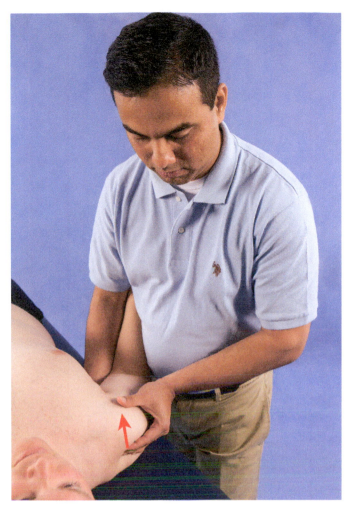

Figure 5.31 Anterior drawer test for anterior shoulder instability.

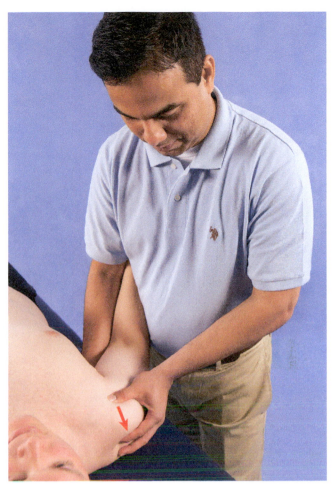

Figure 5.32 Posterior drawer test for posterior shoulder instability.

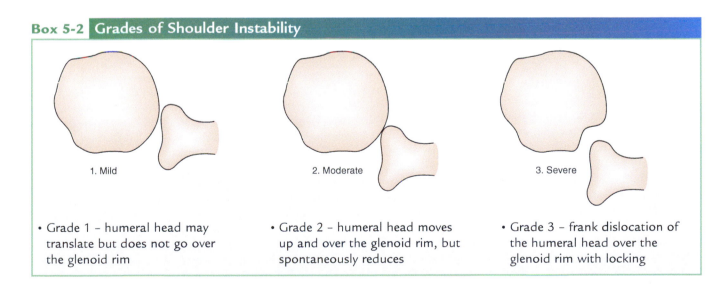

Box 5-2   Grades of Shoulder Instability

1. Mild

2. Moderate

3. Severe

- Grade 1 – humeral head may translate but does not go over the glenoid rim

- Grade 2 – humeral head moves up and over the glenoid rim, but spontaneously reduces

- Grade 3 – frank dislocation of the humeral head over the glenoid rim with locking

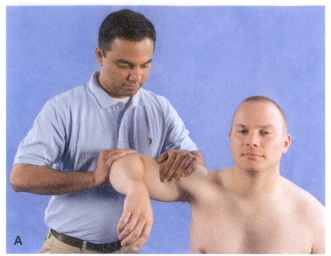

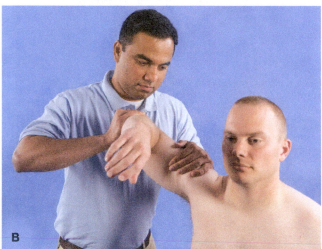

Figure 5.33 Kim test for posterior shoulder instability, posteroinferior shoulder instability, or labral tear. The examiner applies an axial force with the shoulder at 90° abduction (A) then further abducts the shoulder with a posteroinferior glide (B).

and inferior translation of the humeral head. Anterior instability is assessed by gliding the humeral head anteriorly while slightly extending the shoulder. Posterior instability is assessed by gliding the humeral head posteriorly while slightly flexing the shoulder. Inferior instability is assessed by applying a traction force inferiorly and checking for a sulcus sign.[35] A positive test is indicated by excessive movement inferiorly or in more than one direction. See Figure 5.35.

Common Interventions

For TUBS Dislocator

After traumatic dislocation, a patient will often be immobilized in a sling for about 2 weeks. In this early protective phase, the focus of therapy is to decrease pain and muscle guarding, protect the joint from further harm, and minimize loss of motion and strength caused by immobilization. Modalities may be used to decrease pain

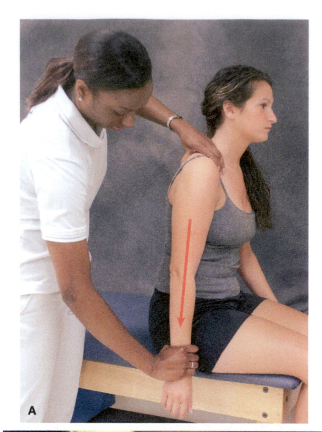

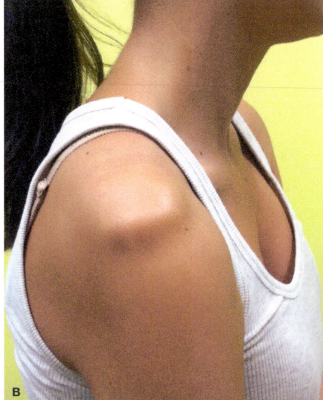

Figure 5.34 Sulcus sign for inferior or multidirectional instability of the shoulder. An inferior distraction force is applied (A). Excessive translation of the humeral head causes a sulcus (B).

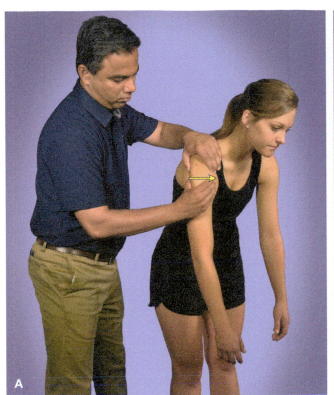

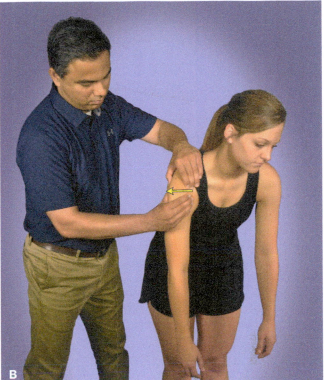

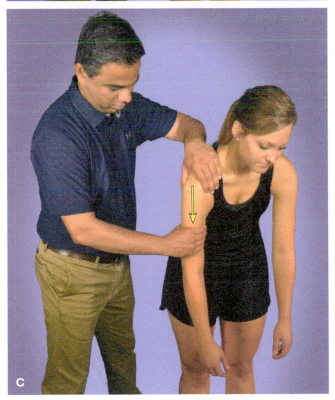

Figure 5.35 Rowe's test for shoulder instability. Anterior glide (A), posterior glide (B), and distraction (C) are assessed with the patient forward flexed.

and inflammation, including cryotherapy and electrical stimulation.

Passive range-of-motion in the patient's pain-free range is usually included in the plan of care initially, along with pain-free AAROM into internal and external rotation. Pendulum exercises may be included to decrease pain and maintain joint ROM. Submaximal isometric exercises to the rotator cuff, deltoids, and scapular stabilizers may be added at this time. Wilk recommends rhythmic stabilization to shoulder ER/IR at 30° scaption to begin recruiting the rotator cuff muscles.[34]

⚑ CLINICAL ALERT!

Patients with an anterior instability are commonly instructed to avoid shoulder external rotation ROM past 60° when the shoulder is abducted to avoid overstressing the anterior capsule.[34] Patients with posterior dislocation should avoid end ranges of shoulder internal rotation with the shoulder abducted and should avoid horizontal adduction. These movements bear a risk of dislocation.

Proprioception in the shoulder has been shown to be decreased after subluxation or dislocation.[36–39] The patient may benefit from proprioceptive retraining for the upper extremity in this phase, including weight-bearing on a ball or balance board (Fig. 5.36).

In the intermediate phase, strengthening is progressed to isotonic exercises, focusing on rotator cuff and scapular muscles to increase the dynamic stability of the shoulder. Proprioceptive retraining is also progressed. In the last phase, consideration is given to the patient's occupation or sport as strengthening, stretching, and proprioceptive training are progressed. Increasing muscle endurance may be a goal of treatment, as some investigators have found that muscle fatigue decreases proprioceptive sense.[40,41]

What's in the Plan of Care? Weight-bearing exercises on the affected side may be contraindicated in patients with a posterior dislocation. They stress the posterior capsule, and in the acute phase, may lead to dislocation.

For AMBRI Dislocator

Rehabilitation for the patient with an AMBRI dislocation has slightly different considerations than that for TUBS. An AMBRI type of instability causes less tissue damage, as frank dislocation is less likely. Because this patient is likely to have had recurring episodes of instability, the focus will be on strengthening of the scapula and rotator cuff, proprioceptive retraining, and neuromuscular control of the scapula and rotator cuff.

It is important to teach the patient to avoid movements and positions that might further stretch the joint capsule and ligaments. Elevation movements should be performed in the scapular plane, rather than the frontal plane, to avoid instability. Rhythmic stabilization to the trunk and

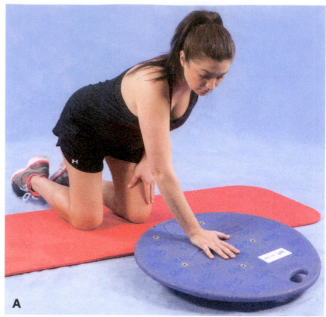

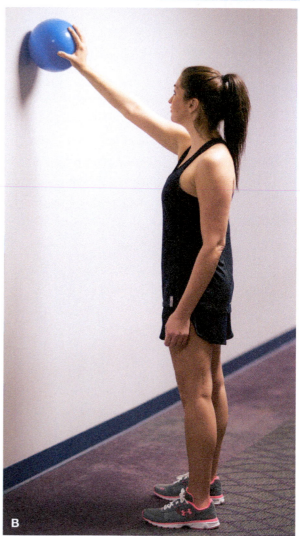

Figure 5.36 Proprioceptive retraining may be included in the POC after shoulder subluxation or dislocation. The patient may be progressed from an unstable surface on the floor (A) to a ball on the wall (B).

extremity may be employed to improve core stability and neuromuscular control.

Weight-bearing exercises may be used to enhance proprioception and obtain co-contraction of the muscles around the joint. For example, plank exercises with the patient on elbows and knees is an early exercise that can be advanced to prone planks on elbows and feet and eventually to prone planks on elbows and feet on an unstable surface.[34]

Scapular and glenohumeral strengthening will likely be included in the plan of care for these patients. The focus of strengthening will often include the scapular upward rotators and rotator cuff muscles, particularly external rotators.

Watch Out For...

Watch out for exercises that position the patient at risk for subluxation or dislocation. As you add exercises to the patient's program, do a final check to make sure the patient isn't going to be in a position of risk. Especially be careful with positions of end range of shoulder internal and external rotation.

Prevention

There are no guidelines to preventing shoulder instability. However, if instability is present, strengthening the rotator cuff and scapular muscles may prevent the problem from becoming worse or requiring surgery.

The Bottom Line:	for patients with instability
Description and causes	Instability of the humeral head due to trauma (TUBS dislocator) or congenital hypermobility syndrome (AMBRI dislocator)
Test	Rowe's test, sulcus sign, anterior drawer test, posterior drawer test, Kim test, apprehension test, surprise test
Stretch	Often not indicated
Strengthen	Rotator cuff muscles, scapular muscles, muscles that act as barrier to movement or counteract destabilizing forces, including pectorals, deltoids, latissimus dorsi, and teres major
Train	Proprioception, neuromuscular control of scapula and rotator cuff muscles
Avoid	Positions of instability, weight-bearing in cases of posterior instability

Interventions for the Surgical Patient

If the patient with a traumatic dislocation has sustained a Bankart lesion, surgery is often indicated to repair the labrum. AMBRI dislocation generally responds to strengthening, but if instability episodes become more frequent or are interfering with daily activities, an inferior capsular shift may be indicated.

Bankart Repair

Surgery. With the goal of surgery to increase stability of the glenohumeral joint, several approaches may be used. The labrum may be anchored back onto the glenoid rim to repair the detachment (Fig. 5.37). If the capsular ligaments are also torn, these are repaired. If there is bone loss on the rim of the glenoid, a bone graft from the iliac crest may be used to rebuild the glenoid.

What's in the Plan of Care? *Postoperative Phase.* Initially after an open Bankart repair it's important to allow the tissues time to heal. The early goals are to decrease pain and to minimize the effects of immobilization. The patient will typically be restricted to 140° of shoulder flexion and 45° of external rotation for 4 weeks.

Early in the rehabilitation process the plan of care will likely include shoulder PROM, advancing to AAROM. External rotation is progressed from neutral up to 45° by the end of four weeks. Submaximal isometric strengthening of the rotators in a neutral position may be used. Do not strengthen internal rotation if the subscapularis muscle was detached in surgery. AROM of the elbow, wrist, and hand are also indicated. Scapular protraction

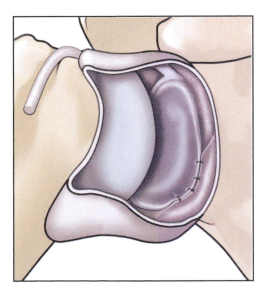

Figure 5.37 Bankart repair is a surgical procedure to reattach the labrum to the glenoid.

in closed- chain and retraction isometrics prone may be used to increase scapular muscle strength.

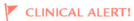

> **CLINICAL ALERT!** ▔▔▔▔▔▔▔▔▔▔
>
> If the subscapularis muscle was detached and reattached in the surgery, the patient should avoid active internal rotation strengthening for 4 to 6 weeks.

By 4 weeks postoperatively, the patient may be gradually allowed to increase external rotation ROM, with a typical goal of full range by 8 weeks. Flexion may be gradually increased to 160°. Resistance bands or light weights may be used to strengthen rotator cuff, deltoid, biceps, and scapular muscles. Proprioceptive retraining, such as PNF techniques, may be added.

Inferior Capsular Shift

Surgery. AMBRI instability is multidirectional, so the surgical approach must be tailored to the instability that is present. If the anterior and inferior capsule is stretched, inferior capsular shift is a common surgical approach. In this surgery, the inferior capsule is tightened, resulting in a doubling of the capsule on the anterior shoulder (Fig. 5.38).

Postoperative Phase. Postoperatively, the patient will be immobilized for 6 weeks, and no shoulder motion is allowed. The patient may perform elbow, wrist, and hand ROM. After this immobilization phase, the plan of care may include AROM of the shoulder with restrictions.

What's in the Plan of Care? Typically, the patient is allowed up to 140° flexion, 70° abduction, 40° external rotation, and internal rotation up to contact with the abdomen. Strengthening with light weights in all planes, avoiding the position of instability, may be initiated. Intervention may include scapular muscle strengthening, such as prone rows and closed chain protraction (Fig. 5.39). By 3 months postsurgery, the patient will be allowed to progress to full shoulder ROM, proprioceptive retraining, and strengthening of the rotator cuff and scapular stabilizers.

Subacromial Impingement Syndrome

Subacromial impingement syndrome (SAIS) is the most common shoulder pathology, and it is estimated to be the source of more than 50% of shoulder pain. In this pathology, the soft tissue structures under the coracoacromial arch are compressed between the humeral head and the arch. The supraspinatus tendon is most commonly affected. In addition, the subacromial bursa and the long head of the biceps tendon are often affected. This compression causes the structures to become inflamed. Figure 5.40 depicts SAIS.

Causes/Contributing Factors

There are many factors that contribute to SAIS. Any narrowing of the subacromial space, either structurally or functionally, may lead to pressure on the structures under the coracoacromial arch. Structural changes include acromial shape, subacromial spurs, and swelling of the rotator cuff tendons or the coracoacromial ligament due to overuse or repetitive overhead activities.

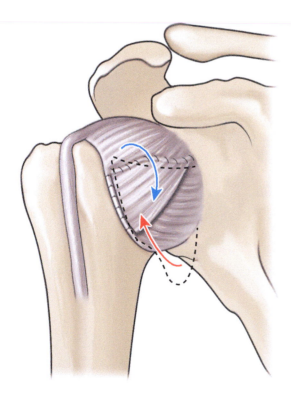

Figure 5.38 Inferior capsular shift is a surgical procedure to tighten the anterior capsule.

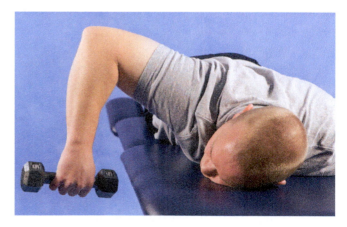

Figure 5.39 Prone rows (A) and closed-chain scapular protraction (B) may be included in the POC after inferior capsular shift.

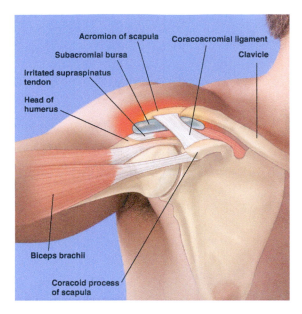

Figure 5.40 Subacromial impingement syndrome involves compression of the soft tissues under the coracoacromial arch. Commonly compressed structures include the supraspinatus tendon, the long head of biceps tendon, and the subacromial bursa.

The effect of acromial shape has been very well studied. It is generally accepted that a hooked-shape acromion is related to SAIS.[42–45] Osteophytic spurs under the acromion or distal clavicle develop with age and have also been linked to SAIS. Repeated or prolonged overhead activity may lead to thickening of the coracoacromial ligament, which narrows the subacromial space. Once the rotator cuff tendon has become inflamed, it swells, further compromising the space. Additionally, blood flow to the supraspinatus is temporarily decreased in the overhead position.

In some cases, it appears that the space is not anatomically limited, but is limited functionally. Causes for this include a tight posterior capsule, weakness of the rotator cuff or scapular muscles, shoulder instability, or abnormal movement (**dyskinesia**) of the scapula.

A tight posterior capsule leads to superior migration of the humeral head during shoulder flexion, causing the space to be temporarily narrowed.[46] Weakness of the rotator cuff may compromise the action of depressing and stabilizing the humeral head. Instability of the shoulder allows the humeral head to elevate into the coracoacromial arch.

Scapular dyskinesia has been linked to SAIS. The most implicated cause of abnormal movement in the scapula leading to SAIS is weakness in the upward rotation force couple. This may lead to a loss of scapular control in the eccentric phase of lowering the arm, with a resulting momentary pressure of the acromion against the humerus. People with SAIS have been shown to have increased downward rotation and anterior tilting of the scapula when compared to normal individuals.[47]

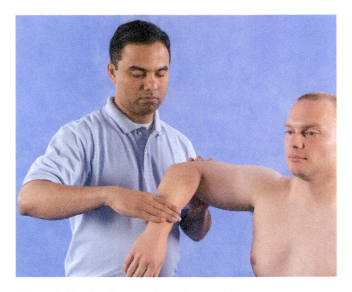

Figure 5.41 Hawkins test for subacromial impingement syndrome.

Symptoms

The hallmark sign of SAIS is a painful arc of motion. Abduction is the most painful movement, with a painful arc typically from 60° to 120° of abduction. The patient will complain of pain with overhead movements. Pain is often worse at night and worse when sleeping on the affected side.

Clinical Signs

There are many tests that may be used to assess SAIS. Often the physical therapy practitioner will use several tests as a cluster to confirm the diagnosis.

Hawkins Test

The patient is sitting while the examiner flexes the arm to 90° with elbow flexion. The examiner then forcibly internally rotates the shoulder. The test may be performed in different degrees of horizontal abduction, moving from the sagittal plane to the frontal plane (Fig. 5.41). A positive test is indicated by reproduction of the patient's pain.

Neer Test

The patient is sitting while the examiner passively internally rotates the shoulder. The examiner then raises the arm to end range of flexion or scaption. Force is applied at end range in an attempt to reproduce the patient's symptoms (Fig. 5.42). A positive test is indicated by reproduction of the patient's pain.

Painful Arc Test

The patient is standing. The examiner instructs the patient to actively abduct the arm on the affected side. A positive test is indicated by a painful arc of motion in the 60° to 120° range or less. Pain outside of this range is considered negative (Fig. 5.43).

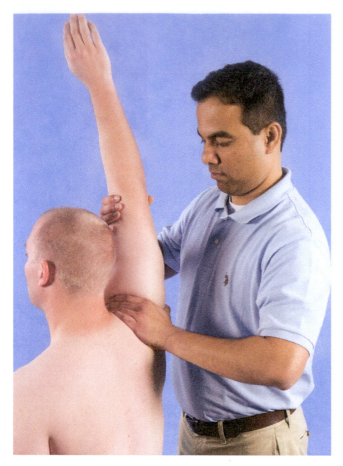

Figure 5.42 Neer test for subacromial impingement syndrome.

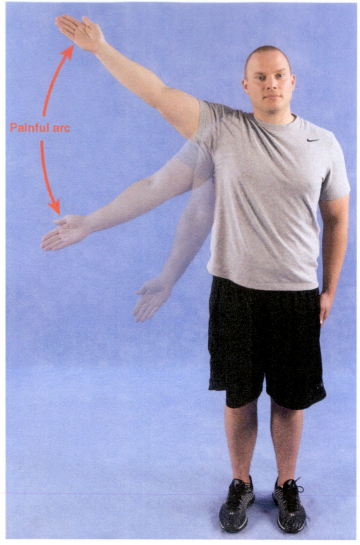

Painful arc

Figure 5.43 Painful arc test for subacromial impingement syndrome. The range between 60° and 120° of shoulder abduction is most painful.

Full Can/Empty Can Test

The patient is standing and actively abducts the arm to 90° with the thumb up (full can position). The examiner provides downward pressure on the arm as if to test the patient's strength (Fig. 5.44A). The patient then elevates the arms to 90° in the scapular plane with thumb down (empty can position). The examiner provides downward pressure as if to test the patient's strength in this position (Fig. 5.44B). A positive test for SAIS is patient complaint of pain while maintaining the empty can test position or with resistance. Weakness may accompany the pain. The full can position should elicit little or no pain. This test may indicate a rotator cuff tear if the patient has pronounced weakness.

Infraspinatus Test

This test is a manual muscle test of infraspinatus. The patient is standing with the arm at the side, elbow bent to 90°, and forearm in a neutral position. The examiner instructs the patient to hold the arm in this position while applying a force to attempt to internally rotate the shoulder (Fig. 5.45). A positive test is indicated by the inability of the patient to resist due to pain or weakness.

Common Interventions

Patients with SAIS will benefit from addressing the causes or contributors to the problem. Typically, the plan of care will include use of anti-inflammatory modalities, such as ice or iontophoresis. Cross-body stretching exercises to the posterior capsule may be indicated (Fig. 5.46). Stretches into shoulder flexion and into shoulder rotation are often included in the plan of care. The patient should be instructed to avoid abduction over 60° and to avoid elevation of the shoulder combined with internal rotation until the pain subsides.

What's in the Plan of Care?

Scapular strengthening for the trapezius, serratus anterior, levator scapulae, and rhomboid muscles may be used to address scapular dyskinesia. Strengthening of the rotator cuff is crucial. Supraspinatus should be strengthened in the "full can" position or with prone

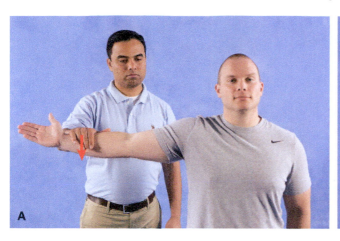

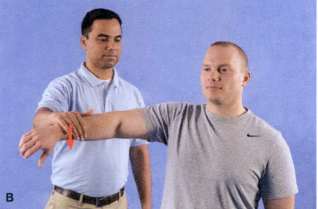

Figure 5.44 Full can/Empty can test for subacromial impingement syndrome. Pain and weakness in the empty can position indicate a positive test.

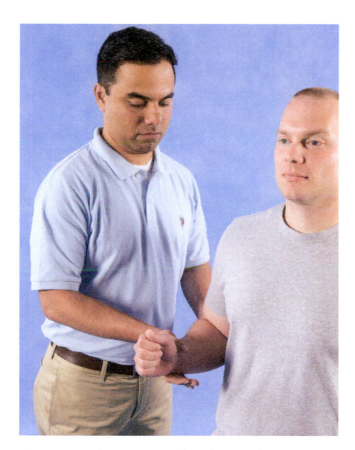

Figure 5.45 Infraspinatus test for subacromial impingement syndrome.

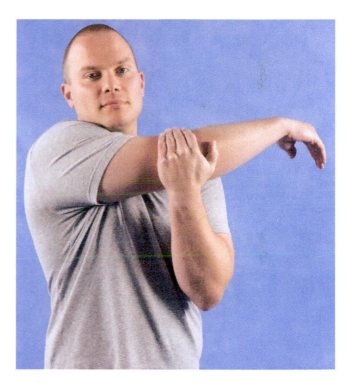

Figure 5.46 Cross-body posterior capsule stretching may be indicated for subacromial impingement syndrome.

horizontal abduction exercises in external rotation at 100° abduction. Focusing on the eccentric phase of this exercise will lead to hypertrophy of the supraspinatus tendon, which counteracts the progression of tendon thinning after inflammation. Strengthening of latissimus dorsi and pectoralis major are often included to further

stabilize the shoulder. Figure 5.47 depicts typical strengthening exercises for SAIS.

Prevention

Maintaining good strength in the shoulder muscles is important in preventing SAIS. If signs of impingement are present, medical attention should be sought to decrease inflammation and increase strength before the changes in the area become irreversible.

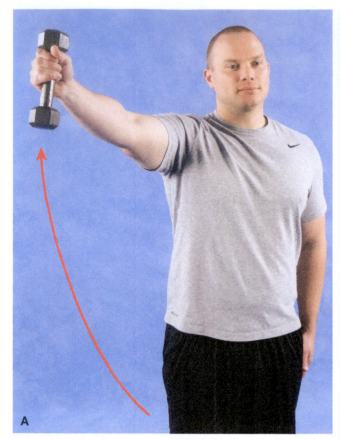

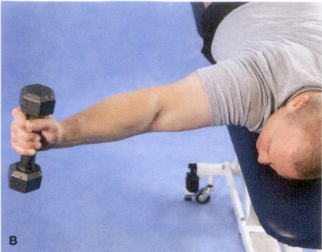

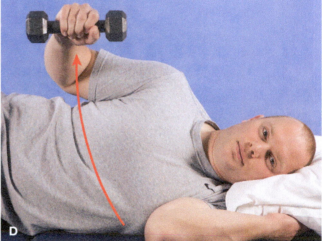

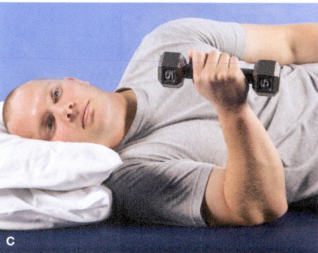

Figure 5.47 Typical exercises in the POC for subacromial impingement syndrome include full-can supraspinatus strengthening (A), prone horizontal abduction (B), and strengthening of internal rotators (C) and external rotators (D).

The Bottom Line: for patients with SAIS

Description and causes	Impingement of the rotator cuff between bones of the shoulder caused by a narrowed space combined with overhead activity
Test	Hawkins test, Neer test, full can/empty can test, painful arc, infraspinatus test
Stretch	Posterior capsule
Strengthen	Rotator cuff, trapezius, serratus anterior, levator scapulae, and rhomboids
Train	Eccentrically to hypertrophy tendon
Avoid	Elevation of the shoulder with internal rotation

Interventions for the Surgical Patient

Subacromial Decompression

If the patient does not respond to conservative therapy, subacromial decompression may be indicated to relieve the pressure on the soft tissues. This procedure may include debridement of the area with removal of the subacromial bursa, **acromioplasty, distal clavicle excision,** and **coracoacromial ligament resection.** In acromioplasty, the underside of the acromion is shaved, removing any spurs and providing more space under the coracoacromial arch. To further decompress the area, the distal end of the clavicle may be removed, with the coracoacromial ligament, if necessary (Fig. 5.48).

Postoperative Phase

After decompression surgery, the patient will often be seen for physical therapy with initial goals of decreasing pain and increasing ROM. The patient may be wearing a sling but gradually weaned off the sling in about 2 weeks. The patient should be instructed to avoid abduction, moving in the scapular plane instead. Pendulum exercises and PROM/AAROM into all planes except abduction and horizontal adduction are typically part of the early plan of care for these patients. Pulleys may be used for AAROM.

Submaximal isometric exercises to internal and external rotators, shoulder flexors, extensors, abductors, and adductors are typically included in the plan of care. Elbow, forearm, wrist, and hand AROM are also common.

By 5 to 6 weeks postsurgery, AROM of the shoulder is initiated with attention to scapular control. Normal scapular movement patterns should be seen. Isotonic rotator cuff strengthening and scapular strengthening

may be added. As the patient progresses, scapular muscle strengthening and rotator cuff strengthening is advanced to use of resistance bands and weights at 90° of abduction.

Rotator Cuff Tendinopathy/Tear

This pathology describes the progression of deterioration that may occur in the rotator cuff tendons. These changes are not necessarily considered to be indicative of inflammation (tendonitis), but of a failed healing response that may lead to rotator cuff tear. The supraspinatus tendon is the most commonly affected of the four rotator cuff tendons.

Rotator cuff tear may be through partial thickness or extend through the full thickness of the rotator cuff. The tear may be small or it may be very large and involve several of the rotator cuff muscles. Full-thickness tears and large tears have less success with conservative treatment and often require surgery. Figure 5.49A depicts a small-to-medium tear within the rotator cuff tendon. Figure 5.49B depicts a large tear at the insertion of the tendon on the greater tubercle.

Causes/Contributing Factors

Many contributing factors have been reported for rotator cuff disease. From a deteriorated state where the muscles are thin, it takes only minimal stress to cause a rotator cuff tear. Some contributors include subacromial impingement, acromial shape, acromial bone spurs, repetitive use, overload of the tendons, abnormal scapular movement, forward head posture, and increased thoracic kyphosis.

Symptoms

Because of the importance of the rotator cuff in shoulder elevation, patients with significant rotator cuff disease or a small tear may have a painful arc of motion as is seen in patients with subacromial impingement syndrome. If the rotator cuff has a medium-to-large tear, the patient will "shrug" the shoulder in an attempt to raise the arm.

Figure 5.50 depicts a patient with a right rotator cuff tear when asked to abduct both arms fully. Note the amount of scapular elevation on the right. The deltoid is normally active, but without the rotator cuff to stabilize and depress the humeral head, the humerus bumps into the acromion and movement is halted. The patient may complain of pain that is worse at night and increases with sidelying on the affected side. The chief complaint, however, will generally be weakness in the arm.

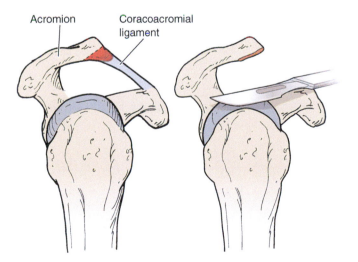

Acromion   Coracoacromial ligament

Figure 5.48 Acromioplasty and coracoacromial ligament resection may be performed to decompress the subacromial space.

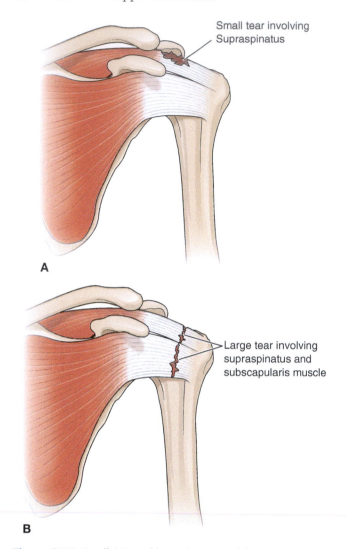

Small tear involving Suprasupatus

A

Large tear involving supraspinatus and subscapularis muscle

B

Figure 5.49 Small (A) and large (B) tear of the rotator cuff.

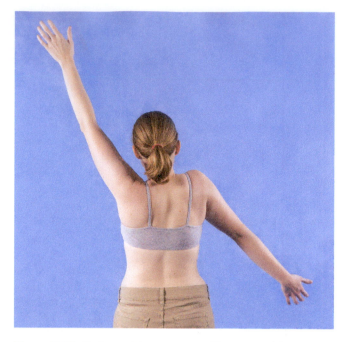

Figure 5.50 Patient with a rotator cuff tear. Resulting weakness leads to elevation of the shoulder girdle with limited abduction motion on attempts to elevate the arm on the affected side.

Clinical Signs

There are many special tests for rotator cuff tendinopathy and tear. These tests may use weakness or pain with muscle contraction as an indicator of tear. Other tests compress the rotator cuff tendons between the humerus and the acromion and are positive if pain results. In addition to special tests for rotator cuff tear, simple muscle testing of the rotator cuff muscles may be used to indicate rotator cuff disease.

Drop Arm Test

The patient is standing with the affected arm hanging by the side. The examiner passively abducts the arm to 90°. The examiner then instructs the patient to slowly lower the arm. The examiner lets go of the patient's arm but remains close enough to provide support if the patient cannot control the arm's descent (Fig. 5.51). A positive test is indicated by the patient's inability to slowly lower the arm, allowing it to drop.

Full Can/Empty Can Test

See previous description (Fig. 5.44AB).

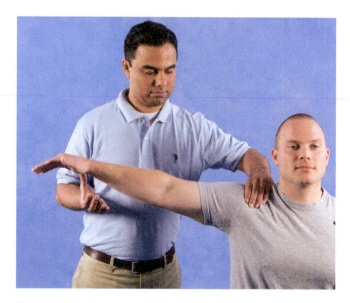

Figure 5.51 Drop arm test for rotator cuff tear.

External Rotation Lag Sign

The patient is sitting with the affected arm supported by the examiner at the elbow. The examiner grasps the patient's wrist, passively flexes the patient's elbow to 90°, and brings the patient's shoulder into a position of 20° of scaption. The examiner then passively moves the patient's shoulder into a position of maximal external rotation. The patient is instructed to hold this position as the examiner releases the patient's wrist (Fig. 5.52). A positive test is indicated by the patient's inability to maintain the shoulder in full external rotation.

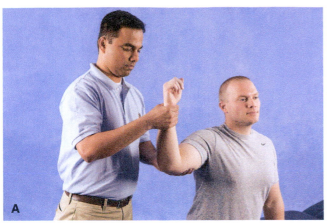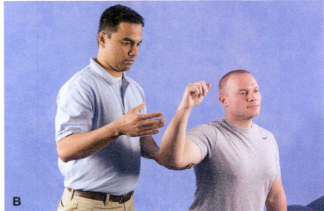

Figure 5.52 External rotation lag sign for rotator cuff tear. The patient is positioned in shoulder external rotation in scaption (A). Upon release, the patient is asked to maintain the position (B).

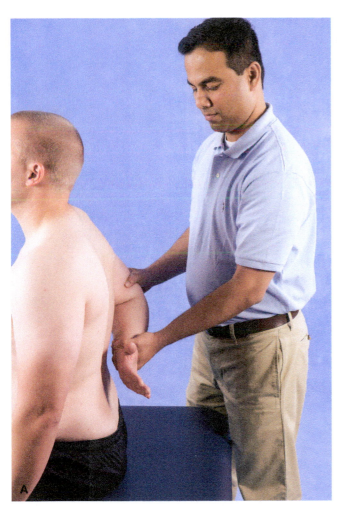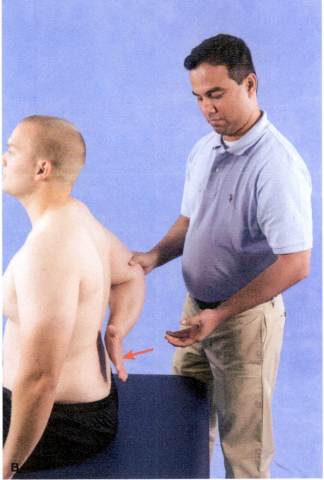

Figure 5.53 Internal rotation lag sign for rotator cuff tear. The patient is positioned in full shoulder internal rotation with the arm behind the back. Upon release, the patient is asked to maintain the position.

Internal Rotation Lag Sign

The patient is seated with the affected arm behind the back. The examiner supports the patient's elbow with one hand, bringing the arm into extension. With the other hand, the examiner grasps the patient's wrist and lifts the patient's hand away from the back. The examiner instructs the patient to maintain this position and then releases the grasp on the wrist (Fig. 5.53). A positive test is indicated by the patient's inability to maintain the hand away from the back.

Common Interventions

The goals of physical therapy are to control pain and inflammation, to protect the rotator cuff tendons, and to restore ROM and strength. Pendulum exercises, PROM, and AAROM of the shoulder are usually included in the plan of care in the early phases. Strengthening of the rotator cuff, scapular stabilizers, deltoids, latissimus dorsi, and pectoralis major may be done using submaximal isometric exercises. The patient is progressed as tolerated using weights and resistance bands. Elbow, forearm, wrist, and hand strengthening may also be part of the plan of care. Stretching of the posterior capsule may be included if tightness is contributing to the pathology.

Prevention

Reducing the likelihood of rotator cuff disease is possible by avoiding repeated overhead positions and maintaining good strength in the rotator cuff and scapular muscles. Maintaining good posture is important, since forward head posture is linked to impingement.[48] Sleeping with the arms overhead should be avoided.

The Bottom Line:	for patients with rotator cuff tear
Description and causes	Gradual deterioration of the rotator cuff leading to tear with contributors including chronic tendinopathy, abnormal posture, acromial shape, and repeated use
Test	Drop arm test, full can/empty can test, external rotation lag test, internal rotation lag test
Stretch	Posterior capsule if it's tight
Strengthen	Rotator cuff, scapular stabilizers, deltoids, latissimus dorsi, and pectoralis major
Train	NA
Avoid	NA

Interventions for the Surgical Patient

If a conservative approach does not restore function or modulate pain, surgical repair may be necessary.

Rotator Cuff Repair

Postoperative Phase

It is estimated to take 8 to 12 weeks after arthroscopic repair of the rotator cuff for healing of the tendon to the bone. Physical therapy after rotator cuff repair is divided into four phases: immediate postsurgical, protected, early strengthening, and advanced strengthening. During phase I (0 to 6 weeks), the patient is restricted from performing AROM and is immobilized in a sling, which is removed only for exercise. The patient is not allowed to lift anything during this phase. Pendulum shoulder exercises, as well as neck, elbow, forearm, wrist, and hand AROM exercises may be included in the plan of care.

What's in the Plan of Care? Supine PROM of the shoulder to 110° flexion and internal and external rotation in the scapular plane with the shoulder in a position of less than 30° scaption may be initiated in the first week. Throughout this phase supine PROM is progressed, resisted exercise to elbow, wrist, and hand are added, and scapular isometrics are initiated.

By phase II (up to week 12), the patient may begin to perform PROM with a pulley. Submaximal isometric exercise to the rotator cuff muscles, scapular strengthening with manual resistance, and AROM of the shoulder may be added in weeks 9 to 12. Full AROM is expected by about 12 weeks.

Phase III is generally 3 to 4 months postsurgery. The patient may still be restricted in how much can be lifted with the affected arm. Until the patient is able to perform shoulder elevation in the scapular plane without shrugging the shoulder, the PT will likely restrict elevation movements to 90°. Prone exercises may be added. By phase IV (up to 5 to 6 months after surgery), the patient may be returning to premorbid functional levels and resuming occupational and sports activities.

Posterior Internal Impingement

Posterior internal impingement (PII) is the compression of supraspinatus and/or infraspinatus between the posterior-superior glenoid rim and the greater tubercle. This occurs in overhead-throwing athletes, in a position of external rotation and abduction such as in the cocking phase of baseball pitching. With repeated stresses, this compression may become symptomatic and be accompanied by tears in the glenoid labrum or posterior-superior rotator cuff muscles (Fig. 5.54).

Causes/Contributing Factors

The cause of PII is still under investigation. It appears that repetitive overhead activity in the position of shoulder external rotation and abduction contributes. Posterior capsule tightness and abnormal movement patterns of the scapula have been implicated.[49,50] Other contributing factors that have been associated with PII include a

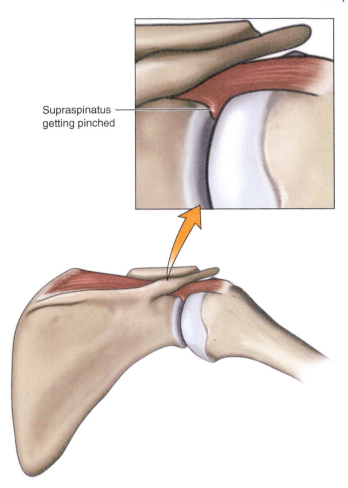

Supraspinatus getting pinched

Figure 5.54 Posterior internal impingement is characterized by compression of the supraspinatus or infraspinatus between the humeral head and glenoid when the arm is abducted and externally rotated.

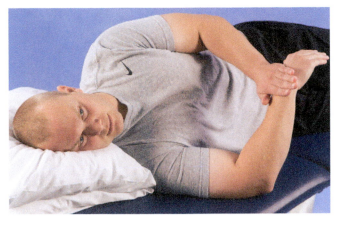

Figure 5.55 The sleeper stretch of the posterior capsule may be indicated for posterior internal impingement.

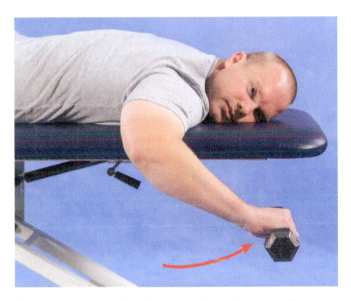

Figure 5.56 Prone shoulder external rotation strengthening for a patient with posterior shoulder impingement.

decrease of shoulder internal rotation ROM, shoulder instability, rotator cuff weakness, and scapular retraction weakness.

Symptoms

The primary symptom of PII is transitory pain in the posterior shoulder in a position of shoulder external rotation with abduction. Pain may be referred into the lateral upper arm.

Clinical Signs

The patient will experience tenderness to palpation underneath the posterior lateral portion of the acromion. There are no special tests to diagnose PII.

Common Interventions

Treatment for PII is aimed at addressing the contributing factors. Often, stretching of the posterior shoulder capsule is indicated. A cross-body horizontal adduction stretch may be used. Internal rotation stretches to the shoulder, such as the sleeper stretch (Fig. 5.55) and PROM in supine may also be used to gain range of motion into

internal rotation. Joint mobilization has been shown to prolong the effect of PROM stretching and may be included in the plan of care.[51]

Strengthening of the rotator cuff and scapular stabilizers is also important for patients who exhibit instability. Rhythmic stabilization into internal rotation and external rotation may be initiated at 20° to 30° of scaption. As the patient progresses, these exercises may be performed at 90° of abduction in the impinging position. The patient may be progressed to use of resistance bands and weight. Strengthening of the shoulder external rotators may be done in the scapular plane standing or in the prone position (Fig. 5.56). Supraspinatus may be strengthened by performing scaption "full can" exercises or prone horizontal abduction exercises in external rotation at 100° abduction. Serratus anterior should also be targeted with punching exercises above 120° of flexion or by having the patient perform push-ups with a "plus."

The Bottom Line:	for patients with posterior internal impingement
Description and causes	Pinching of posterior rotator cuff when the arm is abducted and externally rotated often seen in overhead throwing athletes due to weakness of the rotator cuff or tightness of the posterior capsule
Test	No special tests; tender to palpation below posterolateral acromion
Stretch	Posterior capsule
Strengthen	Rotator cuff, scapular muscles, rhomboids, middle trapezius
Train	NA
Avoid	Impinging motion when acute

Bicipital Tendinopathy

The long head of the biceps tendon originates from the superior glenoid labrum. It runs under the coracoacromial arch as it crosses the top of the humeral head and descends through the intertubercular groove. Because of this anatomical relationship, it is at risk of inflammation (tendonitis) or degeneration without inflammation (tendinosis). Bicipital tendinopathy may occur as an isolated finding but most often accompanies rotator cuff disease, osteoarthritis of the shoulder, glenoid labral tears (Box 5-3), or shoulder instability.

Causes/Contributing Factors

As a primary pathology, bicipital tendinopathy may be caused by overuse of the muscle, particularly in overhead activities. The tendon lies directly in contact with the superior humeral head and between the greater and lesser tubercles, placing it at risk with overhead and repeated movements of the shoulder. Sports that place the arm in a position of extreme shoulder external rotation in an abducted position, such as baseball pitching, volleyball, tennis, and swimming, increase the risk.

As a secondary finding, an impingement in the subacromial space due to rotator cuff disease may lead to impingement of the biceps tendon. Shoulder instability may also contribute to overuse of the long head of the biceps as a shoulder stabilizer.

Symptoms

The most common complaint is pain in the anterior shoulder that is increased with lifting, pushing, and overhead activities. The patient may feel this pain along the bicipital groove.

Clinical Signs

The signs of tendinopathy are pain with palpation, stretch, and contraction. The patient will often complain of tenderness with palpation of the tendon in the bicipital groove. Resisted elbow flexion may elicit pain. Stretch of the tendon by bringing the arm into full shoulder and elbow extension with forearm pronation may also elicit

Watch Out For...

Watch out for signs of musculotendinous pathologies that include pain with palpation, pain with stretch, and pain with contraction. This pattern will be seen in many pathologies of muscle or tendon.

Box 5-3	Superior Glenoid Labral (SLAP) Tears

Tears of the glenoid labrum are reported most commonly in throwing athletes. The tear often involves the anterior, posterior, or superior labrum. Superior labral tears are related to superior instability of the shoulder.[52] Because the long head of the biceps originates from the superior labrum, superior tears are challenging to treat. A tear of the **S**uperior **L**abrum from **A**nterior to **P**osterior (for example, from the 10 o'clock to 2 o'clock position) is called a SLAP lesion. SLAP tears may be caused by and/or impact function in the biceps. The active compression test may be positive in the therapy evaluation of superior glenoid labral tears.

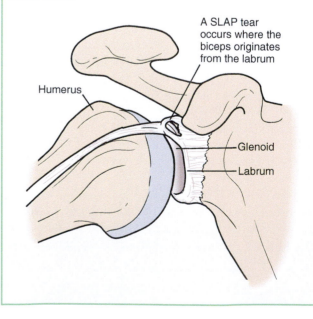

A SLAP tear occurs where the biceps originates from the labrum

Humerus

Glenoid

Labrum

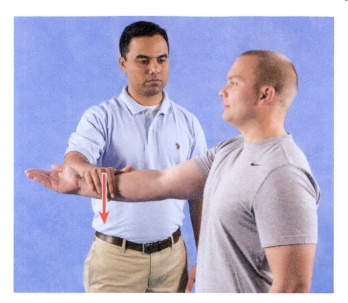

Figure 5.57 Speed's test for bicipital tendonitis.

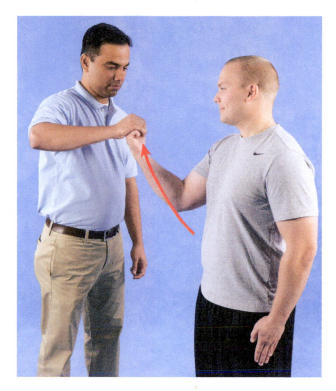

Figure 5.58 Upper cut test for bicipital tendonitis.

pain. In addition, the special tests below may be used to confirm the diagnosis.

Speed's Test

The patient is standing with the shoulder flexed to about 80°, elbow extended, and forearm supinated. The examiner instructs the patient to hold against a downward force into shoulder extension. A positive test is indicated by reproduction of the patient's complaint of pain in the anterior shoulder. See Figure 5.57.

Upper Cut Test

The patient is standing with the shoulder in neutral, elbow flexed to 90°, forearm supinated, and hand in a fist. The examiner covers the patient's fist to resist movement and instructs the patient to quickly bring the hand up across the body toward the chin, doing a boxing "uppercut" maneuver (Fig. 5.58). A positive test is indicated by reproduction of the patient's pain.

Common Interventions

Initially, the goal of treatment for the patient with bicipital tendinopathy is to control pain and inflammation. The patient should avoid overhead activities and heavy lifting. The plan of care may include cryotherapy, pulsed ultrasound, or iontophoresis. As pain subsides, the patient is instructed in gentle stretching into shoulder and elbow extension with forearm pronation to the point of pain. Submaximal isometric strengthening of the biceps may be added.

Gradually the patient is progressed to isotonic biceps, rotator cuff, and scapular strengthening. Rhythmic stabilization in various shoulder and elbow positions can be added. Focusing on eccentric strengthening will help to hypertrophy the biceps tendon, decreasing the likelihood of rupture.

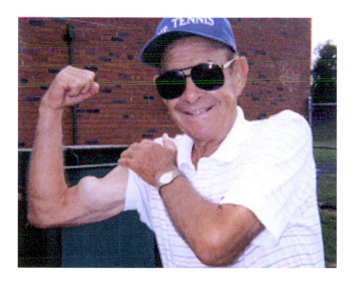

Figure 5.59 Deterioration of the long head of the biceps tendon may lead to rupture. The resulting defect is a "Popeye deformity."

Surgery for bicipital tendinopathy is not usually necessary unless the patient has an associated labral tear or if the biceps tendon ruptures. In the case of rupture, the biceps tendon may be surgically repaired, but this is largely done for cosmetic reasons. Rupture causes a bulge on the anterior upper arm, called a "Popeye" deformity (Fig. 5.59). Functionally, the loss of attachment of one head of the biceps has little impact if not reattached.

The Bottom Line:	for patients with bicipital tendinopathy/tear
Description and causes	Tendon disease or tear due to overuse or in combination with rotator cuff disease
Test	Speed's test, upper cut test, pain with contraction, pain with stretch, tender to palpation
Stretch	Long head of biceps
Strengthen	Long head of biceps, rotator cuff, scapular muscles
Train	Eccentrically when tolerated
Avoid	NA

Acromioclavicular Sprain/Separation

The acromioclavicular (AC) joint is stabilized by the AC ligament and the coracoclavicular ligament. In this pathology, the AC ligament is injured or torn. The coracoclavicular ligament may also be injured. Injury to the ligaments leads to separation of the acromion and the clavicle. This pathology is commonly referred to as a "separated shoulder" and is classified into six types (Box 5-4).

Causes/Contributing Factors

AC injury is frequently caused by either a direct blow to the acromion, pushing the acromion inferiorly on the distal clavicle, or by a fall on an outstretched hand driving the acromion superiorly on the clavicle. A distraction force on the arm may also cause AC injury.

Symptoms

Pain, swelling, and tenderness over the superior shoulder are the chief complaints after AC injury. If the injury is severe enough, you may detect a deformity of lateral clavicular elevation as discussed in Box 5-4. Pain is generally increased with lying on the affected side. ROM may be limited, particularly into elevation and horizontal adduction.

Clinical Signs

There are relatively few special tests for AC injury. One or more of the following tests, in addition to a history of trauma and complaint of superior shoulder pain, is used to diagnose this pathology.

Cross-Body Adduction Stress Test

The patient is in a sitting position with the shoulder flexed to 90°. The examiner supports the upper extremity and horizontally adducts the patient's arm to end range. A positive test is indicated by pain in the AC joint (Fig. 5.60).

Active Compression Test

This is also called O'Brien's Test. The patient is standing with the arm flexed to 90° with elbow extension and 10° of horizontal adduction. The arm is internally rotated so that the thumb points down. The examiner applies a downward force to the arm while instructing the patient to hold against the force (Fig. 5.61A). The arm is then externally rotated and the maneuver is repeated (Fig. 5.61B). A positive test is indicated by pain with the first maneuver that is reduced or eliminated with the second maneuver. Pain that is felt on the top of the shoulder is indicative of AC pathology. Pain that is felt inside the shoulder is indicative of labral pathology.[53]

Acromioclavicular Resisted Extension Test

The patient is sitting with the shoulder in 90° of flexion and internal rotation and elbow flexion to 90°. The examiner, while resisting the motion, instructs the patient to horizontally abduct the arm toward the frontal plane. A positive test is indicated by pain in the AC joint (Fig. 5.62).

Common Interventions

Intervention for AC injury depends upon the degree of separation and tissue damage. With a type I injury, many

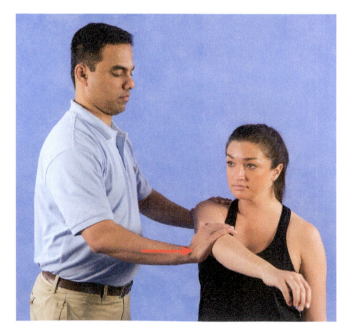

Figure 5.60 Cross-body adduction stress test for acromioclavicular sprain.

Box 5-4   Types of Acromioclavicular Joint Injury[68]

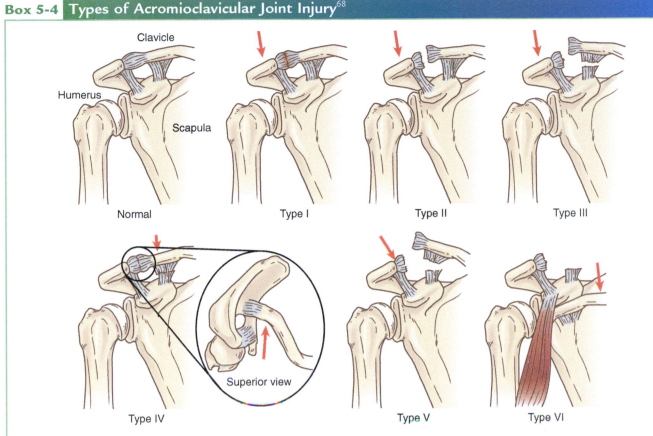

Normal   Type I   Type II   Type III

Type IV   Superior view

Type V   Type VI

Type I – AC ligament sprain with intact coracoclavicular ligament. The AC joint is stable.

Type II – Complete AC ligament rupture with coracoclavicular ligament sprain. Less than 25% elevation of the distal clavicle.

Type III – Complete AC and coracoclavicular ligament rupture. The deltoid-trapezius fascia is damaged. Elevation of the clavicle 25% to 100% (4 mm). The distal clavicle is prominent.

Type IV – Complete AC and coracoclavicular ligament rupture with detachment of the deltoid-trapezius and

posterior displacement of the distal clavicle into the trapezius muscle.

Type V – Complete AC and coracoclavicular ligament rupture. The deltoid-trapezius is detached. Extreme elevation (>100%) of the clavicle, bringing it to a subcutaneous level.

Type VI – Complete AC and coracoclavicular ligament rupture. The fascia above the deltoid-trapezius is detached. The distal clavicle is displaced inferiorly to a subacromial or subcoracoid position.

patients won't seek medical care. This minor injury will generally heal fairly quickly and allow for return to sport in 1 to 2 weeks.

Type II injury takes longer to heal, but good results should be expected within about 4 weeks. The goals of treatment are to decrease pain, minimize loss of motion, and protect the AC and coracoclavicular ligament as scar tissue develops. The patient will often wear a sling initially to decrease pain and inflammation. Cryotherapy may be used for pain control. PROM and AROM activities are initiated as soon as pain allows. Submaximal isometric strengthening of the deltoid, trapezius, rotator cuff, and scapular stabilizers will help to stabilize the

joint. Taping of the AC joint has been shown to decrease pain and allow for functional movement (Fig 5.63).[54] The patient should be progressed to strengthening with resistance bands and weights.

Treatment is the most controversial with type III injury. These patients seem to have equally good outcomes if they are treated conservatively or surgically. Rehabilitation for the nonsurgical type III injury is like that of type II, but on a much slower timetable. Generally, this patient will regain full ROM by 3 weeks and be in rehabilitation for up to 3 months. Proprioceptive retraining, closed-chain stability, and plyometrics are often incorporated in the plan of care.[55]

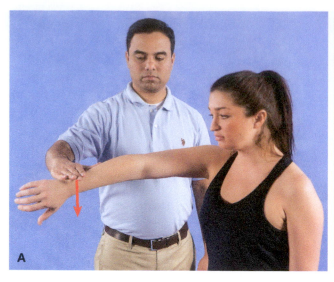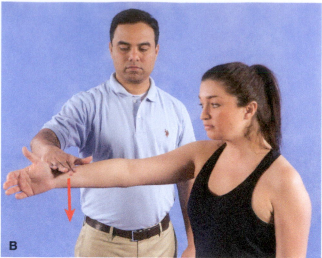

Figure 5.61 Active compression test for acromioclavicular sprain. The examiner applies a downward force with the arm in shoulder flexion and internal rotation (A) and then in shoulder flexion and external rotation (B). A positive test is indicated by pain with the first maneuver that is reduced by the second maneuver.

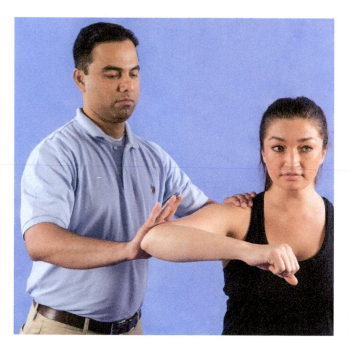

Figure 5.62 Acromioclavicular resisted extension test for acromioclavicular sprain.

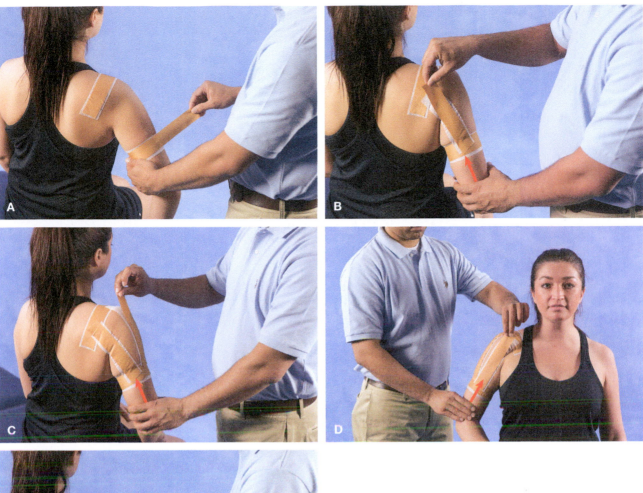

Figure 5.63 Taping may be included in the POC after acromioclavicular sprain. Tape is initially applied across the acromion and the mid-humerus (A). While providing a compressive force, straps are applied from distal to proximal on the posterior arm (B), lateral arm (C), and anterior arm (D). Retaping the acromial and mid-humeral straps (E) ensures the vertical straps are anchored.

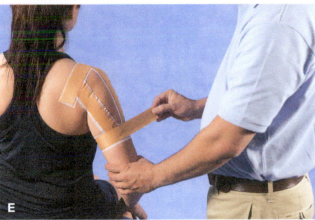

The Bottom Line: for patients with acromioclavicular sprain

Description and causes	Injury to the acromioclavicular, ligament due to trauma
Test	Cross-body adduction stress test, active compression test (O'Brien), acromioclavicular resisted extension test
Stretch	NA
Strengthen	Scapular stabilizers, deltoid, trapezius, rotator cuff, biceps
Train	Proprioception
Avoid	Sleeping on affected side

Interventions for the Surgical Patient

AC Joint Reconstruction

Types IV, V, and VI require surgical intervention in order to correct the alignment and fix the instability. A variety of surgical options is available to reconstruct the AC joint, including use of an allograft to reconstruct the AC[56] or coracoclavicular ligament, wiring the distal clavicle to the acromion or coracoid process, and transferring the coracoacromial ligament from the acromion to the clavicle to act as a stabilizer.

Postoperative Phase

The patient will be wearing a sling after surgery for the first 2 weeks. After this, the sling is used intermittently for pain relief. PROM with restrictions is usually initiated early in the plan of care.

> **CLINICAL ALERT** ————————
>
> The post-surgical patient will have restrictions on arm elevation, generally allowing only 90° of shoulder flexion and abduction. Patients should not perform active movements at the shoulder for 6 weeks. End ranges of internal and external rotation should be avoided.

After 6 weeks, the patient can begin strengthening with light weights or resistance bands. Strengthening scapular stabilizers, rotator cuff muscles, and biceps are often included in the plan of care. Proprioceptive retraining may be added. By 12 to 18 weeks, goals include full ROM and gradual normalization of strength.

Thoracic Outlet Syndrome

Thoracic outlet syndrome (TOS) is a disorder that is the result of compression or irritation of the nerves and/or blood vessels in the neck and anterior chest area. The neurovascular bundle travels from the neck to the axilla, passing through three areas that are very narrow. TOS is believed to be caused by pressure on the nerves in the bundle and possibly on the veins or arteries as well.

The three potential sites of compression are:

- Between the anterior and middle scalene muscles in the neck
- Between the clavicle and first rib
- Between the ribs and pectoralis minor[57]

The most common site of compression appears to be between the clavicle and first rib. Figure 5.64 depicts the three sites of entrapment.

Causes/Contributing Factors

Anything that narrows the passageway for the neurovascular structures may contribute to TOS. This includes

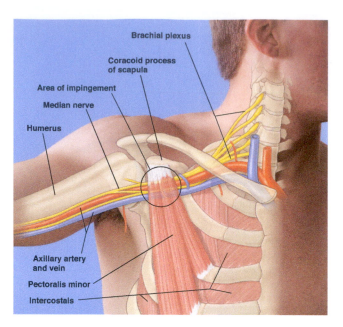

Figure 5.64 Three sites of entrapment of nerves and blood vessels in thoracic outlet syndrome are between the scalene muscles in the neck, between the clavicle and first rib, and under the pectoralis minor.

anatomical abnormalities such as an extra rib (cervical rib) or an enlarged clavicle from a previous fracture. Occupational demands that require overhead, repetitive use of the shoulder may lead to TOS. Sports that place heavy demands on the shoulder, such as baseball pitching and weight lifting, increase the risk. Forward head, rounded shoulders, or sloping shoulders may narrow the space and cause muscle tightness that contributes. Injury to the area may begin the process. Rarely, tumors or enlarged lymph nodes may cause pressure to develop. TOS is more common in women, between the ages of 20 and 50 and may be associated with pregnancy.

Symptoms

Patients complain of pain, numbness, and a tingling sensation in their arm and hand. They may state that their arm feels heavy or weak. There may be circulatory changes as well, including an intermittent bluish color or pallor in their palm. The symptoms will be increased when raising the arm or with repetitive use.

Clinical Signs

Many of the original special tests for TOS were based on the belief that the pathology involved primarily the vascular structures, particularly arteries. However, the incidence of arterial involvement with TOS is low. Tests that are based on this understanding will include an assessment of pulse strength. The examiner palpates the radial pulse to note its strength, not the rate. None of

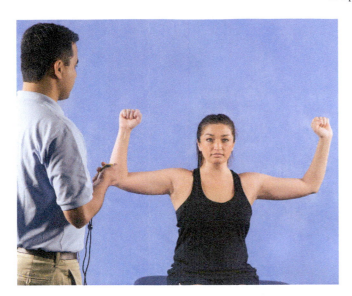

Figure 5.65 Roos test for thoracic outlet syndrome.

the TOS tests has high sensitivity or specificity, so a cluster of tests is often used.

Roos Test

The patient is sitting. The examiner has the patient abduct both shoulders to 90°, fully externally rotate the shoulders, and flex the elbows to 90°. The head is in midline. The patient is instructed to make a fist and then open the hands, repeating slowly and steadily for 3 minutes (Fig. 5.65). A positive test is indicated by reproduction of the patient's symptoms or the inability to complete the full 3 minutes.

Adson's Test

The patient is sitting. The examiner palpates the patient's radial pulse and then has the patient extend and abduct the shoulder with the elbow extended. While monitoring the patient's pulse, the examiner instructs the patient to turn the head toward the arm being tested and hold their breath. This maneuver is repeated with the head rotated away from the side being tested. A positive test is indicated by reproduction of the patient's symptoms or a decrease in pulse strength with head rotation to either side. Figure 5.66 depicts this test.

Hyperabduction Test

The patient is sitting. The examiner palpates the patient's radial pulse and then has the patient abduct the shoulder as far as possible. The pulse is again assessed (Fig. 5.67). A positive test is indicated by reproduction of the patient's symptoms or a decrease in pulse strength.

Wright Test

The patient is sitting. The examiner palpates the patient's radial pulse and then has the patient abduct the shoulder

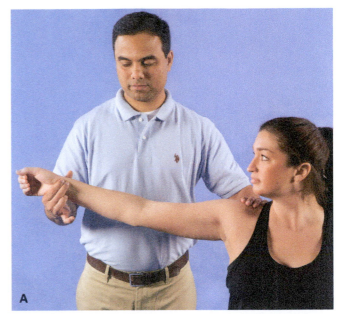

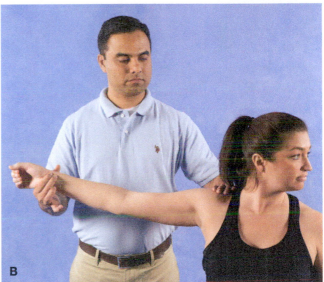

Figure 5.66 Adson's test for thoracic outlet syndrome. This pulse obliteration test is performed with the patient's head rotated toward the affected side (A) and then away (B).

to 90°, externally rotate the shoulder fully, and flex the elbow to 90°. The patient then turns the head away from the affected side and maintains this position for 1 to 2 minutes. The pulse is again assessed (Fig. 5.68). A positive test is indicated by reproduction of the patient's symptoms or a decrease in pulse strength.

Costoclavicular (Military Bracing) Test

The patient is sitting. The examiner palpates the patient's radial pulse and then has the patient retract and depress the shoulder girdle. The pulse is again assessed (Fig. 5.69). A positive test is indicated by reproduction of the patient's symptoms or a decrease in pulse strength.

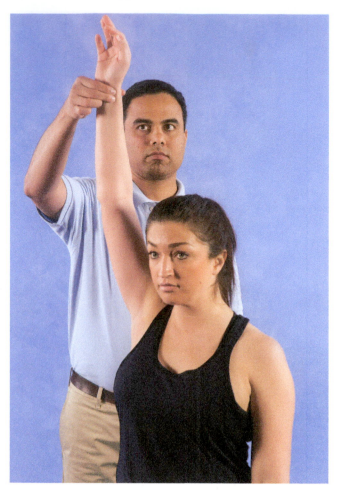

Figure 5.67 Hyperabduction test for thoracic outlet syndrome.

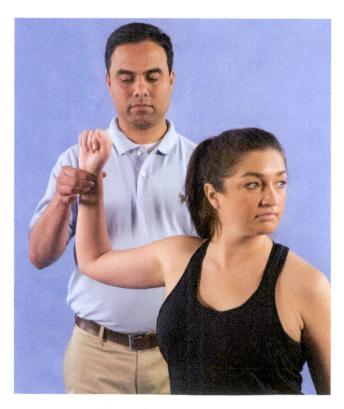

Figure 5.68 Wright test for thoracic outlet syndrome.

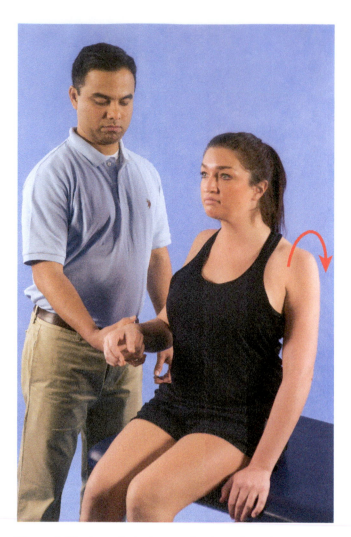

Figure 5.69 Costoclavicular test for thoracic outlet syndrome.

Common Interventions

Because of the multitude of causes for thoracic outlet syndrome, the treatment approach is often multifaceted. In general, the plan of care will include postural retraining, stretching, strengthening, joint mobilization, modalities, and activity modification.[57-59]

Postural retraining is an important aspect of treatment for TOS. Forward head and rounded shoulder posture will contribute to tightness in anterior scalene and pectoralis minor, causing compression of the neurovascular structures. Patients should be instructed in proper posture, including cervical retraction and scapular retraction exercises. Postural retraining should be done frequently throughout the day. In addition, stretching of the pectoralis minor (Fig. 5.70) and the scalenes (Fig. 5.71) is often included in the plan of care.

Modalities such as hot packs, ultrasound, or electrical stimulation prior to exercise may be included in the plan of care. Strengthening the scapular stabilizers, particularly levator scapulae and upper trapezius, may be included if the patient has sloping shoulders. Emphasis should be

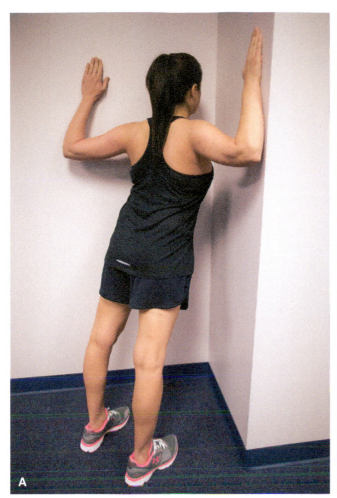 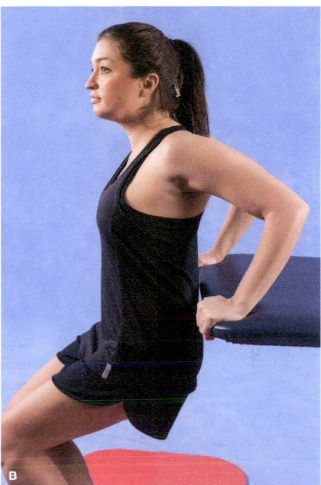

Figure 5.70 Stretching of pectoralis minor using a corner stretch (A) or off the edge of a table (B) may be included in the POC for thoracic outlet syndrome.

on recruiting the muscles and on endurance, rather than strength.

Depending upon the findings on the initial evaluation, joint mobilization of the SC, AC, and scapulothoracic joints, as well as mobilization of the first rib and cervical spine, may be included in the plan of care. Nerve gliding may also be indicated.

Prevention

Maintaining good posture appears to be the key to decreasing the risk of TOS. Carrying heavy bags over the shoulder should be avoided. Since TOS is more common in people who are overweight, maintaining a healthy weight is important.

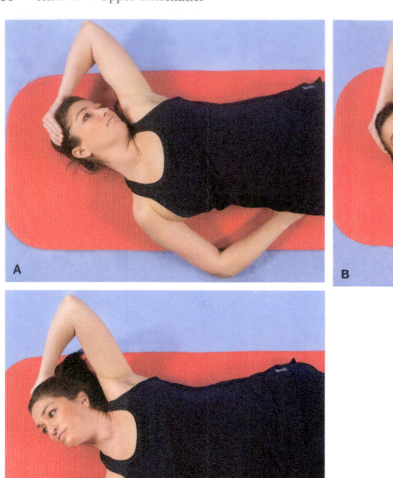

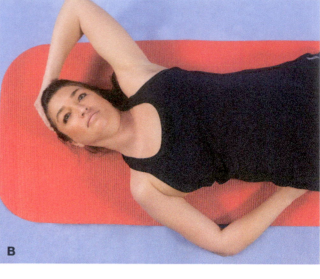

Figure 5.71 Stretch scalenes by side bending away from affected side, with rotation of the head away from affected side (A), in neutral rotation (B), and toward the affected side (C).

The Bottom Line: for patients with thoracic outlet syndrome

Description and causes	Compression on nerves and blood vessels in neck and axillary area related to posture
Test	Roos test, Adson's test, hyperabduction test, Wright test, costoclavicular test
Stretch	Scalenes, pectoralis minor
Strengthen	Upper trap, levator scapulae
Train	Posture, recruitment of muscles, muscular endurance
Avoid	Forward head, rounded shoulders, or sloping shoulder posture

Osteoarthritis of the Shoulder

Osteoarthritis (OA) is the most common type of arthritis. It is also known as degenerative joint disease, or **DJD**. This is a wear-and-tear arthritis, in contrast with rheumatoid arthritis, which is a systemic disease process. To describe it another way, OA is a result of moving parts, in this case the shoulder, wearing out. The manifestations of OA include joint pain, stiffness, loss of range of motion, and deformity. X-rays often reveal decreased joint space, bone spurs (**osteophytes**), and areas of increased bone density (**sclerosis**) displaying as a whitened area.

The two joints in the shoulder most commonly affected by OA are the AC joint and the glenohumeral joint. Figure 5.72 depicts OA of these two joints.

Causes/Contributing Factors

OA of the shoulder is a normal occurrence with aging. However, there are conditions that make it more likely to occur: a history of shoulder instability or rotator cuff tear, increased inclination of the glenoid,[60] and previous trauma to the shoulder. Occupations or leisure activities that involve repetitive overhead movements also increase the risk.

Symptoms

The chief complaints of OA are pain, limited range of motion, and crepitus. The patient may complain of pain at night and stiffness in the early morning. OA of the acromioclavicular joint causes pain on the superior or anterior shoulder, and OA of the glenohumeral joint leads to a diffuse pain in the shoulder area.

Clinical Signs

There are no special tests for OA of the shoulder. Diagnosis is based on x-rays and clinical findings.

Common Interventions

Physical therapy for OA of the shoulder consists of pain relieving and anti-inflammatory modalities, patient education, activity modification, joint mobilization, and

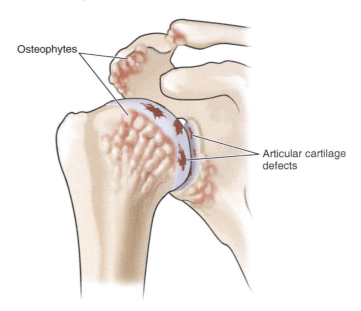

Figure 5.72 Osteoarthritis of the shoulder may involve the glenoid, humeral head, and acromion.

therapeutic exercise.[61] More research is needed in this area, but commonly included in the plan of care are ROM exercises, wand exercises, and pendulum exercises to maintain or improve ROM. PROM and AAROM may be indicated, in a pain-free range. Joint mobilization has been shown to be effective in relieving pain and increasing ROM for shoulder dysfunction. Strengthening exercises have also been used effectively in patient treatment.[62,63]

Prevention

The single best prevention of osteoarthritis of the shoulder is to avoid instability and trauma. Shoulder instability can lead to rotator cuff tear. Rotator cuff tear then leads to joint pathology, with eventual collapse of the humeral head. Maintaining normal range of motion, maintaining a normal balance of strength in the shoulder and scapular muscles, and correcting instability may help prevent osteoarthritis.

The Bottom Line: for patients with shoulder OA

Description and causes	Degeneration caused by wear-and-tear associated with aging and trauma
Test	NA
Stretch	Into all planes in a pain-free range of motion
Strengthen	Weak muscles around shoulder
Train	NA
Avoid	NA

Interventions for the Surgical Patient

If therapy is not successful, surgery may become necessary. The patient may undergo arthroscopic debridement, but if OA is advanced, a total shoulder **arthroplasty** or a reverse total shoulder arthroplasty may be indicated.

Total Shoulder Arthroplasty

Total shoulder arthroplasty is a common treatment option for patients with advanced OA of the shoulder with intact rotator cuff muscles. The prosthetic components consist of a metal humeral component that mimics the rounded humeral head, and a plastic glenoid "socket." The components may be cemented or noncemented into the bone, depending upon the bone quality. Figure 5.73 depicts the prosthetic components of a conventional shoulder arthroplasty and an x-ray of a shoulder after total shoulder arthroplasty.

> **⚑ CLINICAL ALERT**
>
> A common surgical approach is through the anterior shoulder. In this case, the subscapularis tendon with the lesser tubercle are detached to allow the surgeon to get into the joint. After the prosthetic components are inserted, the subscapularis and lesser tubercle are reattached. When this type of approach is used, the patient will be restricted in external rotation ROM and internal rotation strengthening to protect the repair while the bone heals.

Postoperative Phase. After conventional shoulder arthroplasty, the patient will be totally immobilized in a sling for 3 days to 2 weeks. The sling will continue to be worn at night for 4 to 6 weeks. No active shoulder motion is allowed initially, for up to 4 weeks. The patient will be instructed to use ice several times during the day to control inflammation and swelling.

📖 What's in the Plan of Care? Typically, external rotation ROM is restricted to 30° for 4 weeks, and active internal rotation contraction is not allowed for 6 weeks. Typical exercises that are allowed in the plan of care in this early phase are pendulum exercises, active assistive shoulder flexion supine, scapular retraction prone, passive shoulder internal rotation to chest, and neck/elbow/forearm/wrist/hand AROM. Strengthening may include submaximal isometrics into shoulder flexion, abduction, and limited external rotation.

> **⚑ CLINICAL ALERT!**
>
> There is a risk of dislocation after total shoulder arthroplasty. In most cases this occurs due to an anterior instability.[64] The position that places the patient at most risk after conventional total shoulder arthroplasty is in abduction with external rotation. This position should be avoided for at least 6 weeks.

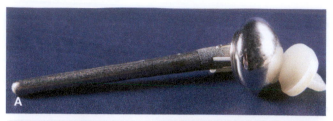
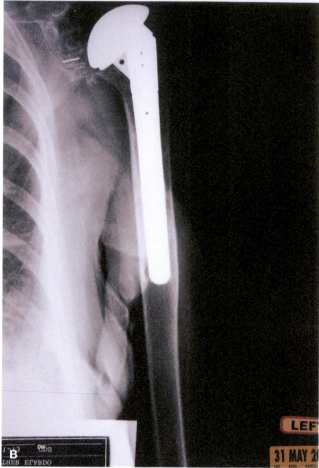

Figure 5.73 Prosthetic components of a conventional total shoulder arthroplasty (A) and radiograph after conventional shoulder replacement (B).

By 4 to 6 weeks after surgery, the patient will often have 90° of shoulder flexion and scaption, nearly full internal rotation, and 30° external rotation. Typically, the plan of care will allow the patient to be progressed to 45° external rotation at this time. Stretching and strengthening exercises can be progressed as well. By 6 to 10 weeks, the patient may be allowed 60° of external rotation. Low resistance, high repetition exercises in flexion, abduction, scaption, extension, and scapular retraction may be initiated. Ultimately, the patient should be expected to achieve up to 160° shoulder elevation and 75° internal and external rotation.

Reverse Total Shoulder Arthroplasty

In reverse total shoulder arthroplasty, the humeral component is concave in shape and the glenoid is

Box 5-5 | Reverse Total Shoulder Arthroplasty

Reverse total shoulder arthroplasty alters the concave-convex relationship of a normal shoulder. Instead of the convex humeral head moving on a concave glenoid, the concave prosthetic component on the humerus moves on the convex prosthetic component of the glenoid. This allows the deltoid to raise the arm without the rotator cuff.

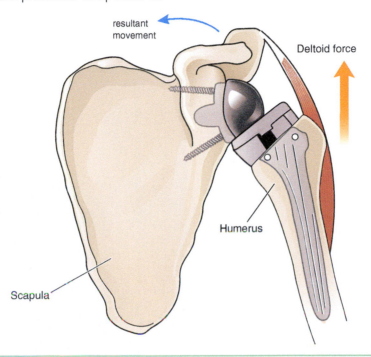

resurfaced with a convex ball, reversing the natural concave-convex relationship of the shoulder. Reverse total shoulder surgery is indicated if the patient has a very deteriorated or torn rotator cuff. Reversing the concave-convex relationship of the glenohumeral joint allows the deltoid to raise the arm without an intact rotator cuff, as shown in Box 5-5. Figure 5.74 depicts the components of a reverse total shoulder arthroplasty and x-rays after a reverse shoulder arthroplasty.

Postoperative Phase. Because of the change in the concave-convex relationship at the shoulder, the lack of an intact rotator cuff, and the position of instability, rehabilitation after reverse total shoulder arthroplasty is quite a bit different from that of a conventional shoulder arthroplasty. The risk of dislocation is higher with a reverse arthroplasty than with a conventional arthroplasty.

⚑ CLINICAL ALERT

The position of dislocation after reverse total shoulder arthroplasty is combined shoulder extension, adduction, and internal rotation. This combined position must be avoided for 12 weeks. Shoulder extension past neutral is also to be avoided for 12 weeks. Patients should be told to keep the elbow within view at all times. Tucking in a shirt or reaching into a back pocket are examples of movements to be avoided.

Initially the patient will be immobilized in a sling for 3 to 4 weeks. When lying supine, a towel should be placed under the elbow to avoid shoulder extension. The plan of care for this patient typically will not allow AROM of the shoulder for 6 weeks nor PROM into internal rotation.

📱 What's in the Plan of Care? The patient may be allowed PROM into flexion to 90° and external rotation to 30°. Submaximal isometrics to scapular muscles and AROM of the neck/elbow/forearm/wrist/hand may be initiated. Around 3 weeks, submaximal isometrics to the deltoids may be added as pain allows. After a reverse total shoulder arthroplasty, deltoids have been made the prime mover for shoulder elevation. The goal will ultimately be to restore the strength of the deltoids to equal or better than that of the unaffected side.

Between 3 to 6 weeks postoperatively, shoulder flexion and scaption will be progressed to about 120°. Shoulder external rotation is performed in the scapular plane as tolerated. At 6 weeks, PROM into internal rotation may be performed in the scapular plane as tolerated up to 50°.

By 6 to 8 weeks, the plan of care will likely include submaximal isometrics for internal and external rotation in the scapular plane. Scapular muscles and the deltoid will be strengthened isotonically, beginning submaximally. The arm may be used for feeding and light ADLs. The patient may be seen as an outpatient for up to 3 to 4

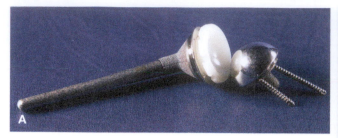

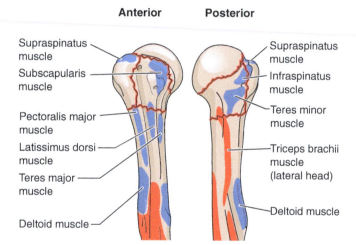

Figure 5.74 Prosthetic components of a reverse total shoulder arthroplasty (A) and radiograph after reverse shoulder replacement (B).

months, with a goal of 120° of shoulder elevation and 20° to 30° of external rotation. Outcomes are directly related to the premorbid health of the rotator cuff, particularly the posterior cuff.[65]

Proximal Humerus Fractures

Fractures of the proximal humerus may occur at the surgical neck, the shaft, the greater tubercle, and the lesser tubercle. The most common area is the surgical neck. The location of the fracture impacts treatment primarily due to muscular attachments. Recall that supraspinatus, infraspinatus, and teres minor insert on the greater tubercle; subscapularis inserts on the lesser tubercle; and pectoralis major inserts on the humeral shaft. Figure 5.75 depicts fracture sites in the proximal humerus and muscular attachments in the area.

Causes/Contributing Factors

Fractures of the proximal humerus are usually caused by trauma. Secondarily, they may occur as a complication of shoulder surgery.

Symptoms

Pain, swelling, and inability to raise the arm are the most common symptoms after fracture.

Figure 5.75 Common locations of fracture of the humeral head. The many muscle attachments in the area impact treatment options.

Clinical Signs

Diagnosis is made by x-ray. No special tests are used to diagnose proximal humerus fracture.

Common Interventions

Because healing of the fracture is the most important consideration, joint motion and strength may become compromised initially due to necessary immobilization. Therapy intervention will focus on maintaining and restoring mobility and strength as the healing process allows.

Most commonly, proximal humeral fractures are simple, nondisplaced fractures. In this case, the patient will be immobilized for a short time to allow healing to begin. Generally after 2 weeks, the patient will begin physical therapy for gentle AROM as pain allows. AROM of the neck, scapula, elbow, forearm, wrist, and hand should also be performed. As the patient progresses, submaximal isometric exercises to the scapular and shoulder muscles may be part of the plan of care. If the fracture involves the tubercles, active contraction of the inserting muscles will likely be restricted for 4 to 6 weeks.

Watch Out For...

Watch out for restrictions of active contraction in pathologies where a muscle is surgically detached and reattached, or where a fracture involves a muscular attachment site. Commonly in these situations, active contraction and resistance exercises are contraindicated until the bone has healed, generally 6 weeks.

Interventions for the Surgical Patient

If the proximal humeral fracture is displaced or comminuted, an open reduction internal fixation (ORIF) may become necessary. In this case, wires, pins, plates, and screws may be used to secure the fragments. If necessary, **hemiarthroplasty** (humeral component only) or total shoulder arthroplasty may be the best surgical option. Rehabilitation after shoulder hemiarthroplasty is similar to that of conventional shoulder arthroplasty (see "Osteoarthritis," above).

Clavicle Fractures

Fractures of the clavicle are very common and most often occur in the middle one-third of the bone.

Causes/Contributing Factors

The common causes of clavicle fracture are a direct blow to the shoulder in a fall and a fall on an outstretched hand. This fracture is also fairly common in newborns, occurring during vaginal delivery.

Symptoms

Pain, swelling, and inability to raise the arm are the most common symptoms after fracture.

Clinical Signs

Diagnosis is made by x-ray. No special tests are used to diagnose clavicle fracture.

Common Interventions

Initially the patient will be put in a sling or a figure-8 splint to immobilize the fracture for 2 to 3 weeks. If range of motion of the shoulder is limited, gentle ROM exercises are usually part of the plan of care after this period of immobility.

> ### ⚑ CLINICAL ALERT! ⎯⎯⎯⎯⎯⎯
>
> The patient should be restricted to less than 90° of shoulder elevation for 6 weeks. The affected arm should not be used to lift objects over 2 pounds for 6 weeks. Pendulum exercises should be avoided, as they tend to inferiorly stress the distal clavicle.[66]

Initially, the plan of care may include supine AAROM into flexion to 90°, isometric shoulder internal and external rotation strengthening with the arm at the side, and strengthening the elbow, forearm, wrist, and hand. After 7 weeks, the plan of care will usually call for strengthening with resistance bands and weights.

Interventions for the Surgical Patient

If the clavicle fracture is displaced or if the patient cannot be immobilized, ORIF of the clavicle is indicated. Rehabilitation after ORIF is similar to that of the nonsurgical patient.

Scapula Fractures

Fractures of the scapula are rare. They can occur in the scapular body, neck, glenoid rim, acromion, coracoid, and spine of the scapula.

Causes/Contributing Factors

The most common cause of scapular fracture is a motor vehicle accident. It can also be due to sports injuries, a direct blow, and as a complication from CPR.

Symptoms

Pain, swelling, and inability to raise the arm are the most common symptoms after scapular fracture.

Clinical Signs

Diagnosis is made by x-ray. No special tests are used to diagnose scapular fractures.

Common Interventions

The patient will usually be immobilized in a sling after scapular fracture for 2 to 14 days. Initially, external rotation is limited to neutral. If the fracture is in the scapular body, the patient may begin ROM and gentle strengthening exercises to the elbow, forearm, wrist, and hand. Submaximal isometric exercise will usually be allowed in the plan of care when tolerated.[67]

SUMMARY

The shoulder is a very complex joint that is often altered by orthopedic pathology. Restoration of lost function is necessary for full independence in activities of daily living and return to work or sports. Pathologies may be due to injury, disease, overuse, biomechanical relationships, loss of motion or strength, or abnormal muscle timing. Treatment interventions must include consideration of all of the factors that are contributing to the pathology.

REVIEW QUESTIONS

1. With your partner, use your hands to represent the scapulae. Move into elevation, depression, protraction, retraction, upward rotation, and downward rotation. Name the muscles that perform each motion.

2. With your partner, use your hands to represent the scapulae again. Move into internal rotation, external rotation, anterior tilt, and posterior tilt. Name the scapular motions that are paired with each of these movements.

3. What scapular movement accompanies each of the following activities of daily living?
   a. Washing your hair
   b. Reaching in your back pocket
   c. Pushing open a door
   d. Reaching the top shelf of a cabinet
   e. Reaching up and back to grasp your seat belt, same hand
   f. Reaching up to grasp your seat belt, opposite hand
   g. Non-weight-bearing gait with axillary crutches, when taking a step with the unaffected leg

4. Describe the importance of upward rotation of the scapula during shoulder abduction in terms of overall shoulder abduction range of motion. What is the contribution of the scapula to abduction range? What is this concept called?

5. During the movement of shoulder abduction, what is the scapula doing to increase the distance between the humeral head and the coracoacromial arch? What is the humeral head doing? Name three structures that lie between the humeral head

and the arch that are protected by these kinematic occurrences.

6. A Clinical Practice Guideline has been created for the pathology of adhesive capsulitis. In what way does this impact your patient education or interventions?

7. When treating a patient with shoulder instability, muscles may be strengthened to provide a barrier or to contract and hold against humeral head translation. Discuss with your lab partner which muscles are barrier muscles, and which are muscles that are antagonists to movement of the humerus in a patient with an anterior instability.

8. On your lab partner, find the three possible sites of entrapment in thoracic outlet syndrome. Appreciate the distance between these three sites.

9. Which muscle of the rotator cuff is most commonly involved in SAIS or tendinopathy/tear? Why is this muscle more predisposed to injury?

10. You are treating a patient who had a reverse total shoulder arthroplasty. What is meant by a reverse total shoulder? Why did the surgeon use the reverse approach? What movements should the patient avoid for the first 12 weeks? Give examples of activities that are to be avoided.

11. For each of the following special tests, name the pathology that yields a positive test:
    a. Adson's test
    b. Anterior drawer test
    c. Apprehension test
    d. Cross-body adduction stress test
    e. Drop arm test
    f. Full can/Empty can test
    g. External rotation lag test
    h. Hawkins test
    i. Hyperabduction test
    j. Kim test
    k. Neer test
    l. Painful arc test
    m. Roos test
    n. Rowe's test
    o. Speeds test
    p. Sulcus sign

PATIENT CASE: Anterior Shoulder Instability

PT Evaluation

Patient Name: XXXXXX XXXXXXXXX   **Age:** 25   **BMI:** 19.1

Diagnosis/History

Medical Diagnosis: Shoulder instability R   **PT Diagnosis:** Anterior shoulder instability R, R shoulder pain

Diagnostic Tests/Results: X-ray- Normal   **Relevant Medical History:** Not remarkable

Prior Level of Function: Patient states that she was able to move her arm fully prior to onset 3 weeks ago. Patient was working out at the gym 4- 6 days a week. She now has modified her workouts for fear of shoulder subluxation.

Patient's Goals: Full ROM without pain, return to gym without restrictions

Medications: None   **Precautions:** Anterior dislocation precautions

Social Supports/Safety Hazards

Patient Living Situation/ Supports/ Hazards: Lives alone

Patient Working Situation/Occupation/ Leisure Activities: Employed as a delivery driver. Her job involves lifting and carrying up to 100 lbs.

Vital Signs

At rest Temperature: 98.2   BP: 110/58   HR: 67   Resp: 13   O2 sat: 99

Subjective Information

Patient is a very active female with 3 week history of right shoulder injury. She states she was opening a door and the wind caught the door and jerked her arm into horizontal abduction. She has had two other episodes of subluxation: once at the gym doing butterflies and once when washing her hair. Chief complaint is of persistent pain and fear of dislocation.

Physical Assessment

Orientation: Alert and oriented   **Speech/Vision/Hearing:** Normal   **Skin Integrity:** Intact. Yellowed bruises noted on anterior shoulder.

ROM: WNL throughout, with exception of R shoulder which is limited actively as follows: 173° flexion, 20° extension, 168° abduction, 30° adduction, 23° external rotation (measured at 90° abduction), 55° internal rotation (measured at 90° abduction). Apprehension on end range of external rotation.

Strength: 5/5 in L UE. R shoulder strength is 4/5 with apprehension; R elbow, wrist, hand 5/5.   **Palpation:** None

Muscle Tone: Normal tone   **Balance/Coordination:** Not tested   **Sensation/Proprioception:** Normal

Endurance: Not tested   **Posture:** Normal   **Edema:** Minimal edema in anterior R shoulder

Pain

Pain Rating and Location: **At best** 1/10 **At worst** 8/10   **Relieving Factors:** Protective posturing, medication

Aggravating Factors: Butterflies at gym, washing hair, putting arm in coat sleeve   **Irritability:** Patient states shoulder is painful after subluxation episodes for 1 day

Functional Assessment

Patient is functionally independent. She has not returned to work due to lifting restriction of 25 lbs.

Special Testing

Test Name: Apprehension test   **Result** Positive   **Test Name:** Rowe's test   **Result** Positive in anterior glide

Assessment

Patient has s/s consistent with anterior instability of the R shoulder

Short-Term Treatment Goals

1. Patient will demonstrate an increase in AROM by 15° in external rotation without a sense of subluxation.
2. Patient will voice and demonstrate an understanding of the precautions for dislocation.
3. Patient will be independent in HEP.

Long-Term Treatment Goals

1. Patient will demonstrate AROM that is within 10° of normal in all cardinal planes.
2. Patient will state that she has had no subluxation/dislocation episodes for 3 weeks.

Treatment Plan

Frequency/Duration: 3 times a week for 1 week, 2 times a week for 2 weeks, 1 time a week for 4 weeks.

Consisting of: Modalities, therapeutic exercise, neuro re-education, patient education

continued

Patient Case Questions

1. Is this patient an AMBRI or a TUBS dislocator?

2. Why is the patient experiencing recurring subluxation/dislocation? How would you instruct the patient to avoid dislocation?

3. What data will you collect the first time you see the patient?

4. If the plan of care does not guide you, what modalities might you use with this patient? Why? Are any modalities contraindicated?

5. If the plan of care does not specifically guide you, describe three therapeutic exercises that are indicated for this patient. Justify your choices

6. How does tissue irritability influence your decision?

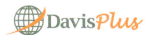 For additional resources, including answers to this case, please visit http://davisplus.fadavis.com

REFERENCES

1. Lippert, L. S. (2017). *Clinical kinesiology and anatomy.* Philadelphia, PA: F.A. Davis Company.

2. Halder, A. M., Kuhl, S. G., Zobitz, M. E., Larson, D., & An, K. N. (2001). Effects of the glenoid labrum and glenohumeral abduction on stability of the shoulder joint through concavity-compression: An in vitro study. *Journal of Bone and Joint Surgery. American Volume.* 83–A, 1062–1069.

3. Lippitt, S., & Matsen, F. (1993). Mechanisms of glenohumeral joint stability. *Clinical Orthopaedics and Related Research*, 20–28.

4. Matsen, F. A., Harryman, D. T., & Sidles, J. A. (1991). Mechanics of glenohumeral instability. *Clinics in Sports Medicine*, 10, 783–788.

5. Edelson, J. G., Taitz, C., & Grishkan, A. (1991). The coracohumeral ligament. Anatomy of a substantial but neglected structure. *The Journal of Bone and Joint Surgery, British Volume*, 73, 150–153.

6. Moorman, C. T., Warren, R. F., Deng, X.-H., Wickiewicz, T. L., & Torzilli, P. A. (2012). Role of coracoacromial ligament and related structures in glenohumeral stability: A cadaveric study. *Journal of Surgical Orthopaedic Advances*, 21, 210–217.

7. Matsen, F. A. (2009). *Rockwood and Matsen's the shoulder, 5th edition*. Philadelphia, PA: Elsevier.

8. Browne, A. O., Hoffmeyer, P., Tanaka, S., An, K. N., & Morrey, B. F. (1990). Glenohumeral elevation studied in three dimensions. *Journal of Bone and Joint Surgery, British Volume*, 72, 843–845.

9. Lawrence, R. L., et al. (2017) Effect of glenohumeral elevation on subacromial supraspinatus compression risk during simulated reaching. *Journal of Orthopaedic Research*, 35, 2329–2337.

10. Inman, V. T., Saunders, J. B., & Abbott, L. C. (1996). Observations of the function of the shoulder joint. 1944. *Clinical Orthopaedics and Related Research*, 330, 3–12.

11. Tamai, K., Akutsu, M., & Yano, Y. (2014). Primary frozen shoulder: Brief review of pathology and imaging abnormalities. *Journal of Orthopaedic Science, Official Journal of the Japan Orthopedic Association*, 19, 1–5.

12. Mullett, H., Byrne, D., & Colville, J. (2007). Adhesive capsulitis: Human fibroblast response to shoulder joint aspirate from patients with stage II disease. *Journal of Shoulder and Elbow Surgery*, 16, 290–294.

13. Wang, K., Ho, V., Hunter-Smith, D. J., Beh, P. S., Smith, K. M., & Weber, A. B. (2013). Risk factors in idiopathic adhesive capsulitis: A case control study. *Journal of Shoulder and Elbow Surgery*, 22, e24–29.

14. Kelley, M. J., Shaffer, M. A., Kuhn, J. E., Michener, L. A., Seitz, A. L., Uhl, T. L. ... (2013). Shoulder pain and mobility deficits: Adhesive capsulitis. *Journal of Orthopaedic and Sports Physical Therapy*, 43, A1–31.

15. Hannafin, J. A., & Chiaia, T. A. (2000). Adhesive capsulitis. A treatment approach. *Clinical Orthopaedics and Related Research*, 95–109.

16. Neviaser, A. S., & Neviaser, R. J. (2011). Adhesive capsulitis of the shoulder. *Journal of the American Academy of Orthopaedic Surgeons*, 19, 536–542.

17. Neviaser, R. J., & Neviaser, T. J. (1987). The frozen shoulder. Diagnosis and management. *Clinical Orthopaedics and Related Research*, 223, 59–64.

18. Binder, A. I., Bulgen, D. Y., Hazleman, B. L., & Roberts, S. (1984). Frozen shoulder: A long-term prospective study. *Annals of Rheumatic Disorders*, 43, 361–364.

19. Cheing, G. L. Y., So, E. M. L., & Chao, C. Y. L. (2008). Effectiveness of electroacupuncture and interferential eloctrotherapy in the management of frozen shoulder. *Journal of Rehabilitation Medicine*, 40, 166–170.

20. Dogru, H., Basaran, S., & Sarpel, T. (2008). Effectiveness of therapeutic ultrasound in adhesive capsulitis. *Joint, Bone, Spine: Revue du Rhumatisme*, 75, 445–450.

21. Jain, T. K., & Sharma, N. K. (2013). The effectiveness of physiotherapeutic interventions in treatment of frozen shoulder/adhesive capsulitis: A systematic review. *Journal of Back and Musculoskeletal Rehabilitation*. doi: 10.3233/BMR-130443.

22. Leung, M. S. F., & Cheing, G. L. Y. (2008). Effects of deep and superficial heating in the management of frozen shoulder. *Journal of Rehabilitation Medicine*, 40, 145–150.

23. Diercks, R. L., & Stevens, M. (2004). Gentle thawing of the frozen shoulder: A prospective study of supervised neglect versus intensive physical therapy in seventy-seven patients with frozen shoulder syndrome followed up for two years. *Journal of Shoulder and Elbow Surgery*, 13, 499–502.

24. Johnson, A. J., Godges, J. J., Zimmerman, G. J., & Ounanian, L. L. (2007) The effect of anterior versus posterior glide joint

mobilization on external rotation range of motion in patients with shoulder adhesive capsulitis. *Journal of Orthopaedic and Sports Physical Therapy, 37*, 88–99.

25. Hovelius, L., Augustini, B. G., Fredin, H., Johansson, O., Norlin, R., & Thorling, J. (1996). Primary anterior dislocation of the shoulder in young patients. A ten-year prospective study. *Journal of Bone and Joint Surgery, American Volume, 78*, 1677–1684.

26. Postacchini, F., Gumina, S., & Cinotti, G. (2000). Anterior shoulder dislocation in adolescents. *Journal of Shoulder and Elbow Surgery, 9*, 470–474.

27. Simonet, W. T., & Cofield, R. H. (1984). Prognosis in anterior shoulder dislocation. *American Journal of Sports Medicine, 12*, 19–24.

28. Neer, C. S. (1985). Involuntary inferior and multidirectional instability of the shoulder: Etiology, recognition, and treatment. *Instructional Course Lectures, 34*, 232–238.

29. Farber, A. J., Castillo, R., Clough, M., Bahk, M., & McFarland, E. G. (2006). Clinical assessment of three common tests for traumatic anterior shoulder instability. *Journal of Bone and Joint Surgery, American Volume, 88*, 1467–1474.

30. Lo, I. K. Y., Nonweiler, B., Woolfrey, M., Litchfield, R., & Kirkley, A. (2004). An evaluation of the apprehension, relocation, and surprise tests for anterior shoulder instability. *American Journal of Sports Medicine, 32*, 301–307.

31. Rowe, C. R., & Zarins, B. (1981). Recurrent transient subluxation of the shoulder. *Journal of Bone and Joint Surgery, American Volume, 63*, 863–872.

32. McFarland, E. G. (2011). *Examination of the shoulder: The complete guide.* New York, NY: Thieme.

33. Buckup, K. (2011). *Clinical tests for the musculoskeletal system: Examinations—signs—phenomena.* New York, NY: Thieme.

34. Wilk, K. E., Macrina, L. C., & Reinold, M. M. (2006). Non-operative rehabilitation for traumatic and atraumatic glenohumeral instability. *North American Journal of Sports Physical Therapy, 1*, 16–31.

35. Magee, D. J. (2013). *Orthopedic physical assessment, 6th edition.* St. Louis, MO: Elsevier Health Sciences.

36. Blasier, R. B., Carpenter, J. E., & Huston, L. J. (1994). Shoulder proprioception. Effect of joint laxity, joint position, and direction of motion. *Orthopaedic Review, 23*, 45–50.

37. Lephart, S. M., Warner, J. J., Borsa, P. A., & Fu, F. H. (1994). Proprioception of the shoulder joint in healthy, unstable, and surgically repaired shoulders. *Journal of Shoulder and Elbow Surgery, 3*, 371–380.

38. Smith, R. L., & Brunolli, J. (1989). Shoulder kinesthesia after anterior glenohumeral joint dislocation. *Physical Therapy, 69*, 106–112.

39. Zuckerman, J. D., Gallagher, M. A., Lehman, C., Kraushaar, B. S., & Choueka, J. (1999). Normal shoulder proprioception and the effect of lidocaine injection. *Journal of Shoulder and Elbow Surgery, 8*, 11–16.

40. Carpenter, J. E., Blasier, R. B., & Pellizzon, G. G. (1998). The effects of muscle fatigue on shoulder joint position sense. *American Journal of Sports Medicine, 26*, 262–265.

41. Myers, J. B., Guskiewicz, K. M., Schneider, R. A., & Prentice, W. E. (1999). Proprioception and neuromuscular control of the shoulder after muscle fatigue. *Journal of Athletic Training, 34*, 362–367.

42. Balke, M., Schmidt, C., Dedy, N., Banerjee, M., Bouillon, B., & Liem, D. (2013). Correlation of acromial morphology with impingement syndrome and rotator cuff tears. *Acta Orthopaedica, 84*, 178–183.

43. Chang, E. Y., Moses, D. A., Babb, J. S., & Schweitzer, M. E. (2006). Shoulder impingement: Objective 3D shape analysis of acromial morphologic features. *Radiology, 239*, 497–505.

44. Natsis, K., Tsikaras, P., Totlis, T., Gigis, I., Skandalakis, P., Appell, H. J., & Koebke, J. (2007) Correlation between the four types of acromion and the existence of enthesophytes: A study on 423 dried scapulas and review of the literature. *Clinical Anatomy, 20*, 267–272.

45. Ogawa, K., Yoshida, A., Inokuchi, W., & Naniwa, T. (2005). Acromial spur: Relationship to aging and morphologic changes in the rotator cuff. *Journal of Shoulder and Elbow Surgery, 14*, 591–598.

46. Harryman, D. T., Sidles, J. A., Clark, J. M., McQuade, K. J., Gibb, T. D., & Matsen, F. A. (1990) Translation of the humeral head on the glenoid with passive glenohumeral motion. *Journal of Bone and Joint Surgery, American Volume, 72*, 1334–1343.

47. Turgut, E., Duzgun, I., & Baltaci, G. (2016). Scapular asymmetry in participants with and without shoulder impingement syndrome; a three-dimensional motion analysis. *Clinical Biomechanics, Bristol Avon, 39*, 1–8.

48. Alizadehkhaiyat, O., Roebuck, M. M., Makki, A. T., & Frostick, S. P. (2017). Postural alterations in patients with subacromial impingement syndrome. *International Journal of Sports Physical Therapy, 12*, 1111–1120.

49. Manske, R. C., Grant-Nierman, M., & Lucas, B. (2013). Shoulder posterior internal impingement in the overhead athlete. *International Journal of Sports Physical Therapy, 8*, 194–204.

50. Spiegl, U. J., Warth, R. J., & Millett, P. J. (2014). Symptomatic internal impingement of the shoulder in overhead athletes. *Sports Medicine and Arthroscopy Review, 22*, 120–129.

51. Manske, R. C., Meschke, M., Porter, A., Smith, B., & Reiman, M. (2010). A randomized controlled single-blinded comparison of stretching versus stretching and joint mobilization for posterior shoulder tightness measured by internal rotation motion loss. *Sports Health, 2*, 94–100.

52. Wilk, K. E., Macrina, L. C., Cain, E. L., Dugas, J. R., & Andrews, J. R. (2013). The recognition and treatment of superior labral (SLAP) lesions in the overhead athlete. *International Journal of Sports Physical Therapy, 8*, 579–600.

53. O'Brien, S. J., Pagnani, M. J., Fealy, S., McGlynn, S. R. & Wilson, J. B. (1998). The active compression test: a new and effective test for diagnosing labral tears and acromioclavicular joint abnormality. *American Journal of Sports Medicine, 26*, 610–613.

54. Shamus, J. L., & Shamus, E. C. (1997). A taping technique for the treatment of acromioclavicular joint sprains: a case study. *Journal of Orthopaedic and Sports Physical Therapy, 25*, 390–394.

55. Ellenbecker, T. S. (2011). *Shoulder rehabilitation: Non-operative treatment.* New York, NY: Thieme.

56. Rushton, P. R. P., Gray, J. M., & Cresswell, T. (2010). A simple and safe technique for reconstruction of the acromioclavicular joint. *International Journal of Shoulder Surgery, 4*, 15–17.

57. Novak, C. B., Collins, E. D., & Mackinnon, S. E. (1995). Outcome following conservative management of thoracic outlet syndrome. *Journal of Hand Surgery, 20*, 542–548.

58. Lindgren, K. A., Manninen, H., & Rytkönen, H. (1995). Thoracic outlet syndrome—a functional disturbance of the thoracic upper aperture? *Muscle & Nerve, 18*, 526–530.

59. Smith, K. F. (1979). The thoracic outlet syndrome: A protocol of treatment. *Journal of Orthopaedic and Sports Physical Therapy, 1*, 89–99.

60. Hawi, N., Magosch, P., Tauber, M., Lichtenberg, S., Martetschläger, F., & Habermeyer, P. (2017). Glenoid deformity in the coronal plane correlates with humeral head changes in osteoarthritis: A radiographic analysis. *Journal of Shoulder and Elbow Surgery, 26*, 253–257.

61. Philadelphia Panel. (2001). Philadelphia Panel evidence-based clinical practice guidelines on selected rehabilitation interventions for shoulder pain. *Physical Therapy, 81*, 1719–1730.

62. Crowell, M. S., & Tragord, B. S. (2015). Orthopaedic manual physical therapy for shoulder pain and impaired movement in a patient with glenohumeral joint osteoarthritis: A case report. *Journal of Orthopaedic and Sports Physical Therapy, 45,* 453–461, A1–3.

63. Guo, J. J., Wu, K., Guan, H., Zhang, L., Ji, C., Yang, H., & Tang, T. (2016). Three-year follow-up of conservative treatments of shoulder osteoarthritis in older patients. *Orthopedics, 39,* e634–641.

64. Moeckel, B. H., Altchek, D. W., Warren, R. F., Wickiewicz, T. L., & Dines, D. M. (1993). Instability of the shoulder after arthroplasty. *Journal of Bone and Joint Surgery, American Volume, 75,* 492–497.

65. Boudreau, S., Boudreau, E. D., Higgins, L. D., & Wilcox, R. B. (2007). Rehabilitation following reverse total shoulder arthroplasty. *Journal of Orthopaedic and Sports Physical Therapy, 37,* 734–743.

66. Johnson, D. H., & Pedowitz, R. A. (2007). *Practical orthopaedic sports medicine and arthroscopy.* Baltimore, MD: Lippincott Williams & Wilkins.

67. Margheritini, F., & Rossi, R. (2011). *Orthopedic sports medicine: Principles and practice.* Milan, Italy: Springer Science & Business Media.

68. Barber, F. A., & Fischer, S. P. (2011). *Surgical techniques for the shoulder and elbow.* New York, NY: Thieme.

Chapter 6

Orthopedic Interventions for the Elbow and Forearm

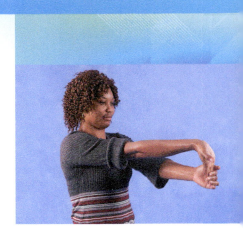

Anatomy and Physiology

Bone and Joint Anatomy and Physiology
Soft Tissue Anatomy and Physiology
    Capsule and Ligaments
    Bursa
    Nerves
    Muscles

Kinematics of the Elbow and Forearm
Joint Mobilization
    Ulnohumeral Joint
    Radiohumeral Joint
    Proximal Radioulnar Joint

Common Pathologies

Lateral Epicondylalgia
    Causes/Contributing Factors
    Symptoms
    Clinical Signs
    Common Interventions
    Prevention
Medial Epicondylalgia
    Causes/Contributing Factors
    Symptoms
    Clinical Signs
    Common Interventions
    Prevention
Cubital Tunnel Syndrome
    Causes/Contributing Factors
    Symptoms
    Clinical Signs
    Common Interventions
    Prevention
Medial Collateral Ligament Sprain
    Causes/Contributing Factors
    Symptoms
    Clinical Signs

    Common Interventions
    Prevention
    Interventions for the Surgical Patient
Radial Head Fracture
    Causes/Contributing Factors
    Symptoms
    Clinical Signs
    Common Interventions
    Interventions for the Surgical Patient
Olecranon Fracture
    Causes/Contributing Factors
    Symptoms
    Clinical Signs
    Common Interventions
    Interventions for the Surgical Patient
Supracondylar Fracture
    Causes/Contributing Factors
    Symptoms
    Clinical Signs
    Common Interventions
    Interventions for the Surgical Patient
Summary

KEY WORDS

Avulsion fracture	Epicondylalgia	Paresthesia
Carrying angle	Epicondylitis	Volkmann's ischemic contracture
Comminuted fracture	Epicondylosis	
Cubital tunnel	Excision	

Anatomy and Physiology

The elbow and forearm joints allow the hand to be positioned in space in a large envelope of functional movement. By the elbow's ability to move in the sagittal plane from full extension to 150° of flexion, and the forearm to move in the transverse plane from palm forward to palm backward, the hand is afforded this remarkable amount of motion. We'll discuss the four joints and three bones of this region and the motions that occur at the elbow (flexion and extension) and throughout the forearm (pronation and supination).

Bone and Joint Anatomy and Physiology

The elbow and forearm complex consists of four joints. At the elbow, the humerus articulates with the radius (radiohumeral joint) and with the ulna (ulnohumeral joint). In the forearm, the radius and ulna articulate at the proximal end (proximal radioulnar joint) and distal end (distal radioulnar joint).

While the elbow functions as a uniaxial hinge-type of joint with one degree of freedom, in reality the ulnohumeral joint is a modified hinge joint, and the radiohumeral joint is a shallow ball-and-socket joint (Fig. 6.1). The elbow has one degree of freedom, allowing flexion and extension in the sagittal plane. The forearm functions as a pivot joint with one degree of freedom, allowing pronation and supination in the transverse plane.

The bones and joints of the elbow and forearm are summarized in Table 6-1.

In anatomical position, the long axis of the humerus forms a valgus angle with the long axis of the ulna. This is referred to as the **carrying angle.** The average carrying angle is reportedly 5° to 15°, with disagreement regarding a gender difference.[1,2]

Soft Tissue Anatomy and Physiology

Capsule and Ligaments

The joint capsule of the elbow encloses all three of the joints of the elbow complex. The capsule is reinforced by three ligaments. The medial collateral ligament (also called the ulnohumeral ligament or ulnar collateral ligament) stabilizes the joint on the medial side. It protects against force that would tend to push the elbow into valgus. The lateral collateral ligament (also called the radiohumeral ligament or radial collateral ligament) stabilizes the joint on the lateral side against a varus force. The annular ligament holds the radial head against the ulna and stabilizes the radius against a distraction force. Distal to the capsule and ligaments of the elbow, the interosseous membrane connects the radius and the ulna throughout the forearm and stabilizes the forearm.

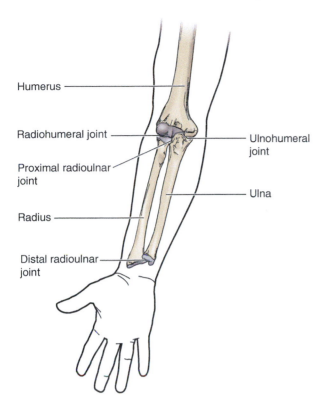

Figure 6.1 The elbow joint consists of the humerus, radius, and ulna. The ulnohumeral joint is a modified hinge joint. The radiohumeral joint is a shallow ball-and-socket joint. The proximal radioulnar joint is a pivot joint.

At the distal end of the forearm the radius and ulna articulate at the distal radioulnar joint. This joint is stabilized by the triangular fibrocartilage complex (TFCC), a soft tissue structure that includes a fibrocartilage meniscus on the distal end of the ulna and several ligaments. This joint and the TFCC will be discussed more completely in Chapter 7.

Bursa

The olecranon bursa lies over the olecranon process on the posterior aspect of the elbow and cushions the triceps brachii tendon from the olecranon to facilitate movement of the tendon over the joint. This bursa cannot normally be felt with palpation over the olecranon but may become palpable and visible when inflamed. (See Box 6-1 on Olecranon Bursitis.)

Figure 6.2 depicts the soft tissue of the elbow. A review of these structures can be found in Table 6-2.

Nerves

Several peripheral nerves innervate the muscles of the elbow or travel through the elbow area to innervate muscles of the forearm and hand. These include the musculocutaneous, the median, the ulnar, and the radial nerves.

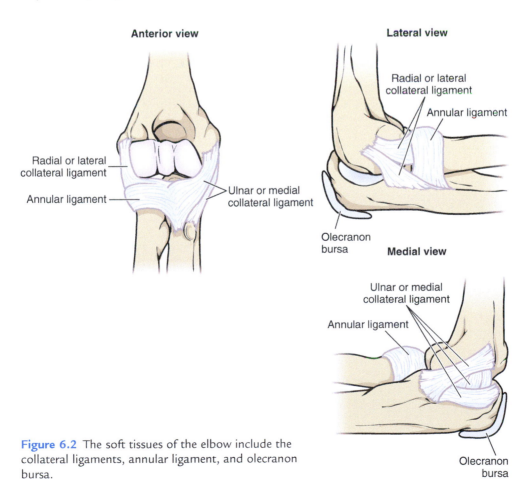

Figure 6.2 The soft tissues of the elbow include the collateral ligaments, annular ligament, and olecranon bursa.

Table 6-1   Bone and Joint Anatomy and Physiology
Of the Elbow and Forearm

Joint	Anatomy	Normal ROM and Movements	Landmarks	Clinical Considerations
Ulnohumeral	Modified hinge shape with 1 degree of freedom. Trochlea on the distal humerus articulates with trochlear notch on the proximal ulna.	Flexion–0–150° Extension–0° Concave ulna slides anteriorly on the spool-shaped trochlea of the humerus during elbow flexion. Ulna slides posteriorly during elbow extension. The convex olecranon process tucks into the olecranon fossa on the posterior humerus.	Olecranon process of ulna on posterior elbow. Medial epicondyle proximal to joint serves as an attachment site for wrist and finger flexors, pronator teres, and ulnar collateral ligament. Cubital tunnel posterior to medial epicondyle is a shallow groove for the ulnar nerve.	Fall onto elbow may lead to olecranon fracture. Ulnar nerve lies in cubital tunnel and is susceptible to entrapment or compression. This joint is not straight, but forms a valgus angle of 5-15°. Close packed position: full elbow extension with forearm supination Loose packed position: about 90° flexion and 10° supination Capsular pattern: greater limitation in flexion than extension
Radiohumeral	Shallow ball-and-socket joint with one degree of freedom. This joint is also referred to as a pivot-hinge joint. In full elbow extension, radial head is not in contact with the humerus.	Concave radial head slides anteriorly on the rounded capitulum of the humerus during elbow flexion and posteriorly during elbow extension.	Lateral epicondyle proximal to the joint serves as an attachment site for wrist and finger extensors, supinator, and radial collateral ligament.	Radial head fracture may result from a fall onto an outstretched hand. Close packed position: 90° elbow flexion with 5° forearm supination Loose packed position: movement away from close packed position. Capsular pattern: greater limitation in flexion than extension
Proximal radioulnar	Also called the superior radioulnar joint. Pivot joint between the radial notch on the proximal ulna and the disc-shaped head of the radius.	Pronation–0–80° Supination– 0–80° Rotation of radial head on proximal ulna to allow for pronation and supination	Radial head is palpated about 1 inch distal to the lateral epicondyle on the posterolateral elbow during pronation and supination.	Radial head fracture may result from a fall onto an outstretched hand. Closed packed position: full pronation and full supination Loose packed position: 70° elbow flexion with 35° supination Capsular pattern: pronation and supination equally limited
Distal radioulnar	Pivot joint between the ulnar notch on the distal radius and the convex distal ulna.	Pronation–0–80° Supination– 0–80° Rotation of the distal radius around the ulna to allow for pronation and supination	Radial styloid process on lateral side of wrist. Distal end of the radius in slight wrist flexion.	Fracture of the distal radius +/- the ulna is common, termed Colles' fracture. Triangular fibrocartilage complex (TFCC) is soft tissue that stabilizes this joint. This complex may contribute to wrist pain (See Chapter 7).

Box 6-1 | Olecranon Bursitis

Bursae are thin pouches of fluid that are found throughout the body. The bursa functions to cushion layers of muscle from each other or from bony prominences. Bursitis is an inflammation or irritation of a bursal sac. It causes warmth, pain, redness, and swelling in the area. Bursitis pain is typically very localized. Swelling may not be noticeable if the bursa is very deep. Because the olecranon bursa is superficial, swelling is very apparent in olecranon bursitis.

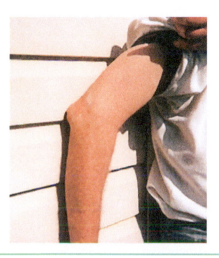

As the musculocutaneous nerve travels through the upper arm it innervates the biceps brachii, brachialis, and coracobrachialis. As its name implies, it then continues into the forearm as a cutaneous nerve, supplying sensation to the skin of the lateral forearm (Fig. 6.3A).

The median nerve travels through the anterior upper arm, crossing the anterior elbow just medial to the brachial artery. As it continues into the forearm, it innervates the two pronator muscles and most of the flexor muscles of the wrist and hand (Fig. 6.3B). At the elbow the median nerve is not prone to injury, but we'll see that as it travels through the carpal tunnel at the wrist it is very vulnerable.

The ulnar nerve lies on the medial side of the upper arm, but runs behind the medial epicondyle coursing through the **cubital tunnel** before coming back to the anterior and medial side of the forearm. It is in this narrowed space of the cubital tunnel that the ulnar nerve is most vulnerable, as it lies against bone and is unprotected. Bumping this area of the elbow elicits pain and tingling, and is commonly referred to as hitting your "funny bone." As the ulnar nerve continues into the forearm, it innervates flexor carpi ulnaris and part of flexor digitorum profundus and then travels into the hand to innervate most of the intrinsic hand muscles (Fig. 6.3C).

The radial nerve lies on the posterior aspect of the upper arm. It provides innervation to the triceps brachii and anconeus, crossing the posterior humerus in the radial or spiral groove. It emerges on the lateral side of the humerus, crossing the elbow anterior to the lateral epicondyle. Below the elbow the radial nerve divides into two branches that innervate the brachioradialis and the extensors of the wrist and hand. The nerve is vulnerable as it runs through the radial groove on the posterior humerus (Fig. 6.3D). Fractures of the humerus in this area can cause damage to the radial nerve.

Watch Out for...

Watch out for places where the nerves might become compressed. Compression of a nerve will impact sensation, strength, and possibly reflexes distal to the site of compression. While a nerve can become compressed or entrapped anywhere along its length, there are places where it is more vulnerable due to the anatomy.

Muscles

The muscles of the elbow and forearm are those which perform elbow flexion, elbow extension, forearm pronation, and forearm supination. An appreciation of the kinematics of the elbow requires an understanding of the kinesiology of the elbow and forearm. A review of muscles with origin, insertion, innervation, action, and clinical relevance is found in Table 6-3.

Kinematics of the Elbow and Forearm

Elbow flexion and extension occur when the concave surfaces of the radius and the ulna slide on the convex distal humerus. Though the humeroradial and humeroulnar joints are distinct, both the radius and ulna move simultaneously due to the abundance of ligaments. Normal elbow flexion range of motion is 150°, with normal extension considered to be 0°.[3]

The main joint of the elbow complex is the ulnohumeral joint. During elbow flexion the concave trochlear notch of the ulna slides anteriorly and superiorly on the convex trochlea of the humerus. At end range the coronoid process of the ulna enters the coronoid fossa on the anterior humerus. In elbow extension, the ulna slides posteriorly and superiorly until the olecranon process of the ulna enters the olecranon fossa on the posterior humerus.

Pronation and supination occur throughout the forearm due to motion at the radiohumeral and proximal radioulnar joints. During the motion of pronation, the radius rolls and crosses over the ulna; in supination the forearm bones are uncrossed. Normal supination and pronation

Table 6-2   Connective Tissue Anatomy and Physiology

Of the Elbow and Forearm

Structure	Anatomy	Function	Clinical Considerations
Joint capsule	Encloses the radiohumeral, ulnohumeral, and proximal radioulnar joints. Inner surface has thin synovial lining		
Medial Collateral (Ulnohumeral) Ligament Also called the ulnar collateral ligament	Three bands: • anterior: from medial epicondyle to coronoid of ulna • posterior: from medial epicondyle to olecranon process of ulna • transverse: runs between the anterior and posterior bands	Stabilizes the joint on the medial side. Protects against force that would tend to push the elbow into valgus.	Overhead-throwing athletes are susceptible to ulnar collateral ligament sprain.
Lateral Collateral (Radiohumeral) Ligament Also called the radial collateral ligament	Two bands: • anterior: from lateral epicondyle to the annular ligament • posterior: from lateral epicondyle posterior to the radial head to the ulna	Stabilizes the joint on the lateral side. Protects against force that would tend to push the elbow into varus, especially in elbow flexion.	
Annular Ligament	Runs from the anterior aspect of the radial notch of the ulna, around the radial head to the posterior radial notch.	Holds the radial head against the ulna and stabilizes the elbow against a distraction force.	The radial head can be pulled out of the annular ligament with a distraction force. This is most common in young children.
Interosseous Membrane	Connects the radius and the ulna throughout the forearm.	Stabilizes the bones of the forearm	
Olecranon Bursae	Several bursae found within, under, or over the triceps brachii tendon at the olecranon process.	Decreases friction between the triceps brachii tendon and the large olecranon process.	May become inflamed and enlarged with noticeable swelling over the olecranon.

range of motion is 80° from the neutral forearm position, allowing a 160° arc of movement.

Joint Mobilization

Elbow joint mobilizations may be used to reduce pain or increase range of motion. Table 6-4 summarizes the movements of the elbow and the glide mobilizations used to increase range of motion.

Ulnohumeral Joint

Anterior and Posterior Glides

Anterior glide of the ulna on the humerus is used to increase flexion of the elbow. Posterior glide of the ulna on the humerus is used to increase extension of the elbow. The patient is positioned in supine with the elbow flexed to about 45°. The examiner stabilizes the humerus with one hand and applies a force on the proximal ulna with the other hand (Fig. 6.4).

Distraction Glide

Distraction of the ulna on the humerus is used to increase flexion and extension of the elbow. The patient is positioned in supine with the elbow flexed to about 45°. The examiner stabilizes the humerus with one hand and applies a distraction force inferiorly (toward the patient's feet) on the proximal ulna as shown in Figure 6.5.

Radiohumeral Joint

Anterior and Posterior Glides

Radiohumeral glides are used to increase flexion and extension. Anterior glides increase flexion, and posterior glides increase extension. The patient is supine or sitting. The examiner stabilizes the humerus with one hand, and grasps the proximal radius with the other hand. An anterior or posterior glide is applied as shown in Figure 6.6.

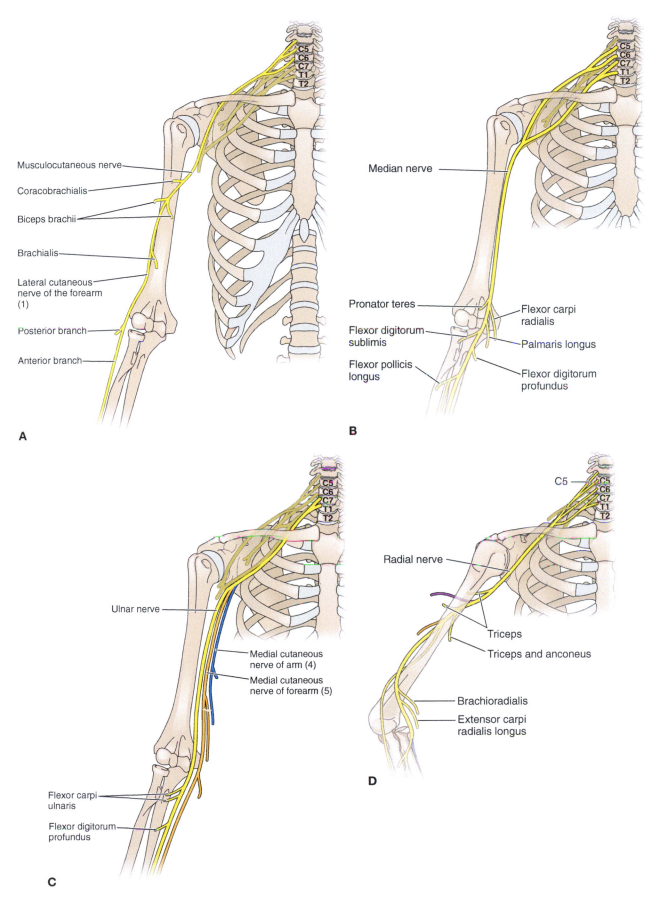

Musculocutaneous nerve
Coracobrachialis
Biceps brachii
Brachialis
Lateral cutaneous nerve of the forearm (1)
Posterior branch
Anterior branch

A

Median nerve
Pronator teres
Flexor digitorum sublimis
Flexor pollicis longus
Flexor carpi radialis
Palmaris longus
Flexor digitorum profundus

B

Ulnar nerve
Medial cutaneous nerve of arm (4)
Medial cutaneous nerve of forearm (5)
Flexor carpi ulnaris
Flexor digitorum profundus

C

C5
Radial nerve
Triceps
Triceps and anconeus
Brachioradialis
Extensor carpi radialis longus

D

Figure 6.3 The musculocutaneous and axillary nerves (A), median nerve (B), ulnar nerve (C), and radial nerve (D) in the upper arm.

Table 6-3   Muscle Anatomy and Kinesiology

Of the Elbow and Forearm

Muscle	Origin	Insertion	Innervation	Primary Action	Clinical Considerations
Biceps brachii	Two-heads: • long head originates from the superior glenoid tubercle of the scapula • short head originates from the coracoid process of the scapula.	Radius	Musculocutaneous nerve	Shoulder flexion, elbow flexion, and forearm supination.	Strongest when used for elbow flexion and forearm supination at the same time.
Brachialis	Deep to biceps brachii, originating from the anterior humerus about midway down the upper arm.	Ulna	Musculocutaneous nerve	Elbow flexion	Larger in cross-section than the biceps brachii and is considered the strongest elbow flexor. It is referred to as the "work horse" of the elbow flexors.
Brachioradialis	Lower part of the lateral humerus	Distal radius near styloid process	Radial nerve	Elbow flexion. Capable of pronating or supinating the forearm to a neutral position.	The greatest strength of the brachioradialis is with the forearm in neutral. Activated with rapid elbow flexion.
Triceps brachii	Three heads: • long head originates from the inferior glenoid tubercle of scapula • lateral head originates from the posterior lateral humerus • medial head originates from the posterior medial humerus	Olecranon process of the ulna	Radial nerve	Elbow extensor. Long head is a shoulder extensor.	
Anconeus	Lateral epicondyle of humerus	Ulna	Radial nerve	Weak elbow extensor, stabilizer during forearm pronation and supination.	Active in initiating the movement of elbow extension. Joint stabilizer during pronation and supination.
Supinator	Lateral epicondyle of humerus	Radius, about midway down	Radial nerve	Forearm supination	Unresisted supination is performed by supinator. Biceps brachii is activated with resistance to the motion. Biceps is four times more powerful than supinator at 90° of elbow flexion.
Pronator teres	Medial epicondyle of humerus	Radius, about midway down	Median nerve	Pronation of forearm	Becomes active with resisted pronation or when quick pronation is required.
Pronator quadratus	Anterior ulna	Anterior radius	Median nerve	Pronation of forearm	Primary pronator. Additionally stabilizes the distal radioulnar joint during pronation.

Table 6-4   Direction of Slide Used to Increase Range of Motion

Limited Range	Direction of Slide in Mobilization
Elbow flexion	Anterior glide of ulna on humerus Distraction
Elbow extension	Posterior glide of ulna on humerus Distraction
Elbow flexion	Anterior glide of radius on humerus
Elbow extension	Posterior glide of radius on ulna
Forearm pronation	Posterior glide of radius on ulna
Forearm supination	Anterior glide of radius on ulna

Proximal Radioulnar Joint
Anterior and Posterior Glides

Proximal radioulnar joint anterior and posterior glides are used to increase forearm pronation and supination. The convex head of the radius articulates with the concave facet of the ulna. Anterior glides of the radius on the ulna increase supination, and posterior glides increase pronation. The patient is positioned supine. The examiner stabilizes the proximal ulna with one hand and with the other hand applies an anterior or posterior force to the head of the radius (Fig. 6.7).

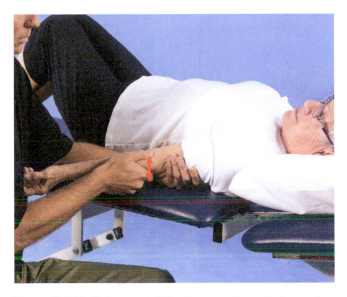

Figure 6.6 Radiohumeral glides increase elbow flexion and extension ROM.

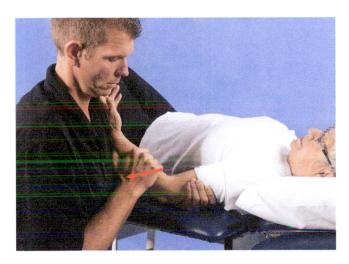

Figure 6.4 Ulnohumeral glides increase elbow flexion and extension ROM.

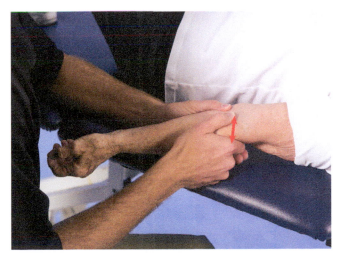

Figure 6.7 Radioulnar glides increase forearm supination and pronation ROM.

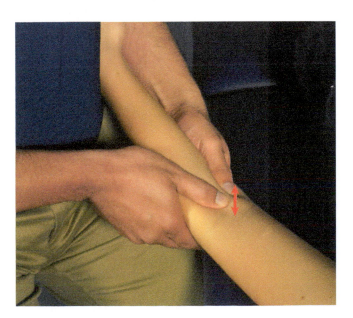

Figure 6.5 Ulnohumeral distraction increases elbow ROM.

Common Pathologies

Lateral Epicondylalgia
Medial Epicondylalgia
Cubital Tunnel Syndrome
Medial Collateral Ligament Strain

Fractures
    Radial Head
    Olecranon
    Supracondylar Fracture of the Humerus

As we have seen, many of the upper extremity muscles insert or originate near the elbow joint. The elbow can be subjected to forces up to three times body weight[4] and can move through speeds of up to 3,000 to 4,500 degrees per second.[5] Due to these anatomical complexities and functional demands, the elbow is a common site of pathology.

Lateral Epicondylalgia

Lateral **epicondylalgia** is a disorder involving the common tendon of the muscles that originate from the lateral epicondyle of the elbow. These muscles are wrist and finger extensors and forearm supinators. Specifically, the origin of the extensor carpi radialis brevis (ECRB) muscle is most commonly involved (Fig. 6.8). The lay term for this pathology is "tennis elbow."

The pathophysiology of epicondylalgia is not well understood. This is reflected in the various terms used to describe the condition. Originally this pathology was termed lateral **epicondylitis,** reflecting a belief that the pain in the diseased tendon was due to inflammation. However, as discussed in Chapter 4, research findings are mixed as to whether inflammation is present in tendon pathologies. For this reason, the currently preferred term is *epicondylalgia,* meaning painful epicondyle, or **epicondylosis,** indicating degeneration without inflammation.[6]

Causes/Contributing Factors

Lateral epicondylalgia is a syndrome caused by overuse of the wrist and finger extensors and forearm supinators. Repeated gripping, resisted wrist extension, and resisted supination of the forearm appear to be risk factors.[7,8] These repeated movements lead to microtearing or macrotearing of the muscles that share a common origin at the lateral epicondyle.

Lateral epicondylalgia occurs primarily between the ages of 35 and 50 in the dominant arm. It is typically work- or sport-related. Although this pathology is not limited to tennis players, up to 50% of tennis players will experience lateral epicondylalgia at some time in their career.[9]

Symptoms

Lateral epicondylalgia will cause tenderness to palpation over the lateral epicondyle area, especially at the origin of ECRB. The patient will complain of pain that is increased with gripping and with movements that require contraction of the wrist extensors and/or forearm supinators. As pain increases, the patient may experience pain with activities of daily living, including turning doorknobs, holding a drinking glass, and drying hair. Additionally, the patient may complain of decreased strength in wrist and hand activities.

Clinical Signs

Diagnosis of lateral epicondylalgia is based on clinical signs and special tests. Because this is a disorder of a contractile soft tissue, the patient will experience pain with palpation, contraction, and stretching of the wrist extensor and/or forearm supinator muscles. Specifically, the patient will complain of discomfort with:

- Palpation
  - at the origin of the ECRB just distal to the lateral epicondyle

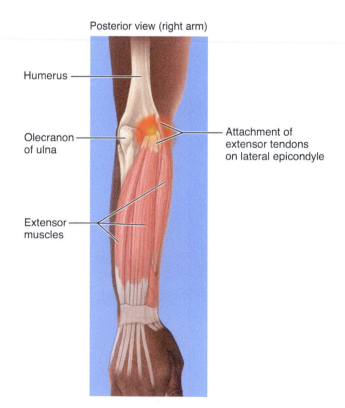

Posterior view (right arm)

Humerus

Olecranon of ulna

Attachment of extensor tendons on lateral epicondyle

Extensor muscles

Figure 6.8 Lateral epicondylalgia involves the common origin of the wrist and finger extensors and forearm supinator.

- Contraction of the common tendon
  - with gripping
  - with resistance of wrist extension
  - with resistance of forearm supination
  - with resistance of extension of the middle finger due to compression of the ECRB by the head of extensor digitorum (Maudsley's test)
- Stretching of the common tendon
  - with passive movement into wrist flexion
  - with passive movement into forearm pronation

Figure 6.9 depicts the some of the clinical tests for lateral epicondylalgia.

Pain-Free Grip

A very common component of the physical therapy evaluation for lateral epicondylalgia is a test of pain-free grip strength of the patient. This is done by having the patient sitting with elbow extended.[10–12] The patient is instructed to squeeze a hand dynamometer for 5 seconds but avoiding discomfort (Fig. 6.10). The patient performs three trials, with a 1-minute rest between attempts. The average of the three attempts is used as a measure of pain-free grip strength and is compared to the unaffected side and to previous measurements.

Common Interventions

The plan of care for lateral epicondylalgia may include modalities, therapeutic exercise, and bracing. Modality interventions that have been recommended in the literature include cryotherapy, ultrasound, laser therapy, high-volt electrical stimulation, iontophoresis, and transverse friction massage.[13–17]

Many programs for lateral epicondylalgia include stretching of the elbow into extension with wrist flexion and forearm pronation to align collage fibers and prevent loss of motion. Strengthening of the wrist extensors and forearm supinators is common. Eccentric strengthening has been shown to yield encouraging results.[18,19] Strengthening the elbow flexors and extensors may also be included in the plan of care.[20] See Figure 6.11 for examples of exercises typically found in the plan of care.

The plan of care may include strengthening of other upper extremity muscle groups as well. Weakness associated with lateral epicondylalgia has been found specifically in the lower trapezius and shoulder rotators[21] and

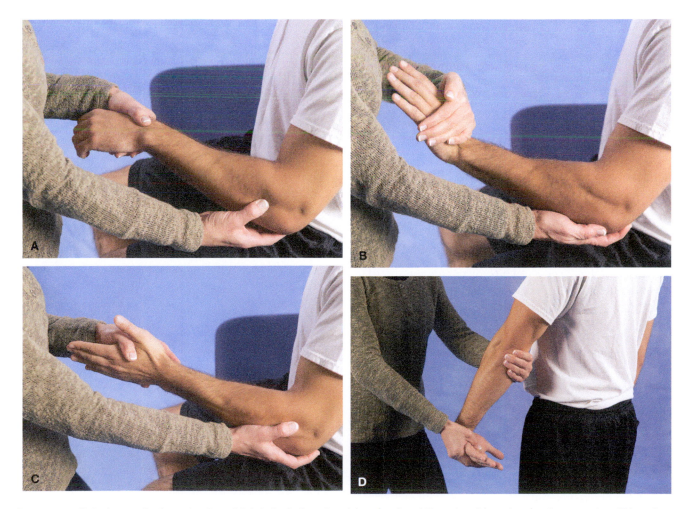

Figure 6.9 Clinical tests for lateral epicondylalgia include pain with palpation (A), pain with resisted wrist extension (B), pain with resisted forearm supination (C), and pain with stretch into wrist flexion with forearm pronation and elbow extension (D).

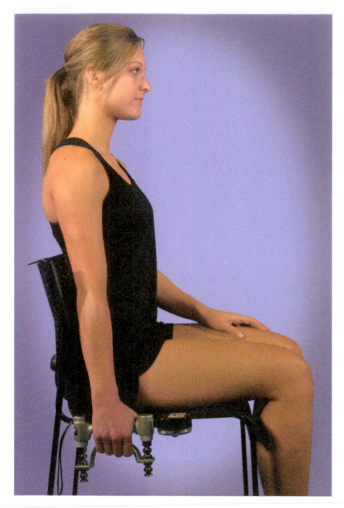

Figure 6.10 Pain-free grip test for lateral epicondylalgia.

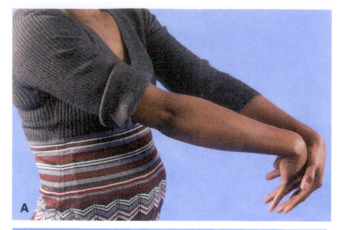

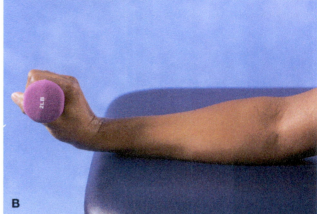

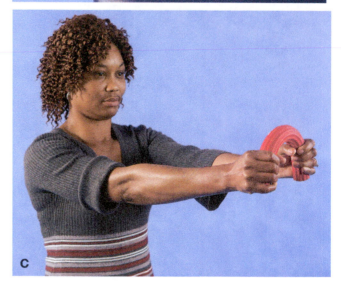

Figure 6.11 The POC for lateral epicondylalgia typically includes stretch (A) and strengthening (B) of the wrist extensors, and strengthening of the forearm supinators (C).

throughout the upper extremity.[22] Therapeutic exercises to address weakness in these areas may be included in the plan of care.

The patient may wear a brace or tape as an adjunct to treatment. The most common brace for lateral epicondylalgia is a counterforce strap that is worn about 1 inch distal to the lateral epicondyle (Fig. 6.12). This type of brace has been shown to distribute the forces in the common extensor tendon and improve pain-free grip strength.[23] Taping the area around the lateral epicondyle in a diamond-shaped pattern is also effective in improving pain-free grip strength (Fig. 6.13).[24] In this technique, the tape is applied from distal to proximal, and the soft tissue is pulled toward the lateral epicondyle with each application. Four pieces of tape create a diamond shape.

Prevention

Avoid high-force and repetitive gripping and resisted wrist extension/forearm supination. Take frequent rest breaks at the first sign of symptoms. Correct faulty upper extremity mechanics.

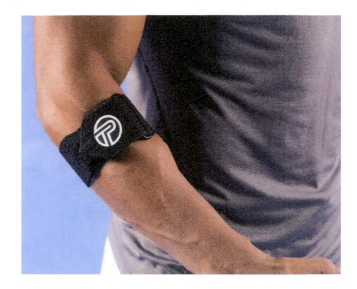

Figure 6.12 A counterforce strap may be effective in the treatment of lateral epicondylalgia.

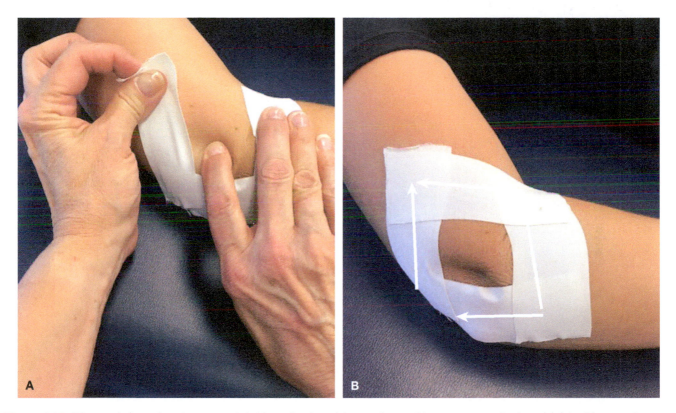

Figure 6.13 Diamond-shaped taping around the lateral epicondyle may be used in treatment of epicondylalgia. The tape is applied distal to proximal, and the soft tissue is pulled toward the epicondyle while taping (A). The result is an "orange-peel" dimpling of the skin over the epicondyle (B).

The Bottom Line: for patients with lateral epicondylalgia

Description and causes	Inflammation or tissue deterioration from overuse (work or sport)
Test	Pain-free grip test, pain with palpation, pain with stretch of affected muscles, pain with contraction of affected muscles
Stretch	Into wrist flexion and forearm pronation with elbow extension
Strengthen	Wrist extensors, forearm supinators, elbow flexors and extensors
Train	Eccentrically
Avoid	Repetitive use of wrist extensors and forearm supinators

Medial Epicondylalgia

Medial epicondylalgia is a disorder involving the common tendon of the muscles that originate from the medial epicondyle of the elbow. Generally, these muscles are wrist and finger flexors and forearm pronators. Specifically, the interface between the pronator teres and flexor carpi radialis origin is most commonly implicated (Fig. 6.14).[9] The lay term for this pathology is "golfer's elbow."

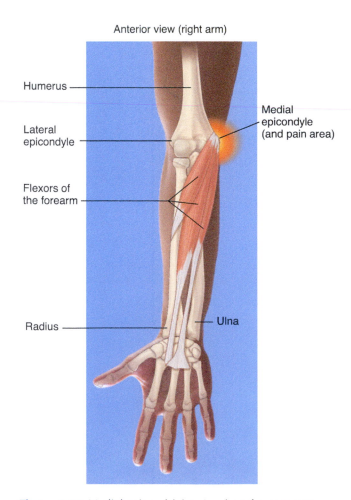

Anterior view (right arm)

Humerus

Lateral epicondyle

Medial epicondyle (and pain area)

Flexors of the forearm

Radius

Ulna

Figure 6.14 Medial epicondylalgia involves the common origin of the wrist and finger flexors and pronator teres.

This pathology is very similar to lateral epicondylalgia. It was formerly termed *medial epicondylitis,* but for the reasons cited in the prior discussion, the currently preferred term is *medial epicondylalgia* or *medial epicondylosis.*

Causes/Contributing Factors

Medial epicondylalgia is an overuse syndrome involving the wrist and finger flexors and forearm pronators. High force and high repetition of gripping, resisted wrist flexion, resisted pronation of the forearm, and hand-arm vibration appear to be risk factors.[7,8] These repeated movements lead to microtearing or macrotearing of the muscles that share a common origin at the medial epicondyle.

Medial epicondylalgia is typically work- or sport-related. Golfers and tennis players are prone to this injury due to the stresses placed on these muscles. In addition, occupations which require repeated and forceful pronation of the forearm or resisted wrist flexion may predispose to medial epicondylalgia.

Symptoms

Medial epicondylalgia will cause tenderness to palpation over the medial epicondyle area. The patient will complain of pain that is increased with gripping and with movements that require contraction of the wrist flexors and/or pronators. As pain increases, the patient may experience pain with activities of daily living. Additionally, the patient may complain of decreased strength in wrist and hand activities.

Clinical Signs

Diagnosis of medial epicondylalgia is based on clinical signs. Because this is a disorder of a contractile soft tissue, the patient will experience pain with palpation, contraction, and stretching of the wrist flexor and/or pronator muscles. Specifically, the patient will complain of discomfort with:

- Palpation
  - at the origin of the common flexor tendon just distal to the medial epicondyle

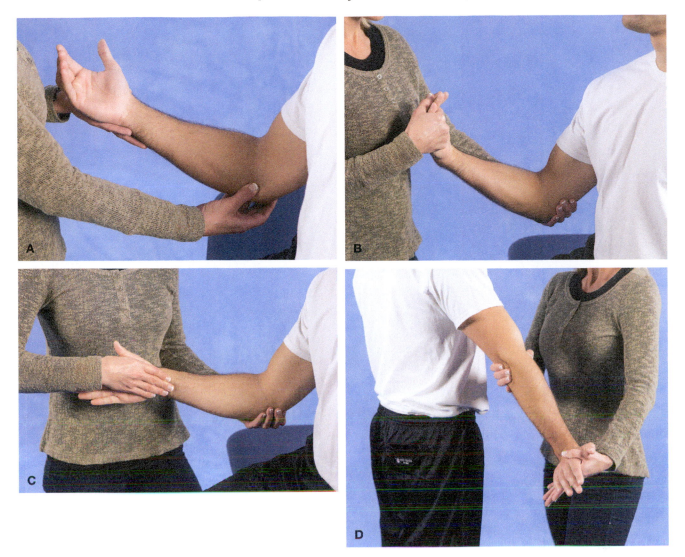

Figure 6.15 Clinical tests for medial epicondylalgia include pain with palpation (A), pain with resisted wrist flexion (B), pain with resisted forearm pronation (C), and pain with stretch into wrist extension with forearm supination and elbow extension (D).

- Contraction of the common tendon
  - with gripping
  - with resistance of wrist flexion
  - with resistance of forearm pronation
- Stretching of the common tendon
  - with passive movement into wrist extension
  - with passive movement into forearm supination

Figure 6.15 depicts the clinical tests for medial epicondylalgia.

Common Interventions

The plan of care for medial epicondylalgia may include modalities, therapeutic exercise, and bracing. Modality interventions that have been recommended are similar to those for lateral epicondylitis and include cryotherapy, ultrasound, laser therapy, high-volt electrical stimulation, and deep transverse friction massage.[13–17]

Many programs for medial epicondylalgia include stretching of the elbow into extension with wrist extension and forearm supination to align collagen fibers and prevent loss of motion. Strengthening of the wrist flexors and forearm pronators is common, specifically eccentric strengthening.[25] Counterforce bracing may also be part of the plan of care. Figure 6.16 shows examples of typical exercises for medial epicondylalgia.

Prevention

Avoid high-force and repetitive gripping, resisted wrist flexion/forearm pronation, and hand-arm vibration. Take frequent rest breaks at the first sign of symptoms. Correct faulty upper extremity mechanics.

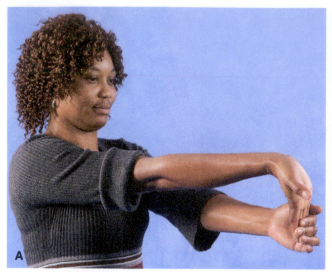

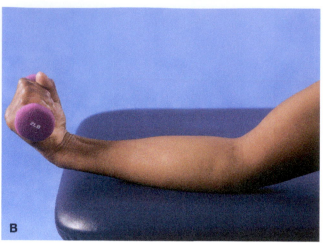

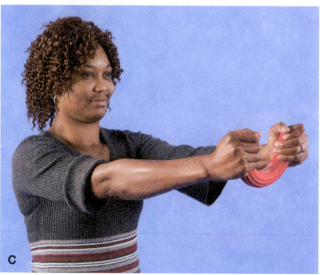

Figure 6.16 Exercises typically found in the POC for medial epicondylalgia include stretching (A) and strengthening (B) of the wrist flexors, and strengthening forearm pronators (C).

The Bottom Line: for patients with medial epicondylalgia

Description and causes	Inflammation or tissue deterioration from overuse (work or sport)
Test	Pain-free grip test, pain with palpation, pain with stretch of affected muscles, pain with contraction of affected muscles
Stretch	Into wrist extension and forearm supination with elbow extension
Strengthen	Wrist flexors, forearm pronators, elbow flexors and extensors
Train	Eccentrically
Avoid	Repetitive use of wrist flexors and forearm pronators

Cubital Tunnel Syndrome

Cubital tunnel syndrome refers to an entrapment of the ulnar nerve at the elbow, specifically as it passes through the **cubital tunnel.** The cubital tunnel is a confined space with the elbow joint capsule as its floor and a ligament as its roof (Fig. 6.17). With nerve swelling or narrowing of the space, the ulnar nerve may be compromised.

Causes/Contributing Factors

Common causes of cubital tunnel syndrome are activities that narrow the cubital tunnel, increasing the pressure on the ulnar nerve. This includes prolonged or repeated flexion of the elbow, pressure over the tunnel, and trauma to the area causing swelling.

The ulnar nerve is stretched up to 3.5 mm during elbow flexion, and the cubital tunnel narrows as much

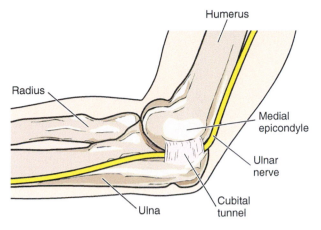

Figure 6.17 Cubital tunnel syndrome results from compression of the ulnar nerve as it runs through the cubital tunnel behind the medial epicondyle.

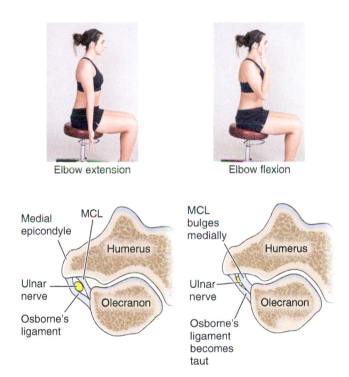

Figure 6.18 The cubital tunnel narrows up to 55% during elbow flexion.

as 55%, as compared to an extended elbow position. Elbow flexion may increase the pressure around the nerve as much as 20 times (Fig. 6.18).[26] Increased risk is associated with prolonged elbow flexion by activities such as sleeping posture or frequent telephone use. For this reason, this pathology may also be known as "cell phone elbow."

Patients who have sustained pressure on the cubital tunnel area by leaning on their elbows are also at risk. This may be found in wheelchair users and desk workers. Overuse of the elbow with repetitive flexion, as may be found in the throwing athlete, also predisposes to cubital tunnel syndrome. Occupations that involve holding a tool in a static position increase the risk.[8]

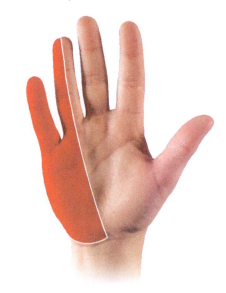

Figure 6.19 Paresthesia, numbness, and tingling in the ulnar nerve distribution may be symptoms of cubital tunnel syndrome.

Symptoms

The most common early complaint with cubital tunnel syndrome is of numbness and tingling in the distribution of the ulnar nerve in the hand, involving the fifth finger, and the ulnar side of the fourth finger (Fig. 6.19). This may be intermittent in nature but may become constant as pressure on the nerve increases. Complaint of **paresthesia,** numbness and tingling symptoms, will usually increase with elbow flexion. Patients may complain of hand weakness, clumsiness, or cramping.

Clinical Signs

The ulnar nerve innervates the flexor carpi ulnaris and flexor digitorum profundus of the fourth and fifth fingers. In the hand it innervates the third and fourth lumbrical muscles, the dorsal and palmar interossei muscles, adductor pollicis, and part of flexor pollicis brevis (Fig.6.3C). Weakness of these muscles may become apparent with advanced cubital tunnel syndrome. Involvement of the interossei muscles often lends the first hard signs of cubital tunnel syndrome as weakness is detected in fifth-finger adduction, and subsequent wasting may be seen around the first dorsal interosseous muscle in the web space on the dorsum of the hand. Additionally, the patient may have a positive elbow flexion test and Tinel's sign over the cubital tunnel.

Elbow Flexion Test

The patient's upper extremity is placed in full elbow flexion with wrist extension. This position is maintained for up to 3 minutes. A positive test is indicated by paresthesia in the ulnar nerve distribution. If the test is not positive, repeating the test while putting pressure on the ulnar nerve at the cubital tunnel should be performed (Fig. 6.20).[27]

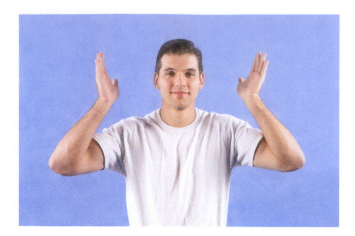

Figure 6.20 Elbow flexion test for cubital tunnel syndrome.

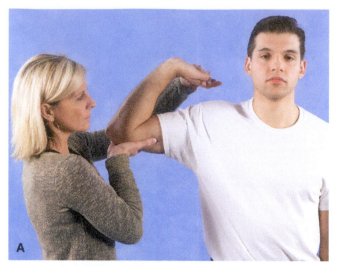

A

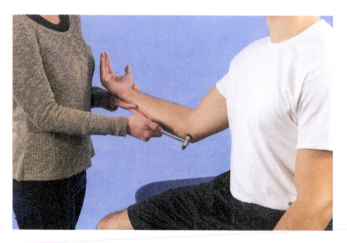

Figure 6.21 Tinel's sign over the ulnar nerve at the elbow for cubital tunnel syndrome.

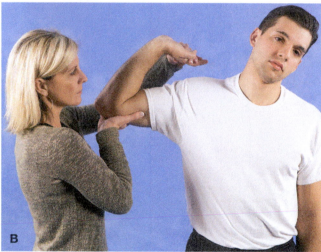

B

Figure 6.22 Ulnar nerve tensioning exercises may be useful in the treatment of cubital tunnel syndrome. If the patient is not experiencing a stretching sensation in position A, neck sidebending (B) may increase the stretch.

Tinel's Sign

Tinel's sign is a test used to detect nerve irritation in multiple sites by tapping on the nerve. For this pathology, Tinel's test is performed by tapping over the ulnar nerve just proximal to the cubital tunnel using a finger or reflex hammer (Fig. 6.21). A positive test is indicated by paresthesia into the hand in an ulnar nerve distribution.

Watch out for the use of Tinel's sign as an indicator of other pathologies. This test is not specific to the ulnar nerve, but can be used to test for nerve irritation in places where the nerve runs superficially.

Common Interventions

Patient education is important in the treatment of this pathology to promote activity modification to avoid prolonged or repeated elbow flexion and cubital tunnel compression. Use of an extension splint at night may be indicated. Patients may be instructed to use a soft elbow pad over the elbow to protect from compression. Hands-free use of the phone should be advised.

Elbow range-of-motion exercises should be done in a pain-free range. Eventually, strengthening exercises may be indicated for muscles innervated by the ulnar nerve. Anti-inflammatory modalities, including cryotherapy, pulsed ultrasound, and iontophoresis, may be included in the plan of care.

Ulnar nerve gliding and tensioning exercises have been shown to be effective for cubital tunnel syndrome.[28] To tense the ulnar nerve, the arm is moved to progressively stretch the ulnar nerve over each joint, to the point of a slight tingling sensation. The patient should be instructed to stop when this sensation occurs. Have the patient begin in a position of wrist and finger extension with arm at the side. Slowly the arm is raised into shoulder abduction and elbow flexion so that the fingers are resting on the shoulder as shown in Figure 6.22A. If the patient is not experiencing any nerve sensation, sidebending the head away from the affected side will increase the stretch (Fig. 6.22B).

Prevention

Avoid prolonged elbow flexion such as sleeping with elbows bent or spending extended time on the phone. Use a hands-free device. Avoid pressure on flexed elbows as occurs when working at a desk.

The Bottom Line:	for patients with cubital tunnel syndrome
Description and causes	Irritation of the ulnar nerve due to prolonged/frequent elbow flexion or pressure on the elbow
Test	Elbow flexion test, Tinel's sign over ulnar nerve
Stretch	Pain-free elbow ROM
Strengthen	Flexor digitorum profundus, flexor carpi ulnaris, hypothenar muscles, lumbricals, and interossei
Train	NA
Avoid	Pressure on elbow, prolonged elbow flexion

Medial Collateral Ligament Sprain

The medial collateral ligament (MCL) of the elbow acts as a restraint to valgus movement. This ligament may become overstretched and sprained with forceful and/or repetitive valgus stress. The MCL may show signs of inflammation, microtears, deterioration, and thinning (Fig. 6.23). The degeneration of the MCL usually occurs over a long time.

Causes/Contributing Factors

This sprain is most commonly seen in the overhead-throwing athlete or after a fall on an outstretched hand. It has been linked to the number of baseball pitches thrown more than the type of pitch or pitch mechanics.[29]

Symptoms

MCL sprain most commonly presents as pain over the area of the medial elbow. Pain will be increased with activity that loads the MCL, such as overhead throwing of a baseball or javelin or hitting of a volleyball.

Clinical Signs

Patient history is often of pain that is increased after activity, especially overhead throwing. Localized tenderness over the MCL indicates the likelihood of MCL sprain. Valgus stress testing at the elbow will usually reproduce pain and will commonly reveal laxity of the MCL.

Valgus Stress Test

This test is performed with the patient's shoulder externally rotated, elbow slightly flexed, and forearm supinated.[30,31] The patient's forearm is stabilized while a force is applied on the lateral elbow in an attempt to open the medial side of the joint (Fig. 6.24).

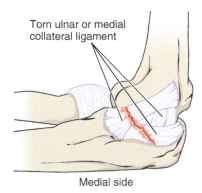

Torn ulnar or medial collateral ligament

Medial side

Figure 6.23 Medial collateral ligament sprain results from valgus stress at the elbow.

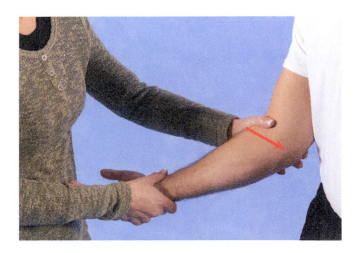

Figure 6.24 Valgus stress test for MCL sprain.

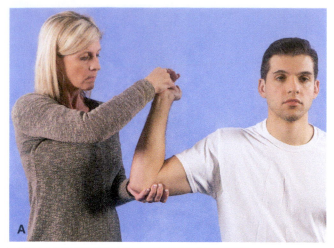

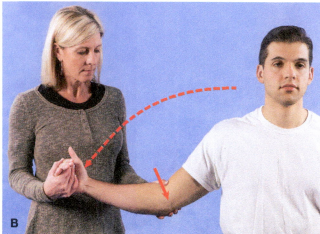

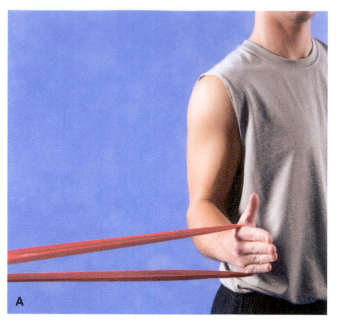

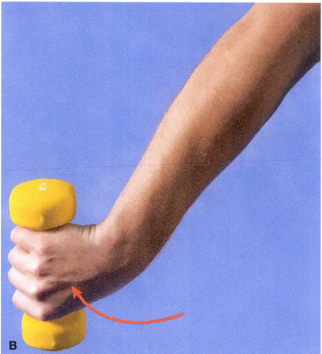

Figure 6.25 Moving valgus stress test for MCL sprain. The examiner applies a valgus force at the elbow in full elbow flexion (A), then quickly extends the elbow to 30° (B).

Moving Valgus Stress Test

This test is performed with the patient in a sitting position. The patient's arm is abducted at the shoulder to 90° and the elbow is fully flexed. A valgus force is applied to the elbow by the examiner while externally rotating the humerus. Maintaining the valgus force, the examiner quickly extends the elbow to 30°. A positive test is indicated by reproduction of the patient's pain in the range between 120° and 70° of elbow flexion (Fig. 6.25).[32]

Common Interventions

Initially, the plan of care for MCL sprain often includes anti-inflammatory and pain-relieving modalities. Ice, pulsed ultrasound, and iontophoresis may be helpful during this time. The patient should be instructed to avoid valgus stresses on the elbow and should avoid pitching. As the patient moves into stages two and three of tissue healing, the plan of care will likely focus on achieving full range of motion of the elbow, generalized strengthening of the muscles around the elbow, and strengthening of the rest of the upper extremity. Focus may be placed on wrist flexors, wrist ulnar deviators, and forearm pronators due

Figure 6.26 Strengthening shoulder internal rotators eccentrically (A) and ulnar deviators (B) may be included in the POC for MCL sprain.

to their ability to help stabilize the medial elbow. Particular emphasis in the throwing athlete may be placed on restoring shoulder external rotation range of motion and eccentric strength of the shoulder internal rotators. Figure 6.26 depicts exercises that are commonly found in the plan of care for MCL sprain.

Prevention

Avoid repetitive overhead throwing. Correct faulty mechanics.

The Bottom Line: for patients with medial collateral ligament sprain

Description and causes	Inflammation of the MCL at the elbow due to overhead throwing
Test	Valgus stress test, moving valgus stress test
Stretch	Maintain ROM in elbow, shoulder external rotation
Strengthen	Wrist flexors, wrist ulnar deviators, and forearm pronators, shoulder internal rotators.
Train	Shoulder internal rotators eccentrically
Avoid	Valgus stress of elbow

Interventions for the Surgical Patient

MCL Reconstruction—Tommy John Surgery

The surgical technique to reconstruct the MCL has been used since the mid-1970s when Dr. Frank Jobe performed a figure-of-eight technique on Tommy John, a major league pitcher. The surgery involves using a graft, usually taken from the palmaris longus or gracilis tendon. This graft is inserted in holes drilled in the distal medial humerus and the proximal ulna.[33,34]

After surgery, the patient will generally be wearing a hinged elbow orthosis that limits elbow ROM. Gradual increases in elbow range of motion are allowed over the first 6 weeks postoperatively. Strengthening exercises may be added after 6 weeks, focusing on the shoulder complex initially.

 CLINICAL ALERT! ————————

Valgus stress on the elbow should be avoided. Care should be taken with shoulder external rotation range of motion or internal rotation strengthening as they may produce a valgus stress on the elbow.

Radial Head Fracture

Fracture of the radial head accounts for 20% to 30% of all elbow fractures. The fracture may be a Type I (nondisplaced), a Type II (slightly displaced), or a Type III (**comminuted**) fracture with three or more fragments of bone (Fig. 6.27).

Causes/Contributing Factors

This is generally a result of a fall on an outstretched hand.

Symptoms

Symptoms include patient complaint of elbow pain and inability to pronate or supinate without increased pain.

Clinical Signs

Clinical signs are history of trauma, swelling over the lateral elbow, and pain with elbow and forearm

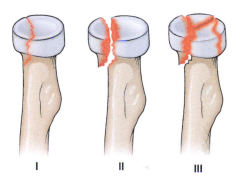

Figure 6.27 Radial head fracture may be nondisplaced, displaced, or comminuted.

movement. Generally, these patients have been diagnosed by x-ray in the emergency room, and are not referred to therapy until after medical treatment for the fracture.

Common Interventions

In a Type I radial head fracture, the patient is generally immobilized with a sling for a few days to weeks. Surgery is not generally necessary. Early AROM or AAROM in the pain-free range has been shown to be effective in terms of improved elbow range of motion and reduced pain.[35] Range-of-motion exercise to the uninvolved joints is also typically included early in the plan of care. Passive range-of-motion exercises **What's in the Plan of Care?** may be included in the plan of care at 4 to 6 weeks. End range of elbow extension is often the most difficult to fully recover.

Strengthening exercises of the scapular and shoulder muscles begins early in the rehabilitation process, generally less than two weeks after fracture. By three to four weeks after injury, isometric strengthening of the elbow may be initiated, and progressed as tolerated. See Figure 6-28 for exercises that might be part of the plan of care by 4 to 6 weeks after injury.[36]

Interventions for the Surgical Patient

Type II radial head fractures will often require an ORIF. Type III radial head fractures are often treated by radial head **excision** or prosthetic implant.[37-39] Physical therapy intervention will depend upon findings on patient evaluation and the surgical approach used.

Olecranon Fracture

Fractures of the olecranon process of the ulna are a fairly common fracture in the elbow (Fig. 6.29). The fracture may be nondisplaced, displaced, or comminuted.

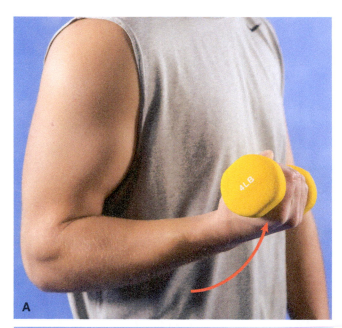

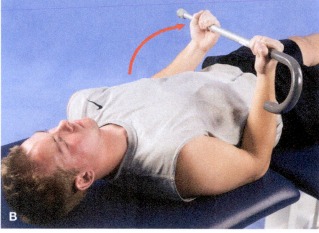

Figure 6.28 Exercises commonly included in the POC after radial head fracture include elbow flexion strengthening (A) and stretching into elbow extension (B).

Causes/Contributing Factors

Olecranon fractures are usually the result of a fall on the bent elbow. They may also occur as an **avulsion fracture**, in the case where a forceful contraction of the triceps brachii avulses the process off the ulna. This may happen in a fall or with sports activities such as weight lifting.

Symptoms

Symptoms include patient complaint of pain, and inability to straighten the elbow without increased pain.

Clinical Signs

Clinical signs are history of trauma, swelling over the posterior elbow, and pain with elbow movement. Generally, these patients have been diagnosed by x-ray in the emergency room, and are not referred to therapy until after medical treatment for the fracture.

Common Interventions

Nondisplaced fractures of the olecranon may not require surgical intervention. The patient may be immobilized in a cast for three to six weeks in slight elbow flexion. When the patient is allowed to begin AROM exercises, compliance with instructions regarding limiting elbow flexion range of motion is very important. Restoring flexion range of motion will proceed slowly, with full flexion generally being allowed after eight weeks. During this early phase, the patient will not be allowed to use the arm to lift.

⚑ CLINICAL ALERT! ────────

Because the triceps brachii inserts on the olecranon, stretching and active contraction of the triceps will likely be restricted. The patient will need to avoid elbow flexion past 90° for six to eight weeks to allow healing to occur. Strengthening exercises can be initiated when bone healing has occurred, but resisted triceps strengthening will generally be avoided for twelve weeks to ensure bone union.

Interventions for the Surgical Patient

Surgical options for patients after olecranon fracture include excision of the olecranon, ORIF with tension wiring, pins, plates and screws, and intramedullary nails.[40-42] Intervention will depend upon the examination findings and surgical approach.

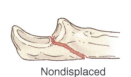

Nondisplaced

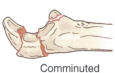

Comminuted

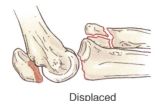

Displaced

Figure 6.29 Olecranon fracture may be nondisplaced, displaced, or comminuted.

Supracondylar Fracture

Supracondylar fracture is a fracture of the distal humerus just proximal to the condyles. This is a fairly common fracture in children, occurring primarily in children under 10 years of age. Fifteen-percent of all pediatric fractures involve the elbow, and fractures of the distal humerus account for 85% of those fractures.[43]

Causes/Contributing Factors

The most common cause of this fracture is a fall on an outstretched hand with the elbow extended.

Symptoms

Symptoms include patient complaint of elbow pain and inability to move elbow without increased pain.

Clinical Signs

Clinical signs are history of trauma, swelling in the cubital fossa, and pain with elbow movement. Generally, these patients have been diagnosed by x-ray in the emergency room, and are not referred to therapy until after medical treatment for the fracture.

Common Interventions

After supracondylar fracture the patient may undergo closed reduction and immobilization for up to six weeks.[44] It is important that the patient be instructed to maintain joint range of motion and strength in the uninvolved joints in both upper extremities. After the period of immobilization, the plan of care may include AROM exercises, gentle painfree PROM, and eventually strengthening of the elbow flexors and extensors.

> ⚑ **CLINICAL ALERT!** ————————
>
> A common complication of supracondylar fracture is arterial compromise of the brachial artery.[45] This artery runs very near a supracondylar fracture site, and may be compromised by the fracture (Fig. 6.30). It is important for physical therapist assistants to recognize signs of arterial compromise in these patients and respond immediately. Signs of ischemia due to brachial artery occlusion include severe pain, discoloration of the hand (white or blue), loss of pulse, and coldness of the hand. If not recognized and treated, this can lead to a **Volkmann's ischemic contracture**, a flexion contracture of the hand resulting in a claw deformity. Pulse oximetry may be a useful tool to ensure that circulation to the hand has not been compromised.[46] See Box 6-2 for information on Volkmann's ischemic contracture.

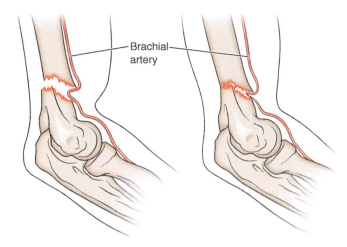

Figure 6.30 Supracondylar fracture of the humerus may lead to vascular compromise due to proximity of brachial artery to fracture site.

Box 6-2	Want to Know More?

Volkmann's ischemic contracture refers to a claw hand deformity that is the result of compromised blood flow and possible nerve damage. The finger and thumb flexors become shortened, pulling the hand into flexion. The median and ulnar nerve may also be affected, and contribute to the deformity. Muscle necrosis becomes irreversible after 4 to 6 hours of ischemia.[47]

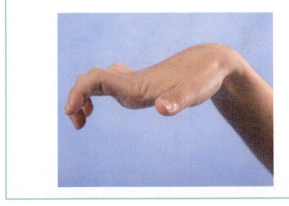

Interventions for the Surgical Patient

Surgical options for patients after supracondylar fracture include ORIF with plates and screws, intramedullary nails, hemiarthroplasty, and total elbow replacement.[46,48–53] Intervention will depend upon the patient findings and surgical approach.

SUMMARY

The elbow and forearm joints serve an important function in hand placement. Normal range of motion, strength, and stability of this area are vital. The configuration of bony and soft tissue structures, redundancy of muscle action, and ability of the muscles to act synergistically ensure the ability of this joint to withstand the forces to which it is subjected and produce smooth movements of the upper extremity. However, we have seen that pathologies are common here, due to the stresses placed on this joint. Frequent consequences of elbow pathology include pain and loss of upper extremity function.

REVIEW QUESTIONS

1. Pathologies of muscle and tendon will lead to pain with palpation, contraction, and stretch.
   a. With your lab partner, discuss the anatomy of the muscles that originate from the lateral epicondyle. What motions will you resist to contract the muscles originating from here? In what position will you put the patient to stretch these muscles?
   b. Discuss the anatomy of the muscles that originate from the medial epicondyle. What motions will you resist to contract the muscles originating from here? In what position will you put the patient to stretch the muscles?

2. With your lab partner, go through the cocking motion in an overhead-throwing athlete. Discuss the relationship between limited external rotation of the shoulder, and increased stress on the MCL.

3. Role-play a simulation of patient education with your lab partner. You are a PTA who is treating a child who has sustained a fracture of the olecranon. Your lab partner is the parent of the child, and you are explaining the reason for an imposed restriction on passive elbow flexion and resisted elbow extension.

4. You are treating a patient with cubital tunnel syndrome. The patient is a 52-year-old female with 4 week history of progressively increasing weakness and numbness into her 4th and 5th fingers. With your lab partner, role-play a patient-education scenario in which you describe the pathology and the precautions you want her to take regarding avoiding pressure on the nerve.

5. For each of the following special tests, name the pathology that yields a positive test:
   a. Elbow flexion test
   b. Moving valgus stress test
   c. Pain free grip test
   d. Tinel's sign
   e. Valgus stress test

PATIENT CASE: Pain Secondary to Lateral Epicondylalgia

PT Evaluation		

Patient Name: XXXXX XXXXXXXXXXX   **Age:** 17   **BMI:** 20.4

Diagnosis/History

Medical Diagnosis: Lateral epicondylalgia R   **PT Diagnosis:** Pain secondary to lateral epicondylalgia R

Diagnostic Tests/Results: None   **Relevant Medical History:** Unremarkable

Prior Level of Function: Unremarkable

Patient's Goals: Decrease pain, return to sport

Medications: ibuprofen 600 mg tid   **Precautions:** None

Social Supports/Safety Hazards

Patient Living Situation/ Supports/ Hazards: Lives with parents, siblings

Patient Working Situation/Occupation/ Leisure Activities: Full-time student; plays tennis competitively at school.

Vital Signs

At rest Temperature: 98.4   BP: 98/60   HR: 68   Resp: 12   O2 sat: 99

Subjective Information

Patient is a female with gradual onset of pain in R lateral elbow, which initially began after playing tennis four weeks ago. Pain began to interfere with sport. She was prescribed NSAID and instructed to decrease playing time, and since has improved.

Physical Assessment

Orientation: Alert and oriented   **Speech/Vision/Hearing:** Normal   **Skin Integrity:** Intact

ROM: WNL, except pain in lateral elbow on end range of elbow extension/forearm pronation/wrist flexion.

Strength: 4/5 MMT in wrist extension, forearm supination with pain   **Palpation:** pain on palpation lateral epicondyle area

Muscle Tone: Normal   **Balance/Coordination:** Not tested   **Sensation/Proprioception:** Normal

Endurance: Not tested   **Posture:** Normal   **Edema:** None

Pain

Pain Rating and Location: At best 0/10   At worst 4/10   **Relieving Factors:** ibuprofen, rest, ice

Aggravating Factors: Tennis, gripping   **Irritability:** With rest, pain is relieved in 15-30 minutes

Functional Assessment

Patient is functionally independent.

Special Testing

Test Name: stretch/contract/palpate   **Result** Positive   **Test Name:**   **Result**

Assessment

Patient has s/s consistent with lateral epicondylalgia R.

Short-Term Treatment Goals

1. Patient will state a 25% decrease in pain.

2. Patient will be independent in HEP.

Long-Term Treatment Goals

1. Patient will state a 75% decrease in pain.

Treatment Plan

Frequency/Duration: 2 times a week for 3 weeks

Consisting of: Modalities, therapeutic exercise, neuro re-education, patient education

continued

Patient Case Questions

1. What factors might be contributing to the patient's lateral epicondylalgia?

2. What would you tell the patient about specific activities to avoid or curtail?

3. What data will you collect the first time you see the patient?

4. If the plan of care does not guide you, what modalities might you use with this patient? Why? Are any modalities contraindicated?

5. If the plan of care does not specifically guide you, describe three therapeutic exercises that are indicated for this patient. Justify your choices.

6. How does tissue irritability/stage of tissue repair affect your choice of modality and exercise?

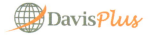 For additional resources, including answers to this case, please visit http://davisplus.fadavis.com

REFERENCES

1. Hoppenfeld, S., & Hutton, R. (1976). *Physical examination of the spine and extremities*. East Norwalk, CT: Appleton-Century-Crofts.
2. Levangie, P. K., Norkin, C. C., & Levangie, P. K. (2011). *Joint structure and function: A comprehensive analysis*. Philadelphia, PA: F.A. Davis Co.
3. Surgeons, American Association of Orthopaedic Surgeons. (1966). *Joint motion: Method of measuring and recording*. Chicago: Churchill Livingstone.
4. An, K. N., Hui, F. C., Morrey, B. F., Linscheid, R. L., & Chao, E. Y. (1981). Muscles across the elbow joint: A biomechanical analysis. *Journal of Biomechanics, 14*, 659–669.
5. Pappas, A. M., Zawacki, R. M., & Sullivan, T. J. (1985). Biomechanics of baseball pitching. A preliminary report. *American Journal of Sports Medicine,13*, 216–222.
6. Chourasia, A. O., Buhr, K. A., Rabago, D. P., et al. (2013). Relationships between biomechanics, tendon pathology, and function in individuals with lateral epicondylosis. *Journal of Orthopaedic and Sports Physical Therapy, 43*, 368–378.
7. Shiri, R., & Viikari-Juntura, E. (2011). Lateral and medial epicondylitis: Role of occupational factors. *Best Practice & Research. Clinical Rheumatology, 25*, 43–57.
8. van Rijn, R. M., Huisstede, B. M. A., Koes, B. W., & Burdorf, A. (2009). Associations between work-related factors and specific disorders at the elbow: A systematic literature review. *Rheumatology, Oxford England, 48*, 528–536.
9. Field, L. D., & Savoie, F. H. (1998). Common elbow injuries in sport. *Sports Medicine, Auckland, NZ, 26*, 193–205.
10. Bisset, L. M., Russell, T., Bradley, S., Ha, B., & Vicenzino, B. T. (2006). Bilateral sensorimotor abnormalities in unilateral lateral epicondylalgia. *Archives of Physical Medicine and Rehabilitation, 87*, 490–495.
11. Dorf, E. R., Chhabra, A. B., Golish, S. R., McGinty, J. L., & Pannunzio, M. E. (2007). Effect of elbow position on grip strength in the evaluation of lateral epicondylitis. *Journal of Hand Surgery, 32*, 882–886.
12. Smidt, N. van der Windt, D. A., Assendelft, W. J., Mourits, A. J., Devillé, W.L., de Winter, A. F., & Bouter, L. M. (2002). Interobserver reproducibility of the assessment of severity of complaints, grip strength, and pressure pain threshold in patients with lateral epicondylitis. *Archives of Physical Medicine and Rehabilitation, 83*, 1145–1150.
13. Bjordal, J. M., Lopes-Martins, R. A., Joensen, J., Couppe, C., Ljunggren, A. E., Stergioulas, A., & Johnson, M. I. (2008). A systematic review with procedural assessments and meta-analysis of low level laser therapy in lateral elbow tendinopathy (tennis elbow). *BMC Musculoskeletal Disorders, 9*, 75.
14. Dingemanse, R., Randsdorp, M., Koes, B. W., & Huisstede, B. M. A. (2014). Evidence for the effectiveness of electrophysical modalities for treatment of medial and lateral epicondylitis: A systematic review. *British Journal of Sports Medicine, 48*, 957–965.
15. Halle, J. S., Franklin, R. J., & Karalfa, B. L. (1986). Comparison of four treatment approaches for lateral epicondylitis of the elbow. *Journal of Orthopaedic and Sports Physical Therapy, 8*, 62–69.
16. Hume, P. A., Reid, D., & Edwards, T. (2006). Epicondylar injury in sport: Epidemiology, type, mechanisms, assessment, management and prevention. *Sports Medicine, Auckland, NZ, 36*, 151–170.
17. Nirschl, R. P., Rodin, D. M., Ochiai, D. H., DEX-AHE-01-99 Study Group (Maartmann-Moe, C., & 2003). Iontophoretic administration of dexamethasone sodium phosphate for acute epicondylitis. A randomized, double-blinded, placebo-controlled study. *American Journal of Sports Medicine, 31*, 189–195.
18. Malliaras, P., Maffulli, N., & Garau, G. (2008). Eccentric training programmes in the management of lateral elbow tendinopathy. *Disability and Rehabilitation, 30*, 1590–1596.
19. Croisier, J.-L., Foidart-Dessalle, M., Tinant, F., Crielaard, J.-M., & Forthomme, B. (2007). An isokinetic eccentric programme for the management of chronic lateral epicondylar tendinopathy. *British Journal of Sports Medicine, 41*, 269–275.
20. Coombes, B. K., Bisset, L., & Vicenzino, B. (2012). Elbow flexor and extensor muscle weakness in lateral epicondylalgia. *British Journal of Sports Medicine, 46*, 449–453.
21. Lucado, A. M., Kolber, M. J., Cheng, M. S., & Echternach, J. L., Sr. (2012). Upper extremity strength characteristics in female recreational tennis players with and without lateral epicondylalgia. *Journal of Orthopaedic and Sports Physical Therapy, 42*, 1025–1031.
22. Alizadehkhaiyat, O., Fisher, A. C., Kemp, G. J., Vishwanathan, K., & Frostick, S. P. (2007). Upper limb muscle imbalance in tennis elbow: A functional and electromyographic assessment.

Journal of Orthopaedic Research, Official Publication of the Orthopaedic Research Society, 25, 1651–1657.

23. Jafarian, F. S., Demneh, E. S., & Tyson, S. F. (2009). The immediate effect of orthotic management on grip strength of patients with lateral epicondylosis. *Journal of Orthopaedic and Sports Physical Therapy, 39,* 484–489.

24. Vicenzino, B., Brooksbank, J., Minto, J., Offord, S., & Paungmali, A. (2003). Initial effects of elbow taping on pain-free grip strength and pressure pain threshold. *Journal of Orthopaedic and Sports Physical Therapy, 33,* 400–407.

25. Hoogvliet, P., Randsdorp, M. S., Dingemanse, R., Koes, B. W., & Huisstede, B. M. A. (2013). Does effectiveness of exercise therapy and mobilisation techniques offer guidance for the treatment of lateral and medial epicondylitis? A systematic review. *British Journal of Sports Medicine, 47,* 1112–1119.

26. Trehan, S. K., Parziale, J. R., & Akelman, E. (2012). Cubital tunnel syndrome: Diagnosis and management. *Medicine and Health Rhode Island, 95,* 349–352.

27. Novak, C. B., Lee, G. W., Mackinnon, S. E., & Lay, L. (1994). Provocative testing for cubital tunnel syndrome. *Journal of Hand Surgery, 19,* 817–820.

28. Oskay, D., Meriç, A., Kirdi, N., Firat, T., Ayhan, C., & Leblebicioğlu, G. (2010). Neurodynamic mobilization in the conservative treatment of cubital tunnel syndrome: Long-term follow-up of 7 cases. *Journal of Manipulative and Physiological Therapeutics, 33,* 156–163.

29. Lyman, S., Fleisig, G. S., Andrews, J. R., & Osinski, E. D. (2002). Effect of pitch type, pitch count, and pitching mechanics on risk of elbow and shoulder pain in youth baseball pitchers. *American Journal of Sports Medicine, 30,* 463–468.

30. Tomberlin, J. P., & Saunders, H. D. (1994) *Evaluation, treatment and prevention of musculoskeletal disorders, Vol. 2, Extremities.* Chaska, MN: The Saunders Group.

31. Safran, M. R., McGarry, M. H., Shin, S., Han, S., & Lee, T. Q. (2005). Effects of elbow flexion and forearm rotation on valgus laxity of the elbow. *Journal of Bone and Joint Surgery. American Volume, 87,* 2065–2074.

32. O'Driscoll, S. W. M., Lawton, R. L., & Smith, A. M. (2005). The 'moving valgus stress test' for medial collateral ligament tears of the elbow. *American Journal of Sports Medicine, 33,* 231–239.

33. Cain, E. L., Jr., Andrews, J. R., Dugas, J. R., et al. (2010). Outcome of ulnar collateral ligament reconstruction of the elbow in 1281 athletes: Results in 743 athletes with minimum 2-year follow-up. *American Journal of Sports Medicine, 38,* 2426–2434.

34. Rohrbough, J. T., Altchek, D. W., Hyman, J., Williams, R. J., 3rd, & Botts, J. D. (2002). Medial collateral ligament reconstruction of the elbow using the docking technique. *American Journal of Sports Medicine, 30,* 541–548.

35. Paschos, N. K., Mitsionis, G. I., Vasiliadis, H. S., & Georgoulis, A. D. (2013). Comparison of early mobilization protocols in radial head fractures. *Journal of Orthopaedic Trauma, 27,* 134–139.

36. Bano, K. Y., & Kahlon, R. S. (2006). Radial head fractures—advanced techniques in surgical management and rehabilitation. *Journal of Hand Therapy, Official Journal of the American Society of Hand Therapy, 19,* 114–135.

37. Duckworth, A. D., McQueen, M. M., & Ring, D. (2013). Fractures of the radial head. *The Bone and Joint Journal, 95–B,* 151–159.

38. Ruchelsman, D. E., Christoforou, D., & Jupiter, J. B. (2013). Fractures of the radial head and neck. *Journal of Bone and Joint Surgery, American Volume, 95,* 469–478.

39. Zwingmann, J., Welzel, M., Dovi-Akue, D., Schmal, H., Südkamp, N. P., & Strohm, P. C. (2013). Clinical results after different operative treatment methods of radial head and neck fractures: A systematic review and meta-analysis of clinical outcome. *Injury, 44,* 1540–1550.

40. Jones, T. B., Karenz, A., Weinhold, P. S., & Dahners, L. E. (2014). Transcortical screw fixation of the olecranon shows equivalent strength and improved stability compared to tension band fixation. *Journal of Orthopaedic Trauma, 28,* 137–142.

41. Liu, Q.-H., Fu, Z. G., Zhou, J. L., et al. (2012). Randomized prospective study of olecranon fracture fixation: Cable pin system versus tension band wiring. *Journal of International Medical Research, 40,* 1055–1066.

42. Raju, S. M., & Gaddagi, R. A. (2013). Cancellous screw with tension band wiring for fractures of the olecranon. *Journal of Clinical and Diagnostic Research, 7,* 339–341.

43. Shrader, M. W. (2008). Pediatric supracondylar fractures and pediatric physeal elbow fractures. *Orthopedic Clinics of North America, 39,* 163–171.

44. Spencer, H. T., Dorey, F. J., Zionts, L. E., Dichter, D. H., Wong, M. A., Moazzaz, P., & Silva, M. (2012). Type II supracondylar humerus fractures: Can some be treated nonoperatively? *Journal of Pediatric Orthopedics, 32,* 675–681.

45. Snyder, A., & Crick, J. C. (2013). Brachial artery injuries in children. *Journal of Surgical Orthopaedic Advances, 22,* 105–112.

46. Soh, R. C. C., Tawng, D. K., & Mahadev, A. (2013). Pulse oximetry for the diagnosis and prediction for surgical exploration in the pulseless perfused hand as a result of supracondylar fractures of the distal humerus. *Clinics in Orthopedic Surgery, 5,* 74–81.

47. *Wheeless' Textbook of Orthopaedics.* Wheeless Online. Retrieved from https://www.wheelessonline.com/ (accessed: September 18, 2017).

48. Aggarwal, S., Kumar, V., Bhagwat, K. R., & Behera, P. (2014). AO extra-articular distal humerus locking plate: Extended spectrum of usage in intra-articular distal fractures with metaphyseal extension—our experience with 20 cases. *European Journal of Orthopaedic Surgery and Traumatology, 24,* 505–511.

49. Argintar, E., Berry, M., Narvy, S. J., Kramer, J., Omid, R., & Itamura, J. M. (2012). Hemiarthroplasty for the treatment of distal humerus fractures: Short-term clinical results. *Orthopedics, 35,* 1042–1045.

50. Ducrot, G., Ehlinger, M., Adam, P., Di Marco, A., Clavert, P., & Bonnomet, F. (2013). Complex fractures of the distal humerus in the elderly: Is primary total elbow arthroplasty a valid treatment alternative? A series of 20 cases. *Orthopaedics and Traumatology, Surgery and Research, 99,* 10–20.

51. Hungerer, S., Wipf, F., von Oldenburg, G., Augat, P., & Penzkofer, R. (2014). Complex distal humerus fractures—Comparison of polyaxial locking and non-locking screw configurations—A preliminary biomechanical study. *Journal of Orthopaedic Trauma, 28,* 130–136.

52. Voigt, C., Rank, C., Waizner, K., et al. (2013). Biomechanical testing of a new plate system for the distal humerus compared to two well-established implants. *International Orthopaedics, 37,* 667–672.

53. Kaźmierczak, M., Pyszel, K. S., & Surdziel, P. H. (2013). Total elbow arthroplasty in complicated distal humerus fracture—A case report. *Polish Orthopedics and Traumatology, 78,* 91–96.

Chapter 7

Orthopedic Interventions for the Wrist and Hand

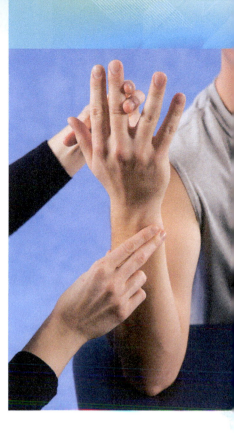

Anatomy and Physiology

Common Pathologies

LEARNING OUTCOMES

At the end of this chapter, the student will:

7.1   Describe the anatomy of the wrist and hand.
7.2   List normal range of motion of the forearm, wrist, and hand.
7.3   Describe normal wrist and hand kinematics.
7.4   Describe the mechanics, and discuss the purposes, of anterior, posterior, inferior, and distraction mobilization techniques of the wrist and hand joints.
7.5   Discuss common wrist and hand pathologies and typical presentation.
7.6   Discuss contributing factors to various wrist and hand pathologies and, when relevant, preventive measures.
7.7   Describe the clinical tests that the physical therapist may have used to diagnose common wrist and hand pathologies and how to administer the tests.
7.8   Explain common treatment interventions for wrist and hand pathologies.
7.9   Describe surgical interventions for the wrist and hand including carpal tunnel release and Dupuytren's release.
7.10 Compare and contrast trigger finger and de Quervain tenosynovitis.
7.11 Describe the manifestations of peripheral nerve injuries in hand deformities.
7.12 Describe the clinical alerts for wrist and hand pathologies.

KEY WORDS

Anatomical snuff box	Fasciectomy	Spica
Ape hand	Fasciotomy	Stenosing tenosynovitis
Benediction hand	Fall on an outstretched hand	Triangular fibrocartilage complex
Boxer's fracture	(FOOSH)	(TFCC)
Carpal tunnel	Guyon's canal	Ulnar claw
Colles' fracture	Paraesthesia	Wrist drop
Extensor expansion	Ray	

Anatomy and Physiology

The distal forearm, wrist, and hand area is structurally and functionally complex. Over 30 joints with various and intricate joint shapes, as well as the many muscles of the wrist and hand, allow for endless positions and motions. While the relatively large movements of the shoulder girdle, shoulder joint, and elbow allow the hand to approach an object, fine movements of the wrist and hand are necessary for most functional purposes.

The complexity of the hand allows great versatility in position and function. It also predisposes the hand to injury and pathology. After reviewing the anatomy, we'll explore the common pathologies of the wrist and hand, including nerve lesions, fractures, and tendon inflammation.

Bone and Joint Anatomy and Physiology

The distal forearm and wrist articulations include the distal radioulnar, the radiocarpal, the midcarpal, intercarpal, and the carpometacarpal joints. The radiocarpal joint and the midcarpal joint collectively are referred to as the wrist joint. Joints of the hand include the metacarpophalangeal and interphalangeal joints. Figure 7.1 illustrates the bones and joints of the wrist and hand.

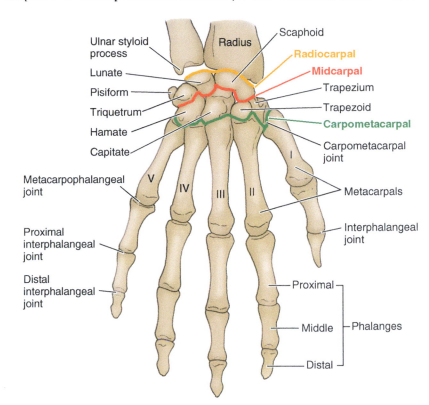

Figure 7.1 Bone and joints of the wrist and hand.

Distal Radioulnar Joint

As described in Chapter 6, rotation of the radius around the comparatively stable ulna results in pronation and supination of the forearm. At the distal radioulnar joint, the concave ulnar notch of the radius articulates with the convex head of the ulna. This is a pivot joint, allowing 1 degree of freedom in the transverse plane. Radioulnar ligaments on the anterior and posterior aspect of the joint provide joint stability. The distal radioulnar joint undergoes more movement than the proximal radioulnar joint during pronation and supination.

Radiocarpal Joint

The radiocarpal joint is formed by the concave distal end of the radius proximally and by the convex scaphoid and lunate bones distally. This articulation is ellipsoidal in shape, allowing wrist flexion and extension as well as radial and ulnar deviation. Nearly all wrist extension and most wrist flexion occurs at this joint.[1]

Midcarpal Joint

The midcarpal joint describes the S-shaped articulation between the proximal and distal rows of carpal bones. It is classified as a plane joint[2] for simplicity, but within the midcarpal joint are saddle-shaped articulations allowing for 2 degrees of freedom. The midcarpal joint contributes to wrist flexion and extension as well as radial and ulnar deviation.[3]

Intercarpal Joints

There are numerous articulations between the carpal bones at the intercarpal joints. Some of the carpal bones are loosely attached to each other, but some are tightly attached, leading movement of one to cause movement of the other. This intricacy allows the carpal area to function efficiently and to easily change shape as needed.

Carpometacarpal Joints

The carpometacarpal (CMC) joints between the distal row of carpals and the five metacarpals contribute to hand flexion and the overall curved shape of the hand. The CMC joints of the thumb and the fifth digit are saddle-shaped.[4] These two are the most mobile of the CMC joints and allow for opposition of these digits. The CMC joints of the index, middle, and ring finger are plane joints and allow very minimal flexion and extension. The index and middle fingers, with the distal carpal bones, form a stable base around which the thumb, little finger, and to some extent the ring finger are able to rotate into opposition.

Metacarpophalangeal Joints

The metacarpophalangeal (MP) joints form the most prominent row of knuckles. The convex distal ends of the metacarpals articulate with the concave proximal phalanx on each digit. These joints allow 2 degrees of freedom, with flexion/extension and abduction/adduction of the proximal phalanx occurring here. The reference point for abduction and adduction is the middle finger. Abduction is movement of the fingers away from the middle finger, and adduction is movement toward the middle finger.

Interphalangeal Joints

The joint between the phalanges is the interphalangeal (IP) joint. In the fingers, there are two IP joints, the proximal interphalangeal joint (PIP) and the distal interphalangeal joint (DIP). In the thumb there is one IP joint between the proximal and distal phalanx. These joints are formed by the articulation of the convex heads of the more proximal phalanx with the concave base of the more distal phalanx. They are hinge joints, allowing for flexion and extension only.

See Table 7-1 for a review of the bones and joints of the wrist and hand.

Soft Tissues

A complete description of the ligamentous anatomy of the wrist and hand is variable and complex, and beyond the scope of this book. We will discuss the major ligaments and soft tissue structures of the wrist and hand, which are summarized in Table 7-2.

Radiocarpal Joint Capsule and Ligaments

The radiocarpal joint has a loose joint capsule but is significantly reinforced by ligaments. Major ligaments of the wrist include radiocarpal ligaments on both the anterior and posterior wrist and collateral ligaments on the medial and lateral sides.

The palmar radiocarpal ligament has several bands that run between the radius and carpal bones on the anterior wrist. It becomes taut at end ranges of wrist extension and serves as a restraint for this movement. The dorsal radiocarpal ligament connects the radius to the carpal bones on the posterior wrist and similarly limits end ranges of wrist flexion. The radial collateral ligament on the lateral wrist limits ulnar deviation, and the ulnar collateral ligament on the medial side limits radial deviation.

Transverse Carpal Ligament or Flexor Retinaculum

The transverse carpal ligament runs across the wrist on the anterior side. It spans the carpal bones on each side of the wrist, forming a tunnel (**carpal tunnel**) through which tendons and nerves enter the hand (Fig. 7.2). In addition to acting as a "roof" of the carpal tunnel, this ligament is an attachment site for the small thenar and hypothenar muscles.

Extensor Expansion

On the posterior aspect, as the tendons of extensor digitorum cross the MP joint on each finger, they flatten out and broaden into a triangular sheet of connective tissue. This aponeurosis is called the **extensor expansion** (or extensor hood) and covers the posterior aspect of each finger (Fig. 7.3). Adding into the extensor expansion are the lumbricals, palmar and dorsal interossei, extensor indicis, and extensor digiti minimi muscles. The extensor expansion terminates on the distal phalanx.

This anatomical arrangement allows all of the muscles that insert into the expansion to extend the PIP and DIP joints of the fingers. The extensor tendon is maintained in the middle of the finger by the widening of the extensor expansion as it crosses the phalangeal joints.

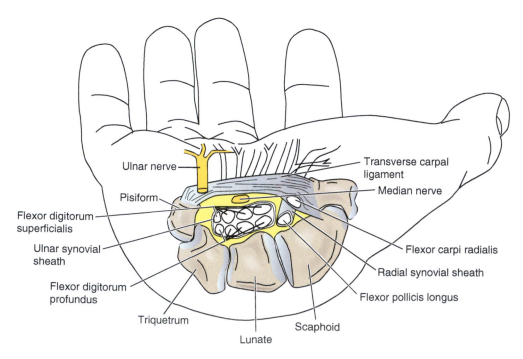

Figure 7.2 The transverse carpal ligament runs across the anterior side of the wrist, forming the roof of the carpal tunnel. The carpal bones form the floor. The median nerve and nine flexor tendons run through the carpal tunnel.

Table 7-1 Bone and Joint Anatomy and Physiology
Of the Wrist and Hand

Joint	Anatomy	Normal ROM and Movements	Landmarks	Clinical Considerations
Distal Radioulnar	Pivot joint between the ulnar notch on the distal radius and the convex distal ulna.	Pronation – 0°–80° Supination – 0°–80° Rotation of the distal radius around the ulna to allow for pronation and supination.	Radial styloid process on lateral side of wrist. Distal end of the radius in slight wrist flexion.	Fracture of the distal radius ± the ulna is common, termed Colles' fracture. Triangular fibrocartilage complex (TFCC) is soft tissue that stabilizes this joint. This complex may contribute to wrist pain.
Radiocarpal	Ellipsoidal joint between the concave distal radius and the convex scaphoid and lunate.	Contributes to wrist extension (0°–70°), wrist flexion (0°–80°), radial deviation (0°–20°), and ulnar deviation (0°–30°).	Radial styloid process on lateral side of wrist. Scaphoid forms floor of anatomical snuff box.	Radiocarpal and midcarpal joints contribute to total motion of wrist. Distal radius and scaphoid fractures are common in this area, leading to limited wrist motion. Closed packed position: wrist extension with radial deviation. Loose packed position: neutral wrist flexion/extension with slight ulnar deviation. Capsular pattern: flexion and extension are equally limited.
Midcarpal	S-shaped joint between proximal and distal rows of carpal bones.	Contributes to wrist extension (0°–70°), wrist flexion (0°–80°), radial deviation (0°–20°), and ulnar deviation (0°–30°).	Entire joint line is not palpable, but distal to Lister's tubercle of the radius is a palpable depression of the capitate. Proximal capitate may be palpated with wrist flexion.	Complex joint that contributes to wrist movements.
Intercarpal	Plane joints between the carpals.			The gliding motions that occur here allow the wrist to change shape easily.
Carpometacarpal (CMC)	Articulation between distal row of carpals and metacarpals. First and fifth digit CMC are saddle-shaped. Digits 2–4 are plane joints.	Thumb abduction 0°–70°, thumb flexion 0°–15°, thumb extension 0°–20°, oppositional rotation to approximate 1st and 5th metacarpals. Often measured in distance between creases at palm.		Saddle shape of CMC 1 and 5 allows for opposition. Plane joints of 2–4 provides stability. CMC joint of the thumb is a common site of osteoarthritis.
Metacarpophalangeal (MP)	Condyloid articulation between convex distal ends of metacarpals with concave proximal phalanx on each digit. Allows 2 degrees of freedom (flexion/extension and abduction/adduction).	Fingers: MP flexion 0°–90°, MP extension 0°–45°. Thumb: MP flexion 0°–50°.	Easily palpated as the proximal and most prominent row of knuckles.	Reference point for abduction and adduction is the middle finger. Ulnar drift of rheumatoid arthritis occurs due to deformity of these joints.
Interphalangeal (IP)	Hinge articulation between the convex heads of the more proximal phalanx with the concave base of the more distal phalanx; allow 1 degree of freedom.	Fingers: PIP flexion 0°–100°, PIP extension 0°, DIP flexion 0°–90°, DIP extension 0°. Thumb: IP flexion 0°–80°, IP extension 0°–20°.	Easily palpated joints of each digit.	

Table 7-2 Connective Tissue Anatomy and Physiology
Of the Wrist and Hand

Structure	Anatomy	Function	Clinical Considerations
Wrist joint capsule	Encases the distal radius and ulna, and the first row of carpals	Provide stability in pronation and supination.	
Palmar radiocarpal ligament	Group of ligaments that connect radius to carpal bones on the anterior wrist	Provides stability. Limits wrist extension.	Wrist sprain may involve this group of ligaments
Dorsal radiocarpal ligament	Group of ligaments that connect radius to carpal bones on posterior wrist	Provides stability. Limits wrist flexion.	Wrist sprain may involve this group of ligaments
Radial collateral ligament	Connects radial styloid process to the scaphoid	Provides stability. Limits wrist ulnar deviation.	Wrist sprain may involve this ligament
Ulnar collateral ligament	Two ligament bands that connect the ulnar styloid process and TFCC to the pisiform and triquetrum.	Provides stability. Limits wrist radial deviation.	Wrist sprain may involve these ligaments
Transverse carpal ligament (Flexor retinaculum)	Spans the carpal bones on the anterior wrist, forming the roof of the carpal tunnel.	Stabilizes the flexor tendons against the anterior wrist. Serves as an attachment site for small thenar and hypothenar muscles.	Relatively stiff structure that forms the roof of the tunnel. With carpal bones forming the floor, the tunnel allows for very limited expansion.
Extensor expansion	Triangular-shaped aponeurosis on the posterior aspect of each finger.	Provides attachment site to finger extensors, palmar and dorsal interossei, and lumbrical muscles. Helps maintain tendon of extensors in the middle of the finger.	Allows the lumbricals and interossei to assist in extension of the IP joints. Damage to the extensor hood may lead to boutonniere deformity of the fingers.
Palmar aponeurosis	Sheath in palm that provides an attachment site for the palmaris longus muscle.	Protects the structures in the palm. Fascial connections form tunnels for flexor tendons.	
Triangular fibrocartilage complex	TFCC consists of a triangular disc (in the distal radioulnar joint), fibrous band attachments to the radius, and a wedge of connective tissue that fills in the space between the distal ulna and the carpals.	Provides a cushion between the ulna and the carpals, and stabilizes the distal radioulnar joint.	Blood flow is minimal, so injuries to the TFCC heal slowly.

Palmar Aponeurosis

A large aponeurosis covers most of the palm, called the palmar aponeurosis. This fascial sheath becomes the attachment site for the palmaris longus muscle and serves to protect the structures in the palm. Fibrous bands from the palmar aponeurosis help to channel the flexor tendons into the fingers. Pathology of this structure results in *Dupuytren's contracture*.

Triangular Fibrocartilage Complex

Between the distal radius, ulna, and carpals lies a structure called the **triangular fibrocartilage complex (TFCC)**. The TFCC is composed of three parts: a triangular meniscal cartilage that lies on the distal end of the ulna, radioulnar ligaments that stabilize the distal radioulnar joint, and the ulnar collateral ligament (Fig. 7.4). This complex provides a cushion between the ulna and the carpals and stabilizes the ulnar side of the wrist joint.[5] Blood flow to this soft tissue structure is minimal, so injuries to the TFCC can be slow to heal.[6] Injuries to this structure often occur in a **fall on an outstretched hand**. These injuries are referred to using the acronym **FOOSH**. The TFCC may be involved in *extensor carpi ulnaris tendinopathy*, as discussed below.

Nerves

Three of the four peripheral nerves that we studied in Chapter 6 continue into the wrist and hand area: the median, ulnar, and radial nerves.

After innervating the pronator teres, the median nerve continues to travel down the anterior forearm innervating

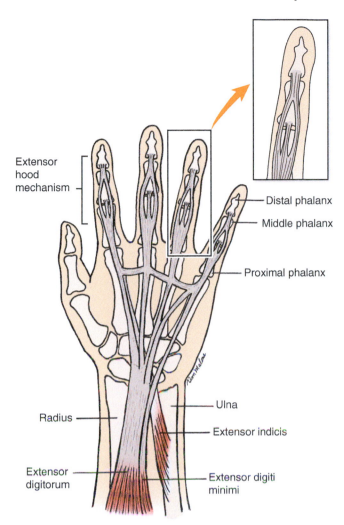

Figure 7.3 The extensor expansion serves as an attachment site for the finger extensors as well as lumbrical and interossei muscles. This hood of connective tissue maintains the extensor tendon in the middle of the finger.

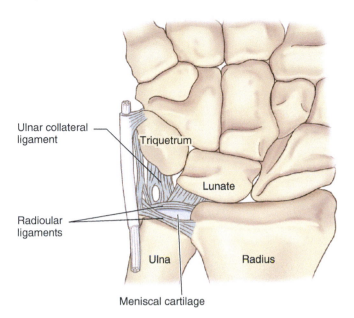

Figure 7.4 Triangular Fibrocartilage Complex (TFCC) includes a meniscal cartilage, the ulnar collateral ligament, and radioulnar ligaments.

most of the extrinsic flexor muscles of the wrist and hand. After innervating pronator quadratus at the wrist, the median nerve passes through the carpal tunnel into the hand. In the hand it innervates the thenar intrinsic muscles and the two lumbricals on the lateral (thumb) side (Fig. 7.5A).

The ulnar nerve enters the anterior side of the proximal forearm after exiting the cubital tunnel. Here it innervates the flexor carpi ulnaris and the medial half of flexor digitorum profundus. It continues into the hand to innervate the hypothenar muscles, the palmar and dorsal interossei, the two medial lumbricals, and adductor pollicis (Fig. 7.5B).

The radial nerve emerges on the lateral side of the humerus, crossing the elbow anterior to the lateral epicondyle. In the forearm, the radial nerve innervates the brachioradialis, supinator and all the extensors of the wrist and hand (Fig. 7.5C). By the time the radial nerve crosses the wrist, it is a sensory nerve only.

Nerves will be discussed in the Pathology section under *carpal tunnel syndrome* and *nerve lesions*.

Muscles

Many of the muscles of the wrist and hand are labeled by their action. For example, muscle names may incorporate the word *flexor*, *extensor*, or *opponens* (muscle of opposition). They also often contain the area of the hand that they affect, such as *carpi* (wrist), *digitorum* (finger), *pollicis* (thumb), *indicis* (index finger), and *digiti minimi* (little finger). Wrist and finger flexor muscles usually originate from the medial epicondyle of the humerus, while wrist and finger extensor muscles often originate from the lateral epicondyle. Muscles that originate proximal to the hand and insert in the hand are called *extrinsic muscles*. If the origin and insertion are within the hand, they are called *intrinsic*.

A review of wrist muscles with origin, insertion, innervation, primary action, and clinical considerations is found in Table 7-3A. A review of extrinsic hand muscles is found in Table 7-3B. A review of intrinsic hand muscles is found in Table 7-3C.

Anatomical Snuff Box

The three "outcropping muscles" on the posterior aspect of the forearm comprise the long thumb extensors and abductor. These muscles are termed the "outcropping muscles" for the way they seem to appear out from under the wrist and finger extensors and travel laterally down into the thumb (Fig. 7.6). Each of these three muscles inserts on one of the three bones in the **ray** of the thumb: the first metacarpal, the proximal phalanx, and the distal phalanx.

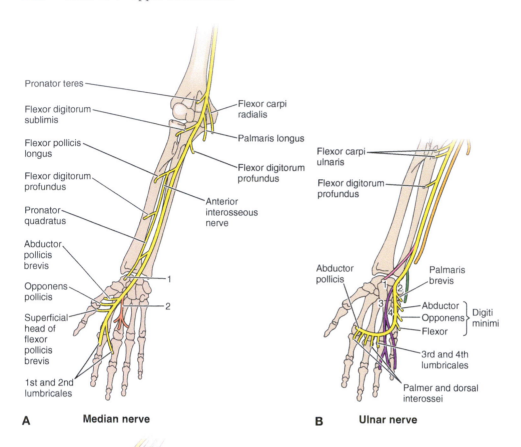

Pronator teres

Flexor digitorum sublimis

Flexor pollicis longus

Flexor digitorum profundus

Pronator quadratus

Abductor pollicis brevis

Opponens pollicis

Superficial head of flexor pollicis brevis

1st and 2nd lumbricales

Flexor carpi radialis

Palmaris longus

Flexor digitorum profundus

Anterior interosseous nerve

1

2

A   Median nerve

Flexor carpi ulnaris

Flexor digitorum profundus

Abductor pollicis

Palmaris brevis

Abductor
Opponens   } Digiti minimi
Flexor

3rd and 4th lumbricales

Palmer and dorsal interossei

B   Ulnar nerve

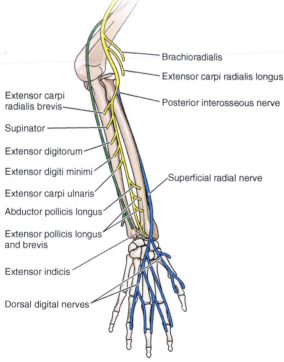

Extensor carpi radialis brevis

Supinator

Extensor digitorum

Extensor digiti minimi

Extensor carpi ulnaris

Abductor pollicis longus

Extensor pollicis longus and brevis

Extensor indicis

Dorsal digital nerves

Brachioradialis

Extensor carpi radialis longus

Posterior interosseous nerve

Superficial radial nerve

C   Radial nerve

Figure 7.5 The median (A), ulnar (B), and radial (C) nerves in the forearm and hand.

Table 7-3A   Muscle Anatomy and Kinesiology
Of the Wrist

Muscle	Origin	Insertion	Innervation	Primary Action	Clinical Considerations
Extensor carpi radialis longus (ECRL)	Lateral epicondyle of the humerus	Base of the second metacarpal	Radial nerve	Wrist extension and radial deviation	
Extensor carpi radialis brevis (ECRB)	Lateral epicondyle of the humerus	Base of the third metacarpal	Radial nerve	Wrist extension	ECRB is a weak radial deviator since it inserts near the middle of the hand with a line of pull near the axis of rotation.
Extensor carpi ulnaris (ECU)	Lateral epicondyle of the humerus and the middle of the shaft of the ulna	Base of the fifth metacarpal	Radial nerve	Wrist extension and ulnar deviation	
Flexor carpi radialis (FCR)	Medial epicondyle of the humerus	Base of the second and third metacarpals	Median nerve	Wrist flexion and radial deviation	
Flexor carpi ulnaris (FCU)	Medial epicondyle of the humerus and the middle of the shaft of the ulna	Base of the fifth metacarpal and the pisiform bone	Ulnar nerve	Wrist flexion and ulnar deviation	
Palmaris longus (PL)	Medial epicondyle of the humerus	On the palmar fascia and transverse carpal ligament	Median nerve	Weak wrist flexor, and a tensor of the palmar aponeurosis	Missing from one or both arms in about 10% of the population, without loss of wrist flexion strength. Because it is an accessory muscle, the tendon of palmaris longus may be harvested and used for ligament reconstruction or eye surgery.

These three muscles form a structure called the **anatomical snuff box.** This depression on the thumb side of the posterior hand is bordered by extensor pollicis brevis and abductor pollicis longus on one side and the extensor pollicis longus on the other side. On the floor of the snuff box lie the scaphoid and trapezium. We'll look at pathology in this area under *de Quervain tenosynovitis.*

Carpal Tunnel
The carpal tunnel is formed by the curved structure of the carpal bones and the transverse carpal ligament that extends across the carpals from medial to lateral. Through this tunnel run the eight tendons of the finger flexors, the long thumb flexor, and the median nerve (Fig. 7.2). The size of the tunnel is unyielding, due to the bony carpal floor and rigid ligamentous roof, which may lead to compression of the structures passing through the tunnel. See *carpal tunnel syndrome.*

Kinematics of the Wrist and Hand

Force Couples
The three primary wrist flexors are flexor carpi radialis, flexor carpi ulnaris, and palmaris longus. With synchronous contractions, the radial deviation of flexor carpi radialis is opposed by the ulnar deviation of flexor carpi ulnaris, leading to straight plane flexion. A maximal effort to flex the wrist will call in the secondary wrist flexors: the flexor digitorum superficialis, flexor digitorum profundus, and flexor pollicis longus.

Likewise, the three primary wrist extensors are extensor carpi radialis longus, extensor carpi radialis brevis, and extensor carpi ulnaris. The radial deviation caused by extensor carpi radialis longus is counteracted by the ulnar deviation of extensor carpi ulnaris, leading to straight

Table 7-3B Muscle Anatomy and Kinesiology

Of the Hand (Extrinsic Muscles)

Muscle	Origin	Insertion	Innervation	Primary Action	Clinical Considerations
Extensor digitorum (ED) (Also called extensor digitorum communis)	Lateral epicondyle of the humerus	Divides into four muscle bellies, and inserts through the extensor expansion onto the posterior aspect of the middle and distal phalanges of the fingers	Radial nerve	Extension of the MP, PIP, and DIP joints of fingers	
Extensor indicis (EI)	Distal ulna	Onto the extensor expansion on the posterior aspect of the index finger	Radial nerve	Extension of the index finger	
Extensor digiti minimi (EDM)	Distal ulna	Onto the extensor expansion on the posterior aspect of the little finger	Radial nerve	Extension of the little finger	
Flexor digitorum superficialis (FDS)	Medial epicondyle of the humerus	Middle phalanx of the fingers	Median nerve	Flexion of the MP and PIP joints of the fingers	The tendons of FDS split and insert on the middle phalanx of the fingers
Flexor digitorum profundus (FDP)	Proximal ulna	Distal phalanx of the fingers	Median nerve (digits 2-3) and ulnar nerve (digits 4-5)	Flexion of the MP, PIP, and DIP joints of the fingers	Runs deep to FDS. After FDS splits, FDP surfaces to run down the anterior fingers and insert on the distal phalanx
Extensor pollicis longus (EPL)	Middle third of the posterior ulna	Distal phalanx of the thumb	Radial nerve	Extend the thumb at the CMC, MP, and IP joints	One of three outcropping muscles that defines the boundaries of the anatomical snuff box
Extensor pollicis brevis (EPB)	Distal third of the radius	Proximal phalanx of the thumb	Radial nerve	Extension of the thumb at the CMC and MP joints	One of three outcropping muscles that defines the boundaries of the anatomical snuff box
Abductor pollicis longus (APL)	Posterior radius and ulna	First metacarpal of the thumb	Radial nerve	Abduction and extension of the CMC joint of the thumb	One of three outcropping muscles that defines the boundaries of the anatomical snuff box
Flexor pollicis longus (FPL)	Middle third of the radius	Distal phalanx of the thumb	Median nerve	Flexion of the CMC, MP, and IP joints of the thumb	

plane extension. If more strength is needed in wrist extension, the long finger extensors (EDC, EDM, EI) will be used as secondary wrist extensors.

There are two primary wrist radial deviators: flexor carpi radialis and extensor carpi radialis longus. As these two muscles contract simultaneously, the flexion moment of FCR is counteracted by the extension moment of ECRL, leading to straight plane radial deviation.

Ulnar deviation is similarly produced by two muscles: flexor carpi ulnaris and extensor carpi ulnaris. The flexion produced by FCU is opposed by the extension

of ECU, allowing these two muscles to produce pure ulnar deviation.

Grasp

In the action of grasping, the flexor digitorum superficialis and profundus are the prime movers. But the wrist extensors are also playing a major role. To oppose the secondary action of FDS and FDP of wrist flexion, the wrist extensors must contract. In doing so, the extensor carpi muscles keep the wrist in an extended position and elongate the finger flexors over the anterior wrist. In this

Table 7-3C Muscle Anatomy and Kinesiology
Of the Hand (Intrinsic Muscles)

Muscle	Origin	Insertion	Innervation	Primary Action	Clinical Considerations
Lumbricals	Four muscles that arise from the tendons of FDP	Extensor expansion on the fingers	Median nerve (digits 2-3) and ulnar nerve (digits 4-5)	Flexion of the MP joints and extension of the PIP and DIP joints of the fingers	The lumbrical muscles allow the hand to perform the grip used to hold a book or plate, called a lumbrical grip.
Palmar interossei	First, second, fourth, and fifth metacarpals. Their action is to adduct the index, ring, and little fingers toward the middle finger. They also assist the lumbricals in MP flexion and PIP and DIP extension. The palmar interossei are innervated by the ulnar nerve.	Base of the first phalanx on their finger of origin and into the extensor expansion	Ulnar nerve	Adduction of the thumb, index, ring, and little finger toward the middle finger. Assist in PIP and DIP extension.	Disagreement over whether the thumb has a palmar interosseous muscle.
Dorsal interossei	Arise from two adjacent metacarpals on the dorsum of the hand	Base of the first phalanx of the index, middle, and ring fingers and into the extensor expansion	Ulnar nerve	Abduction of the index and ring finger away from the midline of the hand, and radial and ulnar deviation of the middle finger. Assist in PIP and DIP extension	
Flexor pollicis brevis	Flexor retinaculum and trapezium	Proximal phalanx of thumb	Median nerve	Flexion of CMC and MP joints of thumb	
Abductor pollicis brevis	Flexor retinaculum, scaphoid and trapezium	Proximal phalanx of thumb	Median nerve	Abduction of the CMC joint of the thumb	
Opponens pollicis	Flexor retinaculum and trapezium	First metacarpal	Median nerve	Opposition of the thumb	
Adductor pollicis	Capitate and second and third metacarpals	Proximal phalanx of thumb	Ulnar nerve	Adduction of the thumb	
Flexor digiti minimi	Flexor retinaculum and hamate	Proximal phalanx of little finger	Ulnar nerve	Flexion of the CMC and MP joints of little finger	
Abductor digiti minimi	Pisiform	Proximal phalanx of little finger	Ulnar nerve	Abducts the MP joint of the little finger	
Opponens digiti minimi	Hook of the hamate	Fifth metacarpal	Ulnar nerve	Opposition of the CMC joint of the little finger	

way, contraction of the wrist extensors prevents active insufficiency of the finger flexors as the fingers become more and more flexed (Fig. 7.7). While it may seem odd that wrist extensors assist finger flexion, an understanding of this relationship explains why gripping may be painful in elbow pathologies such as epicondylalgia, as discussed in Chapter 6.

Joint Mobilization

Joint mobilization in the wrist and hand may be used to increase range of motion or to decrease pain. The loose packed position of the wrist is in 10° of supination (distal radioulnar joint) and neutral flexion/extension with slight ulnar deviation (radiocarpal joint). Table 7-4

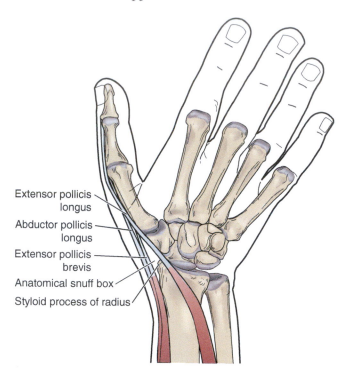

Figure 7.6 The outcropping muscles of the thumb form the anatomical snuff box. Extensor pollicis brevis and abductor pollicis longus form the lateral border of the snuff box, and extensor pollicis longus forms the medial border.

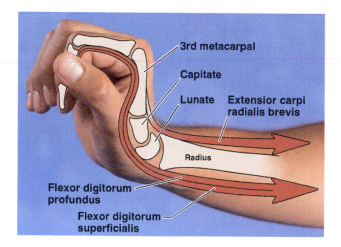

Figure 7.7 Flexor and extensor muscles work synergistically in grasp. The finger flexors rely on wrist extensors to move the wrist into extension, lengthening the flexors. This prevents active insufficiency of the finger flexors as they shorten.

lists the movements of the joints of the wrist and hand with the associated direction of a glide mobilization to increase range of motion.

Distal Radioulnar Joint

Anterior/Posterior Glide

Anterior or posterior glide of the distal radius on the ulna is used to increase range of motion into forearm supination (posterior glide) or pronation (anterior glide).

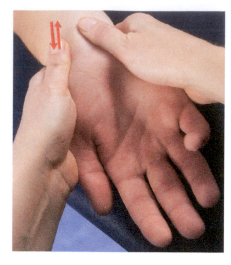

Figure 7.8 Anterior and posterior glide of the radius on the ulna increases forearm pronation and supination ROM.

Table 7-4	Direction of Slide Used to Increase Range of Motion	
Limited Range	**Direction of Slide in Mobilization**
Pronation	Anterior glide distal radioulnar joint
Supination	Posterior glide distal radioulnar joint
Wrist flexion	Posterior glide radiocarpal joint
Wrist extension	Anterior glide radiocarpal joint
Wrist radial deviation	Medial glide radiocarpal joint
Wrist ulnar deviation	Lateral glide radiocarpal joint
General restriction	Distraction radiocarpal joint

The patient may be sitting or supine. The examiner stabilizes the distal ulna with one hand. With the other hand an anterior or posterior force is applied (Fig. 7.8). Alternatively, the radius may be stabilized and the ulna mobilized.

Radiocarpal Joint

Anterior Glide

Anterior glide of the scaphoid and lunate on the radius is used to increase range of motion into wrist extension. The patient may be sitting or supine. The examiner stabilizes the distal radius and ulna with one hand. With the other hand the examiner grasps across the carpals and applies an anterior force (Fig. 7.9).

Posterior Glide

Posterior glide of the scaphoid and lunate on the radius is used to increase range of motion into wrist flexion.

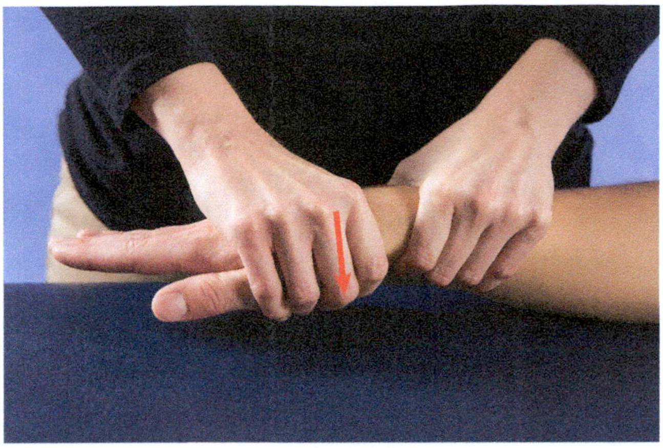

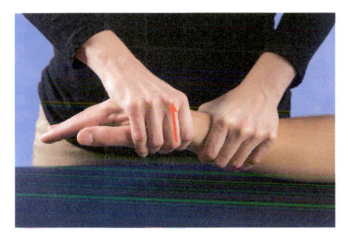

Figure 7.9 Anterior glide of the scaphoid and lunate on the radius increases wrist extension ROM.

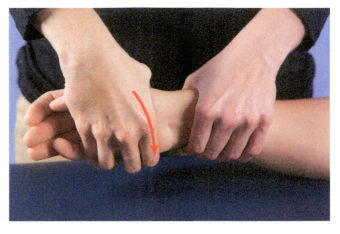

Figure 7.11 Medial glide of the scaphoid and lunate on the radius increases radial deviation ROM.

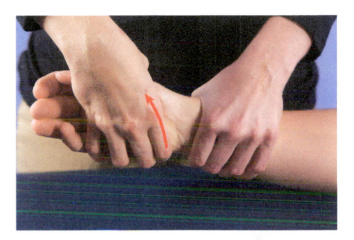

Figure 7.10 Posterior glide of the scaphoid and lunate on the radius increases wrist flexion ROM.

Figure 7.12 Lateral glide of the scaphoid and lunate on the radius increases ulnar deviation ROM.

The patient may be sitting or supine. The examiner stabilizes the distal radius and ulna with one hand. With the other hand the examiner grasps across the carpals and applies a posterior force (Fig. 7.10).

Medial Glide

Medial glide of the scaphoid and lunate on the radius is used to increase range of motion into radial deviation. The patient may be sitting or supine. The examiner stabilizes the distal radius and ulna with one hand. With the other hand the examiner grasps across the carpals and applies a medially directed force (Fig. 7.11).

Lateral Glide

Lateral glide of the scaphoid and lunate on the radius is used to increase range of motion into ulnar deviation. The patient may be sitting or supine. The examiner stabilizes the distal radius and ulna with one hand. With the other hand the examiner grasps across the carpals and applies a laterally directed force (Fig. 7.12).

Distraction

Distraction of the carpals away from the radius is used for general joint restrictions. The patient may be sitting or supine. The examiner stabilizes the distal radius and ulna with one hand. With the other hand the examiner grasps across the carpals and pulls distally (Fig. 7.13).

Carpal Joints

Intercarpal joints may be mobilized using an anterior-posterior glide. The examiner uses the thumb and index finger of one hand to stabilize a carpal bone and with the thumb and index finger of the other hand applies an anterior and posterior glide to an adjacent carpal bone (Fig. 7.14).

Metacarpophalangeal and Interphalangeal Joints

MP and IP joints may be mobilized using the concave-convex rule. The proximal segment of these joints is convex and the distal segment is concave.

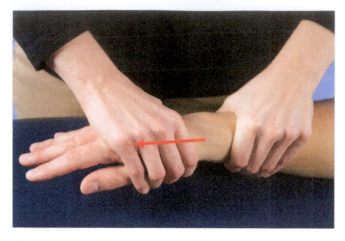

Figure 7.13 Distraction mobilization is used for general joint hypomobility and pain.

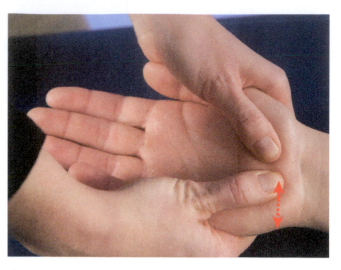

Figure 7.14 Anterior and posterior intercarpal joint mobilization is used for carpal restrictions.

Common Pathologies

Carpal Tunnel Syndrome
De Quervain Tenosynovitis
Extensor Carpi Ulnaris Tendinopathy
Nerve Lesions

Fractures
Dupuytren's Disease (Palmar Fibromatosis)
Hand Tendon Deformities

As we have seen, the wrist and hand area is anatomically complex. By nature of the large number of positions and uses of the hand, it is vulnerable to injury from overuse and trauma. In this section we will discuss the common pathologies of the wrist and hand that are treated with physical therapy.

Carpal Tunnel Syndrome

The carpal tunnel forms a passageway from the anterior forearm into the hand. The tendons of flexor digitorum superficialis, flexor digitorum profundus, and flexor pollicis longus pass through this tunnel. In addition, the median nerve passes through the tunnel as well. Carpal tunnel syndrome (CTS) is a condition of compression of the median nerve in the tunnel (Fig. 7.15).

Causes/Contributing Factors

Recall that the tunnel is unyielding in size, due to the bony floor and ligamentous roof. CTS may be the result of many contributing factors. In general, anything that makes the tunnel smaller, makes the tendons swell or become larger, or makes the nerve larger or more sensitive can lead to CTS.

Women are 3 times more likely to get CTS than men.[7] Diabetes, hypothyroidism, obesity, rheumatoid arthritis, osteoarthritis, gout, lupus, pregnancy, wrist size, and occupational factors, including use of vibrating hand tools, have all been associated with CTS. Occupations which are computer-intensive have not been linked with CTS, but those placing the wrist in non-neutral positions for large parts of the day or requiring significant hand exertion increase the risk.[8–12] Other factors include repeated wrist and hand movements that may lead to tendon swelling, fractures of the wrist, bone spurs, and tumors or cysts in the area.

Symptoms

The most common symptoms of CTS are pain, numbness, tingling, and weakness in the hand. These symptoms

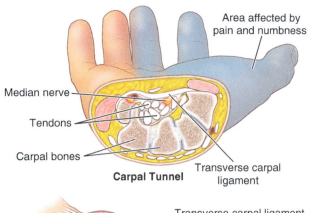

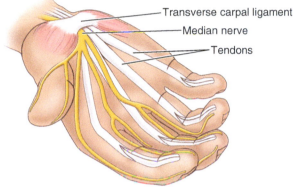

Figure 7.15 In carpal tunnel syndrome, the median nerve is compressed as it runs through the tunnel.

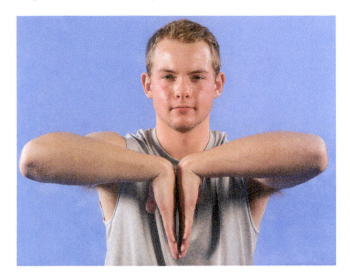

Figure 7.16 Phalen's test for carpal tunnel syndrome.

usually occur specifically in the distribution of the median nerve. Numbness, tingling, and pain are generally felt in the thumb, index, middle, and half of the ring finger. Shaking the hands helps relieve the feeling of pins and needles.[13] Weakness may be noticed in the thenar muscles when gripping small objects. Over time, the thenar eminence may show signs of atrophy. Patients often complain of symptoms that increase at night.

Clinical Signs

Various tests and measures may be used to validate the diagnosis of carpal tunnel syndrome. These include grip and pinch strength, muscle testing of the thenar muscles, observation of hand atrophy, and sensation testing. In addition, special tests are performed that rely on reproducing the patient's symptoms by momentarily increasing nerve compression.

Phalen's Test

Phalen's test is done with the patient sitting or standing. The patient brings the backs of the hands together to position the wrists in end range of flexion. This position can also be accomplished by having the patient rest elbows on a table with the forearms in an upright position and allow gravity to passively flex both wrists. The patient maintains this position for 60 seconds (Fig. 7.16). A positive test is indicated by reproduction of the patient's symptoms in the distribution of the median nerve.

Tinel's Sign

Tinel's sign is a test used to detect nerve irritation in multiple sites by tapping on the nerve. For this pathology, Tinel's sign is performed by tapping over the median nerve at the anterior wrist using a finger or reflex hammer (Fig. 7.17). A positive test is indicated by paresthesia into the hand in a median nerve distribution.

Common Interventions

Often an early intervention is to instruct the patient to wear a wrist splint.[14-17] Many sources recommend a splint that puts the wrist in a neutral position, or one with very slight wrist flexion or extension. The splint may be worn only at night or both day and night.

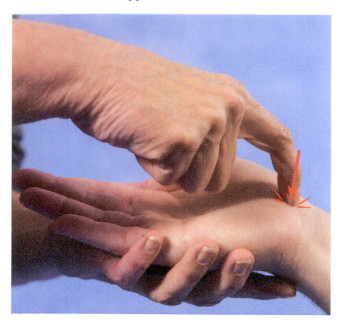

Figure 7.17 Tinel's sign may be performed over the median nerve at the wrist to assess carpal tunnel syndrome. Tapping on the nerve elicits tingling if the test is positive.

Patient education around activity modification for CTS is beneficial. The lowest pressure in the carpal tunnel has been shown to be at 0° wrist flexion/extension with a slightly pronated forearm.[15] Patients should be instructed to avoid prolonged or repeated wrist flexion and extension. As much as possible they should maintain a neutral wrist and forearm position. They should avoid forceful or sustained pinching and gripping.

The physical therapist may prescribe modalities to decrease swelling in the area, or to decrease inflammation. Pulsed ultrasound and laser have been shown to be effective. Soft tissue mobilization may also be used.

The plan of care may include tendon-gliding exercises (Box 7-1).[18,19] This series of movements will glide the flexor tendons and median nerve through the carpal tunnel. The exercises have been shown to be effective

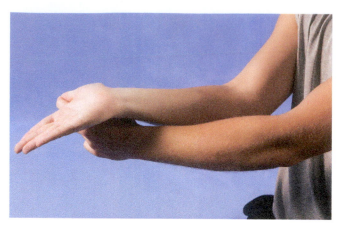

Figure 7.18 Tension exercises for the median nerve may be indicated in treatment of carpal tunnel syndrome.

in reducing the pressure in the carpal tunnel within 1 minute.[19–21] Usually, the patient is instructed to perform five repetitions of each position, holding for 7 seconds, 3 to 5 times a day. The patient may also gently put tension on the median nerve by extending the wrist, supinating the forearm, and stretching the thumb into extension as shown in Figure 7.18.[19] As the patient progresses, gentle strengthening exercises of the thenar muscles may be added to the plan of care. In addition to mobilizing the nerve and tendons, carpal mobilization may be beneficial to decrease pressure on the median nerve.[22]

Prevention

Prevention of CTS aims to decrease the contributing factors. Patients should be advised to avoid prolonged or forceful gripping and wrist positioning at end ranges of flexion or extension as much as possible. If activities and positions that can lead to CTS cannot be avoided, then instruct the patient to take frequent rest breaks or use the other hand. Modify work environments to promote neutral wrist positioning. Encourage the use of large-handle pens for prolonged handwriting.

Box 7-1 Tendon-Gliding Exercises for Carpal Tunnel Syndrome

The Bottom Line: for patients with carpal tunnel syndrome

Description and Causes	Compression of the median nerve due to overuse, anatomically small tunnel, or pregnancy
Test	Phalen's test, Tinel's sign over median nerve
Stretch	Glide the flexor tendons, gently stretch the median nerve
Strengthen	Thenar muscles
Train	NA
Avoid	Repeated wrist flexion and extension, prolonged positioning in end ranges of flexion and extension

Interventions for the Surgical Patient

Carpal Tunnel Release

If conservative measures are not successful and the patient has unrelenting pain, or weakness and atrophy, surgery may be recommended.

Surgery

Carpal tunnel release may be performed using an open technique or an endoscopic technique. Open carpal tunnel release is done through a lengthwise incision on the anterior wrist and hand that is about 2 inches long. Endoscopic release is done using small instruments that are inserted through one or two small incisions at the wrist and hand. In either case, the purpose of the surgery is to cut the transverse carpal ligament to give the median nerve more room. As the area heals, the space between the cut ends of the ligament fills in with scar tissue.

Postoperative Phase

After surgery, the patient may be placed in a splint for 4 to 6 weeks. The patient may be seen for modalities, scar tissue management, nerve- and tendon-gliding exercises, and strengthening. The plan of care may include the use of ultrasound or whirlpool for pain control and tissue extensibility prior to soft tissue mobilization. Gliding exercises as discussed above may be included. The plan of care may include strengthening exercises for the thenar intrinsic muscles. These are usually started after the incision heals and signs of inflammation resolve.

De Quervain Tenosynovitis

De Quervain disease is a pathology that involves painful gliding of the tendons of APL and EPB on the radial aspect of the wrist. The extensor retinaculum on the dorsum of the wrist becomes thickened, restricting the movement of these tendons through the compartment in which they lie. This may or may not be accompanied by inflammation of the two tendons and the synovial sheath that covers them as the tendons pass under the fibrotic retinaculum (Fig. 7.19).[23]

Causes/Contributing Factors

The factors that contribute to de Quervain disease are largely unknown. Repetitive motions or overuse may lead to degenerative changes in the extensor retinaculum and to thickening of the fibrous tunnel through which the tendons travel.[24] There may be an anatomical contributor; study of the anatomy in those with de Quervain syndrome shows a large percentage of two APL tendons and/or the tendon of EPB traveling in a separate sheath.[25] The pathology is 3 to 5 times more common in women than in men. The peak incidence appears to be during pregnancy and menopause, leading some researchers to conclude that hormones may contribute to the pathology.

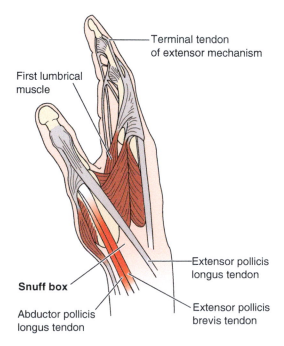

Figure 7.19 De Quervain tenosynovitis involves pathology of the abductor pollicis longus and extensor pollicis brevis on the lateral side of the wrist.

Symptoms

Patients with de Quervain disease usually have pain, tenderness, and swelling over the radial side of the wrist. Crepitus may be present when moving the thumb. Patients may complain of increased pain with gripping, use of the thumb, or moving of the hand into ulnar deviation. Usually the onset of the symptoms is gradual.

Clinical Signs

Pain is increased with palpation, stretch, and active contraction of the APL and EPB tendons.[26,27] The patient may have limited ROM into ulnar deviation, especially when the thumb is kept tucked into the palm. Decreased strength in the thumb or in pinch may be noted. The test for de Quervain disease is Finkelstein's test, but it is often modified as described by Eichhoff. Many clinicians perform it this way and incorrectly refer to the test as Finkelstein's.

Finkelstein Test

The Finkelstein test is done with the patient sitting or standing. The examiner holds the patient's thumb and moves the patient's hand into ulnar deviation (Fig. 7.20).[28] A positive test is indicated by reproduction of the patient's pain over the radial styloid process.

Eichhoff Test

Eichhoff's maneuver is a modification of the Finkelstein test. In this modified test, the patient is asked to flex the thumb into the palm and make a fist around the thumb. The patient is then instructed to slowly ulnarly deviate the wrist (Fig. 7.21). A positive test is indicated by reproduction of the patient's pain over the radial styloid process.

Common Interventions

The plan of care for de Quervain disease frequently involves modalities for pain and inflammation control,

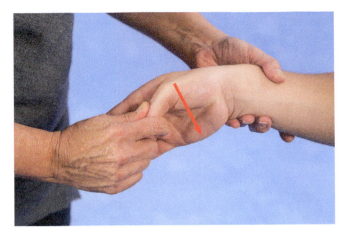

Figure 7.20 Finkelstein's test for de Quervain tenosynovitis.

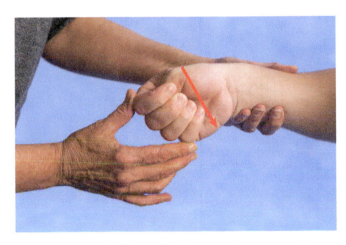

Figure 7.21 Eichhoff's test for de Quervain tenosynovitis.

such as ice massage, iontophoresis, high-volt electrical stimulation, or pulsed ultrasound over the tendons. Splinting of the wrist and thumb MP and IP joints may be used to rest the area. Soft tissue release, friction massage, or myofascial release may be beneficial. Joint mobilization of the thumb CMC and wrist radial glides may also be of benefit.[29] Concentric and eccentric strengthening exercises into wrist radial deviation and all thumb motions should be added to the treatment program as pain subsides.[27,30] Figure 7.22 shows common exercises in the plan of care for de Quervain disease.

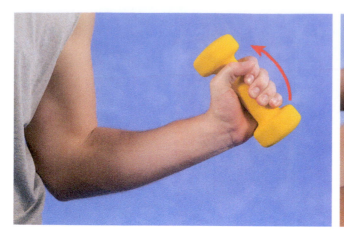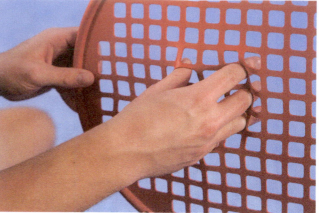

Figure 7.22 Strengthening exercises of radial deviators, and thumb extensors and abductors may be included in the POC for de Quervain disease.

The Bottom Line:	for patients with de Quervain syndrome
Description and Causes	Tendinopathy of APL and EPB caused by overuse or anatomical variance
Test	Finkelstein's test, Eichhoff's test
Stretch	Thumb abductor and extensor, other thumb muscles
Strengthen	Thumb abductor and extensor, wrist radial deviators
Train	NA
Avoid	Repetitive motions of the wrist into radial and ulnar deviation

Extensor Carpi Ulnaris Tendinopathy

This pathology of the tendon of extensor carpi ulnaris (ECU) includes tendonitis, tenosynovitis, tendinosis, and tendon rupture. The ECU tendon is very superficial and easily injured. Similar to the tendons of APL and EPB, the tendon of ECU has a synovial sleeve as it travels through a fibrous sheath under the extensor retinaculum. The tendon or synovial sleeve may become inflamed through overuse. Tendinosis may occur with chronic overloading of the tendon.

Causes/Contributing Factors

Tendonitis or tenosynovitis is often caused by repeated wrist flexion and extension in a supinated position. The most common mechanism for ECU tendinopathy is sports-related, particularly to tennis or golf.[31] Injuries to this area may also involve the TFCC and/or the distal radioulnar joint in addition to the ECU tendon.

Symptoms

The patient will often complain of an ache or pain on the ulnar side of the dorsum of the wrist. Swelling may be present. If the tendon is unstable due to a ruptured sheath, supination may be accompanied by a click or pop and a sensation of pain.

Clinical Signs

Typical of musculotendinous pathologies, pain will increase with palpation, stretch, and active contraction of the muscle.[31] Muscle testing of the ECU by resisting wrist extension and ulnar deviation will usually reproduce the pain. However, because this also compromises the other structures in the area, the ECU Synergy Test is preferred to diagnose ECU tendinopathy.

ECU Synergy Test

The patient is sitting with elbow bent to 90° and resting on a table. The forearm is supinated, and the wrist is kept in a neutral position with the fingers extended. The examiner grasps the patient's middle finger and thumb with one hand and palpates the ECU tendon with the other hand. The patient is instructed to radially abduct (extend) the thumb against resistance (Fig. 7.23). The examiner will feel the ECU tendon bowstring just distal to the ulnar styloid as the muscle contracts. A positive test for tendinopathy is indicated by reproduction of the patient's pain on the dorsal aspect of the ulnar wrist.[32]

Common Interventions

Initially, the patient will be instructed to rest the area. Splinting in a position of slight wrist extension and ulnar deviation may be helpful. Modalities to decrease inflammation may be included in the plan of care, including cryotherapy, pulsed ultrasound, and iontophoresis. Submaximal isometrics may also be included in the plan of care. As pain subsides, the patient may be progressed to isotonic exercise in wrist extension and ulnar deviation in both concentric and eccentric modes.

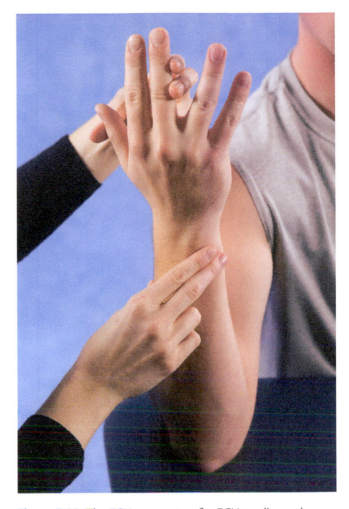

Figure 7.23 The ECU synergy test for ECU tendinopathy.

The Bottom Line:	for patients with extensor carpi ulnaris tendinopathy
Description and Causes	Tendinopathy caused by overuse, especially of wrist flexion/extension with a supinated forearm
Test	ECU synergy test
Stretch	NA
Strengthen	ECU by resisted wrist extension and ulnar deviation
Train	NA
Avoid	Sudden or repeated wrist flexion and extension with a supinated forearm

Nerve Lesions

Lesions of the radial, median, and ulnar nerves may cause weakness and deformity that are displayed in the wrist and hand. Recall the anatomy of peripheral nerves. Nerve axons are covered by myelin, with a connective tissue cover called an endoneurium. These covered axons are bundled in fascicles surrounded by a perineurium. Many fascicles make up the peripheral nerve and are held together by the epineurium.

In Chapter 4, we discussed neurapraxia, axonotmesis, and neurotmesis. Neurapraxia is the mildest form of nerve lesion, which may result from compression or trauma to the nerve. Recovery is full, within about 8 weeks. Axonotmesis is a lesion of the axon with an intact connective tissue sleeve of endoneurium. In this case, the axon may regenerate. However, regrowth is slow at about an inch per month. During the time of regrowth, sensation and motor function distal to the lesion is lost.

Neurotmesis is a complete destruction of the nerve and epineurium covering. Recovery requires surgical repair.

Causes/Contributing Factors

Trauma, compression, motor vehicle accidents, lacerations, falls, and military combat are often causes of peripheral nerve lesions in the arm. There are several contributors to peripheral nerve injury or entrapment.

- *Median nerve* lesions are commonly linked to laceration, blunt trauma to the anterior forearm, and carpal tunnel syndrome due to overuse.
- *Ulnar nerve* lesions are often linked to compression in the cubital tunnel or, in cyclists, at the wrist.[33] The ulnar nerve is vulnerable to laceration or compression at the wrist as it runs through a narrow canal superficial to the transverse carpal ligament called **Guyon's canal.**
- *Radial nerve* lesions may result from humeral fracture and from axillary compression related to improper use of crutches.

Symptoms

General symptoms of nerve lesion may include numbness, tingling, pain, weakness, and deformity. With nerve injury, the symptoms are usually noticed distal to the lesion, although pain may be felt proximal to the lesion. Muscles that are innervated by the nerve distal to the lesion will be weak. Specific symptoms and clinical signs will vary depending upon the nerve that is injured and the location of the lesion, as detailed below.

Clinical Signs

Median Nerve

The most likely site of entrapment or laceration of the median nerve is at the wrist. Sensation will be decreased or absent on the palm side of the hand, in the thumb, index, middle, and half of the ring fingers (Fig. 7.24). **Paresthesia** may be felt here. Muscle testing will reveal weakness of the intrinsic thumb flexor, abductor, opponens, and the first and second lumbricals.

A resting hand deformity that may occur with median nerve lesion at the wrist is an **ape hand.** This deformity is characterized by an inability to abduct or oppose the thumb. The thumb rests in the plane of the fingers instead of the typical resting position anterior to the fingers. The index and middle fingers may be pulled into hyperextension of the MP joints and flexion of the PIP and DIP joints, due to the loss of the lumbricals. The thenar eminence atrophies. See Figure 7.25.

If the median nerve is injured in the upper arm or at the elbow, the patient may display a **benediction hand** or bishop's hand when attempting to make a fist.[34] Because of the weakness of flexor digitorum superficialis and of flexor digitorum profundus of the index and middle fingers, when the patient tries to flex the

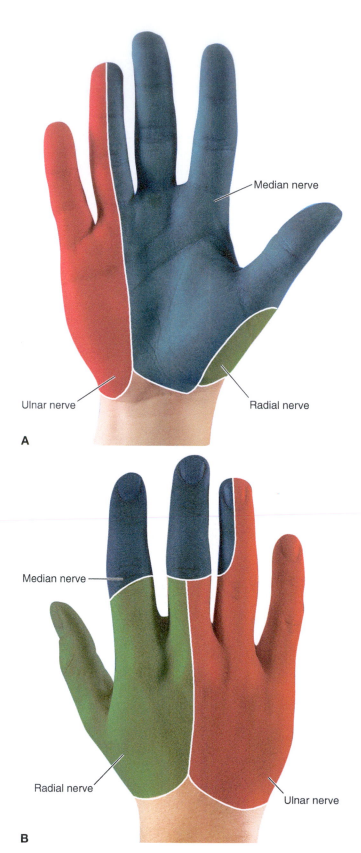

Figure 7.24 Sensory innervation of the hand is provided by the median, ulnar, and radial nerves.

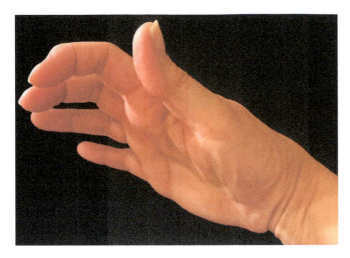

Figure 7.25 Ape hand deformity is caused by a median nerve lesion. The thenar area atrophies and the thumb is pulled into the plane of the fingers.

fingers only the ring and little finger curl. This is not a resting deformity but is seen with an active attempt to make a fist.

Ulnar Nerve

The ulnar nerve is most vulnerable to injury at the elbow as it passes through the cubital tunnel and at the wrist. The ulnar nerve carries sensation from the palm side of the hand in half of the ring finger and the little finger and the dorsum of the ring and little fingers. Sensation in this area may be compromised (Fig. 7.24). Weakness of the intrinsic little finger flexor, abductor, and opponens; the third and fourth lumbricals; and the palmar and dorsal interossei will often be present.

A resting hand deformity that may occur with ulnar nerve lesion at the wrist is an **ulnar claw** (Fig. 7.26). This deformity looks the same as the benediction hand, so it is important to make the distinction that this deformity occurs at rest or on attempts to extend the fingers.[35] It is characterized by extension of the MP joint and flexion of the PIP and DIP joints of the ring and little fingers due to the loss of the third and fourth lumbricals. The hypothenar eminence atrophies.

Watch Out For...

Watch out for the similar appearance of the ulnar claw deformity and the **bishop's hand**. While the position of the fingers is the same, the important difference is that the ulnar claw is a resting hand deformity that is caused by an ulnar nerve lesion, and **bishop's** hand is a position that occurs with attempts to make a fist in the presence of a median nerve lesion.

Injury to the ulnar nerve at the elbow may additionally result in weakness of the flexor digitorum profundus

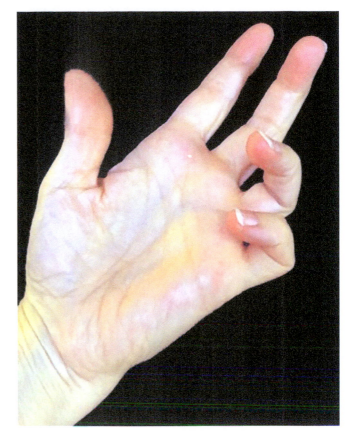

Figure 7.26 An ulnar claw is a result of an ulnar nerve lesion. This is a deformity due to the loss of the 3rd and 4th lumbricals. This deformity resembles the hand position assumed by patients with a median nerve lesion on attempts to make a fist (benediction hand).

to the 4th and 5th digits. While the patient will still demonstrate an ulnar claw deformity, this level of lesion will paradoxically result in less "clawing" of the fingers since the pull into flexion is decreased due to the weakness of FDP.

Radial Nerve

Likely sites of injury of the radial nerve include the posterior humerus (see "Volkmann's ischemic contracture" in Chapter 6), the proximal forearm, and the dorsum of the wrist. Proximal injury may result in sensory loss on the posterior upper arm, forearm, and the dorsum of the index and middle fingers (Fig. 7.24). Muscle testing may reveal weakness of the elbow, wrist, and hand extensors.

A deformity that may occur with radial nerve lesion above the elbow is **wrist drop**.[34] This deformity is characterized by an inability to extend the wrist and fingers (Fig. 7.27). Because of the synergistic action of wrist extensors in grip, the patient will also have decreased grip strength.

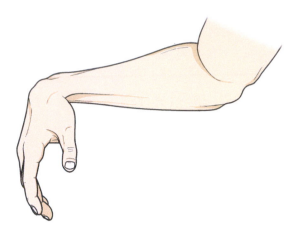

Figure 7.27 A radial nerve lesion results in wrist drop deformity.

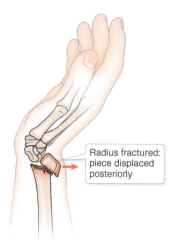

Radius fractured: piece displaced posteriorly

Colles fracture:
commonly due to fall
onto an extended hand

Figure 7.28 Colles' fracture of the distal radius often results in a deformity of the wrist called a dinner fork deformity.

Common Interventions

Physical therapy intervention after nerve injury will depend upon the cause and extent of the injury. Splinting or immobilization in a position of limited nerve stress may be used.[15-18]

 CLINICAL ALERT

Patient education should include information regarding activity modification and return to activity. The plan of care may include modalities to decrease inflammation. Initially, there may be positions, movements, and exercises that are contraindicated due to increased pressure on the nerve.

Mobilization of surrounding tendons and nerves may be beneficial to maintain nerve health.[35,36] Active range of motion exercises may be used to maintain or improve nerve and muscle function.

Fractures

Fractures of the wrist and hand are very common. Although fractures can occur in any of the bones in the wrist and hand, common fractures involve the distal radius and/or ulna, the scaphoid, the fourth and fifth metacarpals, and the phalanges.

A fracture of the wrist often involves the distal radius and/or ulna. This frequently occurs after a FOOSH injury. A distal radius fracture is called a **Colles' fracture.** It often leads to a wrist deformity due to the angle of the fractured segment, called a dinner fork deformity (Fig. 7.28).

The scaphoid is the most commonly fractured bone in the wrist. The bone is shaped like a peanut, with a narrow "waist." This fracture is particularly troublesome, as the blood supply to the scaphoid crosses this waist area and may be compromised in a fracture. This can lead to avascular necrosis of part of the scaphoid.

Metacarpal fractures present an unusual challenge in rehabilitation because the fracture site will be right next to tendons that need to glide to preserve movement. It becomes very important to maintain MP flexion and to ensure extensor digitorum continues to glide across the dorsum of the metacarpals as the fracture heals. A common fracture in this area involves the neck of the fourth or fifth metacarpal. This is called a **boxer's fracture** and may be caused by contact with an object with a closed fist.

Causes/Contributing Factors

Fractures of the wrist and hand are frequently caused by a fall on an outstretched hand, a direct blow, work-related accidents, and sports such as football, wrestling, and basketball. The most common cause is a fall, accounting for nearly half of all wrist and hand fractures.[37]

Symptoms

Pain is the most frequent indicator of a fracture. Pain may be felt at rest and increased with movement or palpation. The patient will also complain of limited motion and possibly a deformity. Swelling is likely to be present immediately after fracture.

Clinical Signs

With a history of trauma, complaint of pain with movement, limited range of motion, and tenderness to palpation, fracture will be suspected. To confirm the diagnosis x-rays are used.

Common Interventions

In general, after fracture the patient will be immobilized by splint, casting, internal fixation, or external fixation. The patient should be instructed to elevate the extremity to minimize swelling. Ice may be used for the first several days. Without compromising the fracture site, mobility of the nearby unaffected joints should be maintained.

Distal Radius or Radioulnar Fracture

If a distal radius or radioulnar fracture is stable and in good alignment, the patient may simply be casted or splinted. For unstable fractures or in instances where alignment is a problem, the patient may undergo a closed reduction, open reduction internal fixation (ORIF), or use of an external fixator.[38]

What's in the Plan of Care? The initial plan of care in the first six weeks may include finger, elbow, and shoulder range-of-motion exercises as are allowed by the splint or cast. Forearm pronation and supination is usually restricted in this phase. Around 6 to 8 weeks, immobilization by cast, splint, or external fixation will be removed. Active assisted range-of-motion exercises to the wrist and forearm may be included in the plan of care. Wrist flexion and extension and forearm supination and pronation may be very limited. After 8 weeks, gentle strengthening of the wrist and fingers may be included in the plan of care.[39,40]

Scaphoid Fracture

Fracture of the scaphoid will usually result in tenderness in the anatomical snuff box. Scaphoid fractures are treated very cautiously with a slow time line, as avascular necrosis and nonunion are common complications. A patient with scaphoid fracture will likely be immobilized in a cast or splint from the elbow to the MP joints. The thumb is usually immobilized by a thumb **spica**. To ensure union of the pieces and to shorten immobilization time, ORIF using a pin or screw may be performed.

If the patient does not undergo ORIF, the initial plan of care will likely include shoulder range of motion as well as mobilization of the finger MP, PIP, and DIP joints. By 6 to 12 weeks, the patient may be allowed to actively move the elbow, and the cast is replaced by a short arm cast. Active range-of-motion exercises may be initiated by about 12 weeks, and strengthening exercises by about 4 months after fracture.

If the patient undergoes ORIF, by 4 to 8 weeks the elbow immobilization is discontinued. Active range-of-motion exercises may be initiated by about 8 weeks and strengthening exercises by about 3 months after fracture.

Metacarpal Fracture

Metacarpal fractures heal very quickly due to good blood supply. However, the location of the fracture, the presence of multiple fractures, and whether the patient underwent surgical repair are important considerations in treatment of hand fractures. Because of these considerations, the patient may be casted or splinted from the wrist with

the fingers freely moveable, immobilized to the MP joints, or fully immobilized to the DIP joints.

It is common with a boxer's fracture for the patient to be casted or splinted with slight wrist extension and MP flexion. The cast will usually immobilize the fingers in relative extension. At 4 weeks, the patient may be splinted to allow restricted exercises but may be required to wear the splint when not in therapy until 6 weeks after fracture.[41]

Dupuytren's Disease (Palmar Fibromatosis)

Dupuytren's disease (Dupuytren's contracture) is a flexion contracture most commonly of the ring and little fingers due to thickening of the palmar fascia. The disorder is characterized by nodules in the palm that proliferate into ropelike collagen cords. The cords shorten, drawing the fingers into flexion.[42] Typically, the MP and PIP joints become contracted in a flexed position, which leads to impaired grip and hand function.

Causes/Contributing Factors

The collagen in the palmar fascia is normally thin, but in Dupuytren's disease it becomes thickened and fibrotic. The reason for this is unknown, but Dupuytren's contracture is up to 10 times more common in men. It has a strong hereditary cause[43] and has been linked to diabetes.[44] Some studies also link it to alcohol consumption, smoking, and occupations that involve hand vibration.[45,46]

Symptoms

The initial sign of Dupuytren's disease is frequently a nodule or dimpling in the palm of one hand. The nodule may initially be tender, but usually the tenderness subsides. As the disease progresses, the patient is likely to experience the contracture of the fourth and fifth digits, and complain of difficulty with activities such as putting on gloves, buttoning a shirt, washing hands, and gripping. Both hands may become involved.

Clinical Signs

The clinical signs of Dupuytren's disease are the findings of a dimple or pit, a hard bump or knot, or a cord of tissue in the palm of the hand, usually proximal to the fourth or fifth digits. In later stages, the fingers begin to draw in in a characteristic fashion (Fig. 7.29).

Common Interventions

At the onset of the process, the patient will benefit from education regarding the disease process and future surgical options. Nonsurgical treatment options include injections of cortisone or collagenase.[47,48] Radiation therapy has been used to treat Dupuytren's

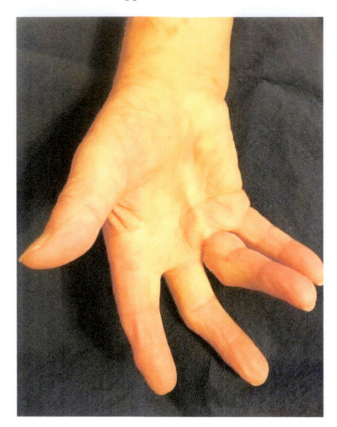

Figure 7.29 Dupuytren's disease is characterized initially by knots or cords in the palm. Eventually it results in flexion contracture of the finger(s).

disease in the early stages. With progression of the deformity, the patient may become a candidate for surgical release.

Interventions for the Surgical Patient
Dupuytren's Release

Several methods are currently used to release the palmar fascia in the patient with Dupuytren's disease. The fascia may be partially or completely removed (**fasciectomy**), the skin and underlying fascia may be removed (**dermo-fasciectomy**), or the fascial layers may be divided (**fasciotomy**) through an open incision or with a closed technique using a blade or needle.[44]

Postoperative Phase

Immediately after surgery the patient may be put in a splint that restricts extension of the MP joints as the palm heals. After the incision heals, the patient may use a night splint that maintains the fingers in extension. A common complication is joint stiffness and loss of flexion ROM. Passive range-of-motion exercises and gentle strengthening may be included in the plan of care when the incision heals. There is a high rate of recurrence of the contracture after surgery.

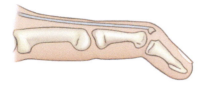

Figure 7.30 Mallet finger is a result of avulsion of the extensor digitorum tendon, with loss of active finger DIP extension.

Hand Tendon Deformities

The following hand deformities are not usually treated in physical therapy. However, they may impact patient function. They are presented here for the purpose of understanding and of communicating deformities of the hand.

Mallet Finger

Mallet finger is caused by the avulsion of the extensor digitorum tendon from the distal phalanx. This is typically due to a sports injury or a blow to the end of the finger. Mallet finger is characterized by an inability to actively extend the DIP joint (Fig. 7.30). The deformity is often corrected by splinting for 6 to 8 weeks but may require surgery to reattach the tendon.

Boutonniere Deformity

This deformity is characterized by flexion of the PIP joint and hyperextension of the DIP joint. It occurs when the middle portion of the extensor hood ruptures at the PIP joint, and the lateral parts of the hood slip anteriorly, pulling the PIP joint into flexion (Fig. 7.31). This may be caused by inflammatory conditions such as rheumatoid arthritis (RA) or by damage to the extensor hood from trauma or burn. The deformity may be lessened or corrected by splinting or surgery.

Swan Neck Deformity

A swan neck deformity is characterized by hyperextension of the PIP joint and flexion of the DIP joint (Fig. 7.31). This deformity may occur in patients with rheumatoid arthritis due to the rupture of the ligament on the anterior aspect of the PIP joint. The patient may benefit from the use of splinting and therapy. Surgical correction includes joint arthroplasty or fusion.

Ulnar Drift Deformity

Ulnar drift deformity, also known as ulnar deviation of the fingers, may occur in patients with rheumatoid arthritis. The MCP joints sublux anteriorly and the fingers are pulled toward the little finger (Fig. 7.31). Splinting, education in joint protection, and physical therapy may be beneficial.

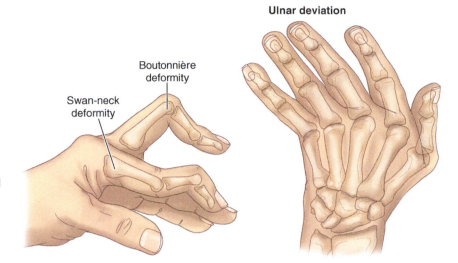

Figure 7.31 Boutonniere, swan neck, and ulnar drift deformities are frequently a result of RA. Boutonniere deformity is characterized by PIP flexion and DIP extension. Swan neck deformity is characterized by PIP hyperextension and DIP flexion. Ulnar drift involves ulnar deviation of the fingers with MCP subluxation.

Trigger Finger

Trigger finger is a **stenosing tenosynovitis** involving a flexor tendon and sheath. Stenosis indicates that the passageway is constricted, either due to an enlargement of the tendon or a narrowing of the opening. Tenosynovitis is an inflammation of the tendon and synovial sheath that covers it. Trigger finger is linked to diabetes, rheumatoid arthritis, and gout.

As a result of the constricted passageway, the finger gets stuck in a flexed position. When further efforts are made to move the finger, the tendon pops through the opening, causing a snapping sensation. At times the patient must use the other hand to straighten the finger. Figure 7.32 depicts a trigger finger due to an enlarged area on the flexor tendon. Patients with trigger finger may benefit from steroid injections into the tendon or surgery to open the constricted tunnel for the flexor tendon.

SUMMARY

In this chapter we have discussed the complexity of the hand. This complexity allows the hand great versatility in position and function. It also predisposes the hand to injury and pathology that significantly impact patients' activities of daily living and occupations. Rehabilitation must be undertaken with thorough knowledge of hand anatomy, function, and pathology.

REVIEW QUESTIONS

1. With your lab partner, review the bones, joints, and muscles in the distal forearm, wrist, and hand area. Discuss the soft tissue structures, including the transverse carpal ligament, extensor expansion, TFCC, and palmar aponeurosis.

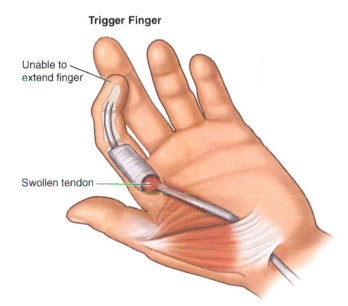

Figure 7.32 Trigger finger is often caused by an enlarged flexor tendon. The finger may get stuck in a flexed position. Attempts to straighten it result in a snapping sensation.

2. With your lab partner, trace the path of the median, ulnar, and radial nerves from above the elbow to the hand. What muscles are innervated along the path of each nerve?

3. Compare and contrast the hand deformity of ulnar claw and benediction hand. What nerve injury is responsible for the deformity? In what ways are they similar? In what ways are they different?

4. You are treating a patient with carpal tunnel syndrome and the plan of care includes instruction in tendon-gliding exercises and stretch of the

median nerve. Simulating with your lab partner, instruct your patient in these exercises.

5. Which two tendons are involved in de Quervain tenosynovitis? How would you stretch these muscles/tendons? How would you strengthen them?

6. Compare and contrast ape hand, benediction hand, and carpal tunnel syndrome. What nerve is involved in each?

7. For each of the following special tests, name the pathology that yields a positive test:
   a. ECU synergy test
   b. Eichhoff's test
   c. Finkelstein's test
   d. Phalen's test
   e. Tinel's sign

PATIENT CASE: Carpal Tunnel Syndrome

PT Evaluation

Patient Name: XXX XXXXXXXXX   **Age:** 39   **BMI:** 23.8

Diagnosis/History

Medical Diagnosis: Carpal tunnel syndrome R

PT Diagnosis: Pain, paresthesia, weakness secondary to carpal tunnel syndrome R hand

Diagnostic Tests/Results: EMG/NCV – positive for CTS

Relevant Medical History: Hypothyroidism, depression

Prior Level of Function: Previous fracture of R scaphoid 8 years ago

Patient's Goals: Decrease pain in hand

Medications: Levothyroxine 100 mcg daily, celexa 20 mg daily

Precautions: Wears night splint

Social Supports/Safety Hazards

Patient Living Situation/ Supports/ Hazards: Recently divorced

Patient Working Situation/Occupation/ Leisure Activities: Employed as physician's assistant for an orthopedic surgeon.

Vital Signs

At rest Temperature: 98.6   BP: 124/76   HR: 78   Resp: 14   O2 sat: 98

Subjective Information

Patient is a male with gradual onset of paresthesia in R hand, esp. at night. This has been interfering with sleep for four weeks. Patient has been using a wrist splint at night with some benefit. Notes pain and paresthesia while at work as well.

Physical Assessment

Orientation: Alert and oriented   **Speech/Vision/Hearing:** wears glasses   **Skin Integrity:** Intact

ROM: WNL

Strength: 4/5 MMT in FPB, OP, and APB, 1&2 lumbricals   **Palpation:** No pain on palpation

Muscle Tone: Not tested   **Balance/Coordination:** Not tested   **Sensation/Proprioception:** Decreased over thumb and digits 2&3

Endurance: Not tested   **Posture:** Rounded shoulders   **Edema:** None

Pain

Pain Rating and Location: At best 0/10   **At worst** 5/10   **Relieving Factors:** Wrist splint, repositioning wrist

Aggravating Factors: Sleeping, prolonged positioning   **Irritability:** After repositioning, he gets relief after about 15 minutes.

Functional Assessment

Patient is functionally independent. He continues to work full-time.

Special Testing

Test Name: Phalen test   **Result** Positive   **Test Name:**   **Result**

Assessment

Patient has s/s consistent with carpal tunnel syndrome R.

Short-Term Treatment Goals

1. Patient will state a 25% decrease in episodes of pain at night.
2. Patient will voice and demonstrate an understanding of the contributing factors of CTS.
3. Patient will be independent in HEP.

Long-Term Treatment Goals

1. Patient will state a 75% decrease in pain.

Treatment Plan

Frequency/Duration: 3 times a week for 3 weeks

Consisting of: Modalities, therapeutic exercise, neuro re-education, patient education

continued

Patient Case Questions

1. The patient asks you to describe the cause of his symptoms. What would you tell him?

2. What factors might be contributing to the patient's CTS?

3. What would you tell the patient about specific activities to avoid?

4. What data will you collect the first time you see the patient?

5. If the plan of care does not guide you, what modalities might you use with this patient? Why? Are any modalities contraindicated?

6. If the plan of care does not specifically guide you, describe three therapeutic exercises that are indicated for this patient. Justify your choices.

7. What other special tests might you use to monitor the patient's progress?

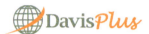 For additional resources, including answers to this case, please visit
http://davisplus.fadavis.com

REFERENCES

1. Kaufmann, R. A., Pfaeffle, H. J., Blankenhorn, B. D., Stabile, K., Robertson, D., & Goitz, R. (2006). Kinematics of the midcarpal and radiocarpal joint in flexion and extension: An in vitro study. *Journal of Hand Surgery, 31,* 1142–1148.

2. Lippert, L. S. (2017). *Clinical kinesiology and anatomy.* Philadelphia, PA: F.A. Davis Company.

3. Kaufmann, R. A., Pfaeffle, H. J., Blankenhorn, B. D., Stabile, K., Robertson, D., & Goitz, R. (2005). Kinematics of the midcarpal and radiocarpal joints in radioulnar deviation: An in vitro study. *Journal of Hand Surgery, 30,* 937–942.

4. Levangie, P. K., Norkin, C. C., & Levangie, P. K. (2011). *Joint structure and function: A comprehensive analysis.* Philadelphia, PA: F.A. Davis Co.

5. Palmer, A. K., & Werner, F. W. (1981). The triangular fibrocartilage complex of the wrist—Anatomy and function. *Journal of Hand Surgery, 6,* 153–162.

6. Bednar, M. S., Arnoczky, S. P., & Weiland, A. J. (1991). The microvasculature of the triangular fibrocartilage complex: Its clinical significance. *Journal of Hand Surgery, 16,* 1101–1105.

7. McDiarmid, M., Oliver, M., Ruser, J., & Gucer, P. (2000). Male and female rate differences in carpal tunnel syndrome injuries: Personal attributes or job tasks? *Environmental Research, 83,* 23–32.

8. Hlebs, S., Majhenic, K., & Vidmar, G. (2014). Body mass index and anthropometric characteristics of the hand as risk factors for carpal tunnel syndrome. *Collegium Antropologicum, 38,* 219–226.

9. Kiani, J., Goharifar, H., Moghimbeigi, A., & Azizkhani, H. (2014). Prevalence and risk factors of five most common upper extremity disorders in diabetics. *Journal of Research in Health Sciences, 14,* 92–95.

10. Mediouni, Z., de Roquemaurel, A., Dumontier, C., Becour, B., Garrabe, H., Roquelaure, Y., & Descatha, A. (2014). Is carpal tunnel syndrome related to computer exposure at work? A review and meta-analysis. *Journal of Occupational and Environmental Medicine, 56,* 204–208.

11. You, D., Smith, A. H., & Rempel, D. (2014). Meta-analysis: Association between wrist posture and carpal tunnel syndrome among workers. *Safety and Health at Work, 5,* 27–31.

12. Zyluk, A. (2013). Carpal tunnel syndrome in pregnancy: A review. *Polish Orthopedics and Traumatology, 78,* 223–227.

13. Wainner, R. S., Fritz, J. M., Irrgang, J. J., Delitto, A., Allison, S., & Boninger, M. L. (2005). Development of a clinical prediction rule for the diagnosis of carpal tunnel syndrome. *Archives of Physical Medicine and Rehabilitation, 86,* 609–618.

14. Brininger, T. L., Rogers, J. C., Holm, M. B., Baker, N. A., Li, Z. M., & Goitz, R. J. (2007). Efficacy of a fabricated customized splint and tendon and nerve gliding exercises for the treatment of carpal tunnel syndrome: A randomized controlled trial. *Archives of Physical Medicine and Rehabilitation, 88,* 1429–1435.

15. Michlovitz, S. L. (2004). Conservative interventions for carpal tunnel syndrome. *Journal of Orthopaedic and Sports Physical Therapy, 34,* 589–600.

16. O'Connor, D., Marshall, S., & Massy-Westropp, N. (2003). Non-surgical treatment (other than steroid injection) for carpal tunnel syndrome. *Cochrane Database of Systematic Reviews, 1,* CD003219.

17. Werner, R. A., Franzblau, A., & Gell, N. (2005). Randomized controlled trial of nocturnal splinting for active workers with symptoms of carpal tunnel syndrome. *Archives of Physical Medicine and Rehabilitation, 86,* 1–7.

18. Kisner, C., & Colby, L. A. (2012). *Therapeutic exercise: Foundations and techniques.* Philadelphia, PA: F.A. Davis.

19. Rozmaryn, L. M., Dovelle, S., Rothman, E. R., Gorman, K., Olvey, K. M., & Bartko, J. J. (1998). Nerve and tendon gliding exercises and the conservative management of carpal tunnel syndrome. *Journal of Hand Therapy: Official Journal of the American Society of Hand Therapists, 11,* 171–179.

20. Seradge, H., Jia, Y. C., & Owens, W. (1995). In vivo measurement of carpal tunnel pressure in the functioning hand. *Journal of Hand Surgery, 20,* 855–859.

21. Wehbé, M. A. (1987). Tendon gliding exercises. *American Journal of Occupational Therapy, 41,* 164–167.

22. Tal-Akabi, A., & Rushton, A. (2000). An investigation to compare the effectiveness of carpal bone mobilisation and neurodynamic mobilisation as methods of treatment for carpal tunnel syndrome. *Manual Therapy, 5,* 214–222.

23. Huissstede, B. M. A., Coert, J. H., Fridén, J., European HANDGUIDE Group. (Hoogvliet, P., & 2014). Consensus on a multidisciplinary treatment guideline for de Quervain disease:

Results from the European HANDGUIDE study. *Physical Therapy, 94*, 1095–1110.

24. Barr, A. E., Barbe, M. F., & Clark, B. D. (2004). Work-related musculoskeletal disorders of the hand and wrist: Epidemiology, pathophysiology, and sensorimotor changes. *Journal of Orthopaedic and Sports Physical Therapy, 34*, 610–627.

25. Kulthanan, T., & Chareonwat, B. (2007). Variations in abductor pollicis longus and extensor pollicis brevis tendons in the Quervain syndrome: A surgical and anatomical study. *Scandinavian Journal of Plastic and Reconstructive Surgery and Hand Surgery, 41*, 36–38.

26. Alexander, R. D., Catalano, L. W., Barron, O. A., & Glickel, S. Z. (2002). The extensor pollicis brevis entrapment test in the treatment of de Quervain's disease. *Journal of Hand Surgery, 27*, 813–816.

27. Howell, E. R. (2012). Conservative care of De Quervain's tenosynovitis/tendinopathy in a warehouse worker and recreational cyclist: A case report. *Journal of the Canadian Chiropractic Association, 56*, 121–127.

28. Elliott, B. G. (1992). Finkelstein's test: A descriptive error that can produce a false positive. *Journal of Hand Surgery, Edinburgh, Scotland, 17*, 481–482.

29. Backstrom, K. M. (2002). Mobilization with movement as an adjunct intervention in a patient with complicated de Quervain's tenosynovitis: A case report. *Journal of Orthopaedic and Sports Physical Therapy, 32*, 86–94; discussion 94–97.

30. Forget, N., Piotte, F., Arsenault, J., Harris, P., & Bourbonnais, D. (2008). Bilateral thumb's active range of motion and strength in de Quervain's disease: Comparison with a normal sample. *Journal of Hand Therapy: Official Journal of the American Society of Hand Therapists, 21*, 276–284.

31. Campbell, D., Campbell, R., O'Connor, P., & Hawkes, R. (2013). Sports-related extensor carpi ulnaris pathology: A review of functional anatomy, sports injury and management. *British Journal of Sports Medicine, 47*, 1105–1111.

32. Ruland, R. T., & Hogan, C. J. (2008). The ECU synergy test: An aid to diagnose ECU tendonitis. *Journal of Hand Surgery, 33*, 1777–1782.

33. Wilmarth, M. A., & Nelson, S. G. (1988). Distal sensory latencies of the ulnar nerve in long distance bicyclists: Pilot study. *Journal of Orthopaedic and Sports Physical Therapy, 9*, 370–374.

34. Barohn, R. J. (2013). *Peripheral neuropathies, An issue of neurologic clinics, e-book.* Philadelphia, PA: Elsevier Health Sciences.

35. Butler, D. S., & Jones, M. A. (1991). *Mobilisation of the nervous system.* United Kingdom: Churchill Livingstone.

36. Elvey, R. L. (1986). Treatment of arm pain associated with abnormal brachial plexus tension. *Australian Journal of Physiotherapy, 32*, 225–230.

37. Chung, K. C., & Spilson, S. V. (2001). The frequency and epidemiology of hand and forearm fractures in the United States. *Journal of Hand Surgery, 26*, 908–915.

38. Wulf, C. A., Ackerman, D. B., & Rizzo, M. (2007). Contemporary evaluation and treatment of distal radius fractures. *Hand Clinics, 23*, 209–226, vi.

39. Brotzman, S. B., & Manske, R. C. (2011). *Clinical orthopaedic rehabilitation: An evidence-based approach.* Philadelphia, PA: Elsevier Health Sciences.

40. Slutsky, D. J., & Herman, M. (2005). Rehabilitation of distal radius fractures: A biomechanical guide. *Hand Clinics, 21*, 455–468.

41. Hardy, M. A. Principles of metacarpal and phalangeal fracture management: A review of rehabilitation concepts. (2004). *Journal of Orthopaedic and Sports Physical Therapy, 34*, 781–799.

42. DiBenedetti, D. B., Nguyen, D., Zografos, L., Ziemiecki, R., & Zhou, X. (2011). Prevalence, incidence, and treatments of Dupuytren's disease in the United States: Results from a population-based study. *Hand, 6*, 149–158.

43. Larsen, S., Krogsgaard, D. G., Aagaard Larsen, L., Iachina, M., Skytthe, A., & Frederiksen, H. (2014). Genetic and environmental influences in Dupuytren's disease: A study of 30,330 Danish twin pairs. *Journal of Hand Surgery, European Volume, 40*, 171–176.

44. Bayat, A., & McGrouther, D. (2006). Management of Dupuytren's disease—Clear advice for an elusive condition. *Annals of the Royal College of Surgeons of England, 88*, 3–8.

45. Becker, K., Tinschert, S., Lienert, A., Bleuler, P. E., Staub, F., Meinel, A., Rößler, J., et al. (2014). The importance of genetic susceptibility in Dupuytren's disease. *Clinical Genetics, 87*, 483–487.

46. Descatha, A., Carton, M., Mediouni, Z., Dumontier, C., Roquelaure, Y., Goldberg, M., Zins, M., et al. (2014). Association between work exposure, alcohol intake, smoking and Dupuytren's disease in a large cohort study (Gazel). *BMJ Open, 4*, e004214.

47. Eaton, C. (2014). Evidence-based medicine: Dupuytren contracture. *Plastic and Reconstructive Surgery, 133*, 1241–1251.

48. Sood, A., Therattil, P. J., Paik, A. M., Simpson, M. F., & Lee, E. S. (2014). Treatment of dupuytren disease with injectable collagenase in a veteran population: A case series at the department of veterans affairs new jersey health care system. *Eplasty, 14*, e13.

PART III

Spine

Chapter 8

Orthopedic Interventions for the Cervical Spine and Temporomandibular Joint

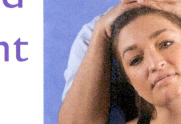

Anatomy and Physiology

Bone and Joint Anatomy and Physiology
    Cervical Spine
    Temporomandibular Joint
Soft Tissue Anatomy and Physiology
    Intervertebral Disc and Vertebral End Plates
    Cervical Spine Ligaments and Joint Capsules
    TMJ Disc, Ligaments, and Joint Capsule
    Nerves
    Blood Supply
Muscular Anatomy and Kinesiology
    Muscular Connection Between the TMJ
      and the Cervical Spine
Posture

Cervical Spine Kinematics
    Effect of Facet Joint Orientation on
      Movement
    Effect of Movement on the Disc,
      Ligaments, and Foramen
TMJ Kinematics

Common Pathologies

Cervicogenic Headache
    Causes/Contributing Factors
    Symptoms
    Clinical Signs
    Intervention
Whiplash
    Causes/Contributing Factors
    Symptoms
    Clinical Signs
    Intervention

Degenerative Joint Disease
Facet Joint DJD
    Causes/Contributing Factors
    Symptoms

    Clinical Signs
    Intervention
Spinal Stenosis (DJD in the Spinal Canal)
    Causes/Contributing Factors
    Symptoms
    Clinical Signs
    Intervention
DJD in the Neural Foramen (Foraminal Stenosis)
    Causes/Contributing Factors
    Symptoms
    Clinical Signs
    Intervention

LEARNING OUTCOMES

At the end of this chapter, the student will:

8.1 Describe the anatomy of the cervical spine and the temporomandibular joint.

8.2 Describe normal range of motion of the cervical spine and temporomandibular joint.

8.3 Discuss normal posture, forward head posture, and cervical retraction in terms of the position of the upper and lower cervical spine.

8.4 Explain normal kinematics of the cervical spine and the temporomandibular joint.

8.5 Discuss the effect of flexion and extension of the spine on the neural foramen and the intervertebral disk.

8.6 Describe common cervical spine and temporomandibular pathologies and typical presentations.

8.7 Discuss contributing factors to various cervical spine and temporomandibular pathologies and, when relevant, preventive measures.

8.8 Describe the clinical tests that may be used to diagnose common cervical spine and temporomandibular pathologies and how to administer the tests.

8.9 Discuss common treatment interventions for cervical spine and temporomandibular pathologies.

8.10 Describe the relationship of whiplash to cervicogenic headache and temporomandibular dysfunction.

8.11 Discuss the importance of normal strength in the deep cervical flexors in the treatment of various cervical pathologies.

8.12 Describe the clinical alert precautions for cervical spine and temporomandibular pathologies.

KEY WORDS

Arthrogenic	Extruded disc	Peripheralization
Bruxism	Flexion bias	Protruded disc
Centralization	Foraminotomy	Radiculopathy
Cervical myelopathy	Forward head posture	Reflex arc
Cervicogenic	Malocclusion	Sequestered disc
Dermatome	Mastication	Shoulder abduction relief sign
Directional preference	Myogenic	Stenosis
Epidural steroid injection	Myotome	
Extension bias	Osteophyte	

Anatomy and Physiology

The spine is a complex region that is a frequent source of pathology. An understanding and appreciation of this area is essential for the PTA. This chapter discusses the cervical spine and the temporomandibular joint. The thoracic and lumbosacral spine will be discussed in Chapter 9.

The cervical region is the most flexible area of the spine. This mobility is necessary to orient the head, eyes, ears, and nose within our environment. Yet, the spinal cord must be protected by a stable structure. The anatomy of this area is designed to accomplish both purposes.

The specialized vertebrae in the cervical spine provide maximum movement into rotation and sidebending. The density of ligaments and intricacy of muscles in the area counteract this mobility.

The temporomandibular joint (TMJ) has muscular connections to the cervical spine and can affect, and be affected by, the cervical spine. An understanding of this relationship, and normal structure and function of the TMJ, is necessary for providing physical therapy interventions.

Bone and Joint Anatomy and Physiology

The spine consists of a column of vertebral bodies separated by intervertebral disks. Many ligaments and muscles support the spine. The vertebrae change in size, features, and facet orientation in each region of the spine, but the essential characteristics remain. The components of the vertebrae can be seen in Figure 8.1.

Cervical Spine

The cervical spine contains seven vertebrae. The first cervical vertebra, atlas, articulates with the occipital condyles at the atlanto-occipital (AO) joint. The second cervical vertebra, axis, articulates with the atlas at the atlanto-axial (AA) joint. Both joints are highly specialized, and the vertebrae bear minimal resemblance to the rest of the cervical vertebrae. The remaining cervical vertebrae resemble the prototype as shown in Figure 8.1. The

Seventh cervical vertebra

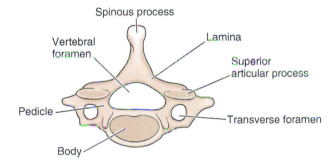

Figure 8.1 Typical features of all vertebrae include the vertebral body, spinous process, transverse processes, pedicles, lamina, superior and inferior articular processes, and spinal canal. In the cervical spine, the vertebrae have a transverse foramen.

vertebral bodies are small, with a relatively large spinal canal.

Facet joints are the point of contact between the superior articular processes of one vertebra with the inferior articular processes of the vertebra above. The alignment of the facet joints in the spine is an important consideration. Most cervical facet joints lie in a plane about 45° between the transverse and frontal plane (Fig. 8.2). The facet joints between atlas and axis lie mostly in the transverse plane. The superior facet joints of atlas are curved surfaces that cup the occipital condyles, lying in a plane midway between the transverse and sagittal. The significance of this will be discussed in "Kinematics" later in this chapter.

Transitional vertebrae at the junction between regions of the spine often have common characteristics of both regions. C7 and T1 are transitional vertebrae. These vertebrae and junction bear special attention, as they are frequently the site of pathology.

Temporomandibular Joint

The TMJ is the synovial articulation between the articular eminence and mandibular fossa of the temporal bone and the condyle of the mandible. The joint surfaces are covered with cartilage, which allows them to withstand stress. A fibrocartilage, S-shaped disc lies in the joint. The joint complex has two distinct joint capsules, dividing the joint into an upper and a lower joint. These two joints must work in unison for the joint to function properly.

The TMJ is moved almost continuously throughout the day as it is involved in chewing, swallowing, talking, and mouth opening and closing. It must be capable of generating significant force for chewing and also fine movements when talking. Figure 8.3 depicts the TMJ.

Table 8-1 summarizes the bony anatomy of the TMJ and the cervical spine and adjacent structures.

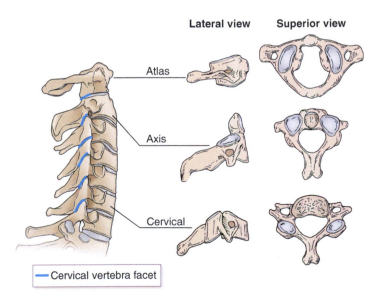

Figure 8.2 The facet joints of the cervical spine lie in a transverse to transverse-sagittal plane.

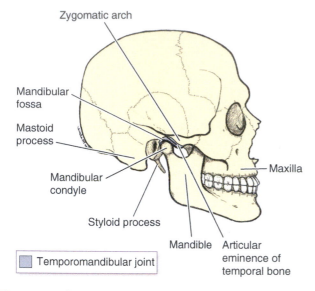

Zygomatic arch

Mandibular fossa

Mastoid process

Mandibular condyle

Styloid process

Maxilla

Mandible   Articular eminence of temporal bone

□ Temporomandibular joint

Figure 8.3 The temporomandibular joint is the articulation of the head of the mandible and the temporal bone.

Soft Tissue Anatomy and Physiology

Intervertebral Disc and Vertebral End Plates

Intervertebral discs are found between the vertebral bodies from C2–3 down, with no discs present in the AO and AA joints. The disc has two parts: the nucleus pulposus and the annulus fibrosus. The nucleus pulposus is the center of the disc and consists of a water-based gel substance. The annulus fibrosus is made up of concentric rings of collagen that contain the nucleus pulposus. Only the outermost rings of the annulus fibrosus are innervated. The inner rings and the nucleus pulposus have neither nerve nor blood supply.

The vertebral end plates are cartilage coverings on the vertebral body. End plates may be considered to be

Table 8-1 Bone and Joint Anatomy and Physiology

Of the Cervical Spine and TMJ

Joint	Anatomy	Normal ROM and Movements	Landmarks	Clinical Considerations
Atlanto-occipital (AO)	Ring-shaped atlas acts as a "washer" between occipital condyles and C2. Facet joints lie between sagittal and transverse plane, facing medially and superiorly.	Flexion 5 Extension 10° Sidebending 5° to each side Rotation 3°–5° to each side	Flat condyles of occiput and superior articular processes of atlas. Transverse foramen. No vertebral body.	Occipital condyles roll on the superior articular processes to move head into flexion and extension. Head and neck rotation occurring here is very minimal.
Atlanto-axial (AA)	Facet joints lie mostly in the transverse plane, facing superiorly and laterally.	Flexion 5° Extension 10° Sidebending none Rotation 40°–45° to each side	Large odontoid process (dens) on C2.	Nearly half of the rotation of the C-spine occurs here. The dens and supporting ligaments are vital to the stability of this joint. Rheumatoid arthritis may lead to erosion of the dens, or subluxation of the dens through the foramen magnum.
C2–3 to C6–7	Facet joints lie at about 45° angle between frontal and transverse plane.	Flexion 35° Extension 70° Sidebending 35° to each side Rotation 45° to each side		Movements of sidebending and rotation always occur together to the same side due to the orientation of the facet joints.
C7–T1	Facet joints lie more toward frontal plane than others in cervical spine.		C7 spinous process is usually most prominent and used as landmark.	
Temporo-mandibular Joint (TMJ)	Articulation between mandibular fossa and articular eminence on temporal bone and mandibular head.	Maximal mouth opening varies by sex and face type, but generally 40–50 mm is normal.	Just anterior to the external auditory meatus on lateral face.	Has a fibrocartilage disc between surfaces.

part of the vertebral body or the intervertebral disc. They are attached to the annulus fibrosus and provide nutrition to the intervertebral disc through diffusion. Figure 8.4 depicts the intervertebral disc and vertebral end plate.

Cervical Spine Ligaments and Joint Capsules

Multiple ligaments support the spinal column. In the cervical spine, the major ligaments are the anterior and posterior longitudinal ligaments, the ligamentum flavum, the intertransverse ligament, and the ligamentum nuchae. The ligamentum nuchae becomes the supraspinous and interspinous ligaments below C7.

The facet joints are synovial joints with a joint capsule. The capsule appears to restrict motion, assisting the ligaments to stabilize the spine. This seems to be of special importance at the transitional junctions of C7–T1 and L4–S1. Table 8-2 summarizes the soft tissues of the cervical spine.

TMJ Disc, Ligaments, and Joint Capsule

An elongated articular disc lies in the TMJ. This disc is biconcave; that is, it is concave over the articular eminence

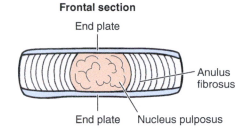

Frontal section

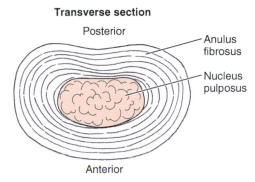

Transverse section

Figure 8.4 Intervertebral disc and vertebral end plates. The fibrous rings of the annulus fibrosus contain the gel substance of the nucleus pulposus.

Table 8-2 Connective Tissue Anatomy and Physiology

Of the Cervical Spine

Structure	Anatomy	Function	Clinical Considerations
Intervertebral disc	Lies between vertebral bodies. Two parts: nucleus pulposus and annulus fibrosus.	Absorbs compressive forces, allows for movement of the spine.	The central nucleus pulposus may break through the fibrous rings that contain it and lead to pressure on spinal nerve roots.
Vertebral end plate	Thin layer of cartilage that covers the top and bottom of the vertebral body. Connected to the annulus fibrosus.	Supplies nutrition to the inner rings of the annulus fibrosus and the nucleus pulposus by diffusion.	The nucleus pulposus may herniate upwardly or downwardly through the end plate (Schmorl's node). Deterioration of the disc, and possibly of the vertebral body, may result.
Ligamentum nuchae	Runs from the occiput to C7.	Limits flexion of the cervical spine.	Ligamentum nuchae becomes the supraspinous and interspinous ligaments below C7.
Ligamentum flavum	Connects the lamina of adjacent vertebrae. Lies posterior to the spinal cord in the spinal canal.	Limits flexion of the spine.	Hypertrophy may lead to spinal stenosis.
Anterior longitudinal ligament	Runs down the length of the spine on the anterior vertebral bodies.	Limits extension of the spine.	
Posterior longitudinal ligament	Runs down the length of the spine on the posterior vertebral bodies, anterior to the spinal cord in the spinal canal.	Limits flexion of the spine.	Hypertrophy may lead to spinal stenosis.
Capsule of the facet joints	Around each facet joint.	Limits flexion and rotation of the spine.	Joint capsules in the cervical spine may be injured and become a source of pain in whiplash injury.
Intertransverse ligament	Runs between adjacent transverse processes.	Limits sidebending to opposite side.	

of the temporal bone superiorly and concave over the condyle of the mandible inferiorly. Essentially, this gives the disc an "S" shape, as shown in Figure 8.5. The disc is attached to the lateral pterygoid muscle anteriorly and to connective tissue posteriorly. It is quite moveable in an anterior-posterior direction.

The disc splits the TMJ into an upper joint and a lower joint. The upper joint is the anterior part of the TMJ, between the articular eminence and the disc. Translation of the disc and condyle occur here. The lower joint is the posterior part of the TMJ between the disc and the condyle of the mandible. Rotation of the condyle occurs here.

The TMJ has a joint capsule composed of fibers that run from the temporal bone to the articular disc and from the disc to the neck of the condyle. The capsule is thin and does not play a role in preventing dislocation of the TMJ.

Ligaments reinforce the capsule and provide strength. The temporomandibular ligament is the primary ligament of the TMJ. It helps to prevent lateral movement of the condyle on the temporal bone.

Table 8-3 summarizes the soft tissues of the TMJ.

Nerves

The largest neural structure in the cervical spine is the spinal cord. The most essential function of the spine is to protect the spinal cord. The cord lies within the spinal canal. Paired sensory nerves enter the spinal cord through the dorsal root. Paired motor nerves exit the cord via the ventral root. The dorsal and ventral roots merge to form the spinal nerve that runs through the neural foramen of the spine. Figure 8.6 illustrates the anatomy of the spinal cord within the foramen of a cervical vertebra.

Although there are seven cervical vertebrae, there are eight pairs of cervical nerves that come off the spinal cord. The cervical nerves are numbered by the vertebral level below the nerve root. In other words, the C1 nerve exits the spinal cord between the occiput and the C1 vertebra. The C2 nerve exits above the C2 vertebra. Likewise, the C7 nerve exits above the C7 vertebra. The nerve below the body of C7 is named the C8 nerve. At this point, the numbering system changes so that the nerve is named for the vertebral level above it. Figure 8.7 depicts this concept.

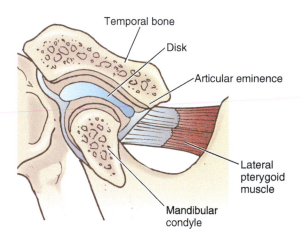

Figure 8.5 The temporomandibular joint has a fibrocartilage disc between the two bony surfaces.

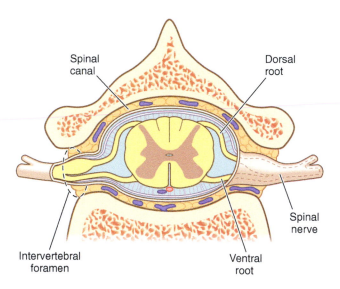

Figure 8.6 The spinal cord lies within the spinal canal. The normal space between the spinal cord and the canal is limited to less than 2.5 mm on the sides and 1 mm on the anterior and posterior aspect.

Table 8-3 Connective Tissue Anatomy and Physiology			
Of the Temporomandibular Joint			
Structure	Anatomy	Function	Clinical Considerations
TMJ articular disc	Lies in the TMJ joint. It is attached to the lateral pterygoid muscle anteriorly. Moves forward with mouth opening, back with mouth closing.	Increases joint congruity. Stabilizes the joint.	Disc derangement may contribute to TMJ pain.
Joint capsule and TM ligament	The capsule is reinforced on the lateral side by the TM ligament. This ligament prevents lateral displacement.	Helps stabilize the TMJ during chewing.	

Spinal nerve roots frequently carry a mixture of sensory and motor neurons. The sensory component of a spinal nerve root provides sensation to an area of skin called the **dermatome.** The motor component provides movement to a group of muscles called the **myotome.** By stimulating the sensory component of a nerve root and eliciting a motor response, the nerve root may be assessed. An example of this is testing of the **reflex arc.** Knowledge of each spinal nerve's corresponding dermatome, myotome, and reflex arc is important in assessment and treatment of spinal pathologies. A summary can be found in Table 8-4. Figure 8.8 illustrates the dermatomes of the cervical nerve roots.

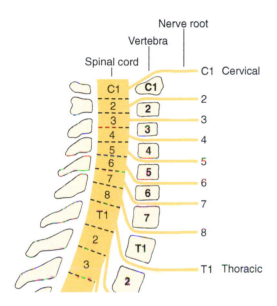

Figure 8.7 Nerve roots are named for the vertebral body that lies below them throughout the cervical spine. The nerve root below the body of C7 is the C8 nerve.

Blood Supply

The major arteries in the neck are the carotid arteries and the vertebral arteries. The carotid arteries split into the internal and external carotid arteries. Internal carotids carry blood flow into the Circle of Willis to supply the brain, while external carotids supply the neck and face. The vertebral arteries travel through the transverse foramen and into the skull. They enter the posterior Circle of Willis to supply the brain.

Muscular Anatomy and Kinesiology

The muscles in the cervical spine have two distinct roles: moving the neck or stabilizing the neck. While the large, superficial muscles can stabilize the spine, their main role is movement. These include the splenius cervicis and splenius capitis, three scalenes, sternocleidomastoid, and erector spinae. The small, deep muscles of the cervical spine are not capable of producing large movements but are important for the stability and proprioception of this region. This muscle group includes the transversospinalis, interspinales and intertransversarii on the posterior neck, and the deep cervical flexors on the anterior neck.

The deep cervical flexors include the longus capitus and longus colli muscles, as well as the very small rectus capitus anterior and rectus capitus lateralis (Fig. 8.9). These muscles play an important role in neck pain and whiplash associated disorders, discussed later in the chapter.

Four muscles largely control the movements of the mandible and are the muscles of **mastication** or chewing. These are the temporalis, the masseter, the medial pterygoid, and the lateral pterygoid (Fig. 8.10). In addition

Table 8-4	Cervical Spine Nerves			
With Associated Dermatome, Myotome, and Reflex				
Level	Dermatome	Myotome	MMT	Reflex
C1	NA	Upper cervical flexion	Sternocleidomastoid	NA
C2	Superior back of the head	Upper cervical extension, neck rotation	Sternocleidomastoid, splenius	NA
C3	Back of the head and anterior neck	Neck side bending	Scalenes	NA
C4	Top of the shoulders, clavicle region	Shoulder shrug	Upper trapezius, levator scapulae	NA
C5	Lateral upper arm	Shoulder abduction	Deltoids	Biceps
C6	Lateral lower arm, thumb and index finger	Elbow flexion, wrist extension	Biceps brachii, wrist extensors	Brachioradialis
C7	Middle finger, posterior forearm	Elbow extension, wrist flexion, finger extension	Triceps brachii, wrist flexors, digit extensors	Triceps
C8	Ring and little finger, medial arm	Finger flexion, thumb extension	Finger flexors, thumb extensor	NA

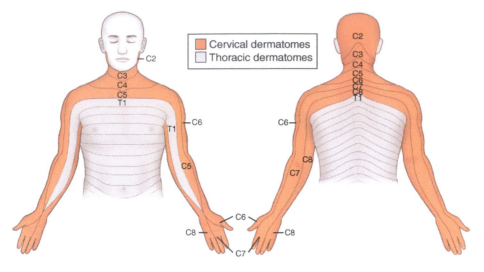

Figure 8.8 Map of cervical spinal nerve dermatomes.

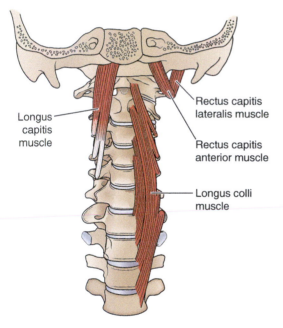

Figure 8.9 The deep cervical flexors include longus colli, longus capitus, rectus capitus anterior, and rectus capitus lateralis.

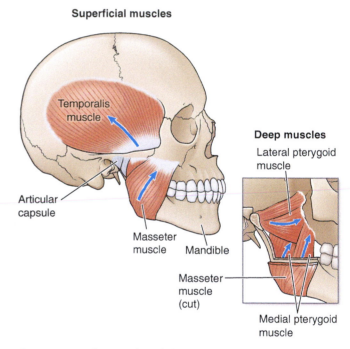

Figure 8.10 The muscles of the TMJ include the temporalis, masseter, medial pterygoid, and lateral pterygoid.

to being the only one of these muscles to depress the mandible, the lateral pterygoid has a second important function through its attachment to the articular disc. During jaw movement, the lateral pterygoid maintains the forward position of the disc on the condyle of the mandible.

Table 8-5 summarizes the muscles of the cervical spine and TMJ, including origin, insertion, innervation, action, and clinical relevance.

Muscular Connection Between the TMJ and the Cervical Spine

Many of the muscles of the TMJ attach, directly or indirectly, to the cervical spine. This allows muscle tightness in the TMJ to affect the posture of the cervical spine. Conversely, cervical spine posture can affect the TMJ. This will be discussed more under *Temporomandibular Dysfunction* later in the chapter.

Posture

The cervical spine is lordotic, or concave posteriorly. In this normal alignment, the head is supported with a minimum of muscle activity. A common postural deviation that occurs in the neck is **forward head posture**. This posture causes the cervical spine to change from a "C" shape to an "S" shape, as the lower cervical vertebrae

Table 8-5 Muscle Anatomy and Kinesiology

Of the Cervical Spine and TMJ

Muscle	Origin	Insertion	Innervation	Action	Clinical Considerations
Sternocleidomastoid	Sternum and clavicle	Mastoid process	Cranial nerve XI (spinal accessory), upper spinal nerves (C2–3)	Bilaterally flexes neck; unilaterally sidebends neck to same side, rotates neck to opposite side.	May be used as an accessory muscle of inspiration.
Scalenes	Transverse processes of cervical vertebrae	Ribs 1 and 2	Lower spinal nerves (C3–7)	Bilaterally assists flexion; unilaterally sidebends neck to same side.	May be used as an accessory muscle of inspiration.
Erector spinae	Spinous processes, transverse processes, ligamentum nuchae	Spinous processes, transverse processes, occiput and mastoid	Adjacent spinal nerves	Bilaterally extends neck and head; unilaterally sidebends neck and head.	The iliocostalis portion of this group is not present in the cervical area.
Splenius cervicis	Spinous processes of T3–T6	Transverse processes of C1–C3	Lower spinal nerves (C2–8)	Bilaterally extends neck; unilaterally rotates and sidebends neck to same side.	Acts on neck only
Splenius capitis	Spinous processes of C7–T3	Lateral occiput and mastoid	Lower spinal nerves (C2–8)	Bilaterally extends head and neck; unilaterally rotates and sidebends head and neck to same side.	Acts on head and neck
Transversospinalis	Transverse processes	Spinous processes above	Adjacent spinal nerves	Neck stabilizer; bilaterally extends neck; unilaterally rotates neck to opposite side.	Important neck stabilizer Includes the semispinalis, multifidus, and rotatores groups.
Interspinales	Spinous process	Spinous process above	Adjacent spinal nerves	Neck stabilizer Neck extension	Important neck stabilizer
Intertransversarii	Transverse process	Transverse process above	Adjacent spinal nerves	Neck side bending	Important neck stabilizer; may have a role in proprioception.
Deep cervical flexors (longus capitus, longus colli, rectus capitus anterior, rectus capitus lateralis)	Atlas, transverse processes of C3–T2	Occiput, transverse processes of C1–C6	Anterior rami C1–C6	Flexing upper cervical spine, i.e., head nodding, chin tuck.	Muscle weakness linked to cervical pathologies.
Temporalis	Temporal bone on side of skull	Mandible	Trigeminal nerve, cranial nerve V	Closes mouth, retrudes jaw; unilaterally deviates jaw to same side.	
Masseter	Zygomatic arch and maxilla	Mandible	Trigeminal nerve, cranial nerve V	Closes mouth; unilaterally deviates jaw to same side.	Very powerful jaw closer used in chewing.
Medial pterygoid	Maxilla and sphenoid	Angle of mandible	Trigeminal nerve, cranial nerve V	Closes mouth, protrudes jaw; unilaterally deviates jaw to opposite side.	
Lateral pterygoid	Sphenoid	Condyle of the mandible	Trigeminal nerve, cranial nerve V	Opens mouth, protrudes jaw; unilaterally deviates jaw to opposite side.	

Protraction

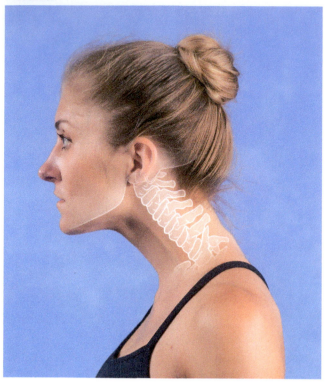

Figure 8.11 In forward head posture, the lower cervical spine is flexed relative to normal alignment.

Retraction

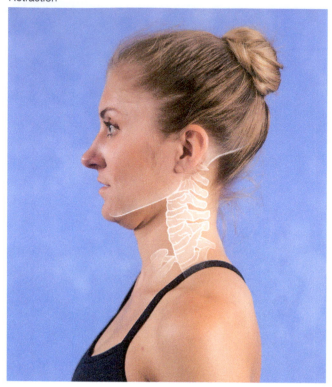

Figure 8.12 When the cervical spine is retracted, the lower cervical spine is extended.

increase in flexion and the upper cervical vertebrae hyperextend (Fig. 8.11).

Cervical retraction exercises are often done to treat problems in the cervical region. In this posture, the cervical spine becomes extended in the lower segments (Fig. 8.12). If extension of the lower cervical spine is desired, having the patient perform retraction before cervical extension ensures that extension is occurring throughout the cervical spine.

Cervical Spine Kinematics

Effect of Facet Joint Orientation on Movement

We have mentioned the importance of facet joint orientation in the cervical spine. While movement in all three planes occurs throughout the spine, orientation of the facet joints provides information about the major movement in any area. The movement of the facet joint that occurs with greatest ease is sliding. By this means, the facet joints act as "steering wheels" of the spine, guiding movement in each area.

The superior articular processes of atlas face medially and superiorly, providing a cupped surface for the occipital condyles to roll the head into flexion and extension. Yet, the amount of rotation and sidebending occurring at the AO joint is almost negligible. At the AA joint, the

Box 8-1	Normal Cervical Spine Range of Motion
Flexion	45°
Extension	90°
Sidebending	40° to each side
Rotation	90° to each side

processes lie almost entirely in the transverse plane. This orientation favors rotation; indeed, almost half of the rotation that occurs in the neck happens at the AA joint. Descending the cervical spine, the facet joints begin to lie more and more toward the frontal plane, favoring sidebending as well as rotation. Table 8-1 summarizes facet joint orientation and movements that occur at each level in the cervical spine. Total cervical spine normal range of motion is found in Box 8-1.

Effect of Movement on the Disc, Ligaments, and Foramen

Movement of the vertebrae affects the nucleus pulposus of the intervertebral disc, causing it to slightly move or deform within the confines of the annular rings. Prolonged positioning or repeated movements are thought to result

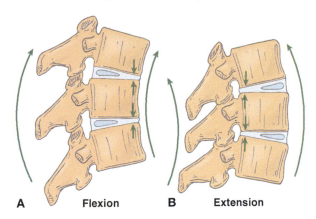

Figure 8.13 Spinal flexion causes the nucleus pulposus to move posteriorly within the annulus fibrosus and opens the neural foramen (A). Spinal extension leads to anterior migration of the nucleus pulposus and closes the neural foramen (B).

in movement of the nucleus.[1] Extension causes the nucleus to move anteriorly; flexion results in posterior movement (Fig. 8.13).

The annular rings are weakest in the posterolateral disc, and pressure of the nucleus against the annulus may result in tearing of the rings, allowing the nucleus to migrate away from the center of the disc.

In addition to the effect on the intervertebral disc, flexion and extension of the cervical spine also affect the neural (intervertebral) foramen as seen in Figure 8.13. The neural foramen are most open with cervical flexion and are smallest during cervical extension. With flexion, the posterior ligaments become taut or tight. In extension, the anterior ligaments are taut.

TMJ Kinematics

Movements of the mandible include elevation, depression, protrusion, retrusion, and lateral deviation.

With mouth opening, mandibular depression occurs by movements in both the upper and lower parts of the TMJ. Anterior rotation of the condyle occurs on the disc while anterior translation or sliding of the disc and condyle occur on the articular eminence of the temporal bone. Normal mouth opening is 40 to 50 mm, or two to three finger breadths at the PIP joint.

Protrusion of the jaw occurs primarily in the upper part of the TMJ. It involves anterior translation of the jaw without rotation. Normal movement of the jaw during protrusion is symmetrical. Motion of 6 to 9 mm is considered normal, allowing the patient to touch upper and lower teeth edge to edge. Retrusion of the jaw occurs by translating the mandible posteriorly. Movement in this direction is very limited. Soft tissues posterior to the condyle allow for only about 3 mm of motion.

Lateral deviation of the jaw occurs by rotation of the ipsilateral TMJ and anterior translation of the TMJ on the contralateral side. Normal lateral deviation is about 8 mm, allowing the patient to move the lower jaw the width of one upper front tooth. The patient should have equal lateral deviation on both sides.

As discussed previously, the TMJ and cervical spine are kinematically interconnected. Forward head posture stretches the muscles inferior to the mandible, which pulls the mandible posteriorly. This may increase compressive forces in the TMJ and cause TMJ pain. Studies have shown that cervical spine pain and TMJ pain often occur together.[2,3]

Common Pathologies

Cervicogenic Headache

Whiplash

Facet Joint DJD

Spinal Stenosis

DJD in the Neural Foramen (Foraminal Stenosis)

Herniated Disc

Temporomandibular Joint Dysfunction

Temporomandibular Muscle Dysfunction

The cervical area is the most vulnerable part of the spine. Its vertebral bodies are small, unlike those of the lumbar spine. Its tremendous mobility places demands on the soft tissue structures that may lead to pathology. The temporomandibular joint is connected by muscles to the cervical spine. Pathologies here impact and are impacted by the cervical spine. Patients may present with pathology in both these related areas. We will look at the common

pathologies of bone, disc, nerve, joint capsule, facet joints, and muscle in these two areas.

Cervicogenic Headache[4,5]   CPG

Cervicogenic headache (CGH) is head pain that comes from soft tissue disorders in the cervical spine. The primary structures that are responsible for producing

Box 8-2 Criteria for Diagnosis of Cervicogenic Headache

All four of the letter categories must be met for a diagnosis of CGH:

A. Pain is localized to the neck and occipital region and may project to forehead, orbital region, temples, vertex, and ears.

B. Pain is precipitated or aggravated by special neck movements or sustained neck posture.

C. At least one of the following:
   1. Resistance to or limitation of passive neck movements
   2. Changes in neck muscle contour, texture, tone, or response to active and passive stretching and contraction
   3. Abnormal tenderness of neck muscles

D. Radiological exam reveals at least one of the following:
   1. Movement abnormalities in flexion/extension
   2. Abnormal posture
   3. Fractures, congenital abnormalities, bone tumors, rheumatoid arthritis, or other distinct pathology except spondylosis and osteochondrosis

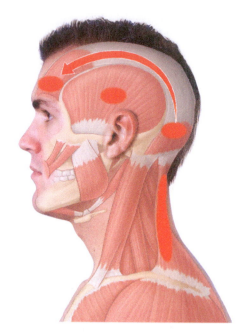

Figure 8.14 Cervicogenic headache starts in the neck and spreads up into the occipital area. It may radiate into the forehead, eye, and temple on the same side.

the symptoms are facet joints, muscles, discs, capsules, and ligaments in the upper cervical spine. Dysfunctions of the facet joints and intervertebral discs above C3 are considered as the primary cause, with the C2–3 facet joints most often implicated.[6–9]

To be classified as CGH, established criteria must be met. These criteria are listed in Box 8-2.[10]

Causes/Contributing Factors

CGH is thought to be due to inflammation or dysfunction of the upper cervical joints, ligaments, and muscles. Contributors include trauma, prolonged neck flexion, and poor posture. CGH may be a result of previous trauma, such as whiplash. There is an association between the likelihood of having CGH and a posture of increased cervical lordosis.[11] Four times as many women as men develop CGH.

CGH is associated with weakness of the deep cervical flexor muscles (longus capitus, longus colli, rectus capitus anterior, and rectus capitus lateralis).[10,12–15] These muscles are responsible for flexion of the head on the cervical spine in a nodding fashion. They also have a role in stabilizing the cervical spine.

Symptoms

Patients with CGH usually complain of pain that is unilateral and doesn't change sides. The pain is felt initially in the neck and spreads to the occipital area. It may radiate into the forehead, eye, and temple on the same

side (Fig. 8.14). The headache is of moderate to severe intensity.[10,16] The onset of headaches may be related to a history of trauma or cervical DJD. Prolonged neck postures or repeated movements may instigate a headache. Other symptoms that patients might experience include dizziness, nausea, and lightheadedness.[17]

Clinical Signs

Patients with CGH often display cervical joint restriction and tenderness in the cervical spine. Weakness in the deep cervical flexors may be present. The following tests are used to assess the patient with CGH.

Cervical Flexion-Rotation Test

The patient is positioned supine, and current symptoms are assessed. The patient is instructed to actively flex the head and neck to end range. The examiner then rotates the patient's head into full rotation bilaterally (Fig. 8.15). The patient is questioned regarding any change in symptoms. A positive test is indicated by a loss of range of motion in rotation of greater than 10° or by reproduction of the patient's headache pain.

Craniocervical Flexion Test

The patient is positioned supine with a pressure-sensing device such as the Chattanooga Stabilizer placed under the lordosis of the neck. With the patient relaxed, the device is set to 20 mm Hg. This test is performed in two steps. In step one the patient is instructed in the movement to be performed. The patient is to slide the head up the table, performing a gentle head nod and decreasing the cervical lordosis. The movement should be small and

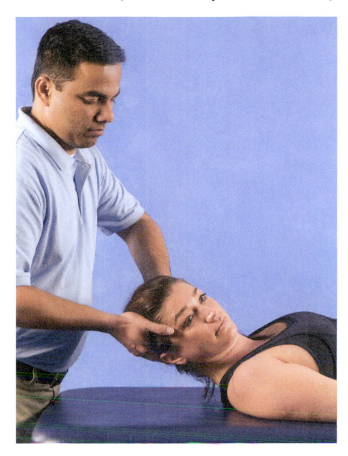

Figure 8.15 Cervical flexion-rotation test for cervicogenic headache.

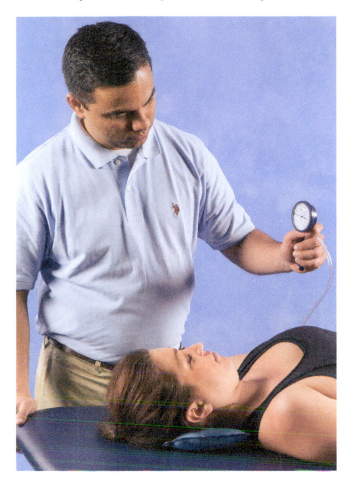

Figure 8.16 Craniocervical flexion test for cervicogenic headache.

controlled to increase the pressure reading to 22 mm Hg. The patient is instructed to hold for 2 to 3 seconds and then relax. The patient continues to perform this motion progressing in 2 mm Hg increments up to 30 mm Hg. The examiner palpates the scalene and sternocleidomastoid muscles with every repetition to ensure that the patient is not using these superficial muscles. If the patient can perform the motion correctly, proceed to step two.

In step two, the strength and endurance of the deep cervical flexors is assessed. The patient is positioned supine with the pressure-sensing device under the neck. The patient is instructed to perform the motion as described in step one, bringing the pressure gauge from 20 to 22 mm Hg, and hold for 10 seconds (Fig. 8.16). Three repetitions are performed at 22 mm Hg. As long as the patient is not contracting the superficial flexors, the test is progressed in 2 mm Hg increments for three 10-second holds. The test is terminated when the patient shows signs of fatigue, such as inability to maintain a steady pressure or the recruitment of superficial neck flexors.

Deep Neck Flexor Endurance Test

The patient is positioned supine, hook-lying on the table. The patient is asked to maximally retract the chin and lift the head and neck 1 inch off the table, keeping the chin retracted. Once in position, the examiner begins keeping time (Fig. 8.17). The examiner draws a line across two approximated skin folds on the patient's neck and places a hand under the patient's head. Verbal commands are given to the patient to maintain the position. The timing is stopped when the subject loses the ability to keep the line edges together or touches the examiner's hand for more than 1 second.[18] Normal values for this test may be related to gender and the presence of neck pain. Generally, females have been shown to have a mean endurance time of about 29 to 32 seconds, and males 35 to 40 seconds.[19,20] Patients with neck pain display a mean endurance time of 24 seconds.[18]

Intervention

Common interventions in the plan of care for the patient with CGH include therapeutic exercises to strengthen the deep cervical flexors, cervical and thoracic spinal joint mobilization, pain-relieving modalities, and stabilization exercises for the cervical spine and scapula.[4]

Several studies have shown either therapeutic exercise or spinal mobilization to be effective, but recent studies

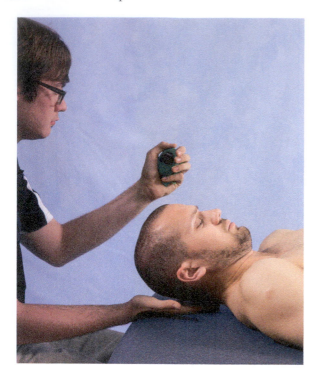

Figure 8.17 Deep neck flexor endurance test for cervicogenic headache.

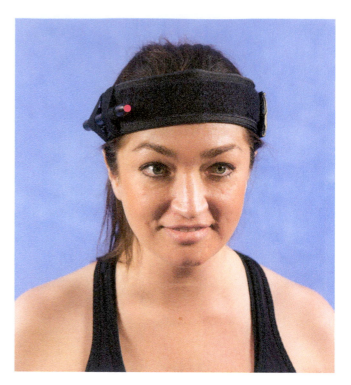

Figure 8.18 Proprioceptive exercise for the cervical spine. Laser pointer is attached to a headband. The patient is instructed to trace letters or point to objects on a wall.

indicate that a treatment program that includes both joint mobilization and exercise to be more effective than either approach in isolation.[17] Therapeutic exercise is likely to include strengthening of the neck flexors, specifically the deep cervical flexors. Neck proprioception exercises may be included.[21] Neck proprioception may be trained using an exercise as shown in Figure 8.18. In

this exercise, the patient traces letters or numbers on a wall with a laser pointer attached to a headband. Scapular strengthening exercises may also be helpful. Modalities commonly include ultrasound, soft tissue mobilization, and electrical stimulation.

The Bottom Line: for patients with cervicogenic headache

Description and causes	Poor posture and weakness of the deep cervical flexors leads to neck pain that radiates into the head
Test	Craniocervical flexion test, cervical flexion-rotation test, deep neck flexor endurance test
Stretch	To restore ideal posture
Strengthen	Deep neck flexors, scapular stabilizers
Train	Neck proprioception
Avoid	Prolonged or repeated cervical postures

Whiplash   CPG

Whiplash refers to an injury to the neck that involves rapid movement of the neck with trauma to the soft tissues and bones of the cervical spine (Fig. 8.19). It commonly occurs after a rear- or side-impact motor vehicle accident but may also be the result of a fall or sports injury. The soft tissues of the neck, including the facet joint capsules, ligaments, muscles, spinal cord, and brain may be affected.

The Quebec Task Force classifies whiplash injuries in categories from 0 to 4.[22] Grade 0 consists of normal findings. Grade 1 is characterized by complaint of pain or stiffness, but no physical findings. Grade 2 is characterized by physical findings such as tenderness or limitation of motion. If the patient has neurological signs such as weakness or decreased reflexes the injury is considered a Grade 3. Grade 4 is characterized by the presence of a fracture or dislocation. These grades are detailed in Box 8-3. Grades 1 and 2 will usually resolve within 6

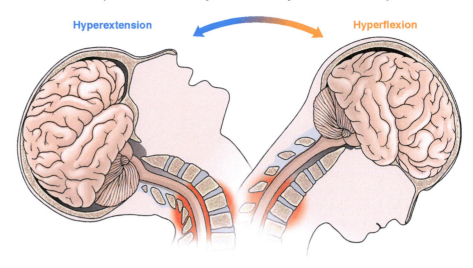

Hyperextension   **Hyperflexion**

Figure 8.19 In whiplash injury, the cervical spine hyperextends and hyperflexes, causing damage to the soft tissues of the cervical spine.

Box 8-3	Quebec Task Force Classification
Grade	**Clinical Presentation**
0	• Patient does not complain of neck pain and no physical signs are observed by the examiner. • These patients are uncommon and will not usually seek assistance, thus going undocumented.
1	• Patient complains of pain to health-care provider. • No physical signs are found. Normal range of motion, normal strength, no swelling. • Usually these patients suffer from small muscle lesions that are not significant enough to cause muscle spasm.

2	• Patient complains of pain to health-care provider.
	• Musculoskeletal signs are found that could include:
	  • Limited range of motion
	  • Spasm or swelling
	  • Point tenderness in neck or shoulders
	• Usually these patients have sprained ligaments in their neck and the muscle tears have caused bleeding and swelling.

3	• Patient complains of pain to health-care provider.
	• Neurological signs are found that could include:
	  • Decreased or absent reflexes
	  • Decreased or limited skin sensation (dermatomes)
	  • Muscular weakness (myotomes)
	• Usually these patients suffer from injuries to the neurologic system because of pressure on nerves or irritation secondary to sustained stretch of neural tissue.
	• These patients will almost always have limited range of motion and other musculoskeletal signs as well.

4	• Patient complains of pain to health-care provider. • X-rays reveal fracture or dislocation.

months of injury, but the concern is that approximately 40% of the patients with whiplash will develop chronic whiplash associated disorder (WAD).[23,24]

Causes/Contributing Factors

Any structure in the cervical spine may be responsible for the pain of whiplash, including the facet joints, capsules, ligaments, discs, muscles, nerves, and bones.

Symptoms

Common symptoms after a whiplash injury are neck pain and/or headache that are constant or related to movement. Symptoms usually occur within 48 hours of injury. In addition, the patient may experience limited motion, dizziness, blurred vision, spinal instability, difficulty sleeping, difficulty concentrating, memory problems, ringing in the ears, temporomandibular joint dysfunction, and fatigue.

Clinical Signs

The clinical signs of whiplash include the musculoskeletal findings as noted above. These findings include limited range of motion of the neck, weakness of neck and arm muscles, and pain. Other findings that may be found include abnormal motor recruitment patterns in the neck and upper trunk, altered balance, decreased proprioceptive

sense in the neck, hypersensitivity to cold and pressure in the neck area, and signs of posttraumatic stress disorder.[23]

Recent studies have shown weakness in the deep cervical flexors and in all of the cervical extensors, including multifidus, rectus capitis muscles, semispinalis, splenii, upper trapezius, longus capitus, and longus colli. In addition to range-of-motion and strength assessment, the **craniocervical flexion test** or **deep neck flexor endurance test** as described earlier under CGH may be helpful in assessing the patient with whiplash and associated disorders.

Intervention

Physical therapy after whiplash commonly involves exercise, patient education, joint mobilization, and modalities.[25,26] Neck-specific exercises, such as neck range-of-motion exercises, strengthening the cervical extensors and deep cervical flexors, and neck proprioception exercises, have been shown to be more effective than general fitness exercise.[27] Patient education, including an explanation of central pain mechanisms and the importance of movement, is often included. Manual therapy, including cervical and thoracic joint mobilizations, may be beneficial in reducing pain and increasing motion and function.

The Bottom Line: for patients with whiplash injuries

Description and causes	Motor vehicle accident or sports injury that involve rapid hyperextension and hyperflexion of the neck, damaging soft tissues
Test	Craniocervical flexion test, deep neck flexor endurance test, neck ROM
Stretch	To improve neck ROM
Strengthen	Deep neck flexors and neck extensors
Train	Neck proprioception
Avoid	Prolonged immobilization or self-immobilizing

Degenerative Joint Disease

Degenerative joint disease (DJD) may occur in several areas in the spine. DJD is also called osteoarthritis (OA). While the Arthritis Foundation recognizes over 100 types of arthritis, DJD is the most common type. In the spine, there are three places where DJD commonly causes symptoms: the facet joints, the neural foramen, and the spinal canal. The following three pathologies are the manifestations of DJD in each of these areas. Often, patients will have DJD in more than one of these locations.

Facet Joint DJD

Osteoarthritis or degenerative joint disease (DJD) of the cervical spine may involve the facet joints. When these joints become arthritic, the articular cartilage begins to deteriorate, and bone spurs or osteophytes form on the joint surfaces. The joint space becomes narrowed (Fig. 8.20).

Causes/Contributing Factors

At each level in the cervical spine, the two facet joints and the intervertebral disc form a joint triad. Under

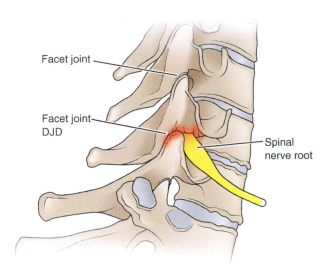

Figure 8.20 Degenerative joint disease of the cervical spine may manifest in degenerative changes in the facet joints and stenosis, or narrowing, of the foramen.

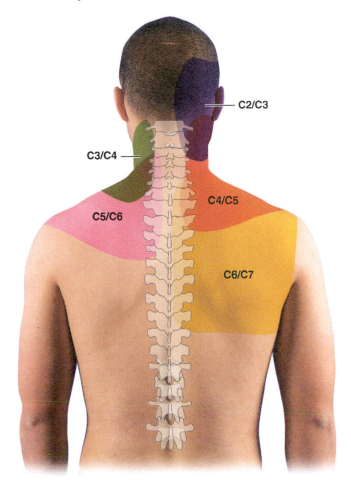

Figure 8.21 The cervical facet joints refer pain into the occiput, scapula, and upper back.

normal conditions, the facet joints bear up to 33% of the load of the spine, with the intervertebral disc absorbing the remaining 67%. Facet joint DJD occurs frequently because of degenerative disc disease (DDD). As the disc deteriorates, the facet joints are made to bear significantly more weight, up to 70% of the load. These small joints begin to wear under this stress, leading to joint wear-and-tear (DJD).

DJD of the facet joints is associated with aging. Although there is no association between developing cervical facet DJD and gender, males with facet DJD have faster progression of the disorder.[28] Obesity is correlated to developing cervical facet DJD. While it is hypothesized that factors such as past trauma and occupational hazards may contribute to facet DJD, these have not been adequately researched.

Symptoms

Extension increases the load-bearing on the facets.[28] Patients with cervical facet DJD will complain of posterior neck pain that is worse with extension and extension with rotation. Pain is usually localized to the neck, but lower cervical spine involvement may refer to the scapular area, and upper cervical facet joints may cause referred pain into the occipital area and cause headache (Fig. 8.21). Neck flexion relieves the pain. The patient may complain of tenderness to palpation over the facet joints.

With advanced facet DJD, the neural foramen may become narrowed, resulting in upper extremity **radiculopathy**. This will be discussed further in this chapter.

Clinical Signs

Cervical range of motion is likely to be limited in extension. Repeated or prolonged extension often increases pain, and repeated or prolonged flexion usually decreases pain. There are no special tests used for cervical facet joint DJD.

Intervention

Patients with cervical facet joint DJD may respond to a flexion approach in the exercise protocol, including deep flexor strengthening. Stretching into cervical flexion or sidebending may relieve the symptoms. Modalities including ultrasound, soft tissue mobilization, and TENS may be useful. Prolonged joint inflammation may lead to chronic pain and central sensitization (Chapter 3). Patients with chronic pain may benefit from therapeutic neuroscience education.[29]

The Bottom Line: for patients with cervical facet joint DJD

Description and causes	Degenerative arthritis of the facet joints associated with aging and degenerative disc disease, causing pain in the posterior neck and upper back
Test	None
Stretch	Into cervical flexion or sidebending
Strengthen	Deep neck flexors
Train	NA
Avoid	Prolonged neck extension

Spinal Stenosis (DJD in the Spinal Canal)

The term **stenosis** means narrowing. The normal space between the spinal cord and the canal is limited to less than 2.5 mm on the sides and 1 mm on the anterior and posterior aspect.[30] In spinal stenosis, the spinal canal is narrowed due to degenerative changes. As the canal becomes more narrowed, the spinal cord gets squeezed. Spinal stenosis is a gradually progressive condition. It may involve any area of the spinal canal, with lumbar and cervical regions being most affected. It may involve only one level or span multiple levels. Figure 8.22 depicts the changes that occur in the spinal canal in spinal stenosis.

Causes/Contributing Factors

Spinal stenosis is most often caused by bony overgrowth into the spinal canal. This may be due to osteoarthritis of the spine associated with aging. It may also be caused by hypertrophy and calcification of the ligaments in the spinal canal, specifically the ligamentum flavum and the posterior longitudinal ligament. In addition, it may be related to a congenitally small spinal canal, to the presence of scoliosis, or to a disc herniation.

Symptoms

Common symptoms of cervical spinal stenosis are bilateral arm pain, fatigue, numbness, tingling, clumsiness, and/or weakness. Pain is increased by extension of the neck and relieved by neck flexion. This is due to a narrowing of the spinal canal in extension and an expansion with flexion. Bilateral arm symptoms of spinal stenosis distinguish this pathology from other cervical pathologies.

As pressure on the spinal cord increases, the patient may experience signs of **cervical myelopathy.** These findings are due to a disruption of nerve impulses through the neck area, and include trunk and lower extremity weakness, gait disturbances, and changes in bowel or bladder. When these signs occur, surgical decompression is required.

Clinical Signs

Clinical signs of spinal stenosis include findings of bilateral pain, weakness, sensory loss, and abnormal reflexes bilaterally. The PTA may assess the effect of prolonged or repeated movements on the patient's symptoms, with the expectation that extension will increase symptoms and flexion will decrease symptoms. There are no special tests for cervical spinal stenosis.

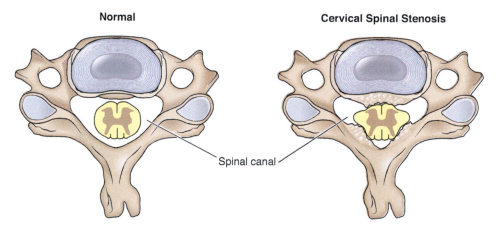

Normal   **Cervical Spinal Stenosis**

Spinal canal

Figure 8.22 In spinal stenosis, degenerative changes in the spinal canal lead to narrowing of the foramen, putting pressure on the spinal cord. Commonly, cervical spinal stenosis leads to neurological symptoms in both arms and may progress to include symptoms in both legs.

Intervention

The plan of care for patients with cervical spinal stenosis may include strengthening of the deep neck flexors and neck extensors to stabilize the cervical spine, strengthening of the scapular stabilizers, and avoiding positions or activities that increase symptoms. Modalities in the plan of care may include cervical traction, TENS, and ultrasound. Patients may benefit from the use of a cervical collar.

The Bottom Line:	for patients with cervical spinal stenosis
Description and causes	Degenerative changes in the spinal canal related to aging that cause narrowing of the foramen and squeezing of the cervical spinal cord
Test	NA
Stretch	NA
Strengthen	Deep neck flexors, neck extensors, scapular stabilizers
Train	NA
Avoid	Activities that increase pain, usually neck extension and retraction

DJD in the Neural Foramen (Foraminal Stenosis)

Osteoarthritis, or degenerative joint disease, may occur in the neural foramen causing a foraminal stenosis. This is more common in the cervical and lumbar areas than in the thoracic spine and may also be called a lateral stenosis. **Osteophytes** slowly overgrow in the foramen, progressively constricting the opening for the spinal nerve. Eventually they may cause the nerve root to become inflamed, a condition known as **radiculopathy**. Figure 8.23 depicts this pathology.

Causes/Contributing Factors

Osteoarthritis of the spine is related to aging. It may be accelerated by hypomobility or hypermobility.

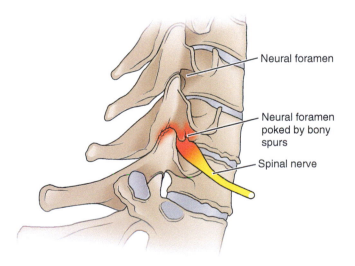

Figure 8.23 DJD in the neural foramen may cause osteophytes to grow into the foramen, leading to narrowing or stenosis.

Symptoms

Many of the arthritic changes in the spine are asymptomatic, but if the nerve root becomes inflamed it can be a significant source of pain. The patient may experience neck pain and upper extremity pain, numbness and tingling, weakness, and loss of reflexes. Specific symptoms depend upon the nerve root that is involved. Symptoms are usually unilateral, occurring on the side of the stenosis.

Because the neural foramen is larger when the spine is flexed, the patient will usually report a decrease in pain in a position of neck flexion. Activities that involve neck flexion are tolerated well. In other words, these patients have a **flexion bias**. With neck extension, pain is increased due to closing down of the neural foramen. Patients will often state that their arm pain is relieved by putting their arm up over their head. This is referred to as the **shoulder abduction relief sign** and is effective because of the decrease in stretch on the nerve roots.

Watch Out For...

Watch out for a change in location of pain in response to position or movement. When the most distal pain moves closer to the spine, it is called **centralization. Peripheralization** refers to the most distal pain moving farther down the arm. The goal in treating radiculopathy pain is symptom centralization. If pain moves farther down the arm, it is a sign of increased pressure on the nerve root. If the most distal pain becomes closer to the spine, it signals decreased pressure on the nerve root.

Sometimes when pain centralizes, it will be perceived as more intense. Conversely, when pain peripheralizes, it may be perceived as less intense. Always the patient and the PTA should be concerned primarily about the location of pain and secondarily about pain intensity.

Box 8-4 **Clinical Signs in C6 Foraminal Stenosis**

Foraminal stenosis may cause pain, numbness, loss of reflexes, and weakness. If the stenosis compresses the C6 nerve root, complaint will be of pain in one upper extremity with numbness in the thumb and index finger. The patient may have loss of brachioradialis reflex. Weakness may be present in the biceps and wrist extensors. Pain in the upper extremity will usually diminish and/or centralize with flexion bias exercises. Extension activities will usually increase and/or peripheralize the symptoms. The patient may complain of increased arm pain, when washing hair in the shower for example, due to cervical extension.

Clinical Signs

The clinical signs of foraminal stenosis in the cervical spine include findings of pain, weakness, sensory loss, and diminished or absent reflexes on the involved side as compared to the uninvolved side. The specific muscles that become weak, area of skin that becomes numb, and reflex that becomes diminished depends upon the nerve root affected (Table 8-4). Refer to Box 8-4 for an application of the clinical signs found in Table 8-4. In addition to these findings, the following tests may indicate irritation of a cervical nerve root.

Spurling's Compression Test

The patient is positioned sitting with the head in a neutral position. The patient's current symptoms are assessed. The patient is then instructed to extend the neck and sidebend to the affected side. Symptoms are again assessed. If there is no increase in radicular symptoms, the examiner places both hands on the top of the patient's head and applies an axial compression force (Fig. 8.24). A positive test is indicated by an increase in the patient's radicular symptoms. If the patient's symptoms increase, the test is stopped and considered positive. Spurling's original test involved cervical sidebending and compression only, but the addition of neck extension described by Anekstein et al. increases the provocation of the test.[31]

Cervical Distraction Test

The patient is positioned supine, and current symptoms are assessed. The examiner cradles the patient's head with one hand under the occiput and one hand on the patient's chin. The examiner then applies a distraction force to the cervical spine (Fig. 8.25). A positive test is indicated by a reduction in the patient's symptoms while the neck is distracted.

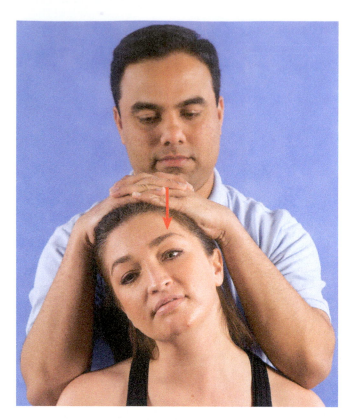

Figure 8.24 Spurling's compression test for cervical radiculopathy.

Upper Limb Tension Test (ULTT), Median Nerve Bias

By putting tension on the median nerve, this test may be useful in ruling out pathology of the nerve roots that contribute to the median nerve, including C5 through T1. The patient is positioned in supine, and current symptoms are assessed. A series of movements are performed passively with the patient's affected arm, with the intention of progressively stretching the nerve. At each step, the patient's symptoms should be assessed. The movements of the patient's arm are as follows:

1. Scapular depression.
2. Abduction of the shoulder to 90°.
3. External rotation of the shoulder.
4. Extension of the wrist and fingers.
5. Supination of the forearm.
6. Elbow extension.
7. Neck sidebending away from the side being tested.

The end position of this test is shown in Figure 8.26. A positive test is indicated by an increase in the patient's symptoms, limitation in range of motion as compared to the unaffected side, increased symptoms

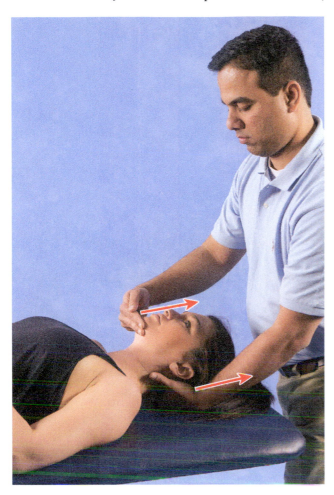

Figure 8.25 Cervical distraction test for cervical radiculopathy.

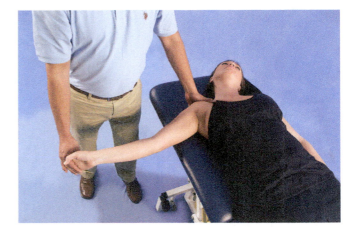

Figure 8.26 End position of the upper limb tension test for the median nerve. This test may be used to determine irritability of the cervical nerve roots from C5–T1.

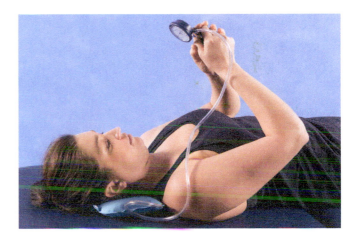

Figure 8.27 Strengthening the deep cervical flexors may be done with a device such as the Chattanooga Stabilizer. The patient is instructed to flatten the cervical lordosis and increase pressure in increments of 2 mm Hg pressure.

with contralateral cervical sidebending, or a decrease with ipsilateral sidebending. If at any point the patient's symptoms increase, the test is stopped and is considered positive. To objectify this test, the range of motion at a restricted joint may be measured. This test is not specific for cervical radiculopathy, but a negative test is a good indication that there is no radiculopathy. In other words, the test is very sensitive but not specific.

Intervention

Treatment for cervical radiculopathy often involves a combination of cervical and thoracic mobilization, nerve gliding, strengthening the deep cervical flexors, strengthening the scapular stabilizers, strengthening the upper extremity, and cervical traction.

Nerve gliding may be done using the same series of movements listed in the ULTT. The patient should be instructed to move to the point of slight neural tension, hold briefly, and then release by allowing the nerve to be on slack over one joint. The physical therapist may perform cervical lateral flexion mobilizations while the PTA holds the extremity at a point of minimum neural tension to glide the nerve.

Strengthening of the deep cervical flexors (longus capitus, longus colli, rectus capitus anterior, and rectus capitus lateralis) may be included in the plan of care. This may be done with a pressure biofeedback device—for example, a blood pressure cuff or a Chattanooga Stabilizer—under the neck as shown in Figure 8.27. The device is inflated to 20 mm Hg. The patient is instructed to perform a gentle head nod, flattening the cervical lordosis, without substituting by using sternocleidomastoid or scalenes. The patient should be instructed to attempt to increase the pressure in 2 mm Hg increments and hold for 5 seconds at each step, up to an increase of 10 mm Hg over baseline.[32] For clarification, the device readings will be 20, 22, 24, 26, 28, and 30 mm Hg, as the patient is able.

Isotonic strengthening of the neck flexors may be included in the plan of care. Figure 8.28 shows isotonic

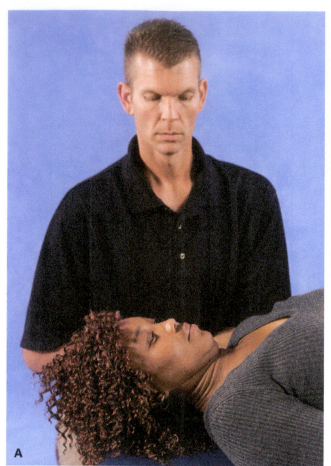

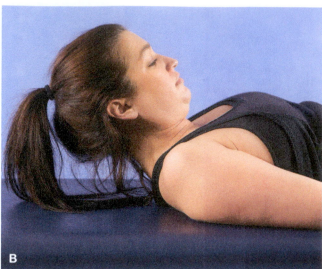

Figure 8.28 Exercises to strengthen the superficial and deep neck flexors. Flexion of the head (A) and flexion of neck and head (B).

exercises for the superficial and deep neck flexors. In the exercise depicted in (A), the patient is instructed to flex the head on the cervical spine, maintaining a neutral neck position.[33] Alternatively, the patient may be instructed to flex the head and the neck on the thoracic spine (B).

 CLINICAL ALERT

The patient should be instructed in the concept of centralization of their pain, and exercises and activities should avoid peripheralization of symptoms.

Strengthening exercises to middle and lower trapezius, serratus anterior, and rhomboids have also been used effectively to treat patients with cervical radiculopathy. The plan of care may also include cervical traction.[34,35]

In addition to physical therapy, patients may receive **epidural steroid injections.** This procedure is done on an outpatient basis and involves a steroid injection around the nerve root to decrease swelling and pain. If therapy and injections are not successful, the patient may undergo a surgical procedure to decompress the nerve root in the foramen, called a **foraminotomy.**

The Bottom Line: for patients with degenerative foraminal stenosis of the cervical spine

Description and causes	Degenerative changes in the neural foramen associated with aging that cause spurs to form, which puts pressure on cervical nerve roots
Test	Spurling's test, cervical distraction test, ULTT
Stretch	The median nerve using the ULTT
Strengthen	Deep neck flexors, scapular stabilizers, upper extremity
Train	Use of deep neck flexors
Avoid	Peripheralization of pain

Herniated Disc

The intervertebral disc (IVD) has two parts: the annulus fibrosus and the nucleus pulposus. The disc is basically circular in shape and the annular rings contain the nucleus in the center. In the pathology of herniated disc, the nucleus pulposus and/or some part of the intervertebral disc is outside the boundaries of the vertebral end plates. The rupture of the disc usually occurs posterolaterally where the annular rings are thinner, potentially leading to pressure on the spinal cord or spinal nerve roots.

The terminology used for the progression of herniated disc varies considerably. The following terminology is in keeping with the most recent recommendations.[36] The term **protruded disc** is used to describe an IVD with minimal displacement outside the boundaries of the end plates. In this case, the annular rings are still intact. **Extruded disc** refers to a progression of herniation in which the displacement of the nucleus is greater and the annular rings are completely torn through. In this case, the disc material remains attached to the disc of origin. **Sequestered disc** is a progression of herniation in which a fragment of disc material breaks away and is not contiguous with the disc of origin. This free-floating mass of disc material is able to migrate away from the parent disc. Figure 8.29 depicts the stages of herniated disc from normal to sequestered.

This pathology may also be called herniated nucleus pulposus (HNP) syndrome. Other terms that may be used to describe this pathology include bulging disc, prolapsed disc, and slipped disc, but these terms are not preferred because they are unclear or misleading.

Causes/Contributing Factors

While the cause of cervical herniated disc is not fully understood, it appears to be largely due to age-related changes in the disc that cause small fissures in the annular rings, allowing the nucleus to migrate through the annulus. As evidence, disc herniation in the cervical spine is unusual before the age of 30.[37] Secondarily, it may be caused by trauma, postural stress, and hypermobility. An area of the cervical spine adjacent to a hypomobile segment is at higher risk due to the hypermobility compensation at this level. Herniated disc over the age of 50 is uncommon but possible.

Herniated disc in the cervical spine occurs primarily in the lower segments, C4–C7. Because herniated disc occurs through the posterior part of the annulus, flexion of the lower cervical spine may increase the risk. Specifically, forward head posture and occupations that involve prolonged neck flexion lead to increased risk.[38]

Symptoms

Symptoms that are associated with cervical herniated disc include neck and arm pain, numbness and tingling, weakness, and loss of reflexes. Patients with a cervical herniated disc may describe an initial onset of posterior neck or scapular pain, later progressing to arm symptoms. The area between the scapulae is often painful, as the cervical discs refer to this area.[39] Specific upper extremity symptoms depend upon the nerve root that is affected by the herniation.

Patients with a cervical herniated disc often demonstrate a **directional preference**. In other words, their

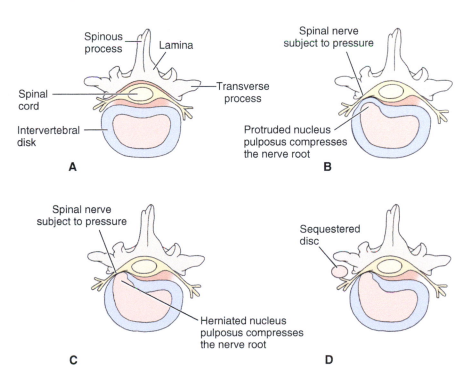

Figure 8.29 The stages of disc herniation. Normal disc (A), protruded disc (B), extruded disc (C), and sequestered disc (D).

symptoms may increase, peripheralize, or both, with certain movements or positions of their neck, and decrease, centralize, or both, with movements in the opposite direction. Most commonly, patients with a herniated disc will complain of increased symptoms with neck flexion and forward head posture. They will commonly get relief from a neutral or extended neck position and cervical retraction. These patients are said to have an **extension bias.**

Clinical Signs

Clinical signs of herniated disc with radiculopathy include findings of pain, weakness, sensory loss, and diminished or absent reflexes in the upper extremity on the involved side as compared to the uninvolved side. Patients often display a decrease in cervical rotation range of motion.[40] In addition, **Spurling's Test,** the **Cervical Distraction Test,** and the **ULTT** discussed above may be used to indicate a cervical radiculopathy.

Intervention

The plan of care for cervical herniated disc often involves a combination of cervical and thoracic mobilization, nerve gliding, strengthening the deep cervical flexors, strengthening the scapular stabilizers, strengthening the upper extremity, and cervical traction.

In addition, cervical retraction exercises are often included. The McKenzie progression for cervical herniated disc begins with cervical retraction in standing or supine, as shown in Figure 8.30. If symptoms centralize, the patient may perform retraction followed by neck extension. If the patient does not respond to these exercises, neck sidebending or rotation toward the affected side may decrease symptoms. McKenzie exercises are performed every hour to two hours throughout the day.

> ⚑ **CLINICAL ALERT** ⎯⎯⎯⎯⎯⎯
>
> The patient should be instructed in the concept of centralization of their pain, and exercises and activities should avoid peripheralization of symptoms.

Strengthening exercises to middle and lower trapezius, serratus anterior, rhomboids, and affected arm muscles have also been used to effectively treat patients with

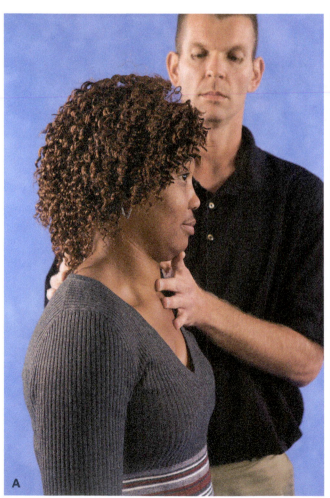
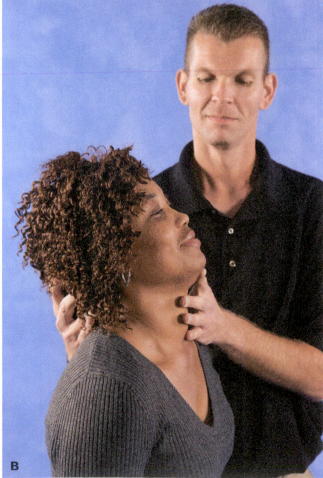

Figure 8.30 McKenzie cervical extension exercises. Retraction (A) and retraction with extension (B).

cervical radiculopathy. Cervical traction may be included in the plan of care.

Postural retraining is important for cervical disc problems. Instruct the patient to assume an ideal posture that reduces lower cervical flexion by retracting the head. This posture should be maintained as long as possible, with frequent reminders to "reset" this position throughout the day.

The Bottom Line:	for patients with herniated disc of the cervical spine
Description and causes	Small tears in the annulus fibrosus associated with aging and forward head posture allowing the nucleus material to migrate posteriorly, putting pressure on a nerve root
Test	Spurling's Test, Cervical Distraction Test, ULTT
Stretch	The median nerve using the ULTT, into cervical retraction/extension
Strengthen	Deep neck flexors, scapular stabilizers, upper extremity
Train	Use of deep neck flexors
Avoid	Peripheralization of pain

Temporomandibular Dysfunction

Temporomandibular dysfunction (TMD) can arise from the joint or from the muscles of mastication. Although they are related, distinguish between temporomandibular joint dysfunction and temporomandibular muscle dysfunction (TM myalgia).

Temporomandibular Joint Dysfunction

Disorders of the temporomandibular joint (TMJ) include joint inflammation, disc displacement, and osteoarthritis (OA). Joint inflammation includes capsulitis and synovitis of the TMJ. Disc displacement (usually anteriorly and medially) generally occurs in the closed mouth position. In some cases, it reduces when the mouth is opened. This is accompanied by a palpable or audible pop or click. Disc displacement may also occur without reduction, meaning that the disc remains displaced when the mouth is open or closed. Osteoarthritis is a deterioration of the TMJ secondary to inflammation.

Causes/Contributing Factors

While contributing factors for **arthrogenic** TMJ pain are controversial, it is widely regarded to be related to trauma, **bruxism** (grinding teeth), and **malocclusion** (malalignment of teeth with jaw closure) or abnormal jaw mechanics. A TMJ that is inflamed or has a displaced disc is at increased risk for OA.

Symptoms

Inflammation of the TMJ causes pain at rest, which is increased with chewing. If the disc is displaced, the patient may or may not experience pain. Disc displacement that reduces when opening the mouth is accompanied by a click or pop. Disc displacement that doesn't reduce with movement will generally cause limited motion into opening or closing and pain with jaw movement. If the disc displacement is on one side, the patient will have jaw deviation on opening and lateral deviation to one side will be restricted.

Clinical Signs

Clinical signs for TMJ dysfunction include limited range of motion, asymmetry of movement, and crepitus in the TMJ during movement. The following special tests may be used in the diagnosis of TMJ dysfunction.

Active Opening

The patient is positioned sitting, with the mouth closed in the resting position. Current symptoms are assessed. The patient performs mouth opening, reporting any recurrence of symptoms (Fig. 8.31). Normal mouth opening is 40 to 50 mm.[41,42] A positive test is indicated by reproduction of the patient's symptoms, by deviation of the jaw to one side, or by limitation of opening to less than 40 mm.

Active Protrusion

The patient is positioned sitting, with the mouth closed in the resting position. Current symptoms are assessed. The patient performs jaw protrusion, reporting any recurrence of symptoms (Fig. 8.32). A positive test is indicated by reproduction of the patient's symptoms or by inability to bring front upper and lower teeth edge-to-edge.

Active Lateral Deviation

The patient is positioned sitting, with the mouth closed in the resting position. Current symptoms are assessed. The patient performs lateral deviation, reporting any

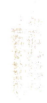

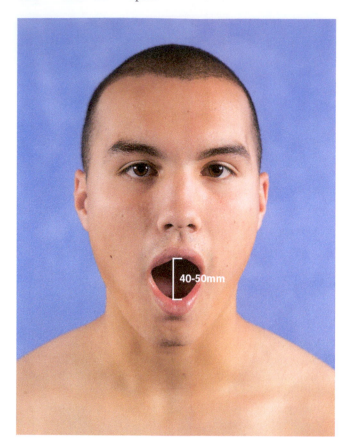

Figure 8.31 Active opening test for TMJ dysfunction.

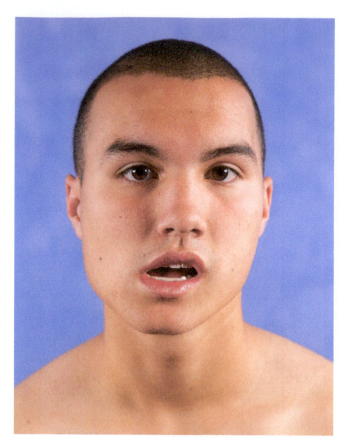

Figure 8.33 Active lateral deviation test for TMJ dysfunction.

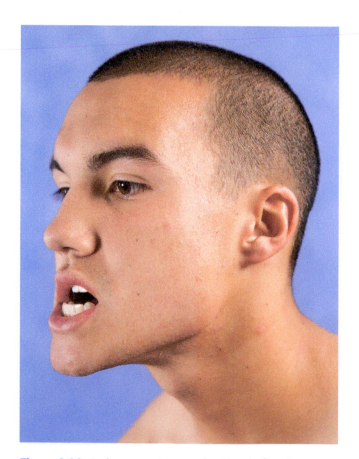

Figure 8.32 Active protrusion test for TMJ dysfunction.

recurrence of symptoms (Fig. 8.33). A positive test is indicated by reproduction of the patient's symptoms, by asymmetry in deviation to one side as compared to the other side, or by inability to move the jaw to each side the width of one top central incisor.

Resisted Movements

The patient is positioned sitting, with the mouth partially open and jaw relaxed. Current symptoms are assessed. The patient performs mouth opening, closing, protrusion, and lateral deviation to each side against resistance (Fig. 8.34). A positive test is indicated by reproduction of the patient's symptoms.

Palpation of the TMJ

The patient is positioned sitting, with the mouth partially open and jaw relaxed. Current symptoms are assessed. The examiner palpates the TMJ by placing the tips of the index fingers into the preauricular region, just anterior to the tragus, hooking the fingers to give slight pressure anteriorly. The patient performs jaw opening and closing (Fig. 8.35). A positive test is indicated by palpation of crepitus during jaw movement.

Stethoscope Assessment of Crepitus of the TMJ

The patient is positioned sitting, with the mouth partially open and jaw relaxed. Current symptoms are assessed.

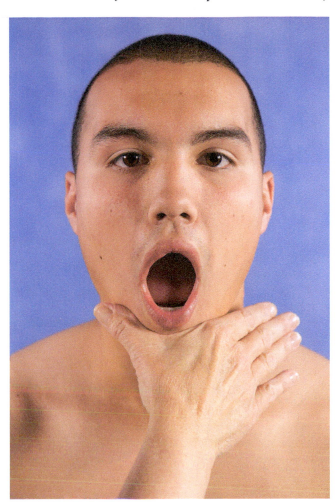

Figure 8.34 Resisted movements test for TMJ dysfunction includes resisted mouth closing.

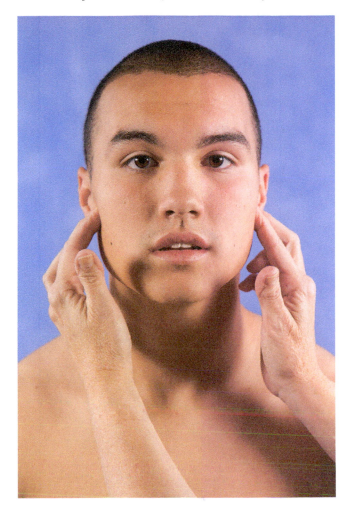

Figure 8.35 Palpation of the TMJ for crepitus indicating TMJ dysfunction.

The examiner places a stethoscope over the TMJ. The patient performs jaw opening/closing, lateral deviation, and protrusion/retrusion (Fig. 8.36). A positive test is indicated by crepitus, popping, or clicking during jaw movement.

Intervention

Patients with arthrogenic TMJ pain may benefit from modalities to decrease pain, including heat, cryotherapy, ultrasound, laser, and electrical stimulation. Passive and active range-of-motion exercises, isometric exercise, and joint mobilization of the cervical spine and TMJ may be included in the plan of care. The patient may be instructed to wear a mouth guard at night to decrease bruxing.

 CLINICAL ALERT ──────────

Initially, activities that cause locking or clicking should be avoided to decrease inflammation.

The patient should be instructed in the proper resting position of the tongue and jaw. The tip of the tongue should be on the roof of the mouth, just behind the top teeth, with the teeth and jaw slightly parted, and lips closed. The patient should become familiar with this position and assume it during normal activities.

As inflammation and joint pain decrease, the patient may be progressed to range-of-motion exercises. If patients have deviation of the jaw to one side when opening, they should be instructed to perform the exercises only in the range in which deviation can be avoided.

Patient education should focus on the self-limiting nature of TMJ. This joint is capable of remodeling, leading to changes in the articular disc. Physical therapy, pain management, and addressing the contributors to TMJ pain help the patient through the painful period.

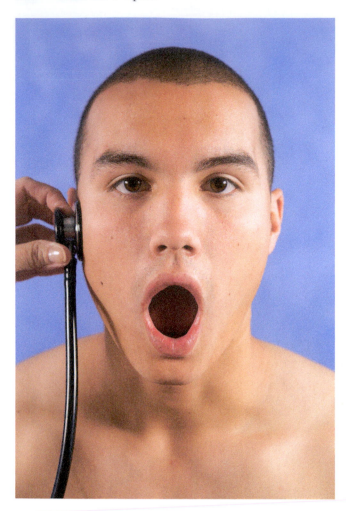

Figure 8.36 Stethoscope assessment of crepitus of the TMJ.

Temporomandibular Muscle Dysfunction

Myalgia, or muscle pain, in the TMJ area is fairly common and accounts for about half of TMD. The patient may have overactive masticatory muscles. This pain is often accompanied by pain in the neck and shoulder area.

Causes/Contributing Factors

It is unclear whether cervical pain predisposes patients to myalgia in the TMJ area, but there seems to be an association. Forward head posture has been associated with temporomandibular myalgia.[3,43–45] Jaw malocclusion and bruxism are also contributors. Bruxism occurring at night may be related to sleeping posture or stress. Fibromyalgia may contribute to temporomandibular myalgia.

Symptoms

Patients with TMD with myalgia may complain of ear, jaw, or facial pain. They may state that their ear feels full. They often report discomfort with chewing. Cervicogenic headache is also common.

Clinical Signs

The special tests listed earlier that assess active and resisted movements are used to assess **myogenic** TMD. The patient will often have pain and limitation of motion with these tests.

Intervention

Patients with myogenic TMJ pain may benefit from modalities to decrease pain and muscle spasm, including heat, cryotherapy, ultrasound, laser, and electrical stimulation. Postural retraining, active range-of-motion exercises, isometric exercise, biofeedback, relaxation exercises, and joint mobilization of the cervical spine and TMJ may be included in the plan of care.

Rocabado advocates six "6 x 6 exercises" for TMD, which are to be done 6 times each, 6 times a day. The patient is initially instructed in the proper resting position of the tongue and jaw, as described above. Instruct the patient to:

1. Assume the proper tongue and jaw position. Perform diaphragmatic breathing through the nose. In the resting position, with mouth slightly open, make a clucking sound.
2. Assume the proper tongue and jaw position. Keeping the tongue on the roof of the mouth, open the mouth until the tongue starts to leave the roof of the mouth. Stop sooner if pain or clicking occurs.
3. Assume the proper tongue and jaw position. Use one or two fingers on the chin to provide resistance to attempted jaw movements. Gently try to open and close the mouth, resisting with your fingers to prevent any movement. Do the same thing gently in a side-to-side direction, preventing lateral deviation. This is a rhythmic stabilization to the jaw.
4. Clasp both hands behind the neck. Without flexing the neck, nod the head by rotating the head on atlas.
5. Retract head back as if to make a double chin. This should cause a feeling of tightness at the back of the neck.
6. Lift lower ribs and chest up and forward, while bringing shoulder blades together.

Patients may be instructed to gently self-stretch into a jaw open position (Fig. 8.37). Talking or singing with a cork in the mouth for 5 to 10 minutes may be used to stretch the muscles, resulting in decreased muscle tension (Fig. 8.38).

Prevention

Patients should be instructed to avoid chewing gum, biting nails, and eating foods that are difficult to chew. They should avoid resting their jaw on their hand.

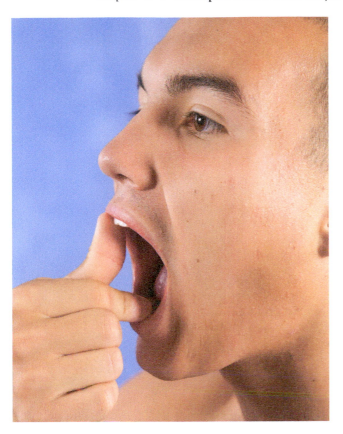

Figure 8.37 Self-stretch into a jaw-open position may be indicated for temporomandibular myalgia.

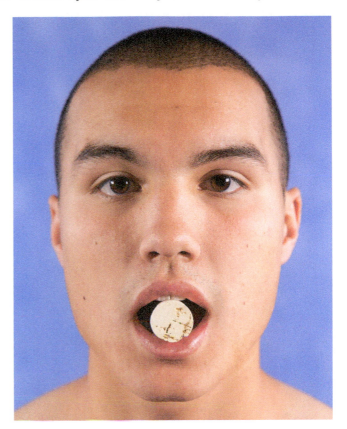

Figure 8.38 The patient may use a cork in the mouth to stretch the muscles of the jaw, resulting in muscle relaxation.

The Bottom Line: for patients with temporomandibular dysfunction

Description and causes	Muscle or joint pain often caused by jaw malocclusion, bruxism, or forward head posture, resulting in pain in the TMJ with or without popping, clicking, and limitation of motion
Test	Range of motion, resisted movement, and palpation tests of the TMJ
Stretch	Into mouth opening and lateral deviation to decrease muscle tension
Strengthen	The muscles of the jaw: temporalis, masseter, and pterygoids
Train	Proper resting tongue position
Avoid	Forward head posture, chewing gum, biting nails, bruxing

SUMMARY

The importance of the cervical spine lies in the ability to protect the spinal cord while still providing maximum mobility. These opposing functions are possible because of the anatomical complexity of the area. However, muscle weakness, muscle imbalance, trauma, and postural abnormalities may lead to a myriad of signs and symptoms, including weakness, loss of reflexes, pain, loss of sensation, and headache. Providing appropriate physical therapy interventions in this region is important to restoring function.

REVIEW QUESTIONS

1. Begin with instructing your lab partner to sit with the neck in good alignment. Using all of your fingers, lightly rest on the cervical spinous processes throughout the cervical spine in this posture. Instruct your partner to move into a forward head posture, while palpating the spinous processes. Have your lab partner repeat the movement several times while you note the flexion of the lower cervical vertebrae and the extension of the upper vertebrae. What movement

of the thoracic spine accompanies forward head posture? What occurs in the thoracic spine with cervical retraction? What occurs in the scapulae?

2. Palpate your lab partner's TMJ. To do this, you may insert your gloved index finger in your partner's ear and curve your finger forward or palpate just anterior to the external auditory meatus. Have your lab partner open and close the mouth and note the downward and anterior movement of the condyle. Have your lab partner move the open jaw from side to side. What do you feel with side-to-side movement? Have your lab partner protrude the lower jaw. How does this feel differently than the movement at the TMJ when opening the mouth?

3. Sit erect and protrude your jaw. Note any difficulties, how much ROM is available, any grinding, and so on. Now assume a forward head posture. In this position, protrude your jaw. Did you notice any changes? What can you conclude?

4. Name the muscles that act as a force couple in cervical rotation to the right.

5. Name the muscles that act as a force couple in cervical sidebending to the right.

6. You are treating a patient with pressure on a cervical nerve root from a disc that is herniated. Explain why the exercises used in the plan of care for this patient may include extending the cervical spine. Would the exercise protocol be likely to change if the nerve pressure was from a bony structure that narrowed the neural foramen? In what way?

7. With your lab partner perform sensation testing, manual muscle testing, and reflex testing associated with a C5 nerve root. Repeat for C6, C7, and C8.

8. You are treating a patient with a history of cervicogenic headaches for the last year, secondary to a whiplash injury. The plan of care specifies that the patient is to be instructed in strengthening exercises for the deep cervical flexor muscles. Describe how this is different from strengthening the sternocleidomastoid and scalene muscles.

9. You are treating a patient with a foraminal stenosis with radiculopathy of C6. The patient states that the pain is increased with neck extension and sidebending toward the affected side. Using your lab partner as a patient simulator, explain to your partner why this is occurring.

10. The plan of care for the patient in question 9 specifies exercises for the neck and for the resulting weakness in the upper extremity. What exercises might you use?

11. You are treating a 35-year-old with a recent history of radicular pain that has been determined to be related to a herniated disc. The patient has a forward head posture. How important is it to correct the forward head? Why or why not?

12. The patient in question 11 relates an increase in posterior neck pain with cervical retraction and abolishment of other arm symptoms. How might you progress this exercise?

13. What activities of daily living would you expect to increase symptoms in a patient with a cervical herniated disc? A cervical foraminal stenosis?

PATIENT CASE: Spondylotic Radiculopathy Cervical Spine

PT Evaluation

Patient Name: XXXXX XXXXX   **Age:** 66   **BMI:** 21.3

Diagnosis/History

Medical Diagnosis: Spondylotic radiculopathy cervical spine   **PT Diagnosis:** L arm pain secondary to cervical spondylosis

Diagnostic Tests/Results: MRI – C7 spondylosis   **Relevant Medical History:** OA, HTN, DM

Prior Level of Function: Not remarkable

Patient's Goals: Decrease pain, return to PLOF

Medications: Procardia ER 60 mg daily, Metformin ER 1000 mg daily   **Precautions:** None

Social Supports/Safety Hazards

Patient Living Situation/ Supports/ Hazards: Lives alone
Patient Working Situation/Occupation/ Leisure Activities: Retired law school professor. Does pro bono work for Legal Aid Clinic.

Vital Signs

At rest   Temperature: 98.6   BP: 130/82   HR: 74   Resp: 14   O2 sat: 98

Subjective Information

Patient is a male with 3-week history of pain in the L arm, with numbness of the middle finger. This began for no apparent reason. Pain interferes with daily activities.

Physical Assessment

Orientation: Alert and oriented   **Speech/Vision/Hearing:** wears hearing aids B.   **Skin Integrity:** Intact

ROM: Cervical spine movements are limited moderately in all planes. c/o pain with prolonged and repeated cervical extension. Most distal pain is below elbow.

Strength: MMT 3/5 triceps, 4/5 wrist flexion.   **Palpation:** Not tested

Muscle Tone: Not tested   **Balance/Coordination:** WNL   **Sensation/Proprioception:** Decreased sensation 3rd digit

Endurance: Not tested   **Posture:** Decreased cervical lordosis   **Edema:** None

Pain

Pain Rating and Location: **At best** 0/10   **At worst** 5/10   **Relieving Factors:** Neck flexion

Aggravating Factors: Neck extension (noted when shaving and using computer)   **Irritability:** Patient can reposition to relieve pain quickly.

Functional Assessment

Patient is functionally independent.

Special Testing

Test Name: Reflex testing/MMT   **Result** Consistent with C7 radiculopathy   **Test Name:**   **Result**

Assessment

Patient has s/s consistent with C7 spondylotic radiculopathy

Short-Term Treatment Goals

1. Patient will state a 25% decrease in pain.
2. Patient will voice and demonstrate an understanding of centralization of pain.
3. Patient will be independent in HEP.

Long-Term Treatment Goals

1. Patient will state a 50% decrease in pain.
2. Patient's most distal pain will be above elbow.

Treatment Plan

Frequency/Duration: 2 times a week for 4 weeks

Consisting of: Modalities, therapeutic exercise, neuro re-education, patient education

continued

Patient Case Questions

1. What factors might be contributing to the patient's spondylosis?

2. What would you tell the patient about specific activities to avoid or curtail?

3. What data will you collect the first time you see the patient?

4. If the plan of care does not guide you, what modalities might you use with this patient? Why? Are any modalities contraindicated?

5. If the plan of care does not specifically guide you, describe three therapeutic exercises that are indicated for this patient. Justify your choices.

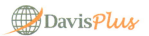 For additional resources, including answers to this case, please visit http://davisplus.fadavis.com

REFERENCES

1. Alexander, L. A., Hancock, E., Agouris, I., Smith, F. W., & MacSween, A. (2007). The response of the nucleus pulposus of the lumbar intervertebral discs to functionally loaded positions. *Spine, 32,* 1508–1512.

2. Marklund, S., Wiesinger, B., & Wänman, A. (2010). Reciprocal influence on the incidence of symptoms in trigeminally and spinally innervated areas. *European Journal of Pain, 14,* 366–371.

3. Olivo, S. A., Bravo, J., Magee, D. J., Thie, N. M., Major, P. W., & Flores-Mir, C. (2006). The association between head and cervical posture and temporomandibular disorders: A systematic review. *Journal of Orofacial Pain, 20,* 9–23.

4. Childs, J. D., Cleland, J. A., Elliott, J. M., Teyhen, D. S., Wainner, R. S., Whitman, J. M., Sopky, B. J., et al. (2008). Neck pain: Clinical practice guidelines linked to the International Classification of Functioning, Disability, and Health from the Orthopedic Section of the American Physical Therapy Association. *Journal of Orthopaedic and Sports Physical Therapy, 38,* A1–A34.

5. Blanpied, P. R., Gross, A. R., Elliott, J. M., Devaney, L. L., Clewley, D., Walton, D. M., Sparks, C., et al. (2017). Neck Pain: Revision 2017. *Journal of Orthopaedic and Sports Physical Therapy, 47,* A1–A83.

6. Bogduk, N. (2001). Cervicogenic headache: Anatomic basis and pathophysiologic mechanisms. *Current Pain and Headache Reports, 5,* 382–386.

7. Bogduk, N., & Marsland, A. (1986). On the concept of third occipital headache. *Journal of Neurology, Neurosurgery, and Psychiatry, 49,* 775–780.

8. Lord, S. M., Barnsley, L., Wallis, B. J., & Bogduk, N. (1994). Third occipital nerve headache: A prevalence study. *Journal of Neurology, Neurosurgery, and Psychiatry, 57,* 1187–1190.

9. Slipman, C. W., Plastaras, C., Patel, R., Isaac, Z., Chow, D., Garvan, C., Pauza, K., et al. (2005). Provocative cervical discography symptom mapping. *The Spine Journal, Official Journal of the North American Spine Society, 5,* 381–388.

10. Petersen, S. M. (2003). Articular and muscular impairments in cervicogenic headache: A case report. *Journal of Orthopaedic and Sports Physical Therapy, 33,* 21–30; discussion 30–32.

11. Farmer, P. K., Snodgrass, S. J., Buxton, A., & Rivett, D. A. (2014). An investigation of cervical spinal posture in cervicogenic headache. *Physical Therapy, 95,* 212–222.

12. Barton, P. M., & Hayes, K. C. (1996). Neck flexor muscle strength, efficiency, and relaxation times in normal subjects and subjects with unilateral neck pain and headache. *Archives of Physical Medicine and Rehabilitation, 77,* 680–687.

13. Nicholson, G. G., & Gaston, J. (2001). Cervical headache. *Journal of Orthopaedic and Sports Physical Therapy, 31,* 184–193.

14. Vernon, H. T., Aker, P., Aramenko, M., Battershill, D., Alepin, A., & Penner, T. (1992). Evaluation of neck muscle strength with a modified sphygmomanometer dynamometer: Reliability and validity. *Journal of Manipulative and Physiological Therapeutics, 15,* 343–349.

15. Watson, D. H., & Trott, P. H. (1993). Cervical headache: An investigation of natural head posture and upper cervical flexor muscle performance. *Cephalalgia: An International Journal of Headache, 13,* 272–284; discussion 232.

16. Nicholson, G. G., & Gaston, J. (2001). Cervical headache. *Journal of Orthopaedic and Sports Physical Therapy, 31,* 184–193.

17. Racicki, S., Gerwin, S., DiClaudio, S., Reinmann, S., & Donaldson, M. (2013). Conservative physical therapy management for the treatment of cervicogenic headache: A systematic review. *Journal of Manual and Manipulative Therapy, 21,* 113–124.

18. Harris, K. D., Heer, D. M., Roy, T. C., Santos, D. M., Whitman, J. M., & Wainner, R. S. (2005). Reliability of a measurement of neck flexor muscle endurance. *Physical Therapy, 85,* 1349–1355.

19. Jarman, N. F., Brooks, T., James, C. R., Hooper, T., Wilhelm, M., Brismée, J. M., Domenech, M. A., et al. (2017). Deep neck flexor endurance in the adolescent and young adult: Normative data and associated attributes. *PM&R: The Journal of Injury, Function, and Rehabilitation, 9,* 969–975.

20. Domenech, M. A., Sizer, P. S., Dedrick, G. S., McGalliard, M. K., & Brismee, J. M. (2011). The deep neck flexor endurance test: Normative data scores in healthy adults. *PM&R: The Journal of Injury, Function, and Rehabilitation, 3,* 105–110.

21. Sharma, D., Sen, S., & Dhawan, A. (2014). Effects of cervical stabilization exercises on neck proprioception in patients with cervicogenic headache. *International Journal of Pharma and Bio Sciences, 5,* B405–B420.

22. Spitzer, W. O., Skovron, M. L., Salmi, L. R., Cassidy, J. D., Duranceau, J., Suissa, S., & Zeiss E. (1995). Scientific monograph of the Quebec Task Force on Whiplash-Associated Disorders: Redefining 'whiplash' and its management. *Spine, 20,* 1S–73S.

23. Elliott, J. M., Noteboom, J. T., Flynn, T. W., & Sterling, M. (2009). Characterization of acute and chronic whiplash-associated disorders. *Journal of Orthopaedic and Sports Physical Therapy, 39*, 312–323.

24. Trippolini, M. A., Dijkstra, P. U., Côté, P., Scholz-Odermatt, S. M., Geertzen, J. H., Reneman, M. F. (2014) Can functional capacity tests predict future work capacity in patients with whiplash-associated disorders? *Archives of Physical and Medicine and Rehabilitation, 95*, 2357–2366.

25. Southerst, D., Nordin, M. C., Côté, P., Shearer, H. M., Varatharajan, S., Yu, H., Wong, J. J., et al. (2016). Is exercise effective for the management of neck pain and associated disorders or whiplash-associated disorders? A systematic review by the Ontario Protocol for Traffic Injury Management (OPTIMa) Collaboration. *The Spine Journal, Official Journal of the North American Spine Society, 16*, 1503–1523.

26. Sutton, D. A., Côté, P., Wong, J. J., Varatharajan, S., Randhawa, K. A., Yu, H., Southerst, D., et al. (2016). Is multimodal care effective for the management of patients with whiplash-associated disorders or neck pain and associated disorders? A systematic review by the Ontario Protocol for Traffic Injury Management (OPTIMa) Collaboration. *The Spine Journal, Official Journal of the North American Spine Society, 16*, 1541–1565.

27. Ludvigsson, M. L., Peterson, G., O'Leary, S., Dedering, A., & Peolsson, A. (2015). The effect of neck-specific exercise with, or without a behavioral approach, on pain, disability and self-efficacy in chronic whiplash-associated disorders: A randomized clinical trial. *Clinical Journal of Pain, 31*, 294–303.

28. Gellhorn, A. C., Katz, J. N., & Suri, P. (2013). Osteoarthritis of the spine: The facet joints. *Nature Reviews, Rheumatology, 9*, 216–224.

29. Louw, A., Diener, I., Butler, D. S., & Puentedura, E. J. (2011). The effect of neuroscience education on pain, disability, anxiety, and stress in chronic musculoskeletal pain. *Archives of Physical Medicine and Rehabilitation, 92*, 2041–2056.

30. Zaaroor, M., Kósa, G., Peri-Eran, A., Maharil, I., Shoham, M., & Goldsher, D. (2006). Morphological study of the spinal canal content for subarachnoid endoscopy. *Minimally Invasive Neurosurgery Journal, 49*, 220–226.

31. Anekstein, Y., Blecher, R., Smorgick, Y., & Mirovsky, Y. (2012). What is the best way to apply the Spurling Test for cervical radiculopathy? *Clinical Orthopaedics and Related Research, 470*, 2566–2572.

32. Jull, G. A., Falla, D., Vicenzino, B., & Hodges, P. W. (2009). The effect of therapeutic exercise on activation of the deep cervical flexor muscles in people with chronic neck pain. *Manual Therapy, 14*, 696–701.

33. O'Leary, S., Jull, G., Kim, M., & Vicenzino, B. (2007). Specificity in retraining craniocervical flexor muscle performance. *Journal of Orthopaedic and Sports Physical Therapy, 37*, 3–9.

34. Cleland, J. A., Whitman, J. M., Fritz, J. M., & Palmer, J. A. (2005). Manual physical therapy, cervical traction, and strengthening exercises in patients with cervical radiculopathy: A case series. *Journal of Orthopaedic and Sports Physical Therapy, 35*, 802–811.

35. Moeti, P., & Marchetti, G. (2001). Clinical outcome from mechanical intermittent cervical traction for the treatment of cervical radiculopathy: A case series. *Journal of Orthopaedic and Sports Physical Therapy, 31*, 207–213.

36. Fardon, D. F., Williams, A. L., Dohring, E. J., Murtagh, F. R., Gabriel Rothman, S. L., & Sze, G. K. (2014). Lumbar disc nomenclature: version 2.0: Recommendations of the combined task forces of the North American Spine Society, the American Society of Spine Radiology and the American Society of Neuroradiology. *The Spine Journal, Official Journal of the North American Spine Society, 14*, 2525–2545.

37. Ikeda, H., Hanakita, J., Takahashi, T., Kuraishi, K., & Watanabe, M. (2012). Nontraumatic cervical disc herniation in a 21-year-old patient with no other underlying disease. *Neurologica Medic-Chirurgica, 52*, 652–656.

38. Wu, M. P., Chen, H. H., Yen, E. Y., Tsai, S. C., & Mo, L. R. (1999). A potential complication of laparoscopy—The surgeon's herniated cervical disk. *Journal of the American Association of Gynecologic Laparoscopists, 6*, 509–511.

39. Cloward, R. B. (1959. Cervical diskography. A contribution to the etiology and mechanism of neck, shoulder and arm pain. *Annals of Surgery, 150*, 1052–1064.

40. Wainner, R. S., Fritz, J. M., Irrgang, J. J., Boninger, M. L., Delitto, A., & Allison, S. (2003). Reliability and diagnostic accuracy of the clinical examination and patient self-report measures for cervical radiculopathy. *Spine, 28*, 52–62.

41. Agerberg, G. (1974). Maximal mandibular movements in young men and women. *Svensk Tandlakare Tidskrift, Swedish Dental Journal, 67*, 81–100.

42. Fatima, J., Kaul, R., Jain, P., Saha, S., Halder, S., & Sarkar, S. (2016). Clinical measurement of maximum mouth opening in children of Kolkata and its relation with different facial types. *Journal of Clinical and Diagnostic Research, 10*, ZC01-05.

43. Munhoz, W. C., & Hsing, W. T. (2014). Interrelations between orthostatic postural deviations and subjects' age, sex, malocclusion, and specific signs and symptoms of functional pathologies of the temporomandibular system: A preliminary correlation and regression study. *Cranio, Journal of Craniomandibular Practice, 32*, 175–186.

44. Rocha, C. P., Croci, C. S., & Caria, P. H. F. (2013). Is there relationship between temporomandibular disorders and head and cervical posture? A systematic review. *Journal of Oral Rehabilitation, 40*, 875–881.

45. Sonnesen, L., Bakke, M., & Solow, B. (2001). Temporomandibular disorders in relation to craniofacial dimensions, head posture and bite force in children selected for orthodontic treatment. *European Journal of Orthodontics, 23*, 179–192.

Chapter 9

Orthopedic Interventions for the Thoracic and Lumbosacral Spine

Anatomy and Physiology

Common Pathologies

LEARNING OUTCOMES

At the end of this chapter, the student will:

9.1   Describe the anatomy of the thoracic, lumbar, and sacral regions of the spine.
9.2   Describe normal range of motion of the lumbar spine.
9.3   Explain normal kinematics of the thoracic and lumbosacral regions, including lumbopelvic rhythm.
9.4   Discuss the significance of the thoracolumbar fascia.
9.5   Describe the effect of flexion and extension on the neural foramen, posterior elements, spinal ligaments, and intervertebral disc.
9.6   Describe common thoracic and lumbar spine pathologies and typical presentation.
9.7   Discuss contributing factors to various thoracic and lumbar spine pathologies and, when relevant, preventive measures.
9.8   Describe the relationship between lumbar facet DJD, spondylosis in the neural foramen, and spinal stenosis.
9.9   Describe the clinical tests used to diagnose common thoracic and lumbar spine pathologies and how to administer the tests.
9.10 Describe the concepts of centralization and peripheralization.
9.11 Discuss common treatment interventions for thoracic and lumbar spine pathologies.
9.12 Describe surgical interventions for thoracic and lumbar spine including laminectomy, discectomy, and vertebral augmentation.
9.13 Describe the relationship between hyperkyphosis and compression fracture.
9.14 Describe the clinical alert precautions for thoracic and lumbar spine pathologies.

KEY WORDS

Ala	Epidural steroid injection	Lateral shift
Bone mineral density (BMD)	Extension bias	Lumbopelvic rhythm
Centralization	Extruded disc	Nutation
Counternutation	Flexion bias	Osteoarthritis
Directional preference	Foraminotomy	Osteochondrosis
Discectomy	Idiopathic	Osteopenia
Electromyography/nerve conduction	Kyphoplasty	Osteophyte
velocity (EMG/NCV)	Laminectomy	Osteoporosis

Anatomy and Physiology

In this chapter, we will continue our discussion of the anatomy of the spine, focusing on the thoracic and lumbosacral regions. Given the stability provided by the ribs, the thoracic spine is unlike the other regions of the spine. It is a common source of postural abnormalities.

The lumbar spine must possess stability to withstand the forces to which it is subjected and yet be mobile to respond to changes in pelvic position. The anatomy of the lumbar spine and SI joint is designed for these purposes. The size and shape of the vertebrae, the density of ligaments, and the interaction of muscles allow this area to bear compressive and shear forces. Dynamic structures, including the intervertebral discs and thoracolumbar fascia, allow the lumbar spine to respond to movements in the pelvis and lower extremities.

The lumbosacral area is a frequent source of pain and pathology. According to the National Institute of Health, low back pain is the most common cause of job-related disability.[1] It is also the most common reason people seek physical therapy. An understanding of the anatomy and physiology of the thoracic and lumbosacral areas is essential for the PTA.

Bone and Joint Anatomy and Physiology

The thoracic spine contains 12 vertebrae. This region is convex when viewed from the posterior. The first thoracic vertebra articulates with C7 and has features common to the cervical and the thoracic spine. From T1 to T11, the facet joints are oriented largely in the frontal plane, providing ease of side bending and rotation. T12 is a transitional vertebra; the body is large like those of the lumbar vertebrae and its inferior facets lie in the sagittal plane.

The most distinguishing characteristic of the thoracic vertebrae is the articulation of each vertebra with a pair of ribs. The thoracic spine has much less range of motion than the cervical spine, due to the rigidity of the ribcage. The ribs articulate both with the vertebral bodies and the transverse processes.

A second distinguishing feature of the thoracic spine is the elongated spinous processes that overlap the vertebra below. The end of the spinous process is approximately at the level of the transverse process of the vertebra below. Figure 9.1 depicts a typical thoracic vertebra. See Table 9-1 for a summary of bone and joint anatomy of the thoracic spine.

The lumbar spine contains five vertebrae. These vertebrae have the largest bodies, which help them withstand the weight-bearing forces to which they are subjected. Each body is somewhat higher anteriorly than posteriorly, resulting in a slight wedge shape. This gives the region a lordotic curve. The spinous processes are broad and square, serving as strong attachment sites for the lumbar ligaments, muscles, and fascia. The facet joints in the lumbar spine lie mostly in the sagittal plane, allowing flexion and extension movements to occur with greatest ease. Figure 9.2 depicts a typical lumbar vertebra.

The fifth lumbar vertebra is atypical in the height of its vertebral body and the orientation of its inferior articular processes. The vertebral body is shorter than that of other lumbar vertebrae. The inferior facets of L5 lie mostly in the frontal plane, which allows them to

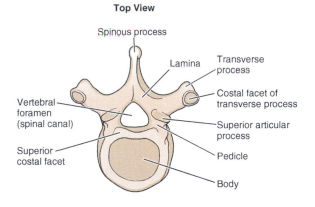

Top View

Spinous process

Lamina

Transverse process

Vertebral foramen (spinal canal)

Costal facet of transverse process

Superior articular process

Superior costal facet

Pedicle

Body

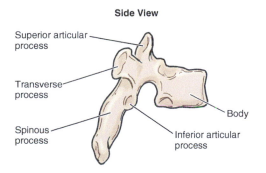

Side View

Superior articular process

Transverse process

Spinous process

Body

Inferior articular process

Figure 9.1 Typical features of a thoracic vertebra include a slender and elongated spinous process and costal facets.

Table 9-1   Bone and Joint Anatomy and Physiology

Of the Thoracic and Lumbosacral Spine

Joint	Anatomy	Normal ROM and Movements	Landmarks	Clinical Considerations
Between vertebral bodies	Intervertebral disc lies between bodies.	ROM is age-related. For people ages 20–35, normal ROM is as follows: Flexion = 35° Extension = 16° Rotation to each side = 18°.		When locating landmarks, knowledge of overlapping of spinous processes is necessary. Spinous processes extend down to level of transverse processes of vertebra below.
Zygapophyseal joint (facet joint)	Superior articular processes articulate with inferior articular processes on vertebra above.			Facet joints lie in frontal plane in thoracic spine, and in sagittal plane in lumbar spine.
Sternocostal joints	Articulation of the ribs with the sternum through the costal cartilage.	Plane joints with very minimal gliding motion.		
Costal facet joints	Articulation of ribs with thoracic vertebrae.	Plane joints with very minimal gliding motion.		
Lumbosacral junction	Promontory at superior end of sacrum articulates with L5. The sacrum is inclined about 30°–40° anteriorly.	Flexion, extension, side bending, and rotation of lumbar spine.		Inclination of the sacrum may lead to anterior slipping of L5 on the sacrum in the presence of pathology.
Sacroiliac joints	Alar wings of sacrum articulate with ilia on each side. Synovial joints, which are irregular and wavy in shape; the shape-matching surfaces interlock the two bones. Stabilized by dense ligaments both anteriorly and posteriorly.	Sacrum can minimally flex (nutate) or extend (counternutate) within the ilia.	Spinous projections on anterior ilium: anterior superior iliac spine (ASIS) and anterior inferior iliac spine (AIIS). Spinous projections on the posterior ilium: posterior superior iliac spine (PSIS) and the posterior inferior iliac spine (PIIS).	Bony landmarks are often used by the physical therapist assistant to determine pelvic symmetry.
Pubic symphysis	Amphiarthrodial joint with a fibrocartilage disc between the two pubic bones. Stabilized by ligaments.		Two rami: the superior pubic ramus and the inferior pubic ramus.	The superior pubic ramus may be used as a landmark by the physical therapist assistant to determine pubic alignment.

serve as a restraint to anterior displacement of L5 on the sacrum.

The sacrum is a triangle-shaped bone that results from the fusion of S1-5. It is tilted anteriorly about 30° to 40° and has a convex curve posteriorly. The top of the sacrum (**sacral promontory**) articulates with L5. The distal end of the sacrum articulates with the coccyx or tailbone. Each side of the sacrum (**ala**) articulates with the ilium at the sacroiliac (SI) joint. The SI joint is a synovial, plane joint with very irregular surface topography. The two bones fit together like puzzle pieces, providing bony stability to the joint.

Table 9-1 summarizes bone and joint anatomy of the thoracic and lumbar spine, sacrum, and ilium.

Soft Tissue Anatomy and Physiology

Intervertebral Disc and Vertebral End Plates

The intervertebral disc has concentric rings of collagen (annulus fibrosus) that encapsulate a water-based gel in

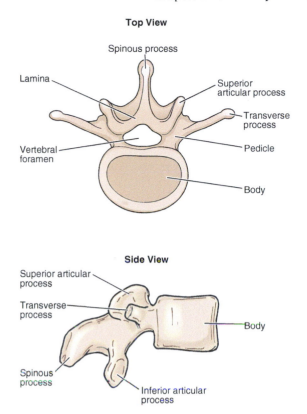

Figure 9.2 Typical features of a lumbar vertebra include a large vertebral body and broad spinous processes.

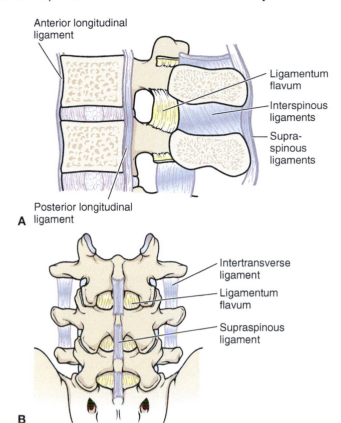

Figure 9.3 Ligaments of the thoracic and lumbar spine.

the center (nucleus pulposus). Only the outermost rings of the annulus fibrosus are innervated. The inner rings and the nucleus pulposus have neither nerve nor blood supply. Vertebral end plates cover the superior and inferior aspect of the vertebral bodies. They are attached to the annulus fibrosus and provide nutrition to the intervertebral disc through diffusion.

Intervertebral discs in the thoracic spine are not commonly a site of pathology due to the relative lack of mobility in the area. However, the intervertebral discs in the lumbar spine are often a site of pathology (see *Herniated Disc* later in this chapter).

Ligaments and Joint Capsules

The ligaments found in the thoracic and lumbar spine are like those in the cervical spine with the exception of ligamentum nuchae. Below C7, ligamentum nuchae becomes the supraspinous and interspinous ligaments. These ligaments limit flexion in the thoracic and lumbar spine.

The other major ligaments include the anterior and posterior longitudinal ligaments, the ligamentum flavum, and the intertransverse ligament. The longitudinal ligaments run the entire length of the spine. The anterior longitudinal ligament is found on the anterior aspect of the vertebral bodies and restricts spine extension. The posterior longitudinal ligament runs down the posterior aspect of the vertebral bodies, inside the spinal canal,

and restricts spine flexion. Very close in location is ligamentum flavum, which runs from the lamina of each vertebra to adjacent vertebrae. It also serves to restrict spine flexion. The intertransverse ligament connects the transverse processes of the vertebrae with those above and below. It restricts spine side bending.

Additional ligaments help stabilize the spine and pelvis. Unique to the lumbar spine, the iliolumbar ligament is a small ligament that runs from the transverse process of L5 to the iliac crest. While it limits motion in all directions, it seems to be most helpful in limiting anterior sliding of L5 on S1. Thick ligaments on the anterior and posterior aspects of the sacroiliac joints enhance the bony stability of the SI joint.

Joint capsules also promote stability of the thoracic and lumbar spine. The facet joint capsules restrict motion, assisting the ligaments to stabilize the spine, particularly from L4 to S1. The sacroiliac joint similarly has a strong fibrous capsule.

Figure 9.3 depicts these ligaments in the spine.

Thoracolumbar Fascia

The thoracolumbar fascia (TLF) is a broad, diamond-shaped connective tissue in the low back. It has three layers: an anterior and middle layer that originate from the transverse processes of the lumbar vertebrae, and the posterior layer that originates from the spinous processes of thoracic, lumbar, and sacral vertebrae. The deeper layers enclose the quadratus lumborum and blend into the transverse abdominis and internal oblique muscles. The posterior layer covers erector spinae and blends with latissimus dorsi and with gluteus maximus, forming a connection between the humerus and the femur. The significance of this important structure will be discussed later in this chapter.

Table 9-2 summarizes the soft tissue structures in the thoracic and lumbosacral spine.

Nerves

As the spinal cord continues through the thoracic spine, it gives off paired spinal nerves at each level. These nerve roots provide both sensation and movement in the trunk. The sensation provided by each nerve root is best appreciated in a dermatome chart (Fig. 9.4). Many of the muscles of the trunk are innervated by motor branches of the thoracic nerves from several levels. For example, the deep transversospinalis muscle group is innervated by branches of T1 to T6 nerves.

The spinal cord continues into the lumbar spine, ending at the L1 vertebral level. In the lower thoracic spine, the nerve roots do not enter and exit the spinal cord at the same level as the neural foramen. Rather, the corresponding neural foramen is progressively more inferior to the nerve root. Below the L1 level, the nerve roots lie outside the spinal cord but remain in the spinal canal for several levels prior to exiting. This bundle of nerve roots resembles a horse's tail and is therefore known as the cauda equina. Figure 9.5 illustrates the anatomy of the spinal cord and cauda equina.

After exiting the neural foramen, lumbar and sacral nerve roots merge to form the lumbosacral plexus. Like the brachial plexus in the upper extremity, this mixing of nerve roots results in representation of several spinal root levels in the peripheral nerves. Figure 9.6 depicts the lumbosacral plexus.

Spinal nerve roots L1 to S2 provide sensation and movement to the lower extremities. S2 to S4 control bowel, bladder, and sexual function. A summary of the dermatome, myotome, and reflex arcs for each level can be found in Table 9-3.

Muscular Anatomy and Kinesiology

Aside from muscles on the back that ultimately move the extremities, the muscular anatomy in the thoracic and lumbar areas consists primarily of the deep stabilizing

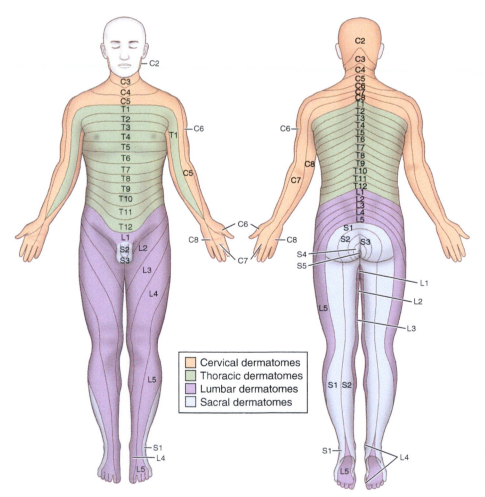

Figure 9.4 Dermatomes of the thoracic, lumbar, and sacral nerve roots.

Table 9-2   Connective Tissue Anatomy and Physiology

Of the Thoracic and Lumbosacral Spine

Structure	Anatomy	Function	Clinical Considerations
Intervertebral disc	Lies between vertebral bodies. Two parts: nucleus pulposus and annulus fibrosus.	Absorbs compressive forces, allows for movement of the spine.	The central nucleus pulposus may break through the fibrous rings that contain it and lead to pressure on spinal nerve roots.
Vertebral end plate	Thin layer of cartilage that covers the top and bottom of the vertebral body. Connected to the annulus fibrosus.	Supplies nutrition to the inner rings of the annulus fibrosus and the nucleus pulposus by diffusion.	The nucleus pulposus may herniate upwardly or downwardly through the end plate (Schmorl's node). Deterioration of the disc, and possibly of the vertebral body, may result.
Ligamentum flavum	Connects the lamina of adjacent vertebrae. Lies posterior to the spinal cord in the spinal canal.	Limits flexion of the spine.	Hypertrophy may lead to spinal stenosis. Highly elastic ligament of the spine, allows for significant motion without rupture.
Supraspinous and interspinous ligament	Found below C7, these ligaments run between spinous processes (interspinous) and along the top of the spinous processes (supraspinous).	Limits flexion of the spine.	
Anterior longitudinal ligament	Runs down the length of the spine on the anterior vertebral bodies.	Limits extension of the spine.	
Posterior longitudinal ligament	Runs down the length of the spine on the posterior vertebral bodies, anterior to the spinal cord in the spinal canal.	Limits flexion of the spine.	Hypertrophy may lead to spinal stenosis.
Capsule of the facet joints	Around each facet joint.	Limits flexion and rotation of the spine.	
Intertransverse ligament	Runs between adjacent transverse processes.	Limits side bending to opposite side.	
Thoracolumbar fascia (TLF)	Three layers that encompass erector spinae and quadratus lumborum with attachments to latissimus dorsi, transverse abdominis and internal oblique, and gluteus maximus muscles.	Supports the lumbar spine and SI joints. Many large muscles of the trunk and extremities insert on the TLF.	May contribute to low back pain. Has role in proprioception. Functionally connects the upper and lower extremities through the muscle attachments.
Iliolumbar ligament	Runs from the transverse process of L5 to the iliac crest.	Limits anterior sliding of L5 on S1.	Important stabilizer in fracture or spondylolysis.
Lumbosacral ligament	Runs from L5 to sacral ala.	Stabilizes the LS junction.	L5 nerve root may run under the ligament and entrap L5.
Anterior sacroiliac ligament	Runs from sacrum to ilium on anterior side.	Prevents anterior opening of the SI joint. Assists the pubic symphysis in resisting separation.	
Posterior sacroiliac ligament	Runs from sacrum to PSIS.	Stabilizes sacrum in load bearing.	
Sacrospinous ligament	Runs from PSIS, sacrum, and coccyx to ischial tuberosity.	Stabilizes sacrum in load bearing.	Biceps femoris and gluteus maximus attach to this ligament.
Sacrotuberous ligament	Runs from lower sacrum to ischial spine.	Stabilizes sacrum in load bearing.	

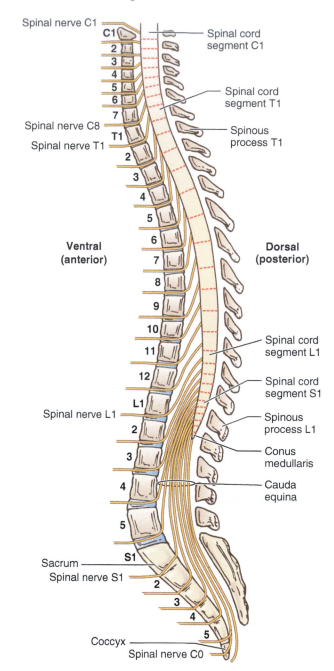

Figure 9.5 The spinal cord ends at the L1 vertebral level. Inferior to this, as the nerve roots travel through the spinal canal, they form the cauda equina.

muscles, muscles of respiration, psoas major, quadratus lumborum, erector spinae, and the abdominals.

The deep stabilizing muscles are the transversospinalis, interspinalis, and intertransversarii. Transversospinalis consists of semispinalis, rotatores, and multifidus. These muscles are small in the upper back and don't make a significant contribution to back strength. Rather they are thought to provide stabilization throughout the thoracic spine. In the lumbar spine the transversospinalis group becomes much larger. Weakness of one muscle of this

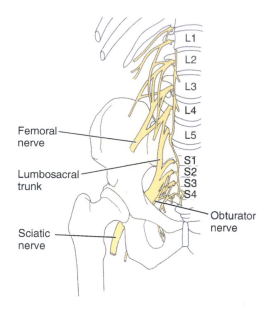

Figure 9.6 The lumbosacral plexus.

group, multifidus, has been linked to low back disc pathology.[2,3]

The muscles of respiration include those involved in inspiration and expiration. The two muscles involved in inspiration are the diaphragm and the external intercostals. The internal intercostals are active in forced expiration.

The erector spinae seen in the cervical area as a neck extensor also continues on the posterior aspect of the thoracic and lumbar spine. It is a powerful trunk extensor and side bender. It is opposed in action by the four muscles of the abdominal group on the anterior trunk. The abdominal muscles are layered with varying fiber orientation.

Psoas major is a hip flexor but also acts as a trunk flexor and lumbar spine stabilizer.[4,5] Similarly, quadratus lumborum is a hip hiker but acts as a lumbar spine side bender.

Muscles of the lumbar spine and trunk play an important role in stabilizing the lumbar spine. The PTA must understand the muscles in the low back and trunk to provide effective intervention. Muscles that affect the thoracic and lumbar spine, with origin, insertion, innervation, action, and clinical relevance are listed in Table 9-4.

Posture

The thoracic spine is kyphotic, or convex, posteriorly. The normal angle of kyphosis has been reported to be 20° to 45°. Females have a greater degree of kyphosis and the curvature in both genders increases with age. Measurement of thoracic kyphosis may be done using a flexicurve ruler as described in Box 9-2 under the pathology of hyperkyphosis. This method obtains similar

Table 9-3 Lumbar and Sacral Spinal Nerves

With Associated Dermatome, Myotome, and Reflex

Level	Dermatome	Myotome	MMT	Reflex
L1	Groin and topmost area of leg	NA	NA	NA
L2	Top of inner thigh	Hip flexion	Iliopsoas	NA
L3	Medial knee	Knee extension	Quadriceps	NA
L4	Big toe, medial malleolus	Ankle dorsiflexion	Anterior tibialis	Quadriceps
L5	Middle three toes and top of foot	Big toe extension	Extensor hallucis longus	NA
S1	Little toe and bottom of foot	Ankle plantarflexion and eversion, hip extension	Gastrocsoleus, fibularis group	Gastrocsoleus
S2	Medial posterior knee	Knee flexion	Hamstrings	NA
S3	Ischial tuberosity	NA	NA	NA
S4	Perianal area	NA	NA	NA
S5	Perianal area	NA	NA	NA

Table 9-4 Muscle Anatomy and Kinesiology

Of the Thoracic and Lumbosacral Spine

Muscle	Origin	Insertion	Innervation	Action	Clinical Considerations
Transverospinalis	Transverse processes	Spinous processes above	Adjacent spinal nerves	Back stabilizer. Bilaterally extend back. Unilaterally rotate back to opposite side.	Important back stabilizer. Includes the semispinalis, multifidus, and rotatores groups.
Interspinales	Spinous process	Spinous process above	Adjacent spinal nerves	Back stabilizer. Back extension.	Important back stabilizer.
Intertransversarii	Transverse process	Transverse process above	Adjacent spinal nerves	Back side bending.	Important back stabilizer. May have a role in proprioception.
Erector spinae	Spinous processes, transverse processes, ligamentum nuchae	Spinous processes, transverse processes, occiput and mastoid	Adjacent spinal nerves	Bilaterally extends back. Unilaterally side bends back.	Group consists of spinalis, longissimus, and iliocostalis groups. The iliocostalis portion of this group is not present in the cervical area.
Rectus abdominis	Pubis	Cartilage of ribs 5-7, xiphoid process	Intercostal nerves (T7-T12)	Flexion of the trunk	May be used as an accessory muscle of respiration, assisting forced expiration. Two straps are separated by the linea alba. The muscles may separate in pregnancy. This is called diastasis recti. Tendinous bands in muscle give the "six-pack" appearance.
External oblique	Lateral side of ribs 5-12	Iliac crest and linea alba	Intercostal nerves 8-12	Bilateral: Flexes the trunk. Unilateral: Rotates the trunk to the opposite side. Side bends trunk to same side.	

Continued

Table 9-4   Muscle Anatomy and Kinesiology—cont'd

Of the Thoracic and Lumbosacral Spine

Muscle	Origin	Insertion	Innervation	Action	Clinical Considerations
Internal oblique	Inguinal ligament, iliac crest, and thoracolumbar fascia	Lowest 3 ribs and linea alba	Intercostal nerves 8–12	Bilateral: Flexes the trunk. Unilateral: Rotates the trunk to the same side. Side bends trunk to same side.	
Transverse abdominis	Ribs 7–12, inguinal ligament, thoracolumbar fascia, iliac crest	Linea alba	Intercostal nerves 7–12	Increases intra-abdominal pressure. Used as a muscle of respiration. Stabilizes the lumbar spine by tensing the thoracolumbar fascia.	
Quadratus lumborum	Iliolumbar ligament and iliac crest	Last rib, transverse processes of lumbar vertebrae	Spinal nerves T12–L4	Hikes hip, side bends trunk to same side	May assist in forced expiration. Easily reverses action.
Diaphragm	Xiphoid process, ribs, lumbar vertebrae	Central tendon of the diaphragm	Phrenic nerve (C3, 4, 5)	Inspiration	Contracts and flattens to expand the thoracic cavity.
External intercostals	Ribs above	Ribs below	Intercostal nerves (T2–T6)	Inspiration	Raises ribs to expand the thoracic cavity.
Internal intercostals	Ribs below	Ribs above	Intercostal nerves (T2–T6)	Expiration	Pulls ribs down to decrease the size of the thoracic cavity.
Psoas major	Vertebral bodies of T12–L5	Lesser trochanter	Spinal nerves L2–3	Hip flexion	Psoas major may reverse action and flex the trunk and stabilize lumbar spine.

results to those obtained by x-ray.[6] Deviations from the normal curve in the thoracic spine are not uncommon. These include hyperkyphosis and scoliosis. Both will be discussed later in this chapter.

When viewed from the side, the lumbar spine is lordotic, or concave posteriorly. In this normal alignment the body is supported with a minimum of muscle activity. The entire spine is seen as a series of gentle curves from cervical spine to sacrum. Alteration of any of these curves will affect the curves above or below and may have consequences on surrounding soft tissues.

Common postural deviations include an increase or decrease in lordosis. With increased lumbar lordosis, the thoracic spine may also assume an increased curvature, accompanied by forward head. Decreased lumbar lordosis may be accompanied by a decrease in thoracic kyphosis, resulting in a flat back posture. Alternatively, decreased lordosis may be accompanied by an increase in kyphosis, hip extension, and forward head, as seen in the swayback posture. A depiction of these postural deviations is shown in Figure 9.7.

Thoracic and Lumbosacral Spine Kinematics

Effect of Facet Joint Orientation on Movement

Motion in the thoracic spine is largely influenced by the orientation of the facet joints and by the ribs. In all directions, movement in the thoracic spine is very limited as compared to the cervical and lumbar regions. Most of the thoracic spine flexion and extension occurs in the lower thoracic area. Side bending is also less restricted in the lower thoracic area, owing mostly to the shortness of the lower ribs. Rotation, on the other hand, occurs primarily in the upper thoracic region. Range of motion in the thoracic spine has not been well investigated and is very dependent upon the position of the lumbar spine when measuring.[7] For this reason, measurements will not be listed in this text.

The lumbar spine allows for movement in all three planes, but facet orientation favors movement in the sagittal plane. In flexion, lumbar spine ROM is limited by the posterior ligaments. In extension, ROM is limited by contact of the **posterior elements** and by the anterior ligaments. However, total range of motion into flexion and extension is increased by movement of the pelvis on the femur.

ROM is also affected by age. For people ages 20–35, normal ROM of the thoracic and lumbar spine has been documented to be 35° flexion, 16° extension, and 18° rotation bilaterally.[8]

Lumbopelvic Rhythm

The interplay of motion occurring throughout the lumbar spine and at the hip during forward bending is called **lumbopelvic rhythm.** During forward bending, the lumbar spine flexes, the sacrum tilts forward (**nutation**), and the pelvis tilts anteriorly (hip flexion). There is disagreement about the timing of the lumbar spine and hip, but in normal movement there would be a contribution from both the spine and the hips. Abnormal lumbopelvic rhythm is associated with low back pain.[9] Figure 9.8 depicts normal lumbopelvic rhythm contrasted with decreased spine and hip contribution to movement.

In the movement of backward bending, the lumbar spine, sacrum, and hip similarly contribute to the total motion. The lumbar spine extends further from its normal lordotic position as the hip joint extends. The superior sacrum tilts posteriorly in a movement called **counternutation.**

For full forward flexion to occur, the hamstring muscles need to be normally long to allow the pelvis to anteriorly tilt. For full extension, the iliopsoas needs to be of normal length to allow posterior tilting. For these reasons, the PTA may see stretching exercises for the hamstrings and hip flexors in the plan of care for patients with low back pathology.

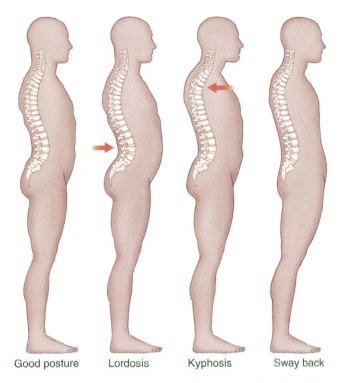

Good posture   Lordosis   Kyphosis   Sway back

Figure 9.7 Deviations from normal posture include increased lordosis, increased kyphosis, and swayback postures.

Figure 9.8 Normal pelvic rhythm (A), forward bending with restricted motion in the hips (B), and forward bending with restricted motion in the lumbar spine (C).

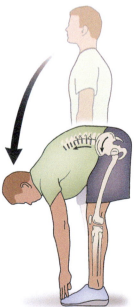
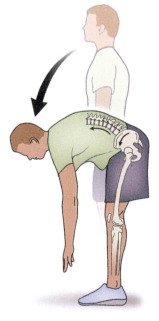
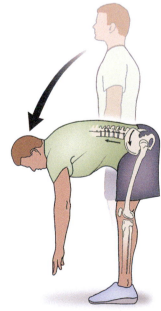

A Normal lumbar and hip flexion

B Limited hip flexion and excessive lumbar flexion

C Limited lumbar flexion and excessive hip flexion

Lumbosacral Kinematics

The lumbosacral junction is the most common site of pathology in the lumbar spine. It is a transitional area from the convex curve of the sacrum to the lordosis of the lumbar spine. Recall that the sacrum is inclined forward and downwardly at a 30° to 40° angle. The wedge shapes of the vertebral bodies in the lumbar spine create a lordosis, reversing this orientation. The vertebral bodies of L4 and L5 are the most wedge-shaped, with a much larger height anteriorly versus posteriorly.

Gravity would tend to cause L5 to slide anteriorly on the sacrum. Bony and soft tissue forces counteract this pull. Particularly, the inferior facets of L5 lie mostly in the frontal plane, increasing the anterior stability of L5 on the sacrum. The iliolumbar, anterior longitudinal, and lumbosacral ligaments help to stabilize this joint as well.

The L5 to S1 junction must withstand both compressive forces and shear forces. Body-weight forces acting on the spine are transmitted through L5-S1 to the SI joints, hips, and lower extremities. In addition, there are compressive forces from contraction of the surrounding muscles. Shear forces at L5-S1 related to the sacral incline exceed body weight.[10]

SI Joint Kinematics

The amount of movement that occurs in the SI joint is controversial. The irregular topography of the joint and the density of ligaments suggest that movement is minimal. Aside from nutation and counternutation, studies show that movements that occur are of a small magnitude.

Nutation occurs when the sacrum rotates anteriorly on the ilium or when the ilium rotates posteriorly on the sacrum. Nutation is accompanied by an increased lordosis of the lumbar spine. Counternutation involves a posterior rotation of the sacrum on the ilium or an anterior rotation of the ilium on the sacrum and is accompanied by a decrease in lumbar lordosis. Figure 9.9 depicts these movements.

Effect of Movement on the Disc, Ligaments, and Foramen

Movement of the vertebrae affects the intervertebral disc, causing it to slightly move or deform within the confines of the annular rings. Prolonged positioning or repeated movements are thought to result in movement of the nucleus.[11] Extension causes the nucleus to move anteriorly; flexion results in posterior movement (Fig. 9.10).

The annular rings are weakest in the posterolateral disc, and pressure of the nucleus against the annulus may result in tearing of the rings, allowing the nucleus to migrate away from the center of the disc.

Flexion and extension of the lumbar spine also affect the neural (intervertebral) foramen, as seen in Figure 9.10. The neural foramen are most open with trunk

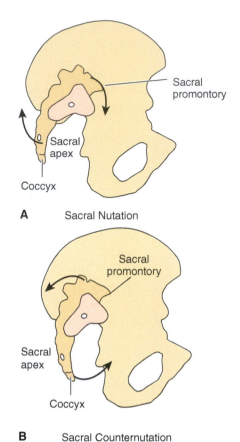

A   Sacral Nutation

B   Sacral Counternutation

Figure 9.9 Nutation and counternutation of the sacrum.

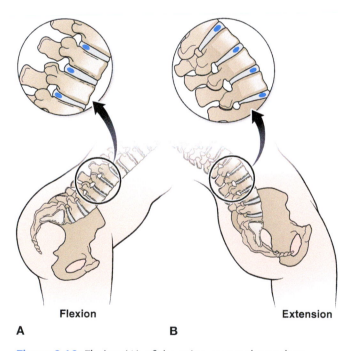

Flexion   **Extension**

A   **B**

Figure 9.10 Flexion (A) of the spine causes the nucleus pulposus to move posteriorly within the annular rings and the neural foramen to increase in size. Conversely, extension (B) causes the nucleus pulposus to move anteriorly within the annular rings and the neural foramen to decrease in size.

flexion and are smallest during trunk extension. With flexion, the posterior ligaments become taut or tight. In extension, the anterior ligaments are taut.

Understanding the changes in the spine with flexion and extension is important in appreciating the rationale for flexion or extension exercises in the plan of care. If a patient has symptoms that are aggravated by flexion, reducing the pressure on the intervertebral disc with **extension bias** exercises may be beneficial. If a patient has symptoms that are aggravated by extension, increasing the size of the neural foramen and decreasing the contact of the posterior elements with **flexion bias** exercises may be indicated.

Function of the Thoracolumbar Fascia

The TLF is a three-layer structure with multiple connections. The anterior and middle layers come from the fascia of the quadratus lumborum muscle and connect to the deep abdominal muscles. Recall that quadratus lumborum inserts on the lumbar vertebrae. The connection of these two muscle groups allows contraction of the transverse abdominis and internal oblique to tense the TLF and support the spine.

The posterior layer of the TLF covers the back muscles from the sacrum to the upper thoracic area. Part of the posterior layer runs from the interspinous ligaments and spinous processes, around erector spinae, to the latissimus dorsi. On the lower trunk, the posterior layer crosses the midline and attaches to the sacrum, ilium, and gluteus maximus. Figure 9.11 depicts these connections.[12–14]

The significance of the TLF lies in the connections of the upper humerus (via the latissimus dorsi), through the lumbar area, to the contralateral upper femur (via the

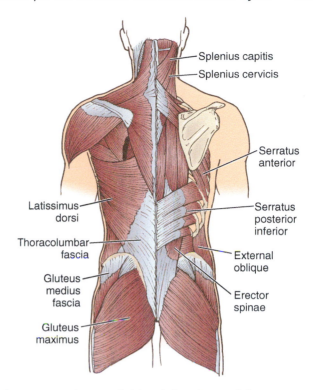

Figure 9.11 The superficial and deep layers of the thoracolumbar fascia connect many of the muscles in the trunk.

gluteus maximus). This network creates an interaction between the arm and leg muscles, and allows for load transmission between arms, legs, and spine. It also appears to have a proprioceptive role and may contribute to back pain.[14]

Common Pathologies

Compression Fracture	**Spinal Stenosis**
Hyperkyphosis	**Degenerative Foraminal Stenosis**
Scoliosis	**Herniated Disc**
Lumbar Sprain/Strain	**Spondylolysis/Spondylolisthesis**
Degenerative Disc Disease	**Ankylosing Spondylitis**
Facet Joint DJD	**Sacroiliac Dysfunction**

A healthy spine requires interplay of the structural and functional components we have described. In this section, we will discuss the common pathologies of the thoracic and lumbar spine.

The thoracic area is the most stable portion of the spine because of the attachment of the ribs. Largely because of this stability, the pathologies of herniated disc and degenerative spondylosis are uncommon in the

thoracic spine. These pathologies are associated with movement. However, the length of the thoracic spine and the influence of gravity lead to problems that are unique to the thoracic area.

The lumbar spine is subjected to extreme loads as it bears the weight of the trunk and upper extremities. The lumbar spine is a frequent source of pain and dysfunction. Indeed, low back pain is the most frequent symptom of patients seeking physical therapy. We will discuss pathologies that involve muscle, disc, joints, nerves, and bone.

Often with spinal pathologies, patients get symptom relief with either flexion or extension and the opposing movement increases symptoms. This is a gross simplification of the spine, but for the sake of clarity we will employ the general patterns for each pathology.

Compression Fracture

Compression fracture is a stable fracture that results in a collapse of the vertebral body. These fractures occur most often in the lower thoracic spine. Compression fractures often cause collapse of the anterior aspect of the vertebral body more than the posterior aspect, resulting in a wedge-shaped body, as shown in Figure 9.12.

Causes/Contributing Factors

The most common cause of compression fracture is **osteoporosis** (see Box 9-1 for osteoporosis information). Secondary causes of compression fracture include trauma, such as a car accident or fall, and cancer. The risk of compression fracture increases with age and is more common in postmenopausal women due to the increased prevalence of osteoporosis. Compression of the vertebrae may occur suddenly or insidiously. Due to an existing weakness of the vertebral body, sudden collapse may occur with lifting or bending. Alternatively, small fractures may occur over time, leading to a compressed vertebra.

Symptoms

When compression fractures occur suddenly, they are accompanied by a sharp pain in the mid to low back.

The pain is increased with sitting, standing, walking, bending, and lifting. Pain is relieved when lying down. Compressive changes that occur gradually are usually less painful and occasionally may occur without pain.

Compression of one vertebral body does not preclude progressive compression of the same vertebra, or compression of other vertebral bodies, resulting in more pain and increasing kyphosis.

With compression and wedging of the vertebral body, the patient may notice an increase in thoracic kyphosis and decrease in height. The ribs may become closer to

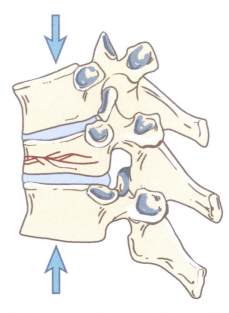

Figure 9.12 Compression fracture results in wedging of the vertebral body.

Box 9-1	Osteoporosis at a Glance

Osteoporosis is a bone disorder characterized by decreased bone mass, compromised bone strength, and changes in bone architecture that increase the risk of fracture. The test for osteoporosis is a **bone mineral density (BMD)** test such as a DEXA scan. Bone mineral density may be classified as normal, osteopenia, or osteoporosis. **Osteopenia** refers to a slight decrease in bone density that is not as advanced as osteoporosis.

Risk factors for developing osteoporosis include lack of exercise, low body mass index (BMI), insufficient dietary calcium/vitamin D intake or production, prolonged use of corticosteroids, smoking, alcohol consumption, female gender, family history, small body frame, advanced age, and Asian or white race.

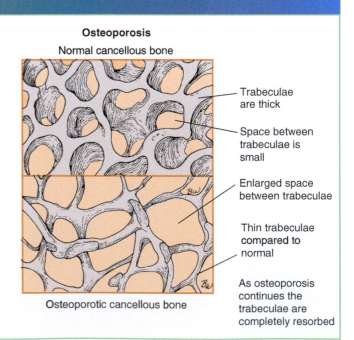

Osteoporosis
Normal cancellous bone

Trabeculae are thick

Space between trabeculae is small

Enlarged space between trabeculae

Thin trabeculae compared to normal

As osteoporosis continues the trabeculae are completely resorbed

Osteoporotic cancellous bone

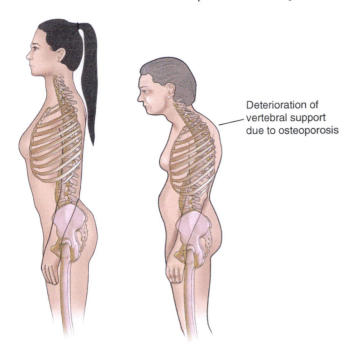

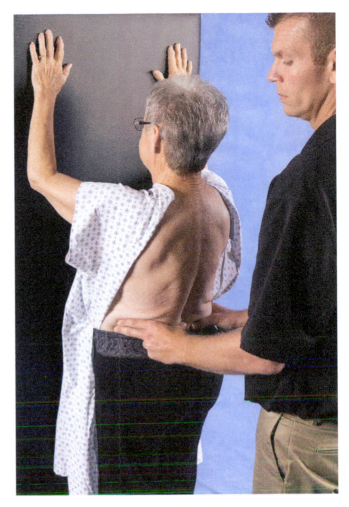

Figure 9.13 Compression fractures often lead to increased thoracic kyphosis and a decrease in the distance between the ribs and the pelvis.

the pelvis, as shown in Figure 9.13. This can lead to compromise of the heart and lungs.

Clinical Signs

The most significant clinical sign of compression fracture is an increased kyphosis. The following tests may be used to objectify the degree of changes in the spine over time.

Rib–Pelvis Distance

The patient is standing with arms raised to shoulder level and braced against a wall. The examiner stands behind the patient and palpates the lower margin of the ribs and the superior surface of the iliac crests at the mid-axillary line (Fig. 9.14). The distance between the ribs and pelvis should be two fingerbreadths. Less than 1 fingerbreadth indicates the likelihood of fracture.

Wall–Occiput Distance

The patient stands with back against a wall, with heels touching the wall. The patient stands as straight as possible and attempts to put the back of his or her head against the wall. The examiner measures the distance between the occiput and the wall (Fig. 9.15). A normal finding is the ability to put the head on the wall. A distance of greater than 7 cm indicates a high likelihood

Figure 9.14 Rib–pelvis distance test for compression fracture.

of thoracic compression fracture.[15] Increased wall–occiput distance also has been shown to correlate with balance and gait speed deficits.[16]

Intervention

A common intervention for patients with compression fractures is strengthening of the spinal extensors. Prone resisted extension of the trunk and arms (Fig. 9.16A, B, C) has been shown to decrease the risk of compression fractures and increase bone mineral density (BMD).[17,18] The patient may begin with simple scapular pinches prone and progress to head and arm raises against resistance, maintaining the cervical and lumbar curves. Instructing the patient in core stabilization can be helpful to minimize trunk flexion when going supine to sit.

Because of their increased risk of fracture, patients may benefit from proprioceptive retraining and balance exercises to decrease the risk of fall-related fracture.[19–21]

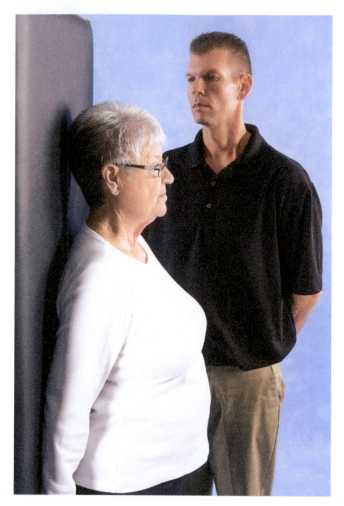

Figure 9.15 Wall–occiput distance test for compression fracture.

This may include exercises on an unstable surface and perturbation exercises. Proprioceptive exercises for the trunk may also be beneficial.

Bracing and modalities may be useful adjuncts to treatment. A brace may be used to decrease pain, increase trunk strength, and limit flexion. Thoracolumbar orthoses (TLO), such as a cruciform anterior spinal hyperextension (CASH), Taylor, or Jewitt brace, may be beneficial for patients with compression fractures. Modalities such as heat, electrical stimulation, and ultrasound may be included in the plan of care to decrease muscle spasm and pain.

Patients with compression fracture may be treated surgically by a vertebral augmentation procedure such as **vertebroplasty** or **kyphoplasty** (see "Interventions for the Surgical Patient").

⚑ CLINICAL ALERT

Stretching into flexion and strengthening trunk flexors should be avoided.[22,23] Patients should be instructed to avoid flexion with increased compressive loading on the spine, such as occurs when bending and lifting a heavy object.

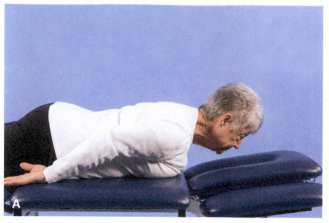

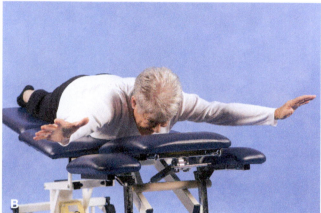

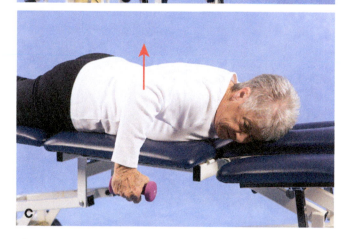

Figure 9.16 Prone scapular pinches (A), prone bilateral arm raises (B), and prone rows (C) may be included in the plan of care for patients with compression fracture.

Prevention

Strengthening back muscles has been shown to decrease the risk of compression fractures.[17] After a compression fracture, the risk for developing another vertebral fracture or hip fracture is increased. Early detection and treatment is crucial to prevent these debilitating consequences of osteoporosis. Resistance training has been shown to increase BMD in the spine, and walking increases BMD in the hips.[24,25] The use of vibration may also be effective in increasing BMD.[26,27]

The Bottom Line:	for patients with compression fractures
Description and causes	Vertebral body collapse and wedging often associated with osteoporosis or trauma
Test	Rib-to-pelvis distance and occiput-to-wall distance
Stretch	Into thoracic extension
Strengthen	Back extensors, core, and extremities
Train	Balance and proprioception of trunk
Avoid	Flexion stretching and strengthening after compression fracture

Interventions for the Surgical Patient

Vertebral Augmentation Procedure

Patients with compression fracture may be candidates for a vertebral augmentation procedure in the form of vertebroplasty or kyphoplasty if pain and tenderness do not decrease within 6 weeks of injury. Vertebroplasty involves injecting bone cement into the vertebral body in order to reinforce the structure of the vertebral body and maintain the vertebral body height. Kyphoplasty is similar, but prior to injecting bone cement, a small, inflatable balloon is placed into the vertebral body and inflated. This compacts the bone and creates a space for the bone cement. Vertebral body height is significantly restored through this step of the procedure. Pain relief after vertebral augmentation generally occurs within 24 hours and is often significant. Figure 9.17 depicts a kyphoplasty procedure.

Hyperkyphosis

The thoracic spine is normally kyphotic. Hyperkyphosis indicates an abnormal increase in the curvature. Normal kyphosis in the thoracic spine varies by age and sex but generally is about 20° at the age of 10 for both sexes. By the age of 65, normal curvature in women is about 45° and in men is about 35°.[28]

Causes/Contributing Factors

Hyperkyphosis may be related to many disorders. Compression fracture may cause wedging of the vertebral body, resulting in hyperkyphosis. Degenerative disc disease leads to more anterior thinning of the disc than posterior, increasing kyphosis. Some disorders, such as cystic fibrosis and chronic obstructive lung disease (COPD) may be contributors.

There are also musculoskeletal factors that contribute to hyperkyphosis. Muscle weakness of the back extensors has been shown to be related, as has decreased proprioceptive sense in the trunk. In addition, people with hyperkyphosis have tightness in hip flexors.

A disease called Scheuermann's disease results in hyperkyphosis in adolescents. This self-limiting disease is characterized by **osteochondrosis** of the vertebral end plates in the spine. Osteochondrosis is a condition of interrupted blood supply to the bone, followed by necrosis and eventual bone rebuilding. In Scheuermann's disease, the vertebral end plates of the thoracic and lumbar spine may be affected. This disorder is more common in males than females by a 2:1 ratio. It is related to a congenital predisposition and a period of rapid growth.

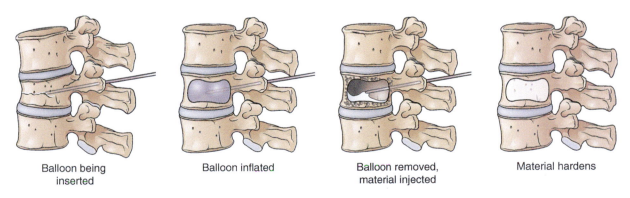

| Balloon being inserted | Balloon inflated | Balloon removed, material injected | Material hardens |

Figure 9.17 Kyphoplasty may be performed on a patient with compression fracture. A balloon is inserted into the vertebral body, inflated to create a space and restore vertebral body height. The space is then filled with bone cement.

Symptoms

Hyperkyphosis is accompanied by complaint of back pain and stiffness. It is associated with increased difficulty with physical activities, such as walking, bending, getting up from a chair, and getting out of the bathtub.[29] With advanced hyperkyphosis, the patient may complain of difficulty breathing.

Clinical Signs

The obvious clinical sign is the increased curvature in the thoracic spine. In addition to the rib–pelvis distance test and occiput-wall distance test that were discussed under "Compression Fracture," the curve may be measured using a flexicurve ruler to monitor progression.

Flexicurve Kyphosis Index

The patient stands in a usual best posture, and the examiner marks C7 and the L5 to S1 joint space. The patient uses a chair or wall as a brace, while the examiner molds a flexicurve ruler to the shape of the patient's thoracic and lumbar curves (Fig. 9.18). The patient removes hand support and the curve is checked to make sure there is no space between the ruler and the patient's skin. Before removing the flexicurve ruler, the markings for C7 and the lumbosacral space are transferred to the ruler. The ruler is placed on graph paper and the curve traced. A kyphosis index is calculated. A resulting value of 13 or greater indicates abnormal kyphosis.[6,30] Box 9-2 details the process for computing the kyphosis index.

Intervention

The keystone intervention for patients with hyperkyphosis is back extensor strengthening. Prone thoracic extension has been shown to reduce kyphosis. Resisted proprioceptive neuromuscular facilitation (PNF) D2 flexion pattern (Fig. 9.19), and weights or exercise bands may be used to strengthen back extensors and scapular retractors. Quadruped arm or leg raises may be beneficial. It is important to strengthen the core stabilizers and instruct patients in supine-to-sit-to-stand activities while performing an isometric contraction of these muscles to minimize trunk flexion.

Stretching exercises are often included in the plan of care. These exercises include stretching into thoracic

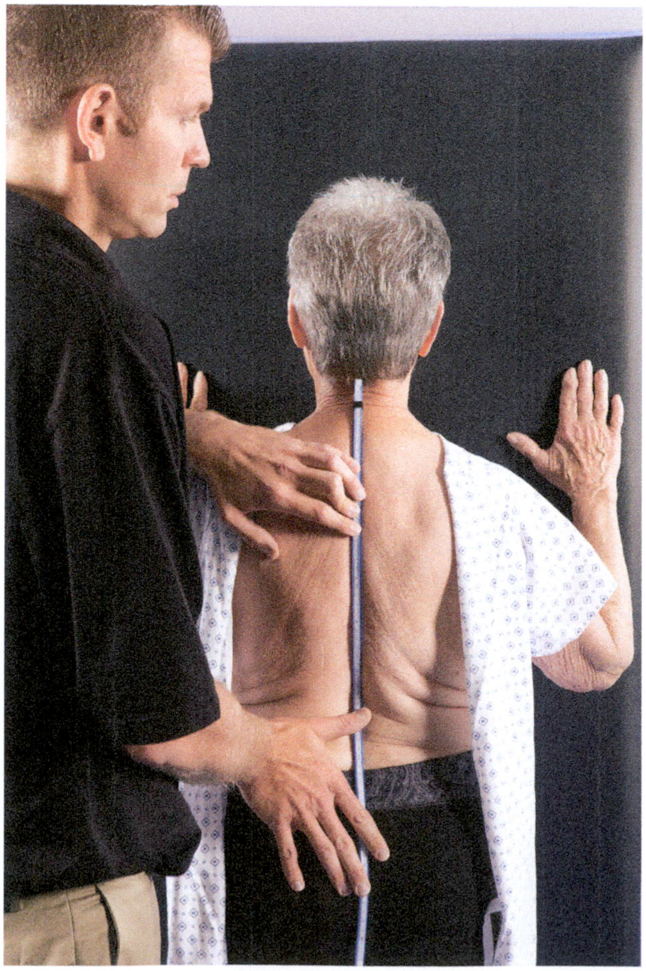

Figure 9.18 Flexicurve kyphosis index for measuring hyperkyphosis.

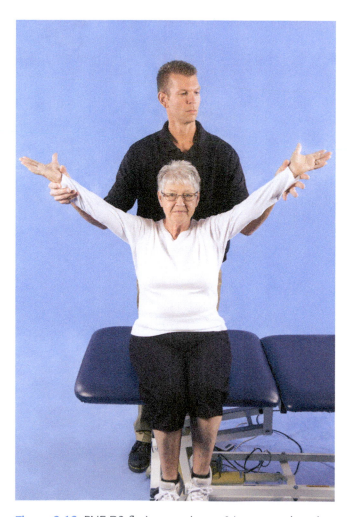

Figure 9.19 PNF D2 flexion may be useful to strengthen the thoracic extensors in a patient with hyperkyphosis.

Box 9-2 Calculating the Kyphosis Index

Step 1. Lay the flexicurve ruler on graph paper, with the two landmarks on the same vertical line.

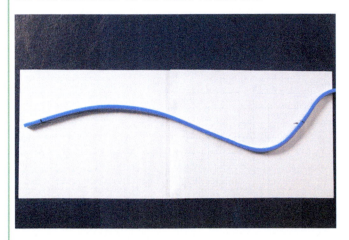

Step 2. Trace the curve onto the paper on the same side of the ruler that contacted the patient's skin.

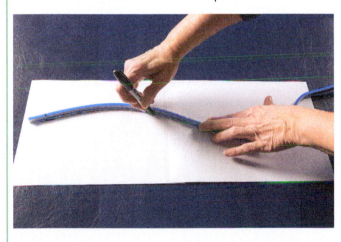

Step 3. Remove the ruler. Mark the paper where the curve crosses the line at the transition from kyphosis to lordosis.

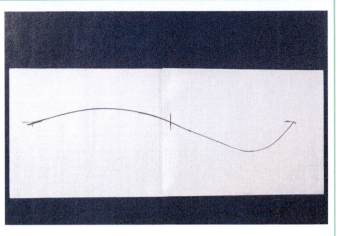

Step 4. Record the greatest distance of the thoracic curve from the vertical line. Record the length of the thoracic curve, from C7 to the cross point.

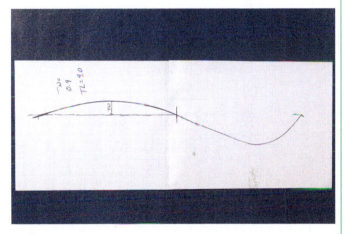

Step 5. Kyphosis index = (thoracic width × 100)/ thoracic length. Kyphosis index of 13 or greater indicates an abnormal kyphosis and is associated with greater difficulty with walking, bending, and chair-to-stand.[29]

extension, shoulder flexion, and hip extension. Lying supine over an exercise ball is useful to stretch the pectoral muscles. Patients may perform self-mobilization lying supine on a foam roll (Fig. 9.20).

Bracing or taping may be used as an adjunct to exercise. Both have been shown to be effective in reducing pain and normalizing the curvature.[31,32] Postural retraining and breathing exercises may be included in the treatment plan.

▶ CLINICAL ALERT

As in the case of compression fractures, stretching and strengthening into flexion should be avoided.[22,23] Patients should avoid flexion with compressive loading on the spine, such as occurs when lifting or carrying a heavy object.

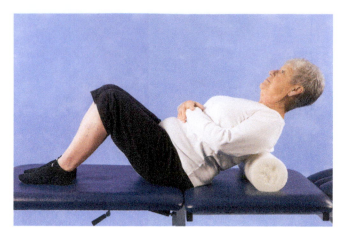

Figure 9.20 Thoracic self-mobilization into extension may be used in the treatment of hyperkyphosis.

Prevention

Prone extensor strengthening exercises have been shown to decrease the kyphosis and improve posture in normal women.[33] Because of the relationship between kyphosis and physical function, elderly patients and postmenopausal women should be encouraged to maintain back extensor strength.

The Bottom Line:	for patients with hyperkyphosis
Description and causes	Increased thoracic kyphosis and pain attributed to compression fracture, degenerative disc disease, and weakness of the trunk
Test	Kyphosis index using flexicurve ruler
Stretch	Into thoracic extension, shoulder flexion, hip extension
Strengthen	Back extensors, scapular retractors, core stabilizers
Train	Posture
Avoid	Flexion stretching and strengthening

Scoliosis

Scoliosis is a curvature of the spine in the frontal plane. When viewed from the posterior, the spine should be straight. In scoliosis, the spine develops an "S" or "C" curvature (Fig. 9.21). The scoliosis curve may be structural or nonstructural. A structural curve is irreversible and fixed. Nonstructural scoliosis is also called functional scoliosis. In this case, the curve can be changed by a change in position. An example of a nonstructural scoliosis is a curve caused by a leg length difference, which can be corrected by a shoe lift. Nonstructural scoliosis may progress to a structural deformity.

Scoliosis curves are named for the side of the convexity at the location of the apex of the curve. In the illustration in Figure 9.21, the major curve is in the thoracic spine, with the convexity toward the right. The lumbar curve is convex to the left. This curve would be termed a right thoracic-left lumbar curve.

Scoliosis has a rotational component toward the side of convexity. In the case depicted, the thoracic vertebrae are rotated toward the right and lumbar vertebrae toward the left. Because of the rotational nature of scoliosis, it is sometime referred to as **rotoscoliosis**. With rotation of the vertebral body, the ribs are prominent posteriorly

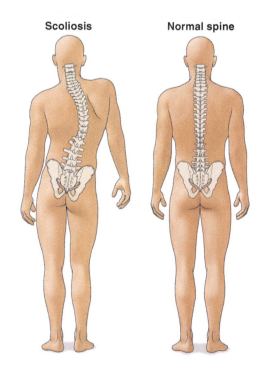

Figure 9.21 Scoliosis involving the thoracic and lumbar spine.

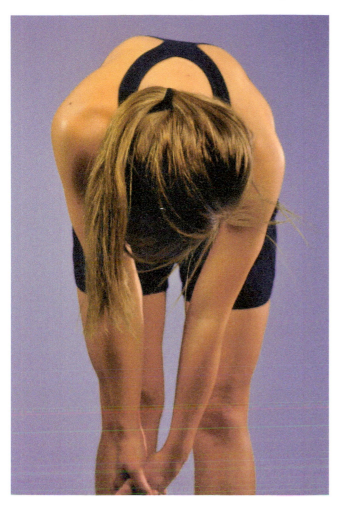

Figure 9.22 The rotational component of scoliosis causes a rib hump to become apparent in forward bending.

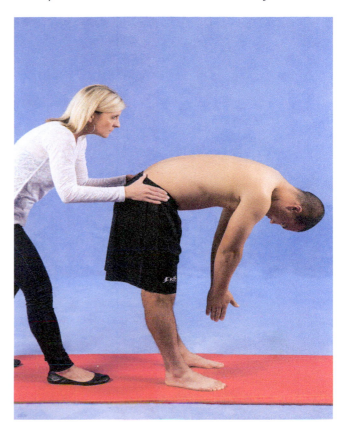

Figure 9.23 Adams forward bend test for scoliosis.

on the side of the convexity, creating a **rib hump** that is apparent when the patient bends forward, as shown in Figure 9.22.

Causes/Contributing Factors

Scoliosis may be attributable to neuromuscular disorders such as cerebral palsy, muscular dystrophy, and spinal cord injury. However, in most instances the scoliosis is **idiopathic,** having no known cause. There is recent evidence that idiopathic scoliosis is largely congenital.[34,35]

Symptoms

Mild scoliosis is often asymptomatic. The patient may not experience any pain or notice asymmetry. As the curve becomes more pronounced, the patient may complain of back pain. It may be obvious that one shoulder is higher, and clothing may not fit well due to the asymmetry. In curves that are very large, the patient may notice compromised cardiopulmonary function or neurological symptoms.

Clinical Signs

Clinically, the patient will often display asymmetry in the iliac crest, PSIS, ASIS, and acromion processes. The curve may be confirmed by the following test.

Adams Forward Bend Test

The patient is standing with feet together. The examiner stands behind the patient and observes the shoulder and iliac crest heights for symmetry. The examiner then instructs the patient to place the palms of the hands together and slowly bend forward at the waist. The examiner observes the symmetry of the back as the thoracic spine comes into the horizontal plane (Fig. 9.23). A positive test is indicated by the presence of asymmetry, specifically a rib hump.

Intervention

Most sources agree that bracing and physical therapy are important components in the conservative treatment of scoliosis. Although it is largely felt that decreasing the curvature with exercise is not possible, some researchers have found improvement in the curvature with exercise and bracing.[36–38]

Typical exercises in the plan of care include stretching of the paraspinals on the concave side of the curve and

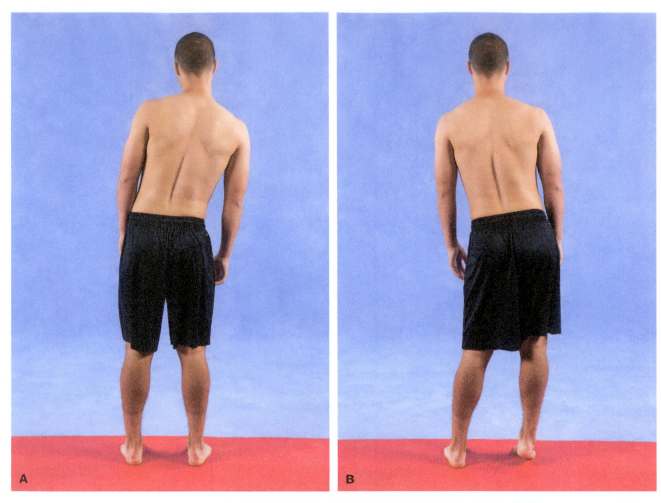

Figure 9.24 Side-shift and hitch exercises in a patient with left thoracic–right lumbar scoliosis. In the side-shift exercise (A), the patient shifts toward the side of the thoracic concavity. In the hitch exercise (B), the patient lifts the heel on the convex side of the lumbar curve, keeping the hip and knee straight. Both positions are held for 10 seconds. These maneuvers reduce the curves.

strengthening those on the convex side. These may be done in prone, quadruped, side-lying, or standing positions. Single arm raises elevating the arm on the concave side in prone or quadruped is an example of stretching. Side-lying stretching over a bolster, lying with the convex side down, may also be used.

Strengthening the paraspinals muscles on the convex side may be done by having the patient perform lateral situps in side lying. Side-shift and hitch exercises have also been shown to be effective (Fig. 9.24).[36,37]

 CLINICAL ALERT

Exercises and activities that promote spinal movement in the direction of the curve should be avoided.

The Bottom Line: for patients with scoliosis

Description and causes	Curvature of the spine in the frontal plane which is usually idiopathic or due to other neuromusculoskeletal disorders
Test	Adam's forward flexion test
Stretch	The paraspinals on the side of the concavity
Strengthen	The paraspinals on the side of the convexity
Train	NA
Avoid	Activities that promote spinal movement in the direction of the curve

Interventions for the Surgical Patient

In cases where the scoliosis curve progresses to greater than 50°, the patient may be a candidate for spinal fusion.

Spinal Fusion

Surgery for severe cases of scoliosis involves fusion of the spine to stop the curve from progressing and partially correct the curve. Typically, this surgery involves straightening the spine as much as possible and immobilizing it with rods, wires, and screws. Small chips of bone are placed between the joints that will eventually create a bony fusion.

After surgery, the patient will generally be restricted from sports or physical education activities for 6 months or longer. It takes about 1 year for the fusion to be fully healed.

Lumbar Sprain/Strain

Muscle strain and ligament sprain in the low back are possible sources of pain. Strain/sprain is graded I (micro-tearing), II (partial tear), or III (complete tear). Injury of a back ligament or muscle may lead to pain and spasm. Because muscle spasms may occur in the presence of pain regardless of the cause, the occurrence of spams doesn't mean the muscle is the primary cause. Bone, disc, ligament, and nerve injuries may also be accompanied by muscle spasm.

Causes/Contributing Factors

Sprain/strain is often attributed to trauma or stressful postures. Trauma commonly results from improper lifting, sudden eccentric loading, a fall, or a motor vehicle accident. Stressful postures, such as prolonged slouched-sitting or repetitive bending, may lead to tissue overload.

Symptoms

Common symptoms of muscle strain or ligament sprain are increased pain with stretch of the muscle or ligament and increased pain with contraction of the muscle. The patient may complain of pain that is increased in sitting or rising from sitting.

Clinical Signs

Patients with lumbar sprain/strain will be tender to palpation over the area. The pain may refer into the legs above the knees. Forward bending may be painful at end ranges, and returning from a forward bent position may increase the pain.

Intervention

The plan of care may include modalities such as cryotherapy, heat, electrical stimulation, or ultrasound to decrease pain and muscle spasm. Stretching exercises are usually part of the initial plan of care, progressing to strengthening, core stabilization, and postural retraining.

Instruction in avoiding prolonged postures and postures that stress the ligaments and muscles of the back is often included in the POC. Instruct the patient to avoid slouched sitting and rounded shoulder postures.

Prevention

Patients should be instructed to prevent postural sprain/strain by avoiding prolonged positioning. For those with occupations that involve prolonged postures, a work site assessment may reveal ergonomic changes that may be beneficial.

The Bottom Line: for patients with lumbar sprain/strain

Description and causes	Muscle or ligament injury from poor posture or injury
Test	NA
Stretch	Into flexion of the spine
Strengthen	Core stabilizers, back extensors
Train	Postural retraining
Avoid	Prolonged positioning

Degenerative Disc Disease

Degenerative disc disease (DDD) includes disc space narrowing, disc desiccation (drying) or fibrosis, and/or fissures or small tears in the annulus fibrosus. It is usually accompanied by **osteophytes**, or bone spurs, that extend out from the vertebral body in many directions. The vertebral end plate is usually eroded. Figure 9.25 shows the changes that occur in DDD.

The intervertebral disc bears the weight of the body on the anterior side of the spine. Together with the facet joints posteriorly, these three joints form a stable triad (Fig. 9.26). Under normal circumstances, the disc bears about two thirds of the weight of the body, with the

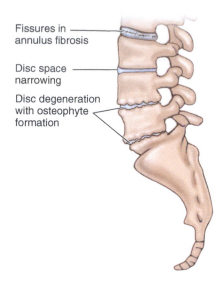

Fissures in annulus fibrosis

Disc space narrowing

Disc degeneration with osteophyte formation

Figure 9.25 Signs of degenerative disc disease include fissures in the annulus fibrosus, disc space narrowing, and osteophytes extending from the vertebral body.

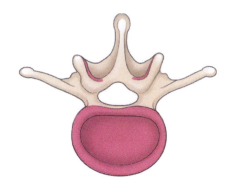

Figure 9.26 The spine has three weight-bearing areas: the intervertebral disc bears about two thirds of the weight and the facet joints bear the other one third.

facet joints together assuming the other one third of the load. Bearing the majority of the forces on the spine often takes a toll on the intervertebral disc.

Causes/Contributing Factors

The intervertebral disc may be compared to a waterbed with foam sides containing the water center. The water in the center absorbs and distributes forces, while the annulus acts like the foam sides to restrain the nucleus. As the nucleus begins to dry with age, the annular rings must absorb the forces. Small fissures in the annular rings make this difficult, and add to further deterioration of the disc.

Lumbar degenerative disc disease has been strongly linked to hereditary factors.[39] It has also been linked to aging, with reports of over 90% of those over 65 having some degree of DDD. There seems to be an association with trauma or inflammatory conditions.[40] There has been conflicting evidence on the effect of occupational stress or overloading on the lumbar discs, with some evidence that this plays a minor role.[41]

Symptoms

There is a strong correlation between DDD and complaints of generalized low back pain. The more severe the DDD, the more likely the person is to have chronic low back pain.

Clinical Signs

There are no special tests for DDD. It should be suspected in older adults with a complaint of chronic low back pain without referral to the lower extremities.

Intervention

There is little evidence for effective intervention for DDD. However, patients with low back pain benefit from general coordination, strengthening, and endurance exercises. In this population, the plan of care is likely to incorporate progressive, low-intensity, submaximal fitness and endurance activities. This may include core strengthening with lumbar stabilization exercises,[42,43] general lower extremity strengthening, walking, and bicycling. Patients should be instructed to avoid prolonged sitting with a flexed posture.[44] Stabilization exercises include instruction in maintaining a neutral spine in progressively more challenging positions, such as supine, sitting, standing, and quadruped.

What's in the Plan of Care?

The Bottom Line: for patients with lumbar degenerative disc disease

Description and causes	Age- and heredity-related changes in the intervertebral disc that leads to fissures, thinning, and bone spurs
Test	NA
Stretch	For general flexibility
Strengthen	Core stabilizers, lower extremities
Train	Aerobically on bicycle or treadmill
Avoid	Prolonged sitting

Degenerative Joint Disease (DJD)

Degenerative joint disease may occur in several areas in the spine. DJD is also called **osteoarthritis** (OA). The Arthritis Foundation recognizes over 100 types of arthritis; DJD is the most common. In the spine, there are three places where DJD commonly causes symptoms: the facet joints, the neural foramen, and the spinal canal. The following three pathologies are the manifestations of DJD in each of these areas. Many times patients will have DJD in more than one of these locations.

Facet Joint DJD

Degenerative joint disease (DJD) of the spine may involve the facet joints. These synovial joints and their articular cartilage show signs of DJD with deterioration of the articular cartilage and bony overgrowth of the joint (Fig. 9.27). Facet joint DJD is linked to DDD.

Causes/Contributing Factors

The facet joints in the lumbar spine form two of the three joints in the joint triad, as discussed earlier. Under normal conditions, the facet joints bear up to 33% of the load of the spine. Extension increases the load bearing.[45] Facet joint DJD occurs frequently as a result of disc degeneration, or DDD. As the disc deteriorates, the facet joints are made to bear significantly more weight, up to 70% of the load. These small joints begin to wear under this stress, leading to joint wear-and-tear (DJD).

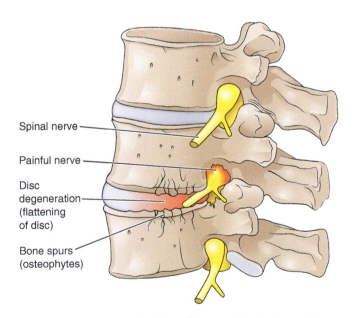

Spinal nerve

Painful nerve

Disc degeneration (flattening of disc)

Bone spurs (osteophytes)

Figure 9.27 Degenerative joint disease of the lumbar spine may manifest in degenerative changes in the facet joints and stenosis, or narrowing, of the foramen.

DJD of the facet joint is associated with aging. It is more common in women. High BMI increases the risk of lumbar facet DJD by three to five times.[45] There seems to be a contribution from hereditary factors, as facet joint orientation may increase the likelihood of developing DJD. African Americans have a lower risk of facet DJD as compared with white Americans.

Symptoms

Patients with lumbar facet DJD will complain of low back pain that is worse with extension, extension with rotation, or straightening from a flexed position. Pain is usually localized to the back but may refer to the lower extremity above the knee. Flexion or sitting relieves the pain. The patient may complain of tenderness to palpation over the facet joint. It is thought that generalized low back pain in older adults is often attributable to facet DJD.

With advancing facet DJD, the neural foramen may become narrowed, resulting in lower-extremity **radiculopathy**. This will be discussed further in this chapter.

Clinical Signs

The physical therapist will likely have assessed repeated movements on the patient's symptoms. In addition, the following test may be helpful.

Extension-Rotation Test

The patient is positioned sitting. The examiner passively guides the patient into lumbar extension and rotation to each side (Fig. 9.28). A positive test is indicated by reproduction of the patient's symptoms.

Intervention

Patients with lumbar facet DJD may respond to a flexion approach in the exercise protocol including core trunk strengthening. Cycling may be included in the plan of care to increase aerobic endurance. Modalities including ultrasound and TENS may be useful. Traction is not recommended to treat back pain without radicular symptoms.[46]

> ⏵ **CLINICAL ALERT**
>
> Extension of the spine will usually exacerbate the patient's symptoms. The patient should be instructed to minimize extension past neutral until pain subsides. This includes avoiding prolonged standing and backward bending.

Prevention

Weight loss may help prevent or slow facet degeneration. A BMI over 25 increases the risk of facet DJD three times, and BMI over 30 carries a five-fold risk.

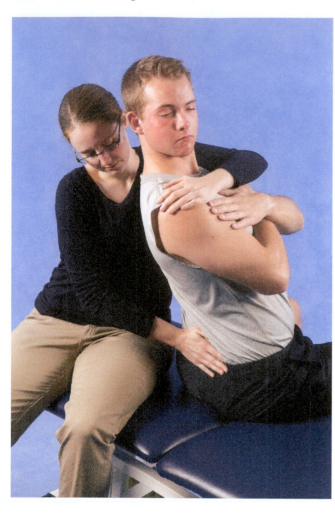

Figure 9.28 Extension-rotation test for facet joint DJD.

The Bottom Line:	for patients with lumbar facet joint DJD
Description and causes	Deterioration of the lumbar facets linked to aging and obesity, which causes pain in the low back
Test	Extension-rotation test
Stretch	Into flexion of the spine
Strengthen	Trunk flexion
Train	Aerobically on bicycle
Avoid	Prolonged standing, backward bending

Spinal Stenosis

The term **stenosis** means "narrowing." In spinal stenosis, the narrowing occurs in the spinal canal. As the canal becomes more narrowed, the spinal cord gets squeezed. Spinal stenosis is a gradually progressive condition. It may involve any area of the spinal canal, with lumbar and cervical regions being most affected. It may involve only one level or span multiple levels. Figure 9.29 depicts the changes that occur in the spinal canal in lumbar spinal stenosis.

Causes/Contributing Factors

Spinal stenosis is most often caused by bony overgrowth into the spinal canal. This may be due to osteoarthritis of the spine associated with aging. It may also be due to hypertrophy and calcification of the ligaments in the spinal canal, specifically the ligamentum flavum and the posterior longitudinal ligament. In addition, it may be related to a congenitally small spinal canal, to the presence of scoliosis, or to a disc herniation.

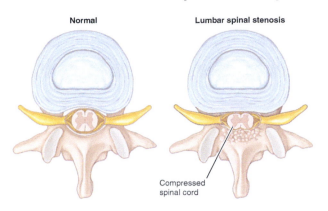

Figure 9.29 In spinal stenosis, degenerative changes in the spinal canal lead to narrowing of the foramen, putting pressure on the spinal cord. Commonly, this leads to neurological symptoms in both legs.

Symptoms

Common symptoms of spinal stenosis are bilateral leg pain, fatigue, numbness, tingling, and/or weakness. Pain is increased by extension of the spine, due to a narrowing of the spinal canal of up to 60% in extension.[47,48] Flexion increases the diameter of the spinal canal[49] and will relieve pain. Patients will generally complain of symptoms that are increased with standing, walking, and backward bending. Pain relief is achieved by sitting or forward bending.

Cook et al. reported that the following symptoms in people over the age of 48 are very likely due to lumbar spinal stenosis: bilateral symptoms, leg pain more than back pain, and pain during walking or standing that is relieved upon sitting.[50] This provides a descriptive portrayal of a patient with spinal stenosis. The bilateral leg symptoms of spinal stenosis distinguish this pathology from other lumbar pathologies.

Watch Out For...

Watch out for similar complaints in patients with claudication. This is an arterial condition that causes pain in both legs with walking or biking. Pain is relieved by rest. The physical therapist will rule out claudication as the cause of bilateral leg pain when diagnosing spinal stenosis.

Clinical Signs

Clinical signs of spinal stenosis include findings of weakness, sensory loss, and diminished or absent reflexes bilaterally. To objectify the patient's signs, the PTA may use one of the following tests.

Two-Stage Treadmill Test

In the two-stage treadmill test, the patient is instructed to ambulate on a treadmill without incline. The speed is set at the patient's comfortable walking speed. The patient ambulates until symptoms occur in the lower extremities, and the time to first symptoms (TFS) is noted (Fig. 9.30A). After the completion of this stage, the patient rests for 10 minutes. The treadmill is set with a 15° incline, which increases the patient's lumbar spine flexion (Fig. 9.30B). The patient ambulates at the same speed as in the first stage, and again the TFS is noted. A positive indicator of spinal stenosis is a longer time before symptoms with the treadmill at an incline.

Bicycle Test

This test is also a two-stage test. The patient is instructed to use a bicycle ergometer with the seat set high, sitting with a normal lumbar lordosis (Fig. 9.31A). The TFS is noted. After a rest period, the test is repeated with the seat lower and the lumbar spine flexed (Fig. 9.31B). A positive indicator of spinal stenosis is a longer time before symptoms with lumbar spine flexion.

Intervention

The plan of care for patients with lumbar spinal stenosis is likely to include flexion bias exercises and strengthening for the trunk and lower extremity muscles. The patient may be instructed to wear a lumbosacral corset when walking to increase the time walked before symptoms.[49] Progressive walking, with a goal of decreased pain with increased walking time or distance, may also be included. Cycling may be used to increase aerobic endurance.

Modalities that are commonly used include TENS, traction, and ultrasound. The research to support these modalities is not conclusive in terms of effectiveness.

CLINICAL ALERT

Extension of the spine will usually exacerbate the patient's symptoms. The patient should be instructed to minimize extension past neutral until pain subsides. This includes avoiding prolonged standing and backward bending.

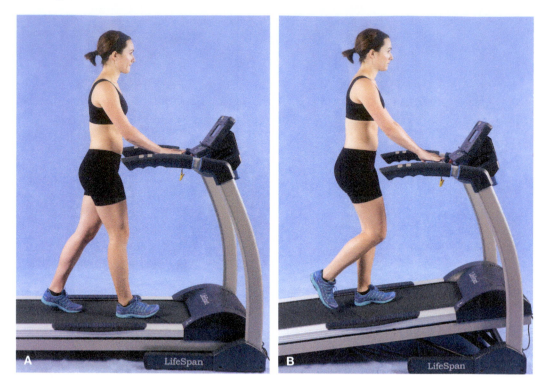

Figure 9.30 Two-stage treadmill test for spinal stenosis. The patient ambulates on a treadmill without incline (A) and then repeats with a 15-degree incline (B). Time to first symptoms is compared in both positions.

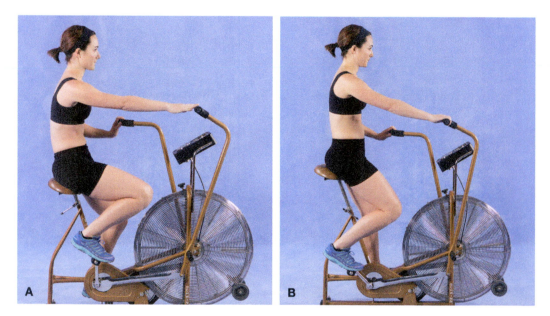

Figure 9.31 Bicycle test for spinal stenosis. The patient pedals a bike with the seat position low (A) and then repeats with the seat high (B). Time to first symptoms is compared in both positions.

The Bottom Line:	for patients with lumbar spinal stenosis
Description and causes	Degenerative changes in the spinal canal related to aging that cause narrowing of the foramen, squeezing the lumbar spinal cord
Test	Two-stage treadmill or bicycle test
Stretch	Into flexion of the spine
Strengthen	Trunk flexion, lower extremities
Train	Aerobically on bicycle
Avoid	Activities that increase pain, commonly lumbar extension, prolonged standing and walking

Degenerative Foraminal Stenosis

Degenerative joint disease may occur in the neural foramen, causing foraminal stenosis. This is also called lateral stenosis. Osteophytes overgrow in the foramen, making the opening smaller. Coupled with degenerative disc disease, the foramen may become so small that the nerve root becomes pinched. This may lead to a pathological nerve root called a radiculopathy.

Degenerative changes in the spine do not occur quickly. The arthritic spurs in the foramen will have been present prior to the onset of symptoms. But with movement, the nerve may become compressed and irritated. Nerve swelling makes it more difficult for the nerve to avoid the arthritic spurs, leading to more constant symptoms.

Causes/Contributing Factors

Osteoarthritis of the spine is related to aging. It may be accelerated by hypomobility or hypermobility.[51] Wear-and-tear on the posterior elements may be increased by hyperlordotic postures.

Symptoms

While spinal osteoarthritis is often asymptomatic, if it leads to radiculopathy it can become a significant source of pain. The patient may experience low back pain, and lower-extremity pain, numbness and tingling, weakness, and loss of reflexes. Specific symptoms depend upon the nerve root that is involved.

Because the neural foramen is bigger when the spine is flexed, the patient will usually report a decrease in pain in flexion or sitting. In standing and walking, pain is increased due to narrowing of the neural foramen, increasing pressure. These patients are said to have a flexion bias.

Watch Out For...

Watch out for a change in location of pain rather than, or in addition to, a change in pain intensity. When the most distal pain moves closer to the spine, it is called **centralization. Peripheralization** refers to the most distal pain moving farther down the leg. It is very important that patients understand this concept. Always the patient and the PTA should be concerned primarily about the location of pain, and secondarily about pain intensity. The goal is symptom centralization. If pain moves farther down the leg, it is a sign of increased pressure on the nerve root, regardless of intensity. If the most distal pain moves closer to the spine, it signifies decreased pressure on the nerve root.

Sometimes when pain centralizes, it will be perceived as more intense. Conversely, when pain peripheralizes, it may be perceived as less intense.

Clinical Signs

Clinical signs of foramen spondylosis with radiculopathy include findings of weakness, sensory loss, and diminished or absent reflexes on the involved side as compared to the uninvolved side. See Table 9-3 for a review of the dermatomes, myotomes, and reflexes in the lumbosacral spine.

In addition to clinical findings of weakness, numbness, or decreased reflexes, the following tests may be useful in indicating radiculopathy.

Straight Leg Raise (SLR) Test

In the straight leg raise test, the patient is placed in a supine position. The examiner passively flexes the patient's leg at the hip, keeping the knee extended (Fig. 9.32). A positive test is indicated by reproduction of the patient's symptoms or asymmetry of range of motion as compared to the unaffected side. More acute pathology is associated

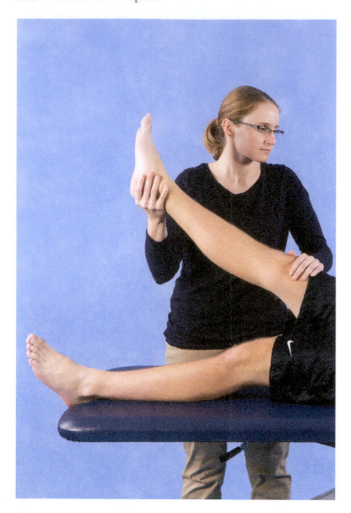

Figure 9.32 Straight leg raise test for lumbar radiculopathy.

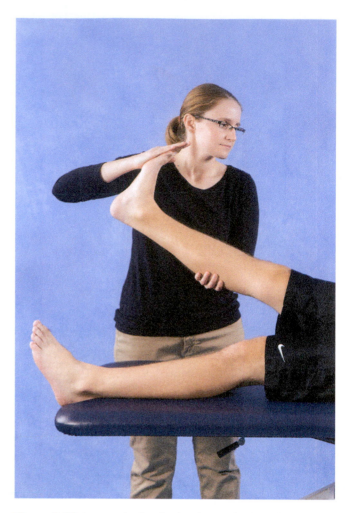

Figure 9.33 Lasegue's sign for lumbar radiculopathy.

with symptom reproduction earlier in the range of motion.[46] Boyd et al. clarified this test by noting that the position of the ankle affects the amount of hip motion, so the ankle should be intentionally immobilized and the position noted for reassessment purposes. They also recommend, for clarification, that the stop point is at the onset of symptoms.[52]

Lasegue's Sign

This modification of the SLR test begins with the same maneuver as in the SLR test and is meant to further confirm nerve root signs. In this test, the examiner passively flexes the patient's leg at the hip, keeping the knee extended as in the SLR test. At the point of symptomatic response, the examiner lowers the patient's leg ½ to 1 inch. At this point, symptoms should be lessened. Maintaining this leg position, the examiner then dorsiflexes the patient's foot (Fig. 9.33). A positive test is indicated by reproduction of the patient's symptoms with dorsiflexion of the foot.

Crossed Straight Leg Raise Test

This test is also called the Well Leg Raise Test and is performed in a manner similar to that of the SLR test.

The patient is placed in a supine position. The examiner passively flexes the patient's uninvolved leg at the hip, keeping the knee extended. A positive test is indicated by reproduction of the patient's symptoms on the opposite, affected side.

Slump Sit Test

The patient is positioned in the sitting position, with hands clasped behind the back. The patient is instructed to slump or slouch into full trunk flexion. The examiner applies slight overpressure to maintain this position. The patient then performs neck flexion, and the examiner maintains this position. The patient's knee is then extended, monitoring for reproduction of patient's symptoms. Further stretch is provided by having the patient dorsiflex the ankle. In each position, the examiner monitors the patient's symptoms. From this position of maximal stretch on the nervous tissues, the patient is instructed to bring the neck back to a neutral position. A positive test is indicated by asymmetrical findings or reproduction of the patient's symptoms in a stretch position with relief with neck extension. Figure 9.34 depicts the steps in this test.

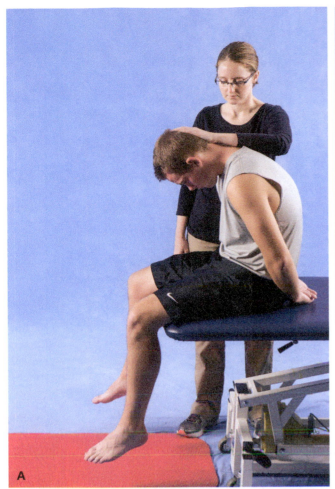

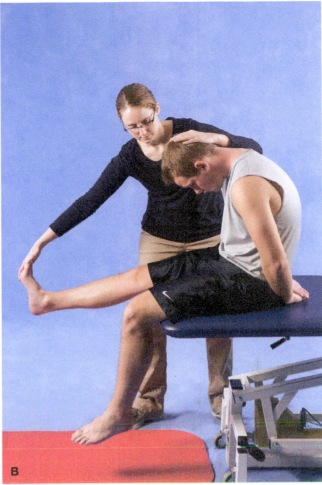

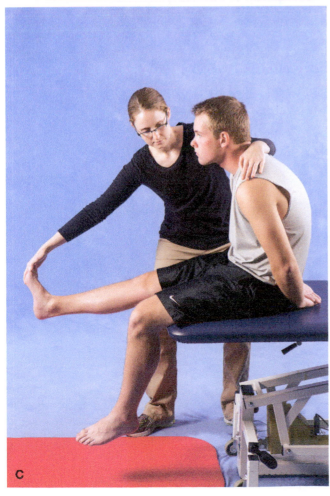

Figure 9.34 Slump sit test for lumbar radiculopathy. With the patient seated, the examiner has the patient flex the lumbar spine and neck (A) and then extend the knee (B). At the point of pain, the patient is asked to extend the neck to neutral (C) to assess the effect on symptoms.

Watch out for the special tests for radiculopathy due to foraminal stenosis to be positive regardless of the cause of the radiculopathy. These tests indicate pressure on the nerve root, but not the *cause* of the pathology. We'll use the same tests for radiculopathy due to disc pathology.

Intervention

It is important that patients with spondylotic radiculopathy understand that even though their symptoms came on quickly, osteophytes form slowly. Normally, there is excess room in the neural foramen. If pressure on the nerve can be relieved and nerve swelling can subside, the patient may again be symptom-free.

Exercises to open the neural foramen decrease nerve root pressure. Therefore, patients with foraminal stenosis will usually respond to flexion bias exercises, including posterior pelvic tilt and knee to chest stretching/positioning. Figure 9.35 depicts common flexion bias exercises.

Abdominal strengthening, core strengthening, and gluteal strengthening are usually included in the plan of care to encourage a flatter lumbar spine. Stretching of the hip flexors and iliotibial (IT) band are also often beneficial.

The patient should be instructed to walk as tolerated without peripheralization of the pain. Nerve mobilization exercises, including the slump sit maneuver and straight leg raising to the point of pain may be helpful.[46] Lumbar traction in a flexed position may be added to the plan of care.

Extension of the spine will usually exacerbate the patient's symptoms. The patient should be instructed to minimize extension past neutral until pain subsides. This includes avoiding prolonged standing and backward bending.

In addition to physical therapy, patients may receive **epidural steroid** injections. This is done as an outpatient procedure and involves a steroid injection around the nerve root to decrease swelling and pain. If therapy and injections are not successful, the patient may undergo a surgical procedure to decompress the nerve root in the foramen, called a **foraminotomy.**

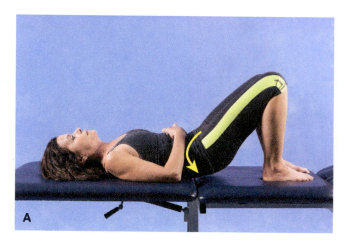
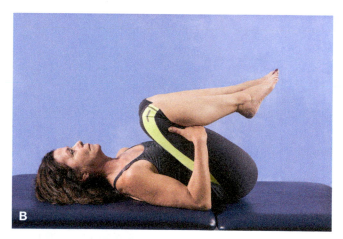
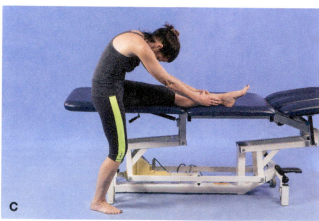
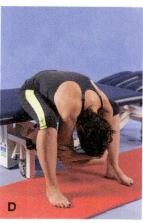

Figure 9.35 Examples of flexion bias exercises. Posterior pelvic tilt (A), knee-to-chest (B), hamstring stretch (C), and flexion sitting (D).

The Bottom Line:	for patients with degenerative foraminal stenosis of the lumbar spine
Description and causes	Degenerative changes in the neural foramen associated with aging that cause spurs to form, which put pressure on nerve roots in the thoracic or lumbar spine
Test	SLR, Lasegue's, crossed SLR, slump sit test
Stretch	Into flexion of the spine
Strengthen	Trunk flexion, lumbar stabilization, lower extremities
Train	Aerobically on a bicycle
Avoid	Prolonged standing, backward bending, peripheralization of pain

Herniated Disc

The intervertebral disc (IVD) has two parts: the annulus fibrosus and the nucleus pulposus. The disc is basically circular in shape and the annular rings contain the nucleus in the center. In the pathology of herniated disc, the nucleus pulposus and/or some part of the intervertebral disc is outside the boundaries of the vertebral end plates. This usually occurs posterolaterally where the annular rings are thinner, potentially leading to pressure on the spinal cord or spinal nerve root.

The terminology used for the progression of herniated disc varies considerably. The following terminology is in keeping with the most recent recommendations.[53] The term **protruded disc** is used to describe an IVD with minimal displacement outside the boundaries of the end plates. In this case, the annular rings are likely still intact. **Extruded disc** refers to a progression of herniation in which the displacement of the nucleus is greater and the annular rings are likely completely torn through. In this case, the disc material remains contiguous with the disc of origin. **Sequestered disc** is a progression of herniation in which a fragment of disc material breaks away and is not attached to the disc of origin. This free-floating mass of disc material can migrate away from the original location. Figure 9.36 depicts the stages of herniated disc from normal to sequestered.

This pathology is frequently referred to as herniated nucleus pulposus (HNP). It may also be called a bulging disc, prolapsed disc, or slipped disc, but these terms are not preferred as they are unclear or misleading.

Causes/Contributing Factors

While the cause of herniated disc is not fully understood, it appears to be largely due to age-related changes in the disc that cause small fissures in the annular rings, allowing the nucleus to migrate through the annulus. Secondarily, it may be caused by trauma. Contributing factors include poor posture, faulty body mechanics, stressful or prolonged back positioning, decreased flexibility, lack of aerobic fitness, obesity, and heredity. Most disc herniation occurs between the ages of 20 and 50. Herniated disc over the age of 50 is uncommon.

Because herniated disc occurs through the posterior part of the annulus, flexion of the lumbar spine increases the risk. Specifically, flat back postures, lifting with a rounded back, occupations that involve repeated lifting or prolonged sitting, and tightness in hamstrings tend to increase risk.

Symptoms

Changes in the intervertebral disc may be asymptomatic. This may be attributed to the lack of innervation of the inner annular rings. It may also occur in instances where the disc is not putting pressure on sensitive structures,

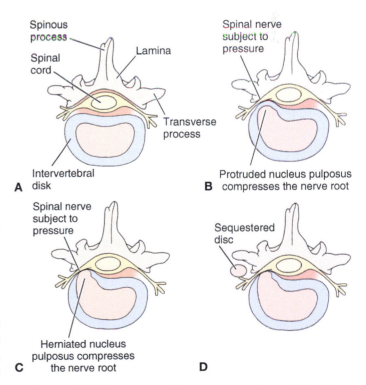

Figure 9.36 The stages of disc herniation. Normal disc (A), protruded disc (B), extruded disc (C), and sequestered disc (D).

or in the absence of inflammation. Indeed, studies have found that 20% to 76% of normal subjects have some degree of disc herniation on MRI.[46,54–57]

Symptoms that are associated with lumbar herniated disc include pain in the low back and lower extremity, numbness and tingling, weakness, and loss of reflexes. Commonly, patients with a lumbar herniated disc describe an initial onset of low back pain, later progressing to lower-extremity symptoms. Pain may be increased with coughing or sneezing. Pressure on sacral nerves may lead to changes in bowel or bladder control. Specific symptoms depend upon the nerve root that is affected by the herniation. Symptoms in the lower extremity indicate radiculopathy.

Patients with a herniated disc often demonstrate a **directional preference**. In other words, their symptoms may increase, peripheralize, or both, with certain movements or positions and decrease, centralize, or both, with movements in the opposite direction. Most commonly, patients with a herniated disc will complain of increased symptoms with flexion, sitting, rising from sitting, forward bending, and lifting. They will commonly get relief from extension, standing, walking, and backward bending. These patients commonly have an extension bias. Figure 9.37 depicts common exercises for patients with an extension bias.

Clinical Signs

Clinical signs of herniated disc with radiculopathy include findings of weakness, sensory loss, and diminished or absent reflexes on the involved side as compared to the uninvolved side. Patients often display a decrease in lumbar extension range of motion.[51]

The patient may also display a **lateral shift.** This may also be referred to as a sciatic scoliosis. With a lateral shift, the patient may move toward (ipsilateral shift) or away from (contralateral shift) the side of leg pain. The shift is named by the direction in which the patient's shoulders shift. Figure 9.38 depicts a right lateral shift. In this case, the patient's pain was in the left leg, so the shift is a contralateral right lateral shift.

In addition to these clinical findings, the PTA may use the straight leg raise test, Lasegue's test, crossed straight leg raise test, and slump sit test in the assessment of patients with a radiculopathy. These tests have been described earlier and are very appropriately applied in cases of herniated disc. Additionally, the following test may be used.

Repeated Movement Testing

The patient is positioned in a standing or prone position. Prior to testing, the patient is questioned regarding the

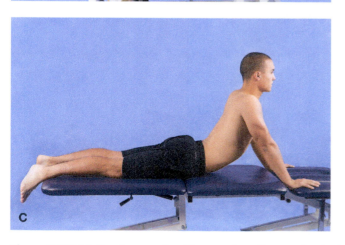

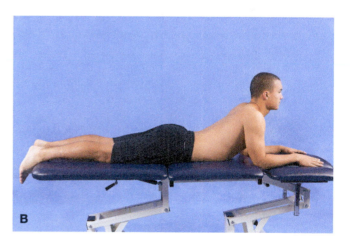

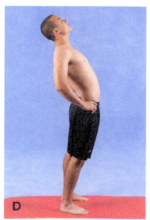

Figure 9.37 McKenzie extension bias exercises. Progression includes prone lying (A), prone-on-elbows (B), prone-on-hands (C), and standing back bends (D).

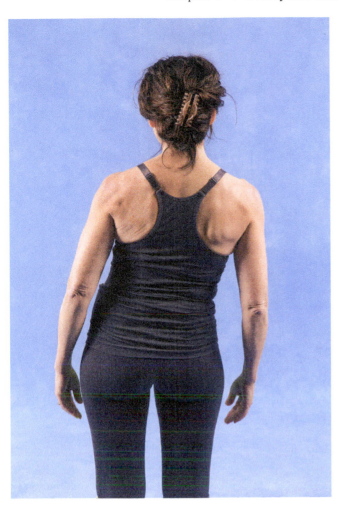

Figure 9.38 Right lateral shift.

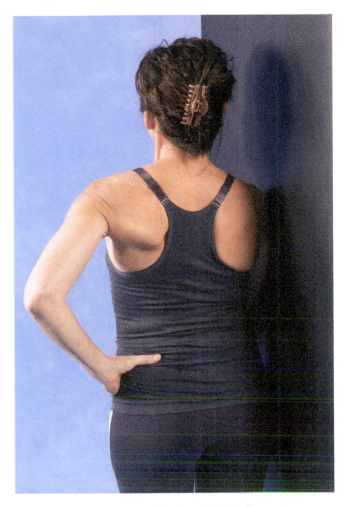

Figure 9.39 To correct a right lateral shift, the patient may stand with the right shoulder against a wall and gently push hips to the right until touching the wall.

intensity and location of pain. The patient is instructed to repeatedly flex or extend up to 20 repetitions. The test is stopped if the patient complains of peripheralization of symptoms. A positive test is indicated by a directional preference. With herniated disc, the patient will commonly complain of increased symptoms with flexion and decreased symptoms with extension.

Intervention

The classic signs of herniated disc, as described above, include low back pain with radiating pain into one leg. Pain is usually increased with flexion activities and improved with extension. Symptoms may include weakness, numbness, and loss of reflexes. The goal in the plan of care will be to centralize the pain, improve mobility, and reduce symptoms.

Typical interventions for this patient include an extension approach, such as McKenzie's protocol. The patient should be instructed to perform as much extension as possible without peripheralizing the pain. A typical progression is shown in Figure 9.38. The patient should be instructed to perform these exercises frequently throughout the day, typically every 1 to 2 hours.

If the patient has a lateral shift, the plan of care is likely to focus on lateral shift correction instead of extension. The patient may perform side glides in a prone or standing position (Fig. 9.39). The physical therapist may use manual techniques to reduce the lateral shift. The shift should be corrected prior to initiating extension exercises.

⚑ CLINICAL ALERT

It is important to avoid peripheralization of the patient's symptoms during exercise.

Patients with subacute and chronic pain may benefit from nerve mobilization techniques. This includes stretching or flossing the sciatic nerve by performing the straight leg raise maneuver or the slump sit maneuver. Patients are instructed to stretch to the point of pain and then relax. This has been shown to be beneficial for patients who have referred pain that doesn't respond to either flexion or extension.[58,59]

Some evidence supports the use of traction for patients with radicular symptoms. Consider performing the traction in the position that centralizes the patient's pain, which is likely to be prone. Traction has been shown to be especially effective for patients who experience peripheralization of their pain in extension and have a positive crossed straight leg raise test.[46]

Patients should be instructed in the importance of remaining active and avoiding bed rest.[60] Education should focus on the neuroscience of pain perception to decrease fear and catastrophizing.[61]

Prevention

Maintaining hamstring flexibility and a normal lumbar lordosis appear to be key to preventing herniated disc. There is a strong positive correlation between lack of aerobic fitness, obesity, and herniated disc. Proper lifting to minimize the stress on the disc is important.

The Bottom Line:	for patients with lumbar herniated disc
Description and causes	Small tears in the annulus fibrosus associated with aging and flat back or flexed posture allowing the nucleus material to migrate posteriorly, putting pressure on a nerve root
Test	SLR, Lasegue's, crossed SLR, slump sit test, repeated movement testing
Stretch	Into extension of the spine
Strengthen	Trunk extension, lumbar stabilization, lower extremities
Train	Aerobically by walking on ground/treadmill or elliptical
Avoid	Prolonged sitting, poor posture, bad body mechanics, peripheralization of pain

Intervention for the Surgical Patient

Discectomy

Discectomy is the surgical removal of the herniated disc. This may be done in a traditional approach or through a smaller incision in an approach called a *microdiscectomy*. The procedure involves removal of the lamina to access the nerve root and disc. This part of the surgery is called a **laminectomy**.

> ⚑ **CLINICAL ALERT** ──────
>
> After surgery the patient is generally instructed to avoid bending, lifting more than 5 pounds, twisting, and sitting for prolonged periods. The patient should be taught to log roll to avoid trunk rotation.

Therapy during the first 4 weeks often includes gentle nerve stretching or flossing, hamstring stretching, modalities for pain control including TENS or cryotherapy, isometric abdominal, gluteal, and back extensor strengthening, and postural retraining. **What's in the Plan of Care?** From weeks 4 through 8, the patient may be progressed to trunk coordination, strengthening, and endurance exercises. Instruction in neutral spine and lumbar stabilization exercises may be added.[62] Walking, biking, or aquatic exercises are often included in the plan of care. Instructions in proper lifting should be provided. After 8 weeks, proprioceptive activities and running may be incorporated.

Spondylolysis/ Spondylolisthesis

It's helpful to understand the medical terminology used for these related pathologies. "Spondylo" means spine; "lysis" is an erosion; "listhesis" means tilting or slipping. Spondylolysis is a defect or erosion in the posterior elements of the vertebra, specifically in the pars interarticularis, which lies between the superior and inferior articulating processes (Fig. 9.40). This defect may involve a congenital thinning, a stress fracture, or a traumatic fracture of the vertebra at this location. Spondylolysis occurs most commonly at L5.

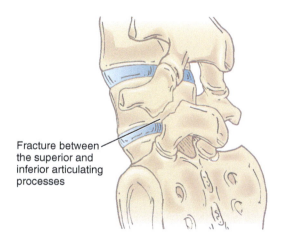

Fracture between the superior and inferior articulating processes

Figure 9.40 In spondylolysis, the area between the superior and inferior articulating processes is thin or fractured.

Box 9-3 Grades of Spondylolisthesis

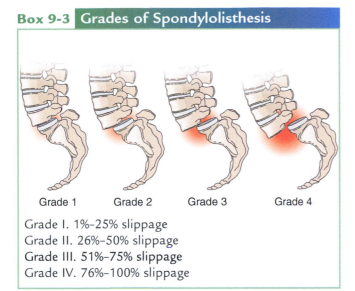

Grade 1   Grade 2   Grade 3   Grade 4

Grade I. 1%–25% slippage
Grade II. 26%–50% slippage
Grade III. 51%–75% slippage
Grade IV. 76%–100% slippage

Spondylolysis leads to an associated condition, spondylolisthesis, in about 25% of cases. Spondylolisthesis is the anterior slippage of one vertebral body on the vertebra below, most commonly L5 on the sacrum. Bilateral spondylolysis causes the inferior facets and spinous process to lose the connection to the rest of the vertebra, allowing the vertebral body to slide forward. Spondylolisthesis is graded from I to IV, as shown in Box 9-3.

Causes/Contributing Factors

Spondylolysis is two to three times more common in males than females. The cause may be hereditary or environmental. With an inherited malunion of the pars interarticularis, there is a link to spina bifida occulta. Some sports increase the likelihood of spondylolysis: gymnasts, weight lifters, football players, wrestlers, and divers are at higher risk. It is felt that the lysis of the pars often occurs due to repetitive stress on the posterior elements from sports.

Symptoms

Spondylolysis is often asymptomatic. When symptomatic, the most common presentation is a teen-aged athlete with a complaint of localized low back pain that is increased with extension or extension-rotation. Occasionally, the pain may radiate into the buttocks or proximal lower extremities. The onset is generally gradual, with complaint of increased pain related to an acute event. Most patients with spondylolysis will not progress to a spondylolisthesis, and the risk of slippage is greatest during the growth spurt related to puberty.[63]

With spondylolisthesis, the symptoms of pain are often felt in the low back and into the legs. The slippage may cause neurological compromise of the nerve roots or cauda equina, resulting in numbness, tingling, weakness,

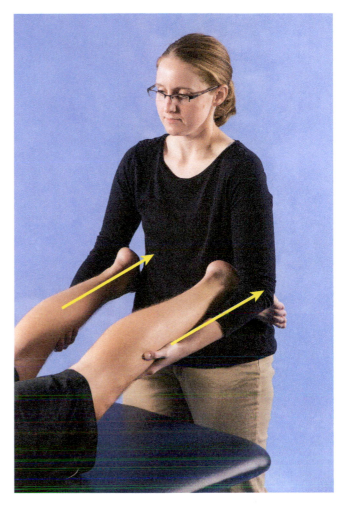

Figure 9.41 Passive lumbar extension test for spondylolysis or spondylolisthesis.

and a feeling of fatigue in the legs. These symptoms are increased in standing and walking.

Clinical Signs

The patient with spondylolysis/spondylolisthesis will often have an increased lumbar lordosis. Hamstring tightness is commonly seen. A step-off may be palpable in the lumbar spine. Patients will complain of increased pain in lumbar extension, with relief of pain in sitting. The patient may display neurological signs in higher grades of slippage. In addition, the following test may be useful in assessing the patient.

Passive Lumbar Extension Test

The subject is instructed to lie prone. The examiner passively elevates both legs about 12 inches from the exam table, keeping the patient's knees extended and gently pulling the legs (Fig. 9.41). A positive test is indicated by complaint of strong pain or instability in the low back.

Intervention

The plan of care for patients with spondylolysis or spondylolisthesis will center around activities that reduce the stress on the posterior elements. Flexion approach exercises, lumbar stabilization exercises, hamstring and hip flexor stretching, and general conditioning are common. Focusing on the muscles that attach into the thoracolumbar fascia, such as latissimus dorsi, internal oblique, and transverse abdominis, will increase muscular support. Myofascial techniques and modalities may be used to decrease muscle spasm.

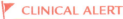

CLINICAL ALERT

Activities that increase pain are to be restricted. Specifically, activities that require end range of lumbar extension should be avoided.

Prevention

While we know little about how to prevent spondylolysis or spondylolisthesis, we do know that when it's related to sports, early detection and intervention may prevent a bony defect from developing and decrease the magnitude of symptoms.

The Bottom Line:	for patients with lumbar spondylolysis/spondylolisthesis
Description and causes	Non-union of pars interarticularis with/without anterior slipping of vertebra due to hereditary factors (associated with spina bifida occulta) and sports that require excessive extension
Test	Passive lumbar extension test
Stretch	Into flexion of the spine, hamstrings, and hip flexors
Strengthen	Trunk flexion, lumbar stabilization, lower extremities
Train	Aerobically on bicycle
Avoid	Prolonged standing, backward bending

Ankylosing Spondylitis

Ankylosing spondylitis is a chronic, progressive, inflammatory arthritis that results in ossification of the soft tissues of the spine and eventual fusion. This condition is also known as "bamboo spine." Generally, inflammatory changes begin in the SI joints, which subsequently fuse. The disease progresses superiorly and may involve the whole spine (Fig. 9.42). Occasionally, hip, knee, or shoulder joints may also be affected.

Causes/Contributing Factors

Ankylosing spondylitis appears to be largely hereditary. It is estimated that greater than 95% of cases are congenital.[64] Environmental contributors are not well understood but may be related to microbial infection.

Males are at least twice as likely to develop ankylosing spondylitis as females. Diagnosis is generally made between the ages of 20 and 40, but many patients have symptoms for a number of years before diagnosis. The disease tends to be milder in women.

Symptoms

The earliest symptoms of ankylosing spondylitis are generally pain in the low back, SI joints, and buttocks. When this is found in conjunction with a complaint of stiffness, limited spine range of motion, and loss of joint space in the sacroiliac joints, ankylosing spondylitis is suspected. Fatigue is a common complaint. Patients will often report that activity decreases pain, which sets this disorder apart from many others. As the disease progresses, the pain may decrease but functional limitation persists.

Clinical Signs

Assessment of the patient with ankylosing spondylitis will include range of motion of the neck and trunk. Patients are often limited in all directions, especially lumbar flexion. The degree of limitation depends upon the severity and progression of the disease. An increase in thoracic kyphosis may be seen. There are no special tests for ankylosing spondylitis.

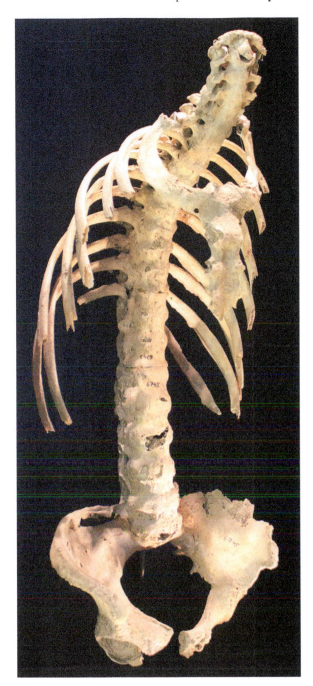

Figure 9.42 Ankylosing spondylitis leads to ossification and eventual fusion of the joints of the spine.

Intervention

The goals of intervention are to decrease pain, and to improve range of motion, activities of daily living, cardiorespiratory function, and overall sense of well-being. Physical therapy has been shown to be effective in the treatment of ankylosing spondylitis. The plan of care often will include education regarding the disease process and avoidance of prolonged flexed postures.

> **⚑ CLINICAL ALERT** ———————
>
> Patients should be instructed to avoid long periods of sitting. Promoting extension by prone lying and use of a lumbar roll in sitting should be encouraged.

Stretching exercises should encourage spinal flexion and extension, as well as hip range of motion.[65] Strengthening exercises for the trunk should favor an extension approach.[66] Cardiorespiratory exercises are an important consideration because cardiopulmonary function may decline as the spine becomes fused. Deep breathing exercises, walking, aerobic exercise, and interval training have all been reported to improve cardiopulmonary function and pain.[67–69] Aquatic exercise may be beneficial for these patients.

The Bottom Line:	for patients with ankylosing spondylitis
Description and causes	Hereditary disorder that causes the soft tissues of the spine to turn to bone, leading to functional decline
Test	NA
Stretch	Into flexion and extension of the spine
Strengthen	Trunk extension, cardiorespiratory system
Train	Aerobically walking on ground/treadmill or elliptical
Avoid	Prolonged positions in flexion

Sacroiliac Dysfunction

There are many dysfunctions that involve the sacroiliac joint; however, a detailed description of sacroiliac dysfunction is beyond the scope of this text. Pathologies of this joint include sacral torsions and rotation of the innominate on the sacrum. Indicators of sacroiliac dysfunction include pain in the SI joint, hip, groin pain, and inner thigh. Asymmetry of the landmarks of the pelvis, including ASIS, PSIS, and pubic symphysis may be indicators of an SI pathology.

SUMMARY

Normal function of the spine relies on the stability and mobility afforded by joints, muscles, ligaments, and intervertebral discs. The thoracic and lumbar spine is complex, and there are many structures in this area that can cause pain in the low back or legs. However, we have known for some time that anatomic pathology and pain are not necessarily correlated. Nowhere, it seems, is this truer than in the spine. While it is important for the PTA to understand common pathologies and treatment approaches, identifying the specific structure that is causing pain is difficult and unnecessary. Combine your knowledge of spine anatomy, physiology, and pathology with an understanding of pain perception for a more holistic approach.

REVIEW QUESTIONS

1. List six muscles that are directly associated with the thoracolumbar fascia.

2. Have your lab partner sit erect in a chair. Measure shoulder flexion. Now have your partner flex the thoracic spine to simulate an increased kyphosis. Measure shoulder flexion in this position. Was there a difference in ROM? Why?

3. You have a patient who has in increased lumbar lordosis. Describe the consequences of this on the neural foramen, facet joints, and intervertebral disc as compared to ideal posture. Is this posture accompanied by an anterior or a posterior pelvic tilt?

4. How does the posture in question 3 affect the shear force on L5–S1?

5. You have a patient who has a flat back. Describe the consequences of this on the neural foramen, facet joints, and intervertebral disc as compared to ideal posture. Is this posture accompanied by an anterior or a posterior pelvic tilt?

6. How does the posture in question 5 affect the shear force on L5–S1?

7. Instruct your lab partner to use both hands to simulate the ilia. Putting your hand between your lab partner's, simulate the sacrum. Perform the motion of nutation. Relative to the sacrum, what type of rotation have the ilia undergone? Now perform the motion of sacral counternutation. Relative to the sacrum, what type of rotation have the ilia undergone?

8. What is the effect of nutation on the lumbar spine? What is the effect of counternutation?

9. With your lab partner perform sensation testing, manual muscle testing, and reflex testing associated with an L4 nerve root. Repeat for L5 and S1.

10. You are treating a 72-year-old patient with neural foramen stenosis. The patient complains of pain that is increased with prolonged standing and decreased with sitting. Are these expected findings? Use a spine model, and any other props necessary, to explain the reason for these symptoms to your lab partner.

11. You are treating a 31-year–old patient with a herniated disc. The patient complains of pain that is increased with prolonged sitting and decreased in lying prone. Are these expected findings? Use a spine model, and any other props necessary, to explain the reason for these symptoms to your lab partner.

12. You are treating a 28-year–old patient with a herniated disc. The patient states that after prolonged standing, pain is temporarily relieved when first sitting or lying down with legs flexed. The MRI shows a very large herniated disc. What could be contributing to the patient's unexpected symptoms? (*Hint:* are there any structures that might be able to immediately relieve pressure in a flexed position?)

13. You are treating a 17-year-old gymnast with low back pain. The diagnosis is spondylolysis with a grade I spondylolisthesis. Use a spine model, and any other props necessary, to explain this pathology to your lab partner.

14. Your patient has had an **EMG/NCV** to determine the level of nerve root involvement. The results show an L4 radiculopathy. What findings might you expect in terms of numbness, weakness, loss of reflexes, functional difficulties?

15. Using a model of a vertebra, locate the three places where DJD becomes symptomatic in the lumbar spine. Note how close the structures are to one another and appreciate why patients with DJD may have symptoms of encroachment in more than one area.

16. You are treating a patient with a herniated disc. The patient states a decrease in pain since the last session. On further questioning, the patient rates the pain at worst a 3 (down from a 4) but describes slight pain in the calf (down to posterior knee on initial visit). Is this an improvement or worsening in the patient's symptoms? Explain the concept of centralization and peripheralization to your lab partner.

17. You are treating a 78-year-old female with recent sudden onset of back pain and a diagnosis of a new compression fracture at T9. The plan of care includes therapeutic exercise. What exercises will you choose for a home program?

18. What activities of daily living would you expect to increase symptoms in a patient with a thoracic compression fracture? A lumbar herniated disc? A lumbar foraminal stenosis?

PATIENT CASE: HNP Syndrome Lumbar Spine

PT Evaluation

Patient Name: XXXXXX XXXXXXXXXXX **Age:** 31 **BMI:** 21.1

Diagnosis/History

Medical Diagnosis: HNP syndrome lumbar spine **PT Diagnosis:** L leg pain secondary to lumbar HNP

Diagnostic Tests/Results: MRI – L4-5 HNP L **Relevant Medical History:** unremarkable

Prior Level of Function: Normally active without pain

Patient's Goals: Decrease pain, return to PLOF

Medications: None **Precautions:** None

Social Supports/Safety Hazards

Patient Living Situation/ Supports/ Hazards: Lives with partner
Patient Working Situation/Occupation/ Leisure Activities: Employed as computer graphics artist. Participates in competitive dog shows.

Vital Signs

At rest Temperature: 98.1 BP: 112/68 HR: 70 Resp: 13 O2 sat: 98

Subjective Information

Patient is a female with 3-week history of pain in the L leg and foot, with numbness of the medial side of the foot. This began for no apparent reason. Pain interferes with work and leisure.

Physical Assessment

Orientation: Alert and oriented **Speech/Vision/Hearing:** Wears glasses **Skin Integrity:** Intact

ROM: Lumbar spine flexion WNL, but c/o pain with prolonged and repeated lumbar flexion. Most distal pain is below knee. Extension is limited to 20°. Hamstring limitation to 40° B.

Strength: MMT 4/5 anterior tibialis. Eversion and plantarflexion 5/5. **Palpation:** No pain with palpation

Muscle Tone: Not tested **Balance/Coordination:** WNL **Sensation/Proprioception:** Decreased sensation medial foot and big toe

Endurance: Not tested **Posture:** Decreased lumbar lordosis **Edema:** None

Pain

Pain Rating and Location: At best 0/10 At worst 6/10 **Relieving Factors:** Lying down flat, walking
Aggravating Factors: Prolonged sitting (riding in car, working at desk) **Irritability:** Patient can lie flat, or get out of car and walk to relieve pain quickly. Pain returns only after assuming positions of discomfort.

Functional Assessment

Patient is functionally independent. However, pain is limiting her ability to participate in dog shows that require driving to attend. She is working from a standing position.

Special Testing

Test Name: Reflex testing/MMT **Result** Consistent with L4 radiculopathy **Test Name:** Lasegue's test **Result** Positive at 40°

Assessment

Patient has s/s consistent with L4 radiculopathy

Short-Term Treatment Goals

1. Patient will state a 25% decrease in pain.
2. Patient will voice and demonstrate an understanding of centralization of pain.
3. Patient will be independent in HEP.

Long-Term Treatment Goals

1. Patient will state a 50% decrease in pain.
2. Patient's most distal pain will be above knee.

Treatment Plan

Frequency/Duration: 2 times a week for 4 weeks
Consisting of: Modalities, therapeutic exercise, neuro re-education, patient education

continued

Patient Case Questions

1. What factors might be contributing to the patient's HNP syndrome?

2. What would you tell the patient about specific activities to avoid or curtail?

3. What data will you collect the first time you see the patient?

4. If the plan of care does not guide you, what modalities might you use with this patient? Why? Are any modalities contraindicated?

5. If the plan of care does not specifically guide you, describe three therapeutic exercises that are indicated for this patient. Justify your choices.

6. What other special tests might you use to monitor the patient's progress?

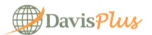

For additional resources, including answers to this case, please visit
http://davisplus.fadavis.com

REFERENCES

1. Low Back Pain Fact Sheet | National Institute of Neurological Disorders and Stroke. Available at: https://www.ninds.nih.gov/Disorders/Patient-Caregiver-Education/Fact-Sheets/Low-Back-Pain-Fact-Sheet (accessed October 29, 2017).
2. Battié, M. C., Niemelainen, R., Gibbons, L. E., & Dhillon, S. (2012). Is level- and side-specific multifidus asymmetry a marker for lumbar disc pathology? *Spine Journal, Official Journal of the North American Spine Society, 12*, 932–939.
3. Fortin, M., Gibbons, L. E., Videman, T., & Battié, M. C. (2015). Do variations in paraspinal muscle morphology and composition predict low back pain in men? *Scandinavian Journal of Medicine and Science in Sports, 25*, 880–887.
4. Neumann, D. A. (2010). Kinesiology of the hip: A focus on muscular actions. *Journal of Orthopaedic and Sports Physical Therapy, 40*, 82–94.
5. Sajko, S., & Stuber, K. (2009). Psoas major: A case report and review of its anatomy, biomechanics, and clinical implications. *Journal of the Canadian Chiropractic Association, 53*, 311–318.
6. Teixeira, F. A., & Carvalho, G. A. (2007). Reliability and validity of thoracic kyphosis measurements using flexicurve method. *Brazilian Journal of Physical Therapy, 11*, 199–204.
7. Nairn, B. C., & Drake, J. D. M. (2014). Impact of lumbar spine posture on thoracic spine motion and muscle activation patterns. *Human Movement Science, 37C*, 1–11.
8. Twomey, L. (1979). The effects of age on the ranges of motions of the lumbar region. *Australian Journal of Physiotherapy, 25*, 257–263.
9. Biely, S. A., Silfies, S. P., Smith, S. S., & Hicks, G. E. (2014). Clinical observation of standing trunk movements: What do the aberrant movement patterns tell us? *Journal of Orthopaedic and Sports Physical Therapy, 44*, 262–272.
10. Khoo, B. C., Goh, J. C., Lee, J. M., & Bose, K. (1994). A comparison of lumbosacral loads during static and dynamic activities. *Australasian Physical and Engineering Sciences in Medicine, 17*, 55–63.
11. Alexander, L. A., Hancock, E., Agouris, I., Smith, F. W., & MacSween, A. (2007). The response of the nucleus pulposus of the lumbar intervertebral discs to functionally loaded positions. *Spine, 32*, 1508–1512.
12. Vleeming, A., Pool-Goudzwaard, A. L., Stoeckart, R., van Wingerden, J. P., & Snijders, C. J. (1995). The posterior layer of the thoracolumbar fascia. Its function in load transfer from spine to legs. *Spine, 20*, 753–758.
13. Vleeming, A., Schuenke, M. D., Danneels, L., & Willard, F. H. (2014). The functional coupling of the deep abdominal and paraspinal muscles: The effects of simulated paraspinal muscle contraction on force transfer to the middle and posterior layer of the thoracolumbar fascia. *Journal of Anatomy, 225*, 447–462.
14. Willard, F. H., Vleeming, A., Schuenke, M. D., Danneels, L., & Schleip, R. (2012). The thoracolumbar fascia: Anatomy, function and clinical considerations. *Journal of Anatomy, 221*, 507–536.
15. Alexandru, D., & So, W. (2012). Evaluation and management of vertebral compression fractures. *The Permanente Journal, 16*, 46–51.
16. Antonelli-Incalzi, R., Pedone, C., Cesari, M., Di Iorio, A., Bandinelli, S., & Ferrucci, L. (2007). Relationship between the occiput-wall distance and physical performance in the elderly: A cross sectional study. *Aging Clinical and Experimental Research, 19*, 207–212.
17. Sinaki, M., Itoi, E., Wahner, H. W., Wollan, P., Gelzcer, R., Mullan, B. P., Collins, D. A., et al. (2002). Stronger back muscles reduce the incidence of vertebral fractures: A prospective 10 year follow-up of postmenopausal women. *Bone, 30*, 836–841.
18. Sinaki, M. (2007). The role of physical activity in bone health: A new hypothesis to reduce risk of vertebral fracture. *Physical Medical and Rehabilitation Clinics of North America, 18*, 593–608, xi–xii.
19. Malmros, B., Mortensen, L., Jensen, M. B., & Charles, P. (1998). Positive effects of physiotherapy on chronic pain and performance in osteoporosis. *Osteoporosis International, 8*, 215–221.
20. Papaioannou, A., Adachi, J. D., Winegard, K., Ferko, N., Parkinson, W., Cook, R. J., Webber, C., & McCartney, N. (2003). Efficacy of home-based exercise for improving quality of life among elderly women with symptomatic osteoporosis-related vertebral fractures. *Osteoporosis International, 14*, 677–682.
21. Bennell, K. L., Matthews, B., Greig, A., Briggs, A., Kelly, A., Sherburn, M., Larsen, J., et al. (2010). Effects of an exercise and manual therapy program on physical impairments, function and quality-of-life in people with osteoporotic vertebral

fracture: A randomised, single-blind controlled pilot trial. *BMC Musculoskeletal Disorders, 11,* 36.

22. Sinaki, M. (2003). Critical appraisal of physical rehabilitation measures after osteoporotic vertebral fracture. *Osteoporosis International, 14,* 773–779.

23. Sinaki, M., & Mikkelsen, B. A. (1984). Postmenopausal spinal osteoporosis: Flexion versus extension exercises. *Archives of Physical and Medicine and Rehabilitation, 65,* 593–596.

24. Martyn-St James, M., & Carroll, S. (2008). Meta-analysis of walking for preservation of bone mineral density in postmenopausal women. *Bone, 43,* 521–531.

25. Martyn-St James, M., & Carroll, S. (2006). High-intensity resistance training and postmenopausal bone loss: A meta-analysis. *Osteoporosis International, 17,* 1225–1240.

26. Gilsanz, V., Wren, T. A., Sanchez, M., Dorey, F., Judex, S., & Rubin, C. (2006). Low-level, high-frequency mechanical signals enhance musculoskeletal development of young women with low BMD. *Journal of Bone and Mineral Research, 21,* 1464–1474.

27. Slatkovska, L., Alibhai, S. M. H., Beyene, J., & Cheung, A. M. (2010). Effect of whole-body vibration on BMD: A systematic review and meta-analysis. *Osteoporosis International, 21,* 1969–1980.

28. Fon, G. T., Pitt, M. J., & Thies, A. C. (1980). Thoracic kyphosis: Range in normal subjects. *AJR American Journal of Roentgenology, 134,* 979–983.

29. Kado, D. M., Huang, M.-H., Barrett-Connor, E., & Greendale, G. A. (2005). Hyperkyphotic posture and poor physical functional ability in older community-dwelling men and women: The Rancho Bernardo study. *Journals of Gerontology, Series A, Biological Sciences and Medical Sciences, 60,* 633–637.

30. de Oliveira, T. S., Candotti, C. T., La Torre, M., Pelinson, P. P., Furlanetto, T. S., Kutchak, F. M., & Loss, J. F. (2012). Validity and reproducibility of the measurements obtained using the flexicurve instrument to evaluate the angles of thoracic and lumbar curvatures of the spine in the sagittal plane. *Rehabilitation Research and Practice, 2012,* 186156.

31. de Mauroy, J., Weiss, H., Aulisa, A., Aulisa, L., Brox, J., Durmala, J., Fusco, C., et al. (2010). 7th SOSORT consensus paper: Conservative treatment of idiopathic & Scheuermann's kyphosis. *Scoliosis, 5,* 9.

32. Weiss, H.-R., Turnbull, D., & Bohr, S. (2009). Brace treatment for patients with Scheuermann's disease—A review of the literature and first experiences with a new brace design. *Scoliosis, 4,* 22.

33. Itoi, E., & Sinaki, M. (1994). Effect of back-strengthening exercise on posture in healthy women 49 to 65 years of age. *Mayo Clinic Proceedings, 69,* 1054–1059.

34. Miyake, A., Kou, I., Takahashi, Y., Johnson, T. A., Ogura, Y., Dai, J., Qiu, X., et al. (2013). Identification of a susceptibility locus for severe adolescent idiopathic scoliosis on chromosome 17q24.3. *PloS One, 8,* e72802.

35. Takahashi, Y., Kou, I., Takahashi, A., Johnson, T. A., Kono, K., Kawakami, N., Uno, K., et al. (2011). A genome-wide association study identifies common variants near LBX1 associated with adolescent idiopathic scoliosis. *Nature Genetics, 43,* 1237–1240.

36. Maruyama, T., Kitagawa, T., Takeshita, K., Mochizuki, K., & Nakamura, K. (2003). Conservative treatment for adolescent idiopathic scoliosis: Can it reduce the incidence of surgical treatment? *Pediatric Rehabilitation, 6,* 215–219.

37. Maruyama, T., Takeshita, K., & Kitagawa, T. (2008). Side-shift exercise and hitch exercise. *Studies in Health Technology and Informatics,135,* 246–249.

38. Negrini, S., Atanasio, S., Fusco, C., & Zaina, F. (2009). Effectiveness of complete conservative treatment for adolescent idiopathic scoliosis (bracing and exercises) based on SOSORT management criteria: Results according to the SRS criteria for bracing studies— SOSORT Award 2009 Winner. *Scoliosis, 4,* 19.

39. Battié, M. C., Videman, T., Kaprio, J., Gibbons, L. E., Gill, K., Manninen, H., Saarela, J., et al. (2009). The Twin Spine Study: Contributions to a changing view of disc degeneration. *Spine Journal, Official Journal of the North American Spine Society, 9,* 47–59.

40. Alkhatib, B., Rosenzweig, D. H., Krock, E., Roughley, P. J., Beckman, L., Steffen, T., Weber, M. H., et al. (2014). Acute mechanical injury of the human intervertebral disc: Link to degeneration and pain. *European Cells and Materials, 28,* 98–110; discussion 110–111.

41. Paul, C. P. L., Schoorl, T., Zuiderbaan, H. A., Zandieh Doulabi, B., van der Veen, A. J., van de Ven, P. M., Smit, T. H., et al. (2013). Dynamic and static overloading induce early degenerative processes in caprine lumbar intervertebral discs. *PloS One, 8,* e62411.

42. Barr, K. P., Griggs, M., & Cadby, T. (2005). Lumbar stabilization: Core concepts and current literature, Part 1. *American Journal of Physical Medicine and Rehabilitation, 84,* 473–480.

43. Barr, K. P., Griggs, M., & Cadby, T. (2007). Lumbar stabilization: A review of core concepts and current literature, Part 2. *American Journal of Physical Medicine and Rehabilitation, 86,* 72–80.

44. Beattie, P. F. (2008). Current understanding of lumbar intervertebral disc degeneration: A review with emphasis upon etiology, pathophysiology, and lumbar magnetic resonance imaging findings. *Journal of Orthopaedic and Sports Physical Therapy, 38,* 329–340.

45. Gellhorn, A. C., Katz, J. N., & Suri, P. (2013). Osteoarthritis of the spine: The facet joints. *Nature Reviews, Rheumatology, 9,* 216–224.

46. Delitto, A., George, S. Z., Van Dillen, L. R., Whitman, J. M., Sowa, G., Shekelle, P., Denninger, T. R., et al. (2012). Low back pain. *Journal of Orthopaedic and Sports Physical Therapy, 42,* A1–A57.

47. Ciricillo, S. F., & Weinstein, P. R. (1993). Lumbar spinal stenosis. *Western Journal of Medicine, 158,* 171–177.

48. Padmanabhan, G., Sambasivan, A., & Desai, M. J. (2011). Three-step treadmill test and McKenzie mechanical diagnosis and therapy to establish directional preference in a patient with lumbar spinal stenosis: A case report. *Journal of Manual and Manipulative Therapy, 19,* 35–41.

49. Genevay, S., & Atlas, S. J. (2010). Lumbar spinal stenosis. *Best Practice and Research, Clinical Rheumatology, 24,* 253–265.

50. Cook, C., Brown, C., Michael, K., Isaacs, R., Howes, C., Richardson, W., Roman, M., et al. (2011). The clinical value of a cluster of patient history and observational findings as a diagnostic support tool for lumbar spine stenosis. *Physiotherapy Research International, 16,* 170–178.

51. Saunders, H. D. (2004). *Evaluation treatment & prevention of musculoskeletal disorders.Volume 1 Spine.* Chaska, MN: Saunders Group.

52. Boyd, B. S., Wanek, L., Gray, A. T., & Topp, K. S. (2009). Mechanosensitivity of the lower extremity nervous system during straight-leg raise neurodynamic testing in healthy individuals. *Journal of Orthopaedic and Sports Physical Therapy, 39,* 780–790.

53. Fardon, D. F., Williams, A. L., Dohring, E. J., Murtagh, F. R., Gabriel Rothman, S. L., & Sze, G. K. (2014). Lumbar disc nomenclature: Version 2.0: Recommendations of the combined task forces of the North American Spine Society, the American Society of Spine Radiology and the American Society of Neuroradiology. *The Spine Journal, 14,* 2525–2545.

54. Kim, S. J., Lee, T. H., & Lim, S. M. (2013). Prevalence of disc degeneration in asymptomatic Korean subjects. Part 1: Lumbar spine. *Journal of the Korean Neurosurgical Society, 53,* 31–38.

55. Lebow, R. L., Adogwa, O., Parker, S. L., Sharma, A., Cheng, J., & McGirt, M. J. (2011). Asymptomatic same-site recurrent disc herniation after lumbar discectomy: Results of a prospective longitudinal study with 2-year serial imaging. *Spine, 36,* 2147–2151.

56. Quiroz-Moreno, R., Lezama-Suárez, G., & Gómez-Jiménez, C. (2008). Disc alterations of lumbar spine on magnetic resonance images in asymptomatic workers. *Revista Médica del Instituto Mexicano del Seguro Social, 46,* 185–190.

57. Rajeswaran, G., Turner, M., Gissane, C., & Healy, J. C. (2014). MRI findings in the lumbar spines of asymptomatic elite junior tennis players. *Skeletal Radiology, 43,* 925–932.

58. Cleland, J. A., Childs, J. D., Palmer, J. A., & Eberhart, S. (2006). Slump stretching in the management of non-radicular low back pain: A pilot clinical trial. *Manual Therapy, 11,* 279–286.

59. George, S. Z. (2002). Characteristics of patients with lower extremity symptoms treated with slump stretching: A case series. *Journal of Orthopaedic and Sports Physical Therapy, 32,* 391–398.

60. Liddle, S. D., Gracey, J. H., & Baxter, G. D. (2007). Advice for the management of low back pain: A systematic review of randomised controlled trials. *Manual Therapy, 12,* 310–327.

61. Louw, A., Diener, I., Landers, M. R., & Puentedura, E. J. (2014). Preoperative pain neuroscience education for lumbar radiculopathy: A multicenter randomized controlled trial with 1-year follow-up. *Spine, 39,* 1449–1457.

62. Hebert, J. J., Marcus, R. L., Koppenhaver, S. L., & Fritz, J. M. (2010). Postoperative rehabilitation following lumbar discectomy with quantification of trunk muscle morphology and function: A case report and review of the literature. *Journal of Orthopaedic and Sports Physical Therapy, 40,* 402–412.

63. Standaert, C. J., & Herring, S. A. (2000). Spondylolysis: A critical review. *British Journal of Sports Medicine, 34,* 415–422.

64. Tsui, F. W., Tsui, H. W., Akram, A., Haroon, N., & Inman, R. D. (2014). The genetic basis of ankylosing spondylitis: New insights into disease pathogenesis. *The Application of Clinical Genetics, 7,* 105–115.

65. Masiero, S., Poli, P., Bonaldo, L., Pigatto, M., Ramonda, R., Lubrano, E., Punzi, L., et al. (2013). Supervised training and home-based rehabilitation in patients with stabilized ankylosing spondylitis on TNF inhibitor treatment: A controlled clinical trial with a 12-month follow-up. *Clinical Rehabilitation, 28,* 562–572.

66. Giannotti, E., Trainito, S., Arioli, G., Rucco, V., & Masiero, S. (2014). Effects of physical therapy for the management of patients with ankylosing spondylitis in the biological era. *Clinical Rheumatology, 33,* 1217–1230.

67. Gyurcsik, Z., Bodnár, N., Szekanecz, Z., & Szántó, S. (2013). Treatment of ankylosing spondylitis with biologics and targeted physical therapy: Positive effect on chest pain, diminished chest mobility, and respiratory function. *Zeitschrigt Für Rheumatologie, 72,* 997–1004.

68. Niedermann, K., Sidelnikov, E., Muggli, C., Dagfinrud, H., Hermann, M., Tamborrini, G., Ciurea, A., et al. (2013). Effect of cardiovascular training on fitness and perceived disease activity in people with ankylosing spondylitis. *Arthritis Care and Research, 65,* 1844–1852.

69. O'Dwyer, T., O'Shea, F., & Wilson, F. (2014). Exercise therapy for spondyloarthritis: A systematic review. *Rheumatology International, 34,* 887–902.

PART IV

Lower Extremities

Chapter 10

Orthopedic Interventions for the Pelvis and Hip

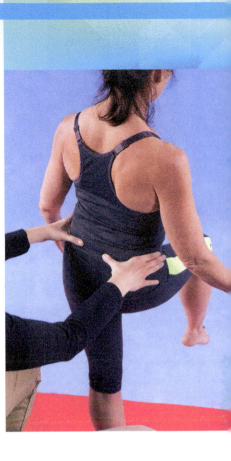

Anatomy and Physiology

Common Pathologies

LEARNING OUTCOMES

At the end of this chapter, the student will:

10.1   Describe the anatomy of the pelvis and hip region.

10.2   List normal hip range of motion.

10.3   Describe normal pelvis and hip kinematics.

10.4   Describe the mechanics, and discuss the purposes, of anterior, posterior, inferior, and distraction mobilization techniques of the hip.

10.5   Describe common hip pathologies and typical presentation.

10.6   Discuss contributing factors to various hip pathologies and, when relevant, preventive measures.

10.7   Describe the clinical tests used to diagnose common hip pathologies and how to administer the tests.

10.8   Discuss common treatment interventions for pelvis and hip pathologies.

10.9   Discuss surgical interventions and postsurgical treatment for the hip including total hip arthroplasty, hemiarthroplasty, and open reduction-internal fixation.

10.10   Explain the relationships between the hip pathologies of labral tear, femoroacetabular impingement, and osteoarthritis.

10.11   Describe clinical alerts for select pelvis and hip pathologies.

KEY WORDS

Angle of inclination	Intertrochanteric fracture	Premorbid
Angle of torsion	Microfracture	Retroversion
Anteversion	Microtearing	Sarcopenia
Avascular necrosis	Neuritis	Sclerosis
Coxa valga	Occult fracture	Subcapital fracture
Coxa vara	Open reduction and internal fixation	Subtrochanteric fracture
Deep vein thrombosis (DVT)	(ORIF)	Total hip arthroplasty
Degenerative joint disease (DJD)	Orthostatic hypotension	Trendelenburg sign/gait, compensated
Dysplasia	Osteoarthritis (OA)	Trendelenburg sign/gait,
Endoprosthesis	Osteophytes	uncompensated
Hemiarthroplasty	Osteoplasty	
Idiopathic	Osteotomy	

Anatomy and Physiology

The hip joint is the most proximal joint in the lower extremity kinematic chain. As such, it is subjected to the compressive and shear forces of body weight, the contraction of the large muscles that cross the joint, and the forces generated by lower extremity movements. The torque felt by the hip can be up to eight times body weight during some activities.[1] As a ball-and-socket joint, the hip has three degrees of freedom. The mobility that results from this bony configuration must be countered by soft tissue structures in order to provide the stability necessary to withstand these extreme forces. The structures that provide this stability are discussed next.

Bone and Joint Anatomy and Physiology

The rounded head of the femur articulates with the acetabulum of the pelvis to form the hip joint. The acetabulum lies at the junction of the ilium, ischium, and pubis, on the lateral side of each innominate bone. This is a deep socket, and it is further deepened by the acetabular labrum. The acetabulum faces anteriorly, laterally, and inferiorly. A horseshoe-shaped cartilage covers the portion of the acetabulum that makes contact with the femoral head and helps distribute the stresses in the joint.[2]

Distal to the femoral head, the bone narrows to become the femoral neck. The narrowing of the bone here makes this an area prone to fracture (see *Subcapital Fracture*). However, if the neck thickens in response to sport, the patient may experience contact of the neck of the femur with the pelvis (see *Femoroacetabular Impingement*). Where the femoral neck meets the shaft there are two large projections: the greater and lesser trochanters. Most of the powerful hip muscles attach to these protuberances. Figure 10.1 depicts the hip joint.

There are two angles that are important in describing normal biomechanics of the hip: the **angle of torsion** and the **angle of inclination**. When the hip is in neutral rotation, the head and neck of the femur do not lie directly in the frontal plane. Rather, they project anteriorly toward the sagittal plane at an angle of about 12° to 15° of the frontal plane. This is called the angle of torsion.

The angle of inclination describes the angle of the femoral neck with the shaft. A normal angle of inclination is 120° to 135°. As this angle becomes less than 120°, the neck and shaft come closer in proximity, creating a varus hip (**coxa vara**). As the angle becomes greater than 135°, the neck and shaft come to form an almost straight bone, creating a valgus hip (**coxa valga**). The implications of the angle of torsion and the angle of inclination will be discussed in more depth later in the chapter. Figure 10.2 illustrates the angle of torsion (A) and the angle of

inclination (B) of the femur. Table 10-1 summarizes bone and joint anatomy.

Soft Tissue Anatomy and Physiology

While the stability of the hip joint is largely due to its ball-and-socket shape, it is enhanced by labrum, capsule, ligaments, and muscles. An understanding of these soft tissues, as well as the bursae, nerves, and blood supply to the hip, is important in understanding pathology.

Labrum

The acetabular labrum (or hip labrum) is a rim of cartilage that extends off the acetabulum and increases the depth of the socket. The depth of the acetabulum plus the labral extension results in the femoral head being mostly covered by the socket. The labrum absorbs shock and distributes pressure, increases joint lubrication, and aids in stability.[3,4]

Capsule and Ligaments

There is one ligament inside the hip joint and multiple ligaments outside the joint. Inside the joint is the ligamentum teres. This ligament has long been regarded as playing an important role in joint stability only in children, but currently it is considered to remain important as a joint stabilizer into adulthood.[5,6] Within the ligamentum teres is a thin artery that supplies blood to a small portion of the femoral head (see "Blood Supply" later).

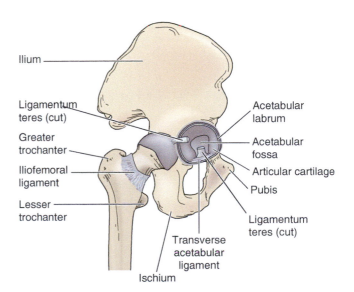

Figure 10.1 The hip joint is a ball-and-socket joint between the acetabulum of the innominate bone and the head of the femur. It is deepened by the acetabular labrum and stabilized by the ligamentum teres inside the joint and three ligaments that blend with the joint capsule.

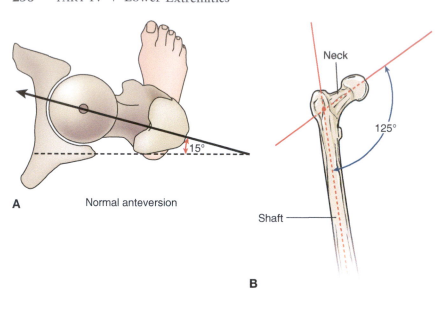

A Normal anteversion

B

Figure 10.2 The femoral head and neck are rotated forward of the frontal plane 12° to 15° in the angle of torsion (A). The femoral neck and shaft form an angle of inclination of 120° to 135°. Both these angles affect biomechanics of the lower extremity.

Table 10-1   Bone and Joint Anatomy and Physiology

Of the Pelvis and Hip

Joint	Anatomy	Normal ROM and Movements	Landmarks	Clinical Considerations
Hip	Ball and socket shape with 3 degrees of freedom Convex femoral head articulates with concave acetabulum of pelvis Angle of torsion of femoral head and neck is normally 12°–15°. Angle of inclination between the neck and shaft of the femur is normally 120°–135°. Horseshoe-shaped acetabular cartilage distributes stresses in joint.	Flexion 0°–125° Extension 0°–20° Abduction 0°–45° Adduction 0°–20° Internal rotation 0°–45° External rotation 0°–45°	Greater trochanter can be palpated on the lateral side of the hip.	Coxa vara (less than 120° angle of inclination) leads to valgus knees. Coxa valga (more than 135° angle of inclination) leads to varus knees. Retroversion of the hip caused by an angle of torsion of less than 8°, leads to out-toeing in stance and gait. Anteversion of the hip caused by an angle of torsion of more than 25° leads to in-toeing in stance and gait. Close packed: full extension with internal rotation. Loose packed: 30° flexion, 30° abduction, slight external rotation. Capsular pattern: internal rotation, flexion, abduction (order varies).

The stability of the hip is increased by a dense joint capsule and three ligaments, one from each of the bones of the pelvis. These ligaments are named by the bones they span: the iliofemoral, ischiofemoral, and pubofemoral. The iliofemoral ligament, also called the Y-ligament, is the strongest ligament in the hip and possibly the strongest in the human body. It is generally accepted that these ligaments, as a whole, limit hip extension.

Iliotibial (IT) Band

Starting at the lateral side of the iliac crest, and running down to the knee, is a broad band called the iliotibial (IT) band. Gluteus maximus, gluteus medius, and tensor

fascia latae insert into the band. The distal end of the IT band inserts into the anterolateral aspect of the tibia and the lateral femoral condyle. Some fibers also blend into the lateral retinaculum of the knee. The IT band will be discussed in more detail in Chapter 11, "Knee Anatomy and Physiology."

Bursae

There are several clinically relevant bursae that are found in the hip area: multiple greater trochanteric bursae, the ischiogluteal bursa, and the iliopsoas bursa.

In the region of the greater trochanter, several bursae cushion the gluteal tendons, the tensor fascia latae and the IT band.[7–9] The anatomy of the bursae in this region is highly variable, but most people have at least three bursae: the subgluteus maximus bursa, the subgluteus medius bursa, and the gluteus minimus bursa. The subgluteus maximus bursa is the largest of the three and is found on the lateral surface of the trochanter, sandwiched between the gluteus maximus and gluteus medius. The other two lie under the smaller gluteal muscles.

The ischiogluteal bursa is found over the ischial tuberosity and cushions the hamstring tendons and gluteus maximus muscle overlying the tuberosity.

The iliopsoas or iliopectineal bursa lies between the anterior hip capsule and the iliopsoas muscle in the anterior hip region. It provides a cushion for iliopsoas as it traverses the front of the pelvis and hip. Table 10-2 summarizes the soft tissues of the hip.

Nerves

The most significant nerve structure in the hip and upper thigh is the sciatic nerve (Fig. 10.3). It is the widest and longest nerve in the body. The sciatic nerve originates from branches of the lumbosacral plexus from L4–S3. It passes under, or occasionally through, the piriformis muscle and travels down the middle of the posterior thigh. As it passes through the posterior thigh, the sciatic nerve innervates most of the hamstring muscles and a portion of adductor magnus. Above the knee, the sciatic nerve splits into its component nerves, the common fibular nerve and the tibial nerve.

The other nerves in hip area are the femoral nerve and the obturator nerve (Fig. 10.4). The femoral nerve arises off of the lumbosacral plexus and contains roots

Table 10-2	Connective Tissue Anatomy and Physiology		
Of the Pelvis and Hip			
Structure	Anatomy	Function	Clinical Considerations
Joint capsule	Dense joint capsule that is reinforced by three ligaments.	Stabilizes the joint. Lined with synovium to produce synovial fluid.	Stability of hip is decreased after hip surgery such as total hip arthroplasty due to opening of capsule.
Ligaments	Three ligaments: • iliofemoral (Y-ligament) • ischiofemoral • pubofemoral	Enhance the stability of the hip joint.	Limit hip extension.
Acetabular Labrum	Rim of cartilage that extends off the acetabulum about 5 mm.[10]	Absorbs shock, distributes pressure across the hip, and deepens the hip socket to increase stability.	Pain in the hip has been found to be related to labral tears.
Ligamentum Teres (Round ligament)	Runs from fovea on femoral head to the acetabulum.	In the child: hip stability. May serve a role in stabilizing the hip in adults. Carries the obturator artery that supplies part of femoral head.	Ligament tears appear to be a cause of nonarthritic hip pain. Dislocation or subluxation of the hip may tear the ligament and artery.
IT Band	Runs from iliac crest, down lateral thigh to tibia and patella. Insertion point for gluteus maximus, gluteus medius, and tensor fascia latae.	Provides stability to the lateral knee.	May become tight, altering biomechanics of lower extremity. Source of pain in IT band friction syndrome (Ch. 11).
Greater trochanteric bursae	Several bursae including one below each of the gluteal muscles: subgluteus maximus bursa, subgluteus medius bursa, and gluteus minimus bursa.	Forms a cushion between each of the gluteal muscles and the structures below.	See *Greater Trochanteric Pain Syndrome.*
Ischiogluteal bursa	Lies on the ischial tuberosity at the origin of the hamstring muscles.	Cushions the hamstring tendons and gluteus maximus from the tuberosity.	See *Ischiogluteal Bursitis.*
Iliopsoas bursa	Lies on the anterior hip under iliopsoas.	Cushions iliopsoas from the anterior hip.	See *Iliopsoas Syndrome.*

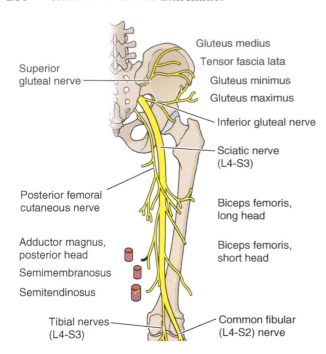

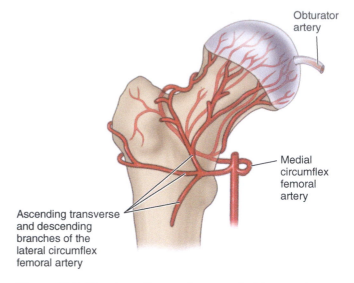

Figure 10.5 The circumflex arteries enter the hip capsule at the femoral neck and run into the head to supply most of the femoral head. A small portion of the head may be supplied by the obturator artery in the ligamentum teres.

Figure 10.3 The sciatic nerve runs through the posterior buttock and thigh. Above the knee, it innervates the hamstring muscles and part of adductor magnus.

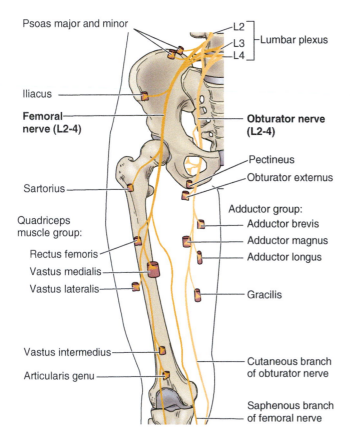

Figure 10.4 The obturator and femoral nerves are on the anterior aspect of the hip. The obturator nerve innervates the adductors of the hip. The femoral nerve innervates the quadriceps group as well as iliacus and sartorius.

from L2–4. It innervates the quadriceps femoris group as well as the pectineus and sartorius muscles. The obturator nerve arises off the same nerve roots and primarily innervates the adductor muscles (part of adductor magnus, adductor longus, adductor brevis, and gracilis).

Blood Supply to the Femoral Head and Neck

Blood supply to the femoral head and neck is derived mostly from the medial and lateral circumflex femoral arteries, which pierce the capsule near its insertion on the femur and run up the neck and into the head. A secondary contributor in some people is a small branch of the obturator artery that enters the head at the insertion of the ligamentum teres (Fig. 10.5). The blood supply to the shaft of the femur is through the nutrient artery. We'll discuss the impact of the circulatory anatomy on surgical treatment after hip fracture later in this chapter.

Muscular Anatomy and Kinesiology

The muscles around the hip can be divided into the following groups: hip flexors, extensors, abductors, adductors, internal rotators, and external rotators. Because the hip abductors are largely responsible for hip internal rotation these actions are paired in the table. A review of hip muscles with origin, insertion, innervation, primary action, and clinical relevance is found in Table 10-3.

Table 10-3   Muscle Anatomy and Kinesiology

Of the Pelvis and Hip

Muscle	Origin	Insertion	Innervation	Primary Action	Clinical Considerations
Iliacus	Iliac fossa	Lesser trochanter	Femoral nerve	Hip flexion	Shortness of the hip flexor leads to an anteriorly tilted pelvis and an increased lumbar lordosis.
Psoas major	Anterolateral sides of T12–L5	Lesser trochanter	Femoral nerve	Hip flexion and trunk flexion. Appears to act as a lumbar spine stabilizer.[11,12]	Iliacus and psoas major are often referred to collectively as iliopsoas due to their common insertion.
Rectus femoris	Anterior inferior iliac spine (AIIS)	Tibial tuberosity	Femoral nerve	Hip flexion and knee extension	
Sartorius	Anterior superior iliac spine (ASIS)	Proximal medial tibia	Femoral nerve	Hip flexion, hip abduction, hip external rotation, and knee flexion	One of three tendons that make up the pes anserine. Bursa lies under this structure.
Semimembranosus	Ischial tuberosity	Medial tibia	Tibial portion of sciatic nerve	Hip extension Knee flexion Tibial medial rotation	Shortness of hamstring muscles leads to posterior pelvic tilt and decreased lumbar lordosis.
Semitendinosus	Ischial tuberosity	Medial tibia	Tibial portion of sciatic nerve	Hip extension Knee flexion Tibial medial rotation	Semitendinosus is one of three pes anserine tendons.
Biceps femoris	Long head: ischial tuberosity Short head: posterior femur	Fibular head	Long head: tibial portion of sciatic nerve Short head: common fibular portion of sciatic nerve	Long head: hip extension and knee flexion Short head: knee flexion Both heads: tibial lateral rotation	Most commonly strained muscle in hamstring group.
Gluteus maximus	Posterior sacrum and ilium	Distal to greater trochanter	Inferior gluteal nerve	Hip extension and hip external rotation	
Gluteus medius	Lateral ilium	Greater trochanter	Superior gluteal nerve	Hip abduction and hip internal rotation	Plays a major role in maintaining a level pelvis during one-legged stance and gait.[13] Weakness results in Trendelenburg gait.
Gluteus minimus	Lateral ilium under gluteus medius	Greater trochanter	Superior gluteal nerve	Hip abduction and internal rotation	

Continued

Table 10-3   Muscle Anatomy and Kinesiology—cont'd

Of the Pelvis and Hip

Muscle	Origin	Insertion	Innervation	Primary Action	Clinical Considerations
Tensor fascia latae	Anterior superior iliac spine (ASIS)	By way of IT band into patella and anterior lateral tibia	Superior gluteal nerve	Hip flexion, hip abduction, hip internal rotation. Stabilizes lateral knee by tightening IT band.	
Adductor magnus	Two heads: Anterior head: ischial ramus Posterior head: ischial tuberosity	Posterior femur	Anterior head: obturator nerve Posterior head: sciatic nerve	Hip adduction. Posterior head also performs hip extension.	In origin, innervation, and action, posterior head of adductor magnus has a kinship with the hamstring muscles.
Adductor longus	Pubis	Posterior femur	Obturator nerve	Hip adduction	
Adductor brevis	Pubis	Posterior femur	Obturator nerve	Hip adduction	
Pectineus	Pubis	Posterior proximal femur	Obturator nerve	Hip adduction and weak hip flexion	
Gracilis	Pubis	Proximal medial tibia	Obturator nerve	Hip adduction. Additionally, it performs weak hip flexion, knee flexion, and is a medial knee stabilizer.	One of three pes anserine tendons
Six deep outward rotators Piriformis Obturator internus Obturator externus Gemellus superior Gemellus inferior Quadratus femoris	Sacrum, ischium, pubis	Greater trochanter	Variable	Hip external rotation Piriformis assists in hip internal rotation when hip is fully flexed.	Piriformis is significant in the role it plays in sciatic nerve entrapment. The sciatic nerve lies very near piriformis, running under it or piercing piriformis as it travels through the buttock region. Other deep rotators act to stabilize the femoral head in the acetabulum. They may be considered the "rotator cuff of the hip."[14,15]

Kinematics of the Pelvis and Hip

Because the hip joint functions in closed chain during the stance phase of gait, and muscles tend to reverse action in closed chain, it is important to consider the effect of the muscles of the hip on both the pelvis (closed chain) and on the femur (open chain). Muscles that flex the femur on the pelvis also have the capability of anteriorly tilting the pelvis on the femur. Muscles that extend the hip also tilt the pelvis posteriorly on the femur. Muscles that abduct the femur become powerful stabilizers of the opposite side of the pelvis in the frontal plane during stance phase. The hip adductors that control the leg in swing phase help stabilize the pelvis in closed chain.

Shortening of the muscles of the hip can affect the position of the spine and pelvis. This is especially true of muscles that span two or more joints. There are several two-joint muscles in this area, including hamstrings, rectus femoris, and gracilis. These muscles impact range of motion of the hip when they become passively insufficient.

Although normal hip flexion is about 125° with knee flexion, it is only 90° with knee extension due to passive insufficiency of the hamstring muscles. While normal hip extension is 20° to 30° with knee extension, it is less with knee flexion due to passive insufficiency of the rectus femoris.

Femur Movement on the Pelvis

The movements of the femur on the pelvis are very familiar and include flexion, extension, abduction, adduction, internal rotation, and external rotation. These motions most easily occur in open chain. Limitation of range of motion in the hip can contribute to lower extremity and/or spine pathology.

Pelvis Movement on the Femur

The position of the neutral pelvis in stance is described as level iliac crests when viewed in the frontal plane and level ASIS and PSIS when viewed in the sagittal plane. In the transverse plane, the pelvis should not be rotated. The pelvis frequently will move on a stable femur during weight-bearing activities, including stance phase of gait. The movements of the pelvis at the hip are anterior tilt, posterior tilt, lateral tilt, and rotation.

Anterior pelvic tilt is the result of flexion of the pelvis on the hip in the sagittal plane. The ASIS moves forward and down and the PSIS moves superiorly. Anterior pelvic tilt is a position of flexion of the hip. This position may be caused by shortening of the iliopsoas, rectus femoris, or erector spinae muscles. The result on the lumbar spine is increased lordosis or extension (Fig. 10.6).

Posterior pelvic tilt is the result of extension of the pelvis on the hip in the sagittal plane. In this case, the ASIS moves up and back relative to its neutral position. The PSIS moves inferiorly. Posterior pelvic tilt is a position of extension of the hip. This position may be caused by shortening of the abdominals, the gluteus maximus, or the hamstring muscles. The effect on the lumbar spine is flattening or flexion (Fig. 10.7).

Lateral pelvic tilt is the result of raising or dropping of the pelvis on one side in the frontal plane. This most frequently occurs in single-leg stance or in gait when one side of the pelvis is not supported. In this position, maintaining a level pelvis depends largely upon the strength in the force couple of gluteus medius on the stance side and quadratus lumborum on the swing side.

With weakness of the lateral pelvic tilt force couple, specifically gluteus medius, the patient is unable to maintain a level pelvis in single-leg stance and/or in gait. If the patient doesn't adopt a compensatory strategy, the pelvis will drop on the unsupported side during stance on the affected side. This is called an **uncompensated Trendelenburg** sign in standing or uncompensated Trendelenburg gait during walking. The patient will usually compensate for the weakness by leaning toward the affected side during stance phase on the affected side. This is called a **compensated Trendelenburg** sign/gait. The position of the stance side hip is one of abduction when the contralateral side of the pelvis is raised and adduction when this side of the pelvis is dropped (Fig. 10.8).

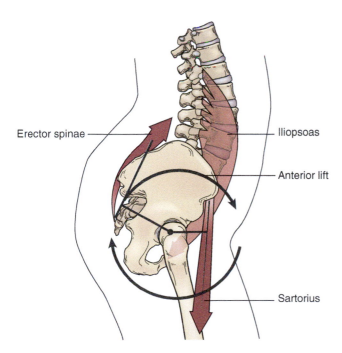

Erector spinae — Iliopsoas — Anterior lift — Sartorius

Figure 10.6 Anterior pelvic tilt may be caused by contraction or shortening of the iliopsoas, rectus femoris, or erector spinae muscles, resulting in lumbar spine extension.

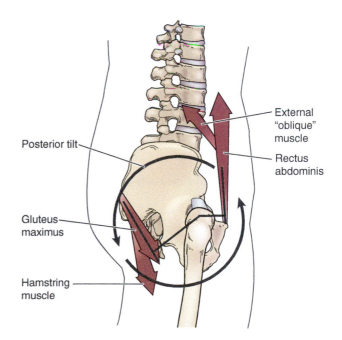

Posterior tilt — External "oblique" muscle — Rectus abdominis — Gluteus maximus — Hamstring muscle

Figure 10.7 Posterior pelvic tilt may be caused by contraction or shortening of the abdominals, gluteus maximus, or hamstring muscles, resulting in lumbar spine flexion.

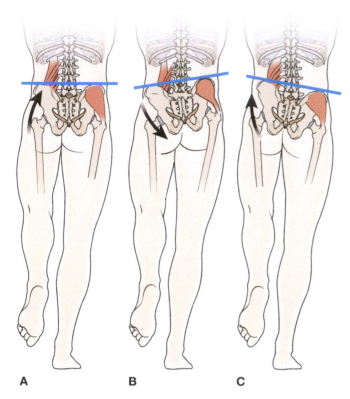

Figure 10.8 Gluteus medius on the stance side and quadratus lumborum on the swing side maintain a relatively level pelvis during gait (A). With weakness of the force couple, the pelvis may drop on the swing side during gait. This is an uncompensated Trendelenburg (B) and is usually caused by gluteus medius weakness on the stance side. The patient may compensate by leaning toward the stance leg and raising the pelvis on the swing side, called a compensated Trendelenburg (C).

Watch Out For...

Watch out for patients adopting a Trendelenburg gait due to hip or knee pain rather than weakness. By leaning toward the affected side, the torque at the hip and knee is significantly decreased, which decreases pain.

Pelvic rotation is movement of the pelvis in the transverse plane. Forward rotation occurs in normal gait as the swing leg advances, and backward rotation increases throughout stance phase. Forward rotation of the pelvis results in internal rotation of the opposite stance leg; backward rotation results in external rotation of the opposite leg (Fig. 10.9).

Anteversion and Retroversion

The femoral head and neck project medially but do not lie directly in the frontal plane. Rather they lie in a plane that runs anteriorly and medially about 12° to 15° of

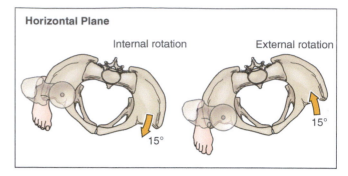

Figure 10.9 Pelvic rotation during gait. The swing leg brings the pelvis into forward rotation, resulting in internal rotation of the stance leg.

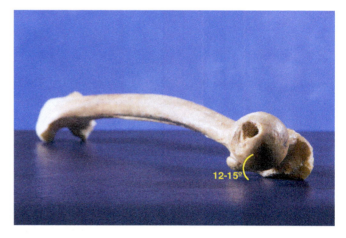

Figure 10.10 With the femoral condyles in the frontal plane, the head and neck project anteriorly and medially, forming the angle of torsion.

the frontal plane, forming an angle of torsion with the shaft of the femur. You can observe this angle by laying a femur on a flat surface and noticing that the neck and head do not lie on the table, but are turned so that the head is raised off the surface (Fig. 10.10).

If the head and neck lie more toward the frontal plane so that the torsion angle is reduced (less than 8°), the femoral shaft must be externally rotated in order to properly seat the head in the acetabulum.[16] The result in this case is that the patient will have increased range of motion into hip external rotation, decreased hip internal rotation range of motion, and will generally walk in a more toe-out position. This position is called hip **retroversion.**

If the head and neck form a torsion angle with the shaft that is greater than normal (more than 25°), the femur must be internally rotated in order to properly seat the femoral head in the acetabulum.[16] The resulting findings are increased hip internal rotation range of motion, decreased external rotation range of motion, and in-toeing during gait. This position is called hip

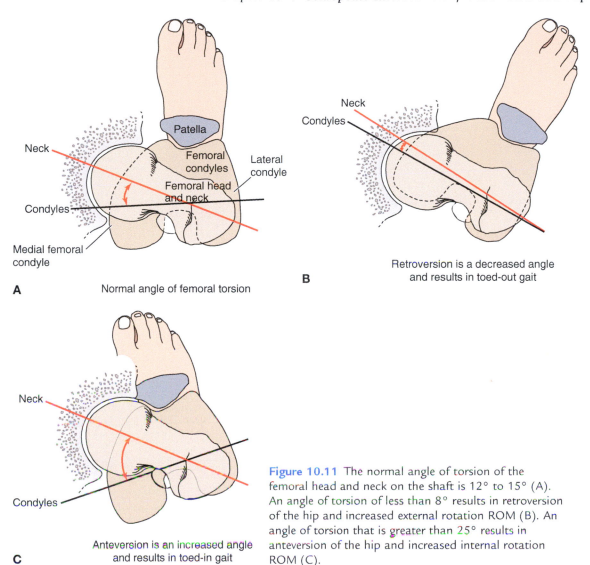

A   Normal angle of femoral torsion

B   Retroversion is a decreased angle and results in toed-out gait

C   Anteversion is an increased angle and results in toed-in gait

Figure 10.11 The normal angle of torsion of the femoral head and neck on the shaft is 12° to 15° (A). An angle of torsion of less than 8° results in retroversion of the hip and increased external rotation ROM (B). An angle of torsion that is greater than 25° results in anteversion of the hip and increased internal rotation ROM (C).

anteversion. Figure 10.11 depicts the normal torsion angle and angles of anteversion and retroversion.

Coxa Vara and Coxa Valga

The angle of inclination of the femoral neck with the shaft is roughly 125°. A varus hip, coxa vara, results when the angle of inclination is less than 120°. A valgus hip, coxa valgus, results from an angle of inclination of greater than 135°. A varus hip is associated with increased valgus at the knee, and a valgus hip is associated with increased varus at the knees. Figure 10.12 depicts the normal anatomy of the femur, coxa vara, and coxa valga. The impact of abnormal hip alignment on the knee can be seen.

Hip Influences in the Kinetic Chain

It is important to understand that the hip exerts a great deal of control over the knee and ankle, not just statically as described above, but dynamically as well. The extensors, abductors, and external rotators of the hip control knee valgus during weight-bearing activities. The powerful muscles of the hip and the joint's position at the top of the kinetic chain afford the hip a tremendous influence.[17,18] This will be discussed in more detail in Chapter 11.

The hip influences the spine as well. Many of the muscles of the hip attach to the pelvis and cause anterior, posterior, or lateral tilting. This influences the position of the lumbar spine. In addition, motion of the hip and spine are intricately connected in the movement pattern of hip and knee flexion. Limitation of motion in the hip can lead to compensatory lumbar spine movement and spine pathology.

Joint Mobilization

To reduce pain or increase range of motion, joint mobilization may be a useful intervention. As a ball-and-socket

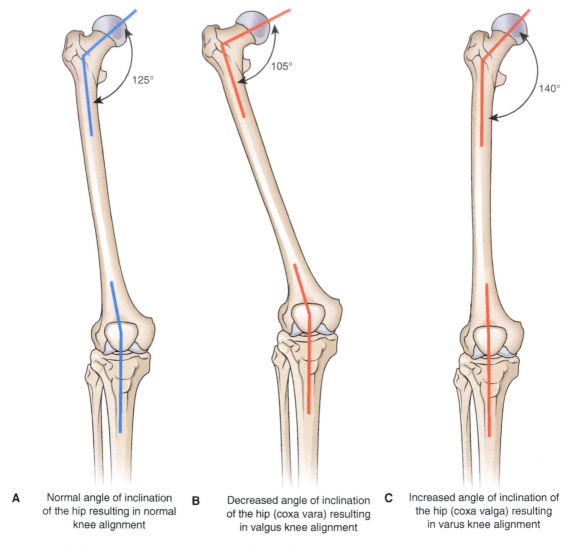

A Normal angle of inclination of the hip resulting in normal knee alignment

B Decreased angle of inclination of the hip (coxa vara) resulting in valgus knee alignment

C Increased angle of inclination of the hip (coxa valga) resulting in varus knee alignment

Figure 10.12 Normal angle of inclination, coxa vara, and coxa valga. Coxa vara is associated with valgus of the knee. Coxa valga is associated with varus of the knee.

joint, movement in the hip joint is accompanied by a slide of the femoral head in the direction opposite the movement of the long bone. The loose-packed position of the hip is 30° hip flexion and 30° abduction with very slight hip external rotation. Table 10-4 lists the cardinal plane motion and the associated direction of mobilization that is used to increase range.

Anterior Glide

Anterior glide is used to increase hip extension and external rotation. With the patient prone, the examiner supports the patient's affected leg. The examiner applies force near the joint in an anterior direction toward the examination table (Fig. 10.13).

Table 10-4	Direction of Slide Used to Increase Range of Motion of the Hip
Limited Range	**Direction of Slide in Mobilization**
Flexion	Posterior and Inferior
Extension	Anterior
Abduction	Inferior
Internal rotation	Posterior
External rotation	Anterior

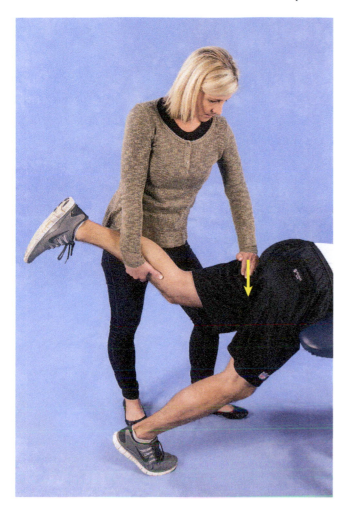

Figure 10.13 Anterior glide of the hip increases hip extension and external rotation.

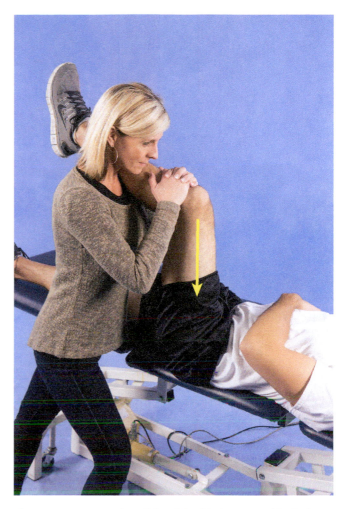

Figure 10.14 Posterior glide of the hip increases hip flexion and internal rotation.

Posterior Glide

Posterior glide is used to increase range of motion into hip flexion and internal rotation. The patient is positioned supine near the edge of the table with the leg in 90° of hip and knee flexion, with slight hip adduction. The examiner stabilizes the patient's affected leg and applies a force downward through the femur (Fig. 10.14).

Inferior Glide

Inferior glide is used to increase range of motion into hip abduction. The patient is positioned supine with the affected leg resting on the examiner's shoulder at about

80° hip and knee flexion. Clasping both hands over the patient's proximal femur, the examiner applies a force toward the patient's feet (Fig. 10.15).

Long Axis Distraction

Long axis distraction is used to alleviate joint pain and stretch the whole capsule. The patient is positioned supine with the affected leg straight. The examiner grasps the patient's leg above the ankle. Force is applied away from the patient's hip by the examiner leaning back and shifting their weight (Fig. 10.16).

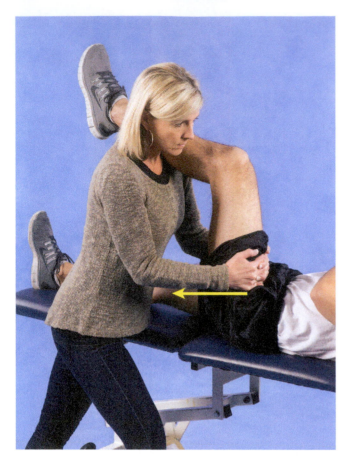

Figure 10.15 Inferior glide of the hip increases hip abduction.

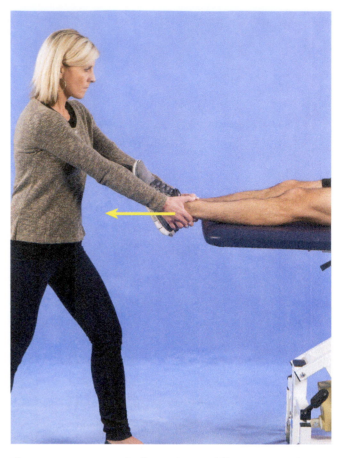

Figure 10.16 Long axis distraction mobilization is used to stretch the hip generally and to decrease joint pain.

Common Pathologies

Osteoarthritis

Hip Fracture

Piriformis Syndrome

Femoroacetabular Impingement Syndrome

Hip Labral Tear

Greater Trochanteric Pain Syndrome

Ischiogluteal Bursitis

Iliopsoas Syndrome (Tendonitis/Bursitis)

Legg-Calvé-Perthes Disease

Hamstring Muscle Strain

Rectus Femoris Muscle Strain

The location, structure, and function of the hip predispose it to injury or pathology. In addition, altered biomechanics in the lower extremity can lead to pain, weakness, inflammation, and damage to the hip joint. In this section we'll discuss hip pathologies that affect people across the age spectrum, from young children to older adults. We'll explore surgical treatments for osteoarthritis and hip fracture. You should notice that the special tests used to diagnose hip pathologies may be indicative of a variety of pathologies.

Osteoarthritis (OA)   CPG

Osteoarthritis (OA) is the most common type of arthritis. It is also known as **degenerative joint disease** or **DJD.** This is a wear-and-tear arthritis, in contrast with rheumatoid

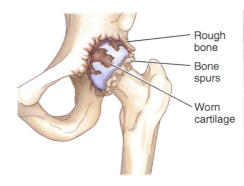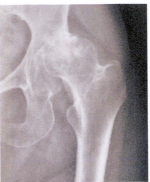

Rough bone
Bone spurs
Worn cartilage

OA hip joint

Figure 10.17 Illustration of hip osteoarthritis and typical x-ray findings of decreased joint space, osteophytes, and sclerosis.

Box 10-1 Developmental Hip Dysplasia

Developmental dysplasia of the hip (DDH) is a condition that is most common in females by a ratio of 8:1. This congenital condition is characterized by a shallow acetabulum and large angle of inclination of the femur. The condition can range from mild to severe. Mild cases may go undetected into adulthood. More severe manifestations lead to dislocation of the hip in newborn children. For mild cases, keeping the baby's hips abducted through splinting will improve the shape of the developing acetabulum. For severe cases, surgery (osteotomy) is performed to relocate the femur, build an acetabulum, and normalize the angle of inclination.

arthritis that is a systemic disease process. Simply put, OA is a result of moving parts, in this case the hip, wearing out. The manifestations of OA include joint pain, stiffness, and loss of range of motion. Muscle atrophy (**sarcopenia**) is often present, as are lax ligaments. X-rays often reveal decreased joint space, bone spurs (**osteophytes**), and areas of increased bone density (**sclerosis**) displaying as a whitened area (Fig. 10.17).

Causes/Contributing Factors

There are many reported risk factors for OA of the hip. It has been linked to increased stresses on the joint from obesity, altered biomechanics, capsular tightness, physically demanding occupations, injury, normal aging,[19–21] leg-length discrepancy, femoroacetabular impingement,[22–25] labral tear,[4] and developmental hip **dysplasia** (Box 10-1). Indeed, the link between hip dysplasia, femoroacetabular impingement, labral tears, and OA of the hip has been described as a continuum of joint disease.[26]

Symptoms

OA often leads to complaints of pain in the anterior hip and groin area and, less commonly, in the lateral hip. Pain may be referred into the medial thigh to the knee. The patient will generally experience increased pain during

or after weight-bearing activities. Morning stiffness lasting less than 1 hour is typical and indicative of OA.[27,28] As the joint further deteriorates, it becomes painful to go from sitting to standing and the joint becomes more limited in range of motion. Limited hip flexion and internal rotation is common. Secondary problems may develop in the lumbar spine due to excessive movement as a compensation for limited hip range of motion.

Clinical Signs

Many sources of information are used to assign the diagnosis of hip OA including x-ray findings, patient complaints, hip range of motion, and special tests. Limitation of motion in three hip movements is highly suggestive of OA.[29,30] The two tests described next are useful in data collection.

FABER Test

The FABER test (also known as the Patrick test) derives its name from the position in which the patient's leg is placed (**F**lexion-**AB**duction-**E**xternal **R**otation). It is used to test for several hip pathologies, including OA. For this test, the patient is placed in a supine position. The examiner places the patient's lower extremity in a position of hip flexion, abduction, and external rotation with the ankle resting just above the knee on the opposite side. Slight downward pressure is applied by the examiner to the flexed knee as well as a stabilizing counterpressure (downward and outward) to the opposite ilium near the anterior superior iliac spine (ASIS) (Fig. 10.18). A positive test is indicated by patient complaint of pain in the hip, buttock, or groin on the flexed leg side. This test also indicates the possibility of labral tear,[31] femoroacetabular impingement,[32] and sacroiliac joint dysfunction.[33]

Hip Scour/Quadrant Test

The hip scour/quadrant test is currently not as supported by the evidence as the FABER test. To perform the hip scour test, the patient is placed in a supine position. The examiner flexes, adducts, and internally rotates the patient's hip and flexes the patient's knee. The patient's hip is passively taken through an arc of motion into hip external rotation, abduction, and increased flexion.[34]

Some sources suggest that, if this does not produce pain, a compressive force may be applied through the femur by downward pressure on the knee while moving the patient into hip internal and external rotation (Fig. 10.19A, B).[29,35] A positive test is indicated by reproducing the patient's complaint of pain in the hip or groin on the side tested.

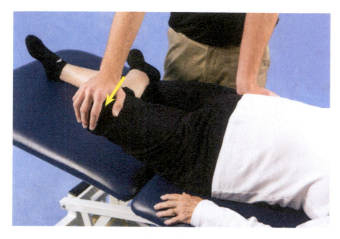

Figure 10.18 FABER test for hip OA. This test may also be used in the diagnosis of FAI and hip labral tears.

Common Interventions

Treatment for OA of the hip will depend upon the severity of symptoms and often will include a combination of physical therapy, pharmacological, and surgical interventions. Patient education consists of information regarding the pathology, progression, and contributing factors. An important component is counseling the patient about a lifestyle change of increased physical activity[36,37] and weight loss, if appropriate.

Therapeutic exercise often includes components of joint range of motion, strengthening, and aerobic exercise in the form of walking or biking.[36–38] Range-of-motion exercises should focus on hip flexion and internal rotation[39] as well as other limited motions. Strengthening exercises are indicated for all the muscles around the hip[40] and knee, particularly hip flexors, hip extensors, hip abductors, hip adductors, and knee extensors.[41] Strengthening these muscles will take stress off the hip joint. Initially, submaximal isometric exercises minimize the joint stresses, but the patient should be progressed to dynamic resistance exercises as tolerated (Fig. 10.20A–C).[42]

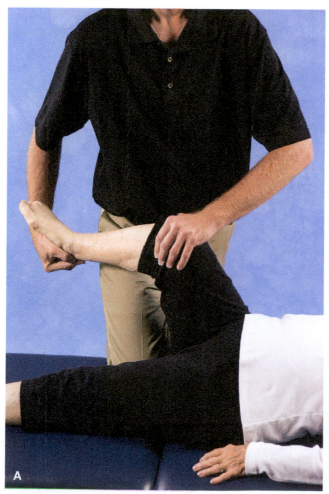
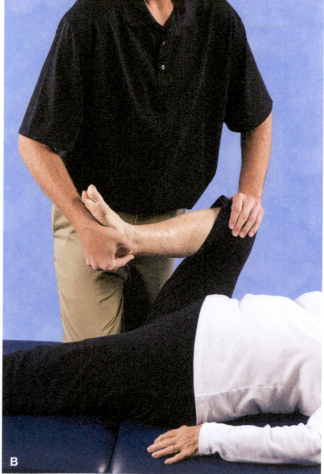

Figure 10.19 Hip scour or quadrant test for hip OA.

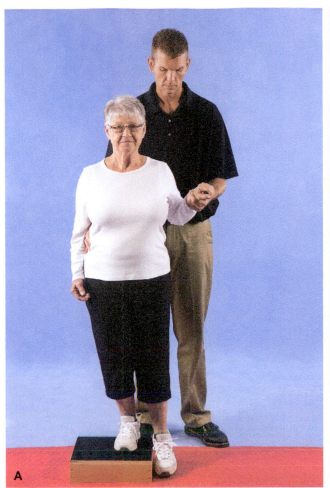

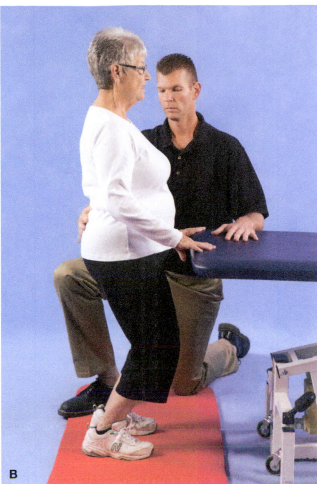

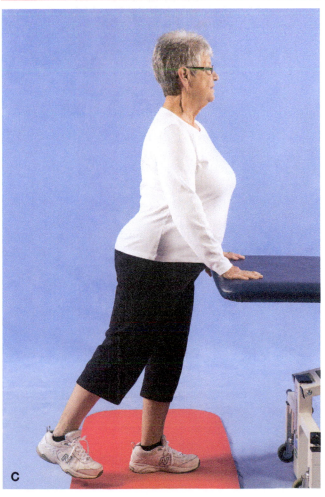

Figure 10.20 Exercises for hip OA may include lateral step-ups (A), mini-squats (B), and standing hip extension exercises (C).

Grade I or II joint mobilizations can be done to decrease hip pain and increase range of motion and function.[35,43] Use of an assistive device will help unload the joint. If there is a leg length discrepancy, correction by use of a shoe lift may be beneficial. The PT or PTA may elect to perform exercises in a pool for the benefits of decreased weight-bearing on the joint.[44]

If the patient is unsuccessful in controlling hip pain and loss of function, a **total hip arthroplasty** may be indicated.

Prevention

Maintaining an active lifestyle will help maintain leg motion and strength and prevent or slow the progression of OA. Leg length discrepancies should be corrected early. Weight loss or maintenance of a healthy body weight minimizes joint stresses.

The Bottom Line:	for patients with OA of the hip
Description and causes	Deterioration of the hip, which may be due to obesity, abnormal biomechanics, normal aging, injury, femoroacetabular impingement, and labral tear
Test	FABER test, hip scouring/quadrant test
Stretch	Into all planes, especially hip flexion and internal rotation
Strengthen	Surrounding muscles, especially hip flexors, extensors, abductors, adductors, and knee extensors
Train	NA
Avoid	Leg length discrepancy, leg weakness, being overweight

Interventions for the Surgical Patient

Total Hip Arthroplasty

There are several surgical options for advanced OA of the hip if the patient has limited function. The most common surgical treatment is total hip arthroplasty (THA), in which the femoral head and neck is replaced by an **endoprosthesis** and the acetabulum is resurfaced with an acetabular component, which is frequently a combination of a metal shell and a plastic liner.[42,45] This surgical option is also used for joint deterioration from other causes such as rheumatoid arthritis, **avascular necrosis** (Box 10-2), fracture, and malignancy.

Seeing the patient preoperatively results in improved strength, function,[46] aerobic capacity,[45] and gait.[47] Preoperative intervention has also been associated with an increased likelihood of patient discharge to home after surgery rather than to a rehabilitation facility.[45,46]

Prior to surgery, the surgeon and patient will decide if the prosthetic components will or will not be cemented into place. By cementing the prosthesis, the patient will usually be allowed to bear weight as tolerated immediately after surgery. However, there is a higher incidence of the prosthesis loosening over time. If the prosthesis is to be noncemented, the implant will have a rough texture, which allows for bone to grow into the prosthesis (Fig. 10.21A, B). This type of fixation lasts longer.

What's in the Plan of Care? In this case, the patient's weight-bearing will likely be restricted for several weeks while bone growth occurs.

Surgery

There are several surgical approaches, each with advantages and disadvantages. The three most common approaches are the posterior (or posterolateral) approach, the anterolateral approach, and the true anterior approach. The posterior/posterolateral approach is most traditional. It involves removing the deep external rotators and possibly gluteus maximus from their insertions and then reattaching after the prosthesis is inserted. This approach has the highest risk of dislocation[48] but surgery time is shorter as compared to that of an anterior approach.

The anterolateral approach is more stable and less likely to dislocate. However, the surgery takes longer to perform. In this approach, the hip abductors are taken off at the insertion and later reattached. Resisted hip abduction may be contraindicated for a few weeks after

Box 10-2 | Avascular Necrosis of the Hip

Bone requires blood flow to stay alive. Avascular necrosis of bone occurs when the blood flow is interrupted to an area of bone. As osteocytes in the bone die, bone formation is halted and the bone collapses. No area of the body is more prone to avascular necrosis than the head of the hip. Blood supply to the hip passes up the neck and into the head and is vulnerable to disruption from dislocation and fracture. Avascular necrosis may also be related to long-term use of steroids and excessive alcohol consumption.

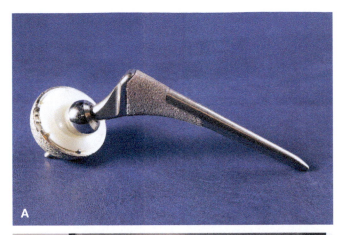

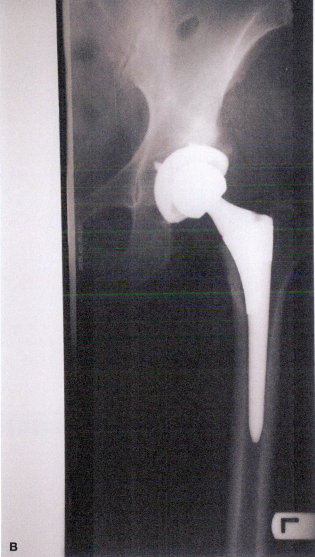

Figure 10.21 The total hip prosthesis consists of a femoral component and an acetabular component. The prosthesis shown is a cementless prosthesis with a metal head (A). Figure B shows a radiograph after total hip replacement.

surgery. This approach may result in weakness of hip abductors after surgery, with a Trendelenburg gait. An uncompensated Trendelenburg gait is characterized by the pelvis dropping on the unaffected side in stance phase on the affected side. A compensated Trendelenburg gait is characterized by leaning toward the affected side in stance phase on the affected side.

CLINICAL ALERT

After an anterolateral approach, active and resisted hip abduction may be contraindicated for several weeks.

In a true anterior approach, the incision is made on the anterior hip. This approach yields the most stable result. No muscles are detached but sartorius, TFL, and rectus femoris are moved out of the way during surgery. Some tightness of these muscles may be seen after surgery.

Postoperative Phase

Following a THA, the patient will be instructed to adhere to dislocation precautions for at least 6 weeks. Some surgeons want the patient to be mindful of these precautions for the rest of their life. Postoperatively, physical therapy intervention will include patient education regarding the risk of hip dislocation. Patients should be able to list the movements to be avoided, and they should be monitored for a demonstration of understanding and adherence. Figure 10.22 shows dislocation precautions after the posterior/posterolateral approach, and Figure 10.23 shows dislocation precautions after the anterior and anterolateral approaches.

CLINICAL ALERT

Dislocation precautions following a posterior or posterolateral approach are to avoid hip flexion greater than 90°, hip adduction past the midline, and hip internal rotation past neutral. While dislocation after an anterior or anterolateral approach is not common, external rotation and extension are the hip positions to be most avoided.

CLINICAL ALERT

During the first few days postoperatively, it is important to teach the patient how to perform "ankle pumps" to prevent **deep vein thrombosis (DVT)**. The risk of DVT is that the clot will dislodge and become a pulmonary embolism, which can be fatal. Signs of a DVT are swelling, pain, or tenderness in the leg that is most noticeable when standing or walking, increased warmth in the area, and red or discolored skin on the leg.[49] Wells' criteria offer a clinical prediction rule that may be used to assess the likelihood of DVT. See Box 10-3 for Wells' criteria.

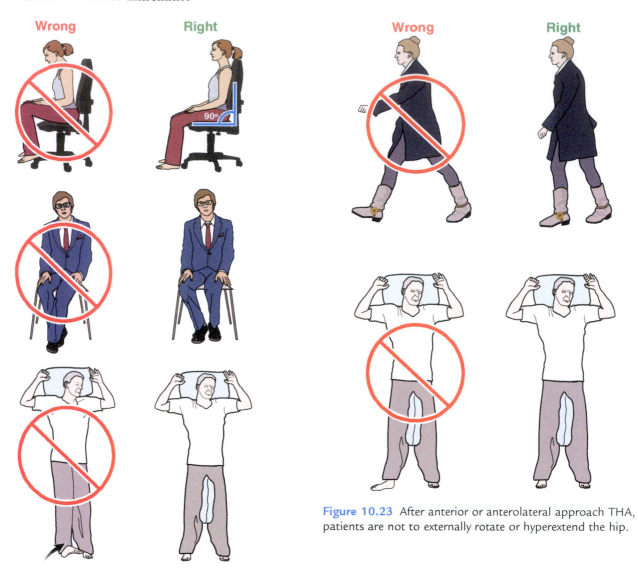

Wrong   **Right**   **Wrong**   **Right**

Figure 10.23 After anterior or anterolateral approach THA, patients are not to externally rotate or hyperextend the hip.

Figure 10.22 After posterior or posterolateral approach THA, patients are not to flex past 90°, adduct past midline, or internally rotate the hip.

Box 10-3	Wells' Criteria for Risk of Deep Vein Thrombosis

Wells' Criteria	Score
Does the patient have active cancer?	+1
Has the patient been bedridden more than 3 days or had major surgery in the last four weeks?	+1
Does the patient have calf swelling of more than 3 cm compared to the other leg?	+1
Does the patient have collateral, nonvaricose, superficial veins?	+1
Is the patient's entire leg swollen?	+1
Does the patient have localized tenderness along the deep venous system?	+1
Is there pitting edema, greater in the symptomatic leg?	+1
Does the patient have paralysis, paresis, or recent immobilization of the LE?	+1
Does the patient have a previous history of DVT?	+1
Is there an alternative diagnosis to DVT that is as likely or more likely?	−2
TOTAL (−2 to 9)	*

*A score of −2 to 9 is obtained using the criteria above. The risk of DVT is considered high if greater than 2, moderate if 1 or 2, and low if less than or equal to 1. From Wells PS et al.[50]

Common components of the rehabilitation plan of care after THA include active assistive range of motion (AAROM) and active range of motion (AROM) of the hip, gentle strengthening of hip muscles without violating dislocation precautions, and gait training. Additionally, the unaffected leg and the upper extremities should be strengthened. As the patient progresses, more aggressive strengthening exercises may be prescribed. Resistance may be added to the exercises. The goals of treatment will usually be to return the patient to their **premorbid** level of function and, if possible, to full range of motion, normal strength, and a normal, symmetrical gait pattern. Figure 10.24 shows exercises that might typically be performed after total hip arthroplasty.

Hip Fracture

Fractures of the femur around the hip area are fairly common in older adults. The classification of hip fractures in this area are **subcapital, intertrochanteric,** and **subtrochanteric.** Subcapital fractures occur through the neck of the femur, intertrochanteric fractures generally occur along a line between the greater and lesser trochanters, and subtrochanteric fractures include any fractures that fall below the lesser trochanter (Fig. 10.25).

Causes/Contributing Factors

According to the Centers for Disease Control and Prevention, 90% of hip fractures are a result of a fall.[51] They can also result from a pathological fracture due to malignancy or other trauma. This is a problem primarily in white, older females, with the incidence increasing each decade of life. Osteoporosis (decreased bone density) and a decline in balance with age may be the greatest contributing risk factors.

Symptoms

Pain in the hip and inability to ambulate are common indicators of hip fracture. Upon fracture, the leg may externally rotate and shorten (Fig. 10.26). Occasionally, hip fracture may not show on an x-ray and remain undiagnosed for a period of time. This is called an **occult fracture.** In this case, the patient may be ambulatory but have an antalgic gait, with decreased time spent in single leg stance on the affected side.

Clinical Signs

The diagnosis is generally made by x-ray. There are no special tests that the PTA would need to employ.

Common Interventions

Surgical intervention to stabilize the fracture will be performed soon after the diagnosis. Physical therapy will be initiated generally on day 1 postoperatively.

Box 10-4 **Fall Prevention Tips**

Instructions to lower risk of falling include:

1. Maximizing visual acuity—using lights at night, keeping eyeglasses clean, and having regular vision checks are recommended.
2. Managing **orthostatic hypotension** if the patient is on blood pressure medication—standing briefly before walking away from a chair to allow the blood pressure to return to normal may be helpful.
3. Keeping the home "fall-proof" as much as possible—by keeping walkways clear, mopping up spills, and minimizing clutter.
4. Using an assistive device if needed.
5. Wearing proper footwear with moderate traction on the sole.

Prevention

Prevention of hip fracture includes prevention and management of osteoporosis through nutrition, exercise, and pharmacological intervention. Exercises to improve balance are beneficial. The Chinese tradition of Tai Chi has been shown to be effective in this regard. Maintaining lower extremity strength and range of motion helps prevent falls. See Box 10-4 for other fall prevention tips.

Interventions for the Surgical Patient

Hip fractures may be surgically treated by **hemiarthroplasty,** which is the replacement of the head of the hip with a femoral prosthesis. Alternatively, the surgeon may repair the patient's fracture by using pins, plates, screws, wires, or nails. This repair is called **open reduction, internal fixation (ORIF).** The region of the fracture will determine the impact on blood supply to the femoral head and thereby dictate surgical options.

Hemiarthroplasty

Fracture through the femoral neck (subcapital fracture) will often disrupt the blood supply to the femoral head. Recall that the arteries to the femoral head travel through the area of the neck of the femur. The risk of loss of blood flow to the femoral head is high with a fracture in this location, which increases the likelihood of avascular necrosis. With subcapital fracture, replacement of the head of the femur is the recommended approach. In this approach, only half of the hip, specifically the femoral half, is replaced. The patient's native acetabulum remains. The femoral component is much larger than a total hip endoprosthesis because it must accommodate the patient's natural acetabulum. Figure 10.27 shows the prosthesis and an x-ray after hemiarthroplasty.

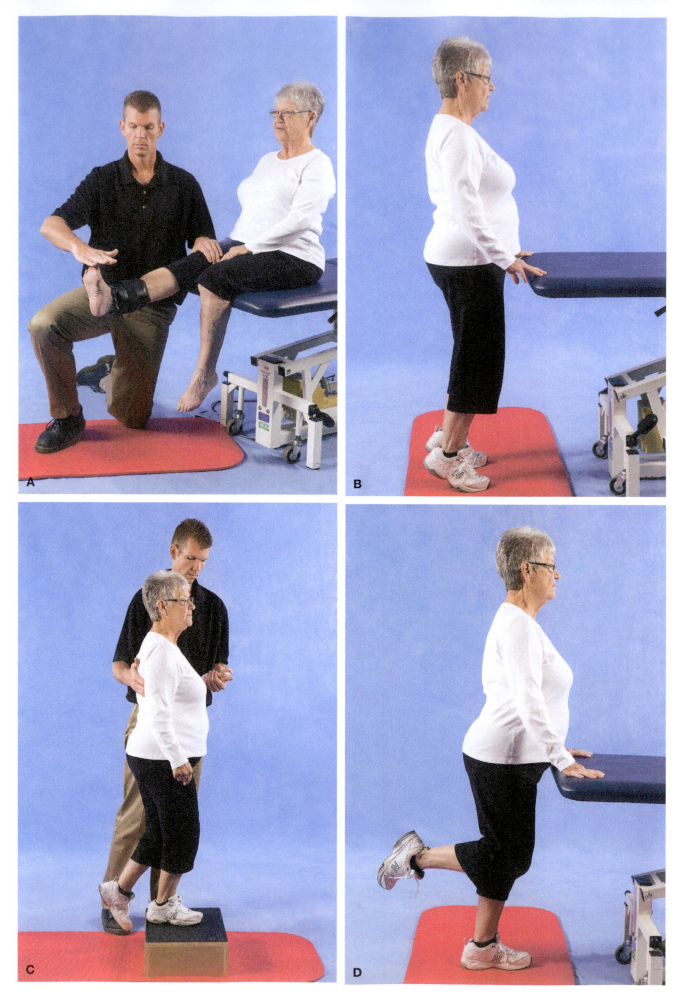

Figure 10.24 Common exercises after total hip arthroplasty include long arc quadriceps strengthening (A), calf raises (B), steps-ups (C), and standing knee flexion (D).

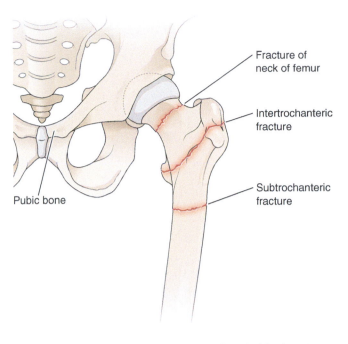

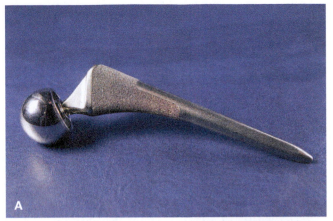

Figure 10.25 Femoral fracture can be classified by location as subcapital, intertrochanteric, or subtrochanteric.

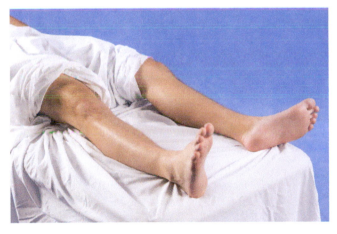

Figure 10.26 A clinical sign of hip fracture is external rotation and shortening of the affected leg.

Postoperative Phase

Physical therapy after hemiarthroplasty is similar to that after total hip arthroplasty. The patient must be educated regarding hip dislocation precautions. Therapeutic exercises may consist of AAROM to AROM of the hip, submaximal isometric or submaximal dynamic hip strengthening exercises,[42,52] and strengthening of the unaffected leg and upper extremities. The patient will usually be allowed to bear weight as tolerated, and the goal of gait training generally will be to restore the patient to the prior level of function.

ORIF of the Hip

Intertrochanteric and subtrochanteric fractures are generally surgically repaired by ORIF since the vascularity of

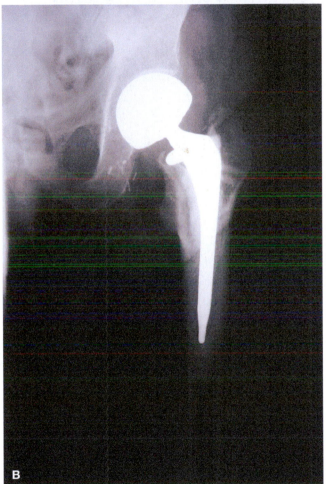

Figure 10.27 The hip hemiarthroplasty prosthesis (A) and an x-ray after hemiarthroplasty (B).

the femoral head has not been compromised, as is the case with subcapital fracture. The fracture site is reduced into alignment through an incision (open reduction), and the fracture is stabilized by pins, plates, screws, wires, or nails (internal fixation). Figure 10.28 is an x-ray of a hip after ORIF.

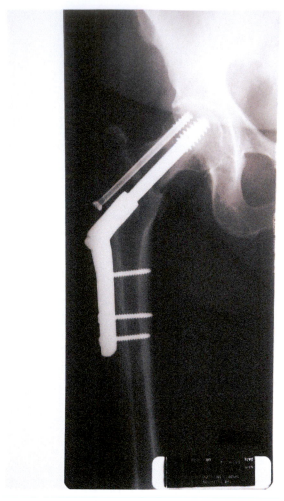

Figure 10.28 Radiograph after ORIF of the hip due to fracture.

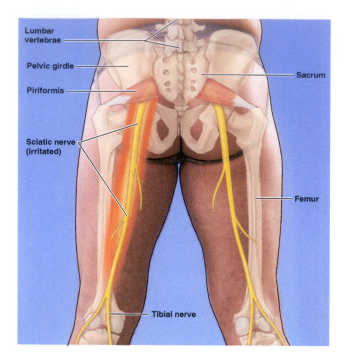

Figure 10.29 A contributor to piriformis syndrome may be the relationship of the sciatic nerve to the piriformis muscle. In piriformis syndrome, part or all of the nerve may exit through the piriformis rather than below it.

Postoperative Phase

Physical therapy after ORIF includes instruction in ankle pumps to prevent DVT. Therapeutic exercise, mobility activities, and gait training are common components of the plan of care. Weight-bearing may be restricted for 3 to 6 weeks. Therapeutic exercises may include AAROM to AROM and gentle strengthening of the hip. The unaffected leg and the upper extremities should be strengthened as well. As the patient progresses, more aggressive strengthening exercises may be prescribed. Resistance may be added to the exercises. The goals are to return the patient to their premorbid level of function and, if possible, to full hip range of motion, normal hip strength, and a normal, symmetrical gait pattern. Recovery from this type of fracture is generally slower than it is from hemiarthroplasty or total hip arthroplasty, because of the need for bone healing and the likelihood that the patient will have restricted weight-bearing.

Piriformis Syndrome

The sciatic nerve forms off the sacral plexus in the pelvis and travels through the buttock region, generally below and sometimes through the piriformis muscle under the gluteus maximus. The nerve continues down the posterior buttock and thigh, passing between the greater trochanter of the femur and the ischial tuberosity. At the piriformis muscle, the sciatic nerve experiences a potential site of entrapment. This can lead to inflammation of the sciatic nerve, or **neuritis**.

Causes/Contributing Factors

The cause of this compression is primarily considered to be spasm or shortening of the piriformis muscle.[53–55] Variations in the anatomical arrangement of the piriformis muscle and the sciatic nerve, specifically instances where the nerve pierces the muscle rather than coursing under it, have long been implicated (Fig. 10.29). However, the incidence of this anatomical configuration does not seem to be higher in patients who electively undergo surgical release of the piriformis than in the general population, both being about 16%.[56] Recently, in a case study an elongated piriformis with poor motor control has been implicated as a contributing factor.[57]

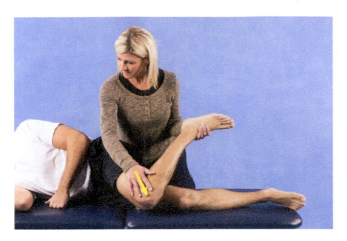

Figure 10.30 FAIR test for piriformis syndrome.

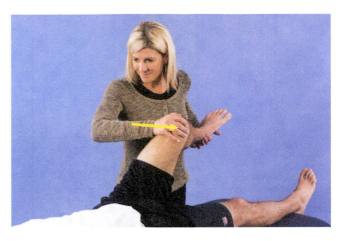

Figure 10.31 FADIR test for piriformis syndrome. This test is also called the anterior hip impingement test. This test may also be used in the diagnosis of FAI and labral tear.

Symptoms

Entrapment of the sciatic nerve leads to pain in the buttock and posterior thigh, which is increased in sitting, squatting, and with deep palpation or prolonged stretch of the piriformis. Pain is generally increased in hip flexion, adduction, and internal rotation.[53,55] The patient may experience numbness and tingling in the buttock and posterior thigh.

Clinical Signs

The patient will often present with limited hip internal rotation and adduction range of motion. The following tests may be useful to diagnose this syndrome.

FAIR Test for Piriformis Syndrome

For the FAIR test, the patient is placed in a sidelying position with the affected side up. The patient's hip is flexed to 90° and the knee is flexed. The patient's hip is then adducted and internally rotated to end range. If the patient has pain in the buttock or a reproduction of symptoms, the test is considered positive (see Fig. 10.30).[29,30,53,55]

FADIR Test for Piriformis Syndrome

In the FADIR test, the patient is placed in a supine position with the hip and knee flexed to 90°. The test is performed similarly to the FAIR test, with the examiner passively moving the hip into flexion, adduction, and internal rotation. A positive test for piriformis syndrome is indicated by pain in the buttock or reproduction of symptoms. This test is also called the anterior hip impingement test. It may be used in the diagnosis of femoroacetabular impingement (FAI) syndrome and labral tears in addition to piriformis syndrome (see Fig. 10.31).

Common Interventions

Treatment of piriformis syndrome involves decreasing the compression of the sciatic nerve. The physical therapist will evaluate for contributors, including postural factors, sacral dysfunction, muscle tightness or weakness, and motor control. Treatment commonly includes stretching of the piriformis and soft tissue mobilization. Strengthening of hip abductors, external rotators, and extensors may be included in the treatment plan, as well as re-education in proper movement patterns. Typical exercises that might be included in the plan of care are found in Figure 10.32.

Watch Out For...

Watch out for the proper way to stretch piriformis. Although piriformis is an external rotator when the hip is extended, as the hip exceeds 90° of flexion it becomes an internal rotator. Exercises to stretch piriformis reflect these biomechanics. Stretch into hip internal rotation if hip flexion is less than 90° but into hip external rotation with increasing hip flexion.

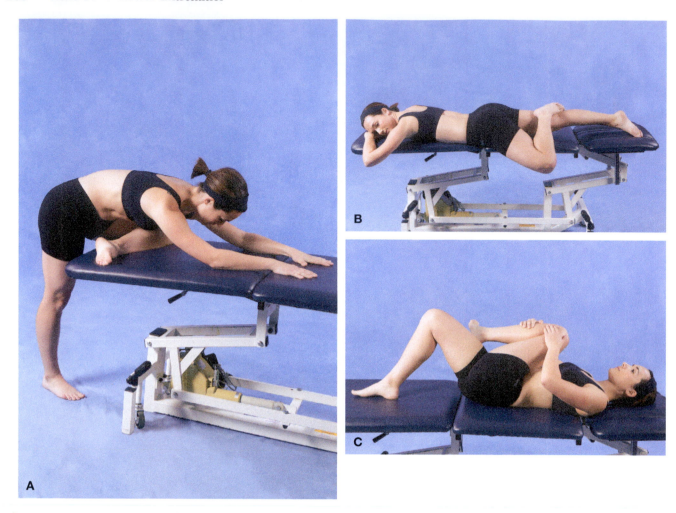

Figure 10.32 Exercises commonly used to stretch piriformis include hip flexion and external rotation supine (A), prone FABER position (B), and supine flexion with adduction (C).

The Bottom Line:	for patients with piriformis syndrome
Description and causes	Compression on the sciatic nerve related to relationship of piriformis to the nerve or spasm of piriformis
Test	FAIR, FADIR, decreased ROM into hip IR
Stretch	Into hip IR with hip extended or external rotation with hip flexion past 90 degrees, soft tissue mobilization of piriformis
Strengthen	Hip abductors, hip external rotators, hip extensors
Train	Proper movement pattern of hip
Avoid	NA

Femoroacetabular Impingement Syndrome   CPG

Femoroacetabular impingement (FAI) syndrome is characterized by abnormal contact between the femur and the rim of the acetabulum. The reason for the abnormal contact is an abnormal shape of the femoral head/neck, or of the acetabulum, or both.

There are three forms of FAI: cam, pincer, and mixed (cam and pincer). The cam anomaly is on the femur; the pincer anomaly is on the acetabulum. In the cam anomaly the femoral head is either not spherical and/or the femoral neck is enlarged. This causes the femur to contact the

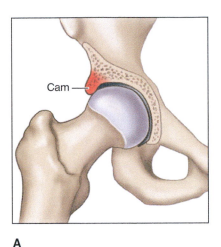
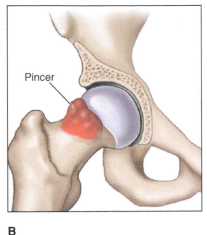
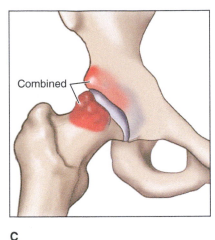

A **B** **C**

Figure 10.33 Femoroacetabular impingement occurs due to thickening of the femoral neck (A), an elongation of the acetabulum (B), or both.

acetabulum at the end range of flexion. In the pincer anomaly, the acetabulum covers more than the usual amount of the femoral head. A mixed type of FAI occurs when both anomalies are present. It is thought that FAI can lead to labral tears and OA.[22–26] Figure 10.33 depicts cam, pincer, and mixed types of anomalies.

Causes/Contributing Factors

Cam-type impingement is about twice as common in males as in females. Pincer anomaly is more common in middle-aged, active women.[58] Recent research into these anomalies indicates that they appear more likely to occur in people who engage in high-impact sports, such as football, hockey, and soccer. The cam deformity in particular appears to be triggered by vigorous sports activity during childhood and adolescence, around the time of closure of the capital growth plate.[59–63]

Research has shown a link between nonarthritic hip pain/FAI and hip muscle weakness, abnormal movement patterns, and joint hypermobility. Harris-Hayes et al.[64] found that patients who have hip pain have weakness in the hip abductors and rotators. Casartelli et al.[65] similarly found that patients with FAI have weakness in the hip flexors, external rotators, abductors, and adductors. Abnormal movement patterns, particularly medial collapse of the knee into valgus during activities such as walking, stair climbing, and sit to stand, have been implicated in FAI (see "Dynamic Valgus" in Chapter 11).[15,66,67]

Congenital joint hypermobility may also contribute to FAI.[68] This can be assessed using the Beighton score.[69] The patient is given a point on each side for thumb abduction to the forearm, 5th finger MCP hyperextension past 90°, elbow hyperextension, and knee hyperextension. Two points are given for being able to touch palms to the floor without knee flexion. This is covered in depth in Chapter 5 under "Shoulder Instability."

Symptoms

The most common symptom of FAI is groin pain of moderate to severe intensity. This pain may be accompanied by buttock pain. Patients complain of pain that is exacerbated by running, sitting, pivoting, and walking.[32] Pain is generally relieved by rest and change of position.

Clinical Signs

The most commonly performed special tests employed in the differential diagnosis of FAI are the FABER, the FADIR, and the resisted straight leg raise test.

FABER Test for FAI

The FABER test may be used in the differential diagnosis of FAI. A positive test is indicated by patient complaint of pain in the hip, buttock, or groin on the flexed leg side. See *Osteoarthritis* for more information on the FABER test.

FADIR Test for FAI

The FADIR test may also be used in the diagnosis of FAI. A positive test is indicated by pain in the anterior hip or groin. See *Piriformis Syndrome* for more information on the FADIR test.

Resisted Straight Leg Raise Test for FAI

The resisted straight leg raise test (also called the Stinchfield test) is performed with the patient in a supine position. The patient flexes the hip to 30° with the knee extended. The examiner applies a downward pressure above the knee, with instruction to the patient to hold the leg in position (Fig. 10.34). A positive test is indicated by pain in the anterior hip or groin.

Common Interventions

Because intervention for FAI prior to surgery is a relatively new area of research, little is known about the effectiveness of therapy prior to surgery. However, early studies indicate possible benefits from strengthening the hip abductors and external rotators. It may be helpful to target the deep hip external rotators in patients with hypermobility. Normalizing movement patterns also appears to have a beneficial result.

Prevention

At this time, it appears that a cam type of anomaly leading to FAI is more likely in adolescents who participate in high-intensity sports. Varying the type of sports activities during this formative time may be recommended while more data is collected.

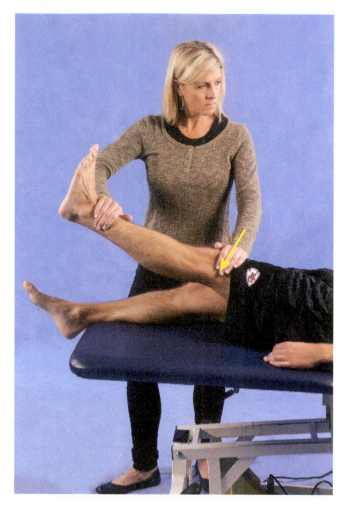

Figure 10.34 Resisted straight leg raise (Stinchfield) test for FAI. This test may also be used in the diagnosis of labral tears.

The Bottom Line: for patients with femoroacetabular impingement

Description and causes	Thickening of the femoral neck and/or elongation of the acetabular rim leading to impingement of the two bones, possibly related to high-impact sports
Test	FAIR, FABER, FADIR, resisted SLR tests
Stretch	NA
Strengthen	Hip external rotators and abductors, deep rotators to stabilize hip
Train	Normal movement patterns, avoiding collapse of knee into valgus
Avoid	Playing high-intensity sports year-round

Interventions for the Surgical Patient

Surgical options for FAI include **osteotomy** and **osteoplasty** to reshape the femoral head, neck, or acetabular rim. This may be accompanied by **microfracture** or abrasion of the articular cartilage to stimulate new cartilage growth. The labrum may be repaired or **resected**.

Rehabilitation after surgery for FAI will depend upon the surgical procedure used and the findings on the initial evaluation.[70,71] Patients will likely be limited in weight-bearing for up to 6 to 9 weeks after microfracture and up to 3 to 4 weeks after osteoplasty. The patient may be placed in a brace to limit hip flexion and abduction. Early modality intervention may include cryotherapy or use of an ice-compression system.

Hip flexion past 90°, extension past neutral, and internal rotation are typically restricted to avoid inflammation of the anterior hip capsule and labrum.[72] Patients should be told to avoid sitting with knees higher than hips, crossing legs, and sitting on their leg to prevent further irritation of the anterior hip structures. Prolonged sitting or standing should initially be avoided.

Range of motion otherwise may be preserved by using a stationary bike with the seat set high, or by continuous passive motion (CPM). Passive circumduction has been shown to be effective. In the early phase of rehabilitation, patients should be instructed to lie in a prone position for 2 hours per day to maintain hip extension ROM to neutral.[70] Gentle stretching in all planes of hip motion may be initiated at 4 weeks postop.[72]

Straight leg raise for the purpose of strengthening quadriceps or hip flexors, or stretching hamstrings may be contraindicated in the early phase of rehabilitation.[71]

Strengthening exercises may begin with submaximal isometrics and gentle AROM. The plan of care 4 to 6 weeks after surgery may include strengthening of quadriceps, hamstrings, gluteus maximus, gluteus medius, and core muscles. See Figure 10.35 for exercises typically included in the plan of care for FAI.

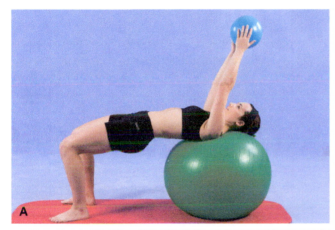
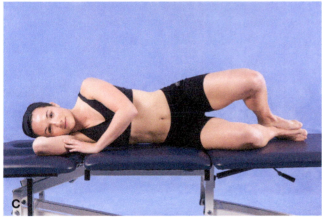
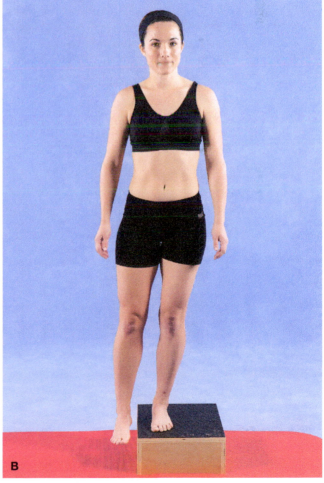

Figure 10.35 Exercises included in the plan of care after surgical intervention for FAI may include core strengthening (A), gluteus medius strengthening (B), and gluteus maximus strengthening (C). Patients should avoid hip extension past neutral and hip flexion greater than 90 degrees.

Hip Labral Tear   CPG

The acetabular labrum absorbs shock, stabilizes and lubricates the hip joint, and serves to distribute the pressures in the joint.[3,4] We have come to appreciate that the labrum is subject to tear and as such can be a source of pain. There is a correlation between labral tear and early onset OA.[4] Figure 10.36 depicts a hip labral tear.

Causes/Contributing Factors

To date, there have been five causes of labral tears that have been identified: trauma, FAI, hip capsule laxity/hypermobility, developmental hip dysplasia, and degeneration of an aging hip.[4,73] Traumatic causes include motor vehicle accidents; hip dislocation; and sports that involve twisting, hyperabduction, or hyperextension with or without external rotation.

Symptoms

The most common symptom is anterior hip and groin pain. Less commonly the patient may complain of pain in the lateral hip or posterior buttock. It's likely that groin pain is associated with an anterior labral tear and that buttock pain is associated with a posterior labral tear.

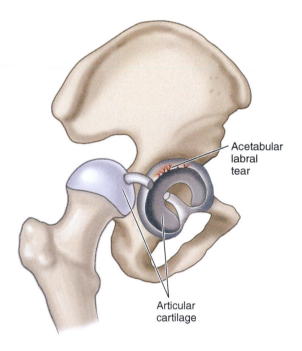

Acetabular labral tear

Articular cartilage

Figure 10.36 Acetabular labral tear may cause pain in the anterior hip or buttock.

Clinical Signs

As in the pathology of FAI, there are several tests that may be used in the diagnosis of hip labral tear. The FABER, FADIR, and resisted straight leg raise have all been shown to be useful. Additionally, the posterior hip impingement test may also yield positive results. In all cases, a positive test is indicated by reproduction of the patient's pain.

Posterior Hip Impingement Test

The posterior hip impingement test is performed with the patient in a supine position with the hip and knee extended. The unaffected limb may be flexed or left lying on the table. The examiner passively extends and externally rotates the patient's hip and lowers the leg off the side or end of the table. A positive test is indicated by anterior or posterior hip pain (Fig. 10.37).

Common Interventions

Initially, treatment for a labral tear often includes rest, anti-inflammatory medication, use of an assistive device to unload the hip, and physical therapy. According to Lewis and Sahrmann,[74] physical therapy treatment of labral tears focuses on reducing anteriorly directed forces on the hip and avoiding pivoting on the affected side. They recommend correction of abnormal muscle recruitment and movement patterns around the hip to minimize hyperextension forces. Particular attention should be paid to normal activation of iliopsoas and gluteus maximus muscles.[75]

According to Yazbek in a case study of four patients with suspected labral tears, a program of hip and lumbar stabilization and correction of muscle imbalance with focus on gluteus maximus, gluteus medius, and iliopsoas muscle strengthening was effective in treatment.[76] Patients were instructed to control knee valgus and hip adduction dynamically.

Instruction to the patient may include sitting with the knees at the level of the hips, avoiding sitting with legs crossed, and sitting on legs, which is often accompanied by hip rotation. The patient should avoid hip hyperextension in gait. Lewis and Sahrmann recommend avoiding weight-training of quadriceps and hamstrings and avoiding exercises that cause hip hyperextension.[74]

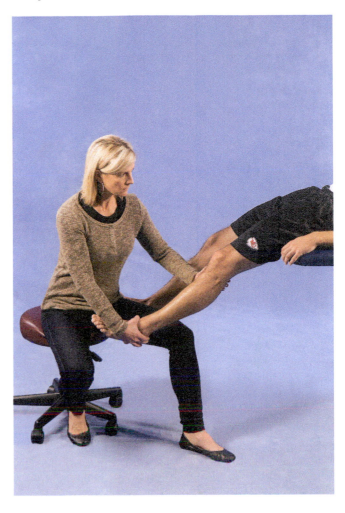

Figure 10.37 Posterior hip impingement test for labral tear.

The Bottom Line:	for patients with hip labral tears
Description and causes	Trauma, FAI, hip capsule hypermobility, developmental hip dysplasia, and degeneration associated with aging
Test	FABER, FADIR, resisted SLR, posterior impingement tests
Stretch	NA
Strengthen	Hip flexors, extensors, abductors
Train	Neuromuscular control of dynamic knee valgus
Avoid	Hip hyperextension, extremes of hip flexion, pivoting, sitting with knees lower than hips or with legs crossed

Interventions for the Surgical Patient

Labral Debridement/Repair/Excision

Surgical intervention for labral tear may be done arthroscopically or through open incision. Options include debridement, repair, or excision of the labrum. With a deeper understanding of the importance of the labrum, efforts to repair it have become more common.

Postoperative Phase

After debridement or repair, the patient will usually be allowed to bear weight as tolerated. Initially, the patient can perform isometric hip strengthening in all directions except hip flexion. Cycling is allowed as tolerated but should not be performed on a recumbent bike in light of the excessive hip flexion.

> ▶ **CLINICAL ALERT** ──────
>
> Exercises are performed as tolerated by the patient, with general instructions to avoid hip extension range of motion past neutral, avoid excessive hip flexion range of motion, and avoid activation of the hip flexors. AROM may begin about 2 weeks postoperatively, but the patient should avoid active straight leg raises. Exercises that require hyperextension of the hip beyond neutral, such as prone hip extension or lunges, should also be avoided.

Typically, 4 to 6 weeks postoperatively, the patient's plan of care will include more strengthening exercises and weight-bearing activities. Strengthening of the gluteal muscles is an important component of this phase. The patient should be told to avoid hip rotation with weight-bearing. Correction of gait faults, especially hip and knee hyperextension, will likely be advised.

In addition to labral debridement and repair, patients may undergo a joint resurfacing, osteoplasty or osteotomy, or a procedure to stimulate new cartilage growth. In these cases, the recovery process is slower. The patient will have limited weight-bearing for about 6 weeks. Active and active-assisted exercises in gravity-minimized positions are typically part of the plan of care for the first 6 weeks postoperatively in these cases.

What's in the Plan of Care?

Greater Trochanteric Pain Syndrome

This regional pain pathology was initially thought to be caused by inflammation of the bursae around the greater trochanter. Recently, following further research, it appears that greater trochanteric pain syndrome (GTPS) is caused by a number of conditions, including tendinopathy of the gluteal insertions, tears in the gluteal muscles, coxa saltans (external snapping hip), as well as inflammation of the bursae around the greater trochanter. There are several bursae around the hip. Couple this with the variability of location, and it explains the difficulty of a differential diagnosis.

Causes/Contributing Factors

There are risk factors that have been identified for GTPS, including age (most cases are diagnosed between the 4th and 6th decades,[7] gender (women outnumber men up to 4:1), tightness of the iliotibial (IT) band, leg length discrepancies, knee OA, low back pain, and obesity. Many of the contributing factors seem to indicate that altered lower limb biomechanics may be a root cause.

Trauma and overuse have long been implicated in the pathology of trochanteric bursitis, yet a significant percentage of patients with presenting symptoms cannot remember a traumatic event. Microtrauma of the gluteal muscles or tendons, or of the IT band, is thought to be a frequent source of the pain. This can occur with or without inflammation of the bursae. In a study by Bird et al., of 24 women with symptoms of GTPS, 11 had a gluteus medius tear, 15 had tendinitis, and 2 had signs of bursitis.[77] The prevalence of tears in the gluteal tendons has not been determined, but some researchers believe that up to 25% of women and 10% of men will have tears by late middle age.[8]

Coxa saltans, or external snapping hip, is another disorder that can contribute to GTPS. External snapping hip is characterized by the IT band moving over the greater trochanter, from posterior when the hip is extended to anterior when the hip is flexed. If snapping hip becomes a frequent occurrence, it is possible that the IT band will become inflamed and the snapping will become painful.

Symptoms

The patient's complaints in GTPS are pain in the lateral hip that may radiate into the lateral thigh to the knee. This pain is increased by lying on the affected side, when moving from a sitting to a standing position, with prolonged standing, by sitting with the affected leg crossed, with stair climbing, and with running. There will likely be tenderness to palpation on the posterior or lateral side of the greater trochanter. The patient may complain of increased pain with certain hip movements, particularly hip external rotation and abduction.

Clinical Signs

The patient will have distinct tenderness to palpation over or posterior to the greater trochanter. Hip abduction against resistance will often reproduce the patient's pain. The patient may have a positive FABER test.[8] If IT band tightness is contributing to the patient's symptoms, the Ober test (a test to evaluate a tight, contracted, or inflamed IT band) may also be positive. Studies have indicated that single-leg standing for 30 seconds may reproduce the patient's pain.[78] If the patient has tears in the gluteus medius or gluteus minimus, there may be weakness on manual muscle testing of hip abduction. The following special tests may be used for patient assessment.

Ober Test

For the Ober test, the patient is positioned in a sidelying position, with the side to be evaluated facing up. The opposite leg is flexed at the hip to 45° and at the knee to 90° to help stabilize the patient. The examiner maintains the position of the pelvis by pushing superiorly and downwardly on the iliac crest. The examiner then passively abducts the patient's leg and extends it to be in line with the trunk. The patient's knee can be flexed to 90° (Ober test) or held extended (modified Ober test). While the examiner continues to stabilize the pelvis, the patient is instructed to relax and allow the leg to adduct

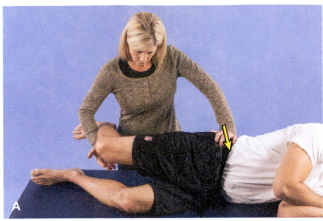

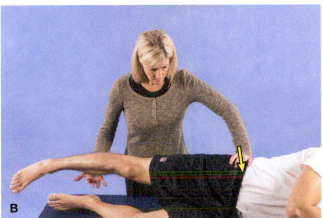

Figure 10.38 A positive Ober test (A) indicates IT band tightness or inflammation, which can contribute to GTPS. Modified Ober test (B) is performed with the knee extended.

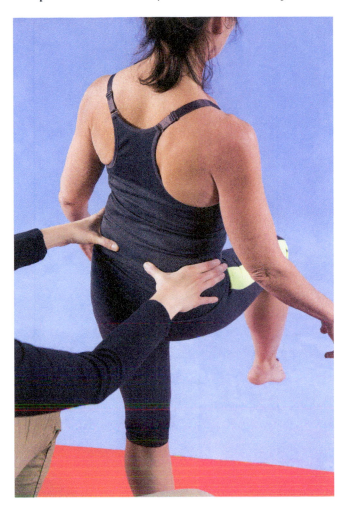

Figure 10.39 A Trendelenburg sign may be used in the diagnosis of GTPS. Pelvic drop indicates weakness of the gluteus medius on the stance leg side.

toward the table. The examiner supports the leg to prevent internal rotation or flexion of the hip (Fig. 10.38). Subjectively, the examiner can note if the tested extremity can adduct to a normal range, or an inclinometer may be used for a more objective measurement.[79] Note that the Ober test and the modified Ober test are not interchangeable. It is important to perform the test in the same manner on retesting as was done initially.

Trendelenburg Sign

A Trendelenburg sign is reproduced by having the patient stand facing away from the examiner. The patient is instructed to stand on one leg. The examiner notes the extent of pelvic drop of the unsupported pelvis (Fig. 10.39). This is compared to results when the patient repeats the test standing on the other leg. Asymmetry is considered a positive test.

Common Interventions

The research on GTPS has been helpful in our understanding of the pathology, but there is very little research on treatment. With an understanding that at least four pathologies can lead to a diagnosis of GTPS, we are left to apply the principles of tissue healing to infer best practice.

If the bursae appear to be inflamed, the treatment plan will likely include some components of stretching of the lateral hip structures, including the IT band. The patient should be instructed to avoid activities that increase pain and to avoid sidelying on the affected side. Because of the frequency of gluteus medius and minimus tears, strengthening of these muscle groups may be beneficial. A focus on eccentric strengthening will hypertrophy muscles and tendons, which should be beneficial. With coxa saltans, it is important to educate the patient on the importance of avoiding movements that cause the snapping. Stretching of the IT band helps to decrease the incidence of snapping.[80] See Figure 10.40 for exercises that are commonly found in the plan of care for GTPS.

Anti-inflammatory modalities may be beneficial in this area, including ultrasound, phonophoresis, iontophoresis,

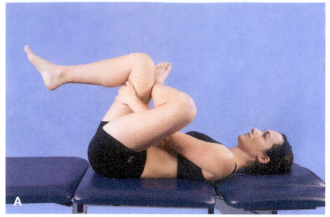

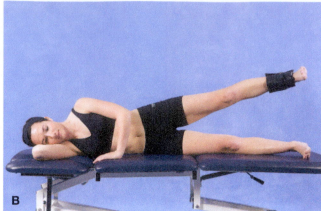

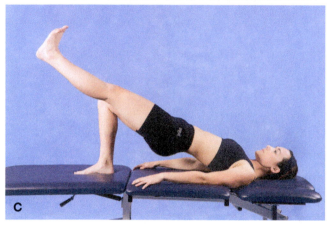

Figure 10.40 Exercises that are commonly included in the plan of care for GTPS include gluteal stretching (A), hip abductor strengthening (B), and hip extensor strengthening (C).

and cryotherapy. Because of the contribution of altered biomechanics of the lower extremity, the plan of care may include gait modification, strengthening of the back and the rest of the lower extremity, and foot orthoses worn in the shoe to limit unwanted movement.

Prevention

Weight loss, correction of leg length differences, and maintenance of hip strength and range of motion are all good measures to counteract the contributing factors for GTPS.

The Bottom Line:	for patients with GTPS
Description and causes	Inflammation of the trochanteric bursae, often accompanied by gluteal insertion tears associated with hip weakness and altered biomechanics
Test	Tenderness to palpation, pain with resisted hip abduction, weakness of hip abduction, FABER, Ober, Trendelenburg sign, single leg standing test
Stretch	IT band
Strengthen	Hip abductors
Train	Hip muscles eccentrically
Avoid	Leg length differences, being overweight, lying on affected side, repeated hip flexion and extension if hip snaps

Ischiogluteal Bursitis

The ischiogluteal bursa overlies the ischial tuberosity and provides a cushion between the tuberosity and the hamstring and gluteus maximus muscles. Inflammation of this bursa is called ischiogluteal bursitis, ischial tuberosity bursitis, or "weaver's bottom."

Causes/Contributing Factors

Ischiogluteal bursitis is frequently caused by trauma, specifically a fall onto the buttocks. It may also be caused by occupations that require prolonged sitting, particularly sitting with vibration such as driving a truck or tractor.[81]

Symptoms

The hallmark sign of ischiogluteal bursitis is buttock pain, which may radiate down the posterior thigh. The area of the bursa will be tender to palpation. Passive hip flexion range of motion will likely be limited due to pain. Pain will be increased with sitting and walking. The patient may complain of increased pain with resisted hip extension with knee extension.

Clinical Signs

Diagnosis of ischiogluteal bursitis is largely made on clinical findings. The Sign of the Buttock test may be performed to rule out sciatic nerve contribution.[82]

Sign of the Buttock Test

To perform the sign of the buttock test, the patient lies in a supine position and the examiner takes the patient's leg up into a straight leg raise position. At the point of limitation of hip flexion, the patient's knee is then flexed and the examiner attempts to gain additional hip flexion range of motion (Fig. 10.41). If no further range is possible, it implicates the ischiogluteal bursa or other problem in the buttock. If further hip flexion is attained, the test is considered negative for ischiogluteal bursitis.

Common Interventions

The plan of care for this patient is likely to include alleviating the contributing factors, rest, and anti-inflammatory

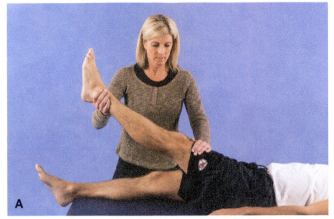

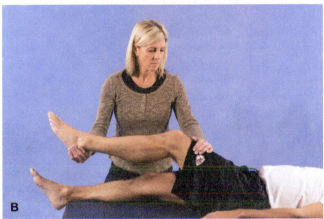

Figure 10.41 The sign of the buttock test for ischiogluteal bursitis. The examiner performs a straight leg raise to the point of pain (A) and then flexes the knee (B). No further increase in hip flexion with knee flexion indicates a positive test.

modalities. Stretching of the hamstring muscles is recommended to reduce compression on the bursa caused by tightness of the hamstrings. Postural correction may also be recommended to decrease anterior pelvic tilt.

Prevention

Avoid prolonged sitting, particularly in instances coupled with vibration, to prevent ischiogluteal bursitis.

The Bottom Line: for patients with ischiogluteal bursitis

Description and causes	Inflammation of the bursa on the ischial tuberosity caused by trauma or prolonged sitting
Test	Sign of the buttock test
Stretch	Hamstrings
Strengthen	NA
Train	Posture to avoid anterior pelvic tilt
Avoid	Prolonged sitting

Iliopsoas Syndrome (Tendonitis/Bursitis)

Iliopsoas is a powerful hip flexor and is made up of two muscles: iliacus and psoas major. Iliopsoas syndrome is a regional pain syndrome of the anterior hip that includes iliopsoas tendonitis (inflammation of the insertion tendon of iliopsoas) and iliopsoas bursitis (inflammation of the bursa that lies under the iliopsoas muscle and anterior to the hip joint).

Causes/Contributing Factors

Iliopsoas syndrome is considered an overuse syndrome that can occur as a result of occupational- or sports-related trauma. It is most prevalent in gymnasts, dancers, and running athletes who perform repeated hip flexion movements. Predisposing factors include strength and flexibility deficits in the hip musculature and muscle imbalances.[83] One study found that all of the patients with iliopsoas syndrome had hip flexor tightness and weakness of hip rotators.[83] It may occur in conjunction with acute or chronic arthritis.[84]

Symptoms

The cardinal sign of iliopsoas syndrome is pain in the anterior hip that is increased with resisted hip flexion and with passive hip extension. The patient may complain of tenderness in this area (Fig. 10.42). Pain is aggravated by activities that require repeated hip flexion movements. It may be associated with a snapping sensation in the anterior hip as the iliopsoas tendon moves over the lesser trochanter or the iliopectineal eminence. This is sometimes referred to as an internal snapping hip as opposed to coxa saltans or external snapping hip.

Clinical Signs

The Thomas test is a test for hip flexor and rectus femoris length, but because it stretches the iliopsoas tendon and puts pressure on the underlying bursa, it is common for patients with iliopsoas syndrome to experience pain, tightness, and limitation of motion with this test.

Thomas Test

To perform the Thomas test, place the patient in a supine position with hips at the end of the plinth. Both hips and knees are flexed to the chest. Holding the unaffected leg flexed to maintain lumbar spine flexion, the patient is instructed to lower the affected side to the table. The examiner looks for limitation of hip extension or reproduction of patient's pain on the affected side (Fig. 10.43).

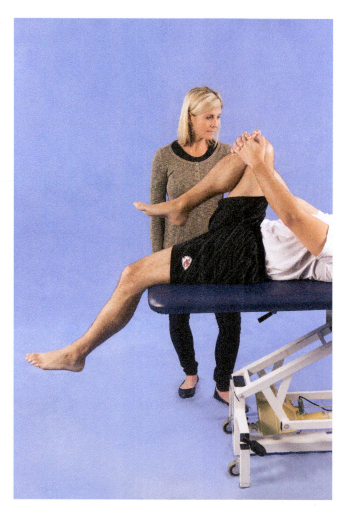

Figure 10.43 Thomas test for hip flexor tightness. Iliopsoas syndrome may cause a positive test indicated by limited motion or pain.

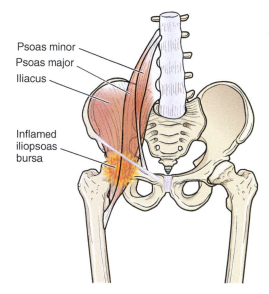

Psoas minor
Psoas major
Iliacus

Inflamed iliopsoas bursa

Figure 10.42 Iliopsoas syndrome is characterized by pain and tenderness in the anterior hip near the insertion of iliopsoas.

Common Interventions

The plan of care for this patient is likely to include stretching of the hip flexors. Additionally, Johnston et al. have shown that stretching of the hip external rotators, quadriceps, and hamstrings is effective.[83] This same study showed improvement in patients with an exercise program that included hip internal rotation (IR) and external rotation (ER) strengthening with elastic bands. As a progression the patients performed hip abduction and ER (clams) against elastic bands and single leg mini-squats on the affected side (Fig. 10.44).

Prevention

Avoiding overuse of hip muscles, maintenance of hip strength and range of motion, and maintenance of muscle balance are all good measures to counteract the contributing factors. This is especially true for athletes whose sport involves repeated hip flexion and for patients with arthritis.

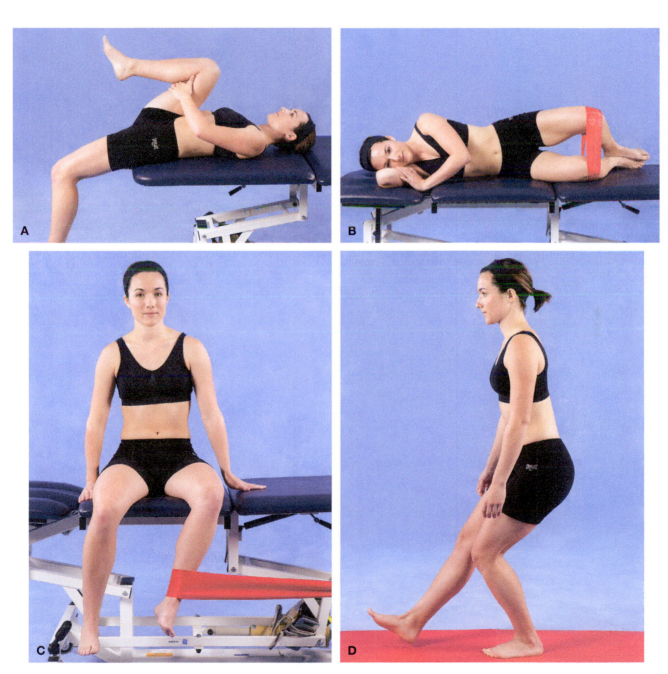

Figure 10.44 Exercises commonly included in the plan of care for iliopsoas syndrome include stretching hip flexors (A), clams (B), strengthening hip external rotators (C), and mini-squats (D).

The Bottom Line: for patients with iliopsoas syndrome

Description and causes	Iliopsoas bursitis or tendinopathy resulting in anterior hip pain, caused by weakness or overuse of the hip flexors
Test	Thomas test
Stretch	Hip flexors, external rotators, quadriceps, hamstrings
Strengthen	Hip rotators, abductors, hip extensors
Train	NA
Avoid	Overuse of hip flexors

Legg-Calvé-Perthes Disease

Legg-Calvé-Perthes (LCP) disease is an avascular necrosis of the femoral head and is **idiopathic** in nature, meaning that is has no known cause. It is seen most commonly in boys (4:1 ratio) between the ages of 4 and 10. The vascular disruption may lead to fracture or flattening of the femoral head (Fig. 10.45). This process is generally self-limiting, and symptoms will improve in 1 to 2 years.

There is a possibility for full recovery with remodeling of the femoral head, with an improved prognosis in patients who develop symptoms at an earlier age. However, continued pain, dysfunction, and development of OA in adulthood is common.[85]

Causes/Contributing Factors

At this time, the cause is unknown. It is thought to be a result of impaired blood flow through the artery of

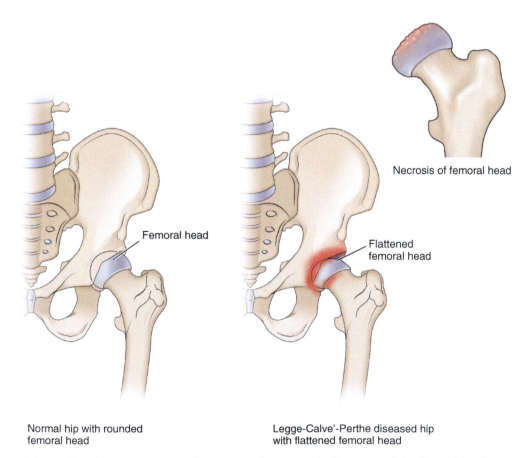

Necrosis of femoral head

Femoral head

Flattened femoral head

Normal hip with rounded femoral head

Legge-Calve'-Perthe diseased hip with flattened femoral head

Figure 10.45 Legg-Calvé-Perthes disease is an avascular necrosis that results in flattening of the femoral head.

the ligamentum teres. This artery in childhood is an important contributor to femoral head circulation.

Symptoms

The initial symptom may be painless limping. Soon after onset the child will complain of pain in the hip, knee, or groin. Pain is increased with hip movements and activities. Hip ROM is usually limited. The patient may have a shortened leg and an altered or antalgic gait pattern.

Clinical Signs

There are no special tests to diagnose LCP disease. The physician will usually make the diagnosis based on x-ray results.

Common Interventions

The major goal in intervention for LCP disease is to promote a normal, spherical shape of the femoral head.

If the flattened shape persists, the patient is more likely to develop OA later in life.[86] Medical intervention may include bracing or casting to maintain the femoral head in the acetabulum in order to re-form the head into a spherical shape, although the need for this is controversial.[87] It has been shown that physical therapy interventions twice a week for 12 weeks has a benefit of improved ROM and strength and decreased joint dysfunction.[88] Therapy consists of:

- Hip stretching
- Isometric strengthening of hip flexors, extensors, abductors and adductors for 4 weeks, then progressing to dynamic strengthening of these muscle groups
- Balance training beginning in week 3 on a stable surface, progressing to an unstable surface

The Bottom Line:	for patients with Legg-Calvé-Perthes disease
Description and causes	Avascular necrosis of the femoral head primarily occurring in young boys that may be caused by decreased circulation from the artery of the ligamentum teres.
Test	NA
Stretch	Hip in all planes
Strengthen	Hip flexors, extensors, abductors, and adductors
Train	Balance
Avoid	NA

Hamstring Muscle Strain

Hamstring strain is a tearing of the fibers of the hamstring muscle. Grade I strain is a mild injury with minimal stretching or tearing of muscle fibers. Grade II strain involves more tearing and possibly a partial tear of the muscle. Grade III strain is a complete tear or rupture of the muscle. The long head of the biceps femoris is biomechanically most prone to injury.[89] The hamstring muscle may be injured at the proximal origin on the ischial tuberosity or in the mid-muscle belly (Fig. 10.46). Injury at the distal attachments are uncommon.

Causes/Contributing Factors

Hamstring strain most frequently occurs during an eccentric contraction due to the high tension developed in the muscle.[90,91] It can also be a result of overstretching

of the muscle at a high velocity or, alternatively, the result of a forceful contraction of the muscle.

Anyone may experience a hamstring strain but it is a condition most common in the athlete. Hamstring strain often becomes a recurrent problem; the best predictor of a hamstring strain is a previous history.[92–96] Research suggests that previously injured players have more than twice as high a risk of another injury.[93,97]

It is still unknown why the risk of recurrent injury is so high, but it may be that hamstring weakness[98–100] or asymmetries between quad and hamstring strength and/or between the hamstrings on one leg as compared to the other are risk factors.[101–103] One study found that electromyographic (EMG) activity in a strained biceps femoris is reduced as compared to that of a normal muscle, possibly indicating an altered neural function in the previously injured muscle.[99]

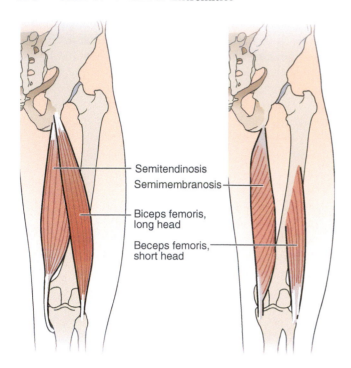

Figure 10.46 Hamstring strain most often occurs in the biceps femoris, long head.

Symptoms

Localized pain, swelling, and bruising may occur on the posterior thigh. The patient may complain of the three signs of muscle injury: pain with palpation, stretch of the injured muscle, and contraction of the muscle. Altered gait may occur, with a shortened stride length on the affected side, or an antalgic gait. In grade III strains, there may be weakness on muscle testing.

Clinical Signs

Provocation tests for hamstring strain include palpation, passive stretch, and active contraction of the hamstrings. These three signs should reproduce the patient's complaint of pain. There are many variations on this theme, including the taking off the shoe test (TOST).

Taking Off the Shoe Test

To perform the TOST, the patient is placed in a standing position, wearing shoes. The patient is instructed to remove the shoe on the affected side with the help of the unaffected leg. To do this, the hip on the affected side should be externally rotated to about 90°, and the patient should use the arch of the unaffected side foot to pry the shoe off (Fig. 10.47). Pain in the biceps femoris area indicates a positive test.[82,104]

Common Interventions

Conventional treatment for a hamstring strain in stage I of tissue healing often includes inflammation control

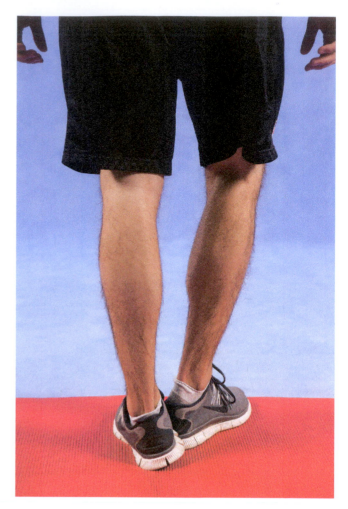

Figure 10.47 The taking off the shoe test for biceps femoris strain.

and gentle PROM (days 0 to 4). During this phase, rest of the muscle may include the use of crutches. Treatment of an injury in stage II of tissue healing often includes components of stretching into hip flexion with knee extension to restore flexibility and to align collagen fibers.[90,105–107] Gentle hamstring strengthening exercises are usually initiated at this time. This may include submaximal isometrics and gentle isotonic strengthening into hip extension and/or knee flexion.[108] The plan of care may include biking.

In stage III of healing, more aggressive stretching and strengthening is often added, including eccentric hamstring strengthening (Fig. 10.48).[90,94,98,99,105,106,108,109] Endurance training may be a component of the treatment plan.[90,105,106] Late in stage III, sport-specific activities and plyometric activities may be added.

Treatment should consider muscle strength imbalances prior to return to sport.[86,101,103,107] Recent research indicates the benefit of agility and trunk stabilization exercises. Nerve stretching in the form of the slump test has been shown to decrease sympathetic activity and thereby

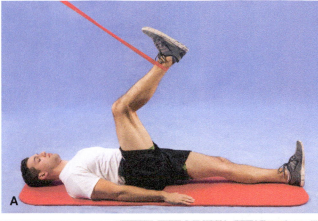

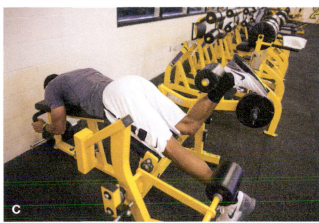

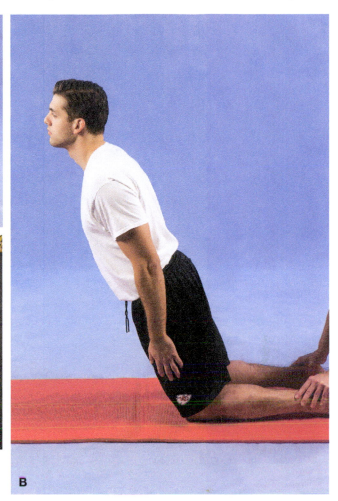

Figure 10.48 Exercises commonly included in the plan of care for hamstring strain include open chain eccentric strengthening (A), closed chain eccentric strengthening (B), and endurance training (C).

increase blood flow to the leg. This may be beneficial in grade I strains.[110]

Prevention

In view of the recurrence of hamstring strain, it is best to prevent strain initially. Although there is some controversy regarding how to best prevent hamstring strain, the best approach seems to include stretching before exercising or playing sports, adequate warm-up, and avoiding fatigue.

It appears important to have good flexibility in the hamstrings and to maximize strength. In a normal relationship of hamstring-to-quad strength, the hamstrings should be about 60% to 80% of the strength of the quadriceps. This may be less important than equalizing the strength of the hamstrings to that of the uninjured side.[101–103] Measures of prevention also include maintaining agility, coordination, and trunk stability.[106,107,111]

The Bottom Line:	for patients with hamstring strain
Description and causes	Microtearing, partial, or complete tear of the hamstring most often involving biceps femoris commonly due to sport
Test	Taking off the shoe test; pain with palpation, stretch, and contraction of the hamstrings
Stretch	Hamstrings, sciatic nerve
Strengthen	Hamstrings (progressing to eccentric exercise), trunk
Train	Agility, sport drills
Avoid	Playing sport without stretching or warm-up, fatigue, return to sport before strength is equal to unaffected leg

Rectus Femoris Muscle Strain

Rectus strain is a tearing of the fibers of the rectus femoris muscle, which is graded I to III based on severity. Grade I involves **microtearing** of the muscle fibers. Grade II is more severe and includes a partial tear of the muscle. Grade III is a complete tear. Of the four heads of the quadriceps, the rectus femoris is most prone to strain because of its long length, crossing over two joints, and potential for force generation. Strains can occur around the central tendon of the rectus or at the proximal or distal ends (Fig. 10.49). Central tendon injuries require a longer time to heal.[112]

Causes/Contributing Factors

The rectus femoris is most prone to injury during kicking, sprinting, and jumping activities. Injury appears to be related to loss of flexibility, loss of strength, and muscle imbalance, including a less-than-optimum hamstring-to-quadriceps ratio and weakness on one side compared with the other.[101–103]

Symptoms

Localized pain, swelling, and bruising may occur on the anterior thigh. The patient may complain of the three signs of muscle injury: pain with palpation, pain with stretch of the injured muscle, and pain with contraction of the muscle. Altered gait may occur, with a shortened stride length on the unaffected side or an antalgic gait.

Clinical Signs

Provocation tests for rectus femoris strain include palpation, passive stretch, and active contraction of the involved muscle. These three signs often reproduce the patient's complaint of pain. In grade III strains, there may be weakness on muscle testing. The Thomas test may be positive. When rectus femoris is the limiting muscle, the patient will extend the knee during the Thomas test with an effort to further extend the hip.

Common Interventions

Conventional treatment for a rectus strain in stage I of tissue healing often includes inflammation control and gentle PROM (days 0 to 4). During this phase, rest of the muscle may include the use of crutches. Treatment of a subacute injury in stage II often includes components of stretching into knee flexion with hip extension to restore flexibility of the rectus and to align collagen fibers. Gentle rectus strengthening exercises are usually initiated during this time. This may include submaximal isometrics and gentle isotonic strengthening into hip flexion and/or knee extension.

In stage III of healing, more aggressive stretching and strengthening are often added, including eccentric quadriceps strengthening. Since there is a paucity of research on rectus femoris strain, we are left to extrapolate from the research involving hamstring strain and knowledge of tissue healing. Doing so, it appears that focusing on endurance training, muscle balance, trunk stabilization, sport-specific activities, agility, and plyometrics would be beneficial.

Prevention

Preventive measures include stretching before exercising or playing sports, adequate warm-up, and avoiding fatigue. It appears important to have good flexibility in the rectus femoris and to maximize strength. In a normal relationship of quad-to-hamstring strength, the quadriceps should be about 1.3 to 1.5 times the strength of the hamstrings. Equalizing the strength of the quadriceps is a good measure, as are agility, coordination, and trunk stability activities.

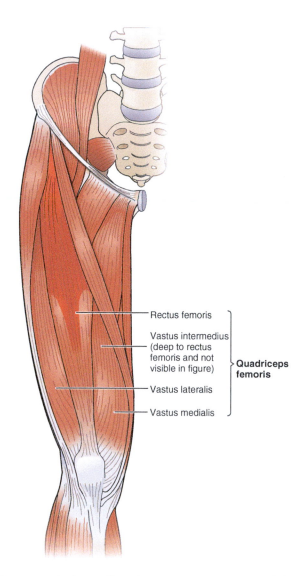

Rectus femoris
Vastus intermedius (deep to rectus femoris and not visible in figure) ⎫
Vastus lateralis   ⎬ Quadriceps femoris
Vastus medialis   ⎭

Figure 10.49 Rectus femoris strain may occur around the central tendon or at either end. Central tendon injuries are most difficult to heal.

The Bottom Line:	for patients with rectus femoris strain
Description and causes	Microtearing, partial, or complete tear of the rectus femoris commonly due to sport
Test	Pain with palpation, stretch, and contraction of the rectus femoris
Stretch	Rectus femoris
Strengthen	Rectus femoris (progressing to eccentric exercise), trunk
Train	Agility, sport drills
Avoid	Playing sport without stretching or warm-up, fatigue, return to sport before strength is equal to that of unaffected leg

SUMMARY

As the most proximal joint in the lower extremity kinetic chain, the hip joint is subjected to tremendous forces. As a result, pathologies of the hip are common in the structures that are responsible for hip stability: the joint itself, the labrum, and the muscles and bursae surrounding the hip. Additionally, the blood supply to the femoral head is precarious, leading to pathologies that involve avascular necrosis. Altered biomechanics of this joint may lead to pathology not just of the hip but of the rest of the lower extremity.

REVIEW QUESTIONS

1. Using your lab partner as a patient simulator, educate the patient in posterior THA dislocation precautions. Put your instructions in terms of functional activities.

2. Using your lab partner as a patient simulator, educate the patient in anterior THA dislocation precautions. Put your instructions in terms of functional activities.

3. Discuss how the blood supply to the hip is impacted by the location of hip fracture and the consequences of this. What pathologies are a result of decreased blood flow to the hip?

4. How does gluteus medius weakness impact the ability to maintain a level pelvis during gait? Describe the difference between a compensated and uncompensated Trendelenburg sign.

5. A Clinical Practice Guideline has been created for non-arthritic hip pain. In what way does this impact your patient education or interventions?

6. Compare and contrast the FAIR test and the FADIR test.

7. Compare and contrast the FADIR test and the posterior hip impingement test.

8. For each of the following special tests, name the pathology that yields a positive test:
   a. FABER test
   b. FAIR test
   c. FADIR test
   d. Hip scour/quadrant test
   e. Ober test
   f. Posterior hip impingement test
   g. Resisted straight leg raise (Stinchfield) test
   h. Sign of the buttock test
   i. Thomas test
   j. TOST
   k. Trendelenburg sign

9. Discuss the relationship among FAI, labral tears, and OA of the hip.

10. Compare and contrast the effect of hamstring strain and rectus femoris strain on stride length.

PATIENT CASE: Degenerative Joint Disease (OA), Hip

PT Evaluation

Patient Name: XXXXX XXXXXXXXXXXX   **Age:** 59   **BMI:** 26.6

Diagnosis/History

Medical Diagnosis: Degenerative Joint Disease (OA), hip   **PT Diagnosis:** Pain in R hip secondary to DJD

Diagnostic Tests/Results: X-rays – moderately severe hip DJD   **Relevant Medical History:** borderline HTN, THA L (9 years ago), osteopenia

Prior Level of Function: Normally active

Patient's Goals: Decrease pain, ambulate without device

Medications: Meloxicam 7.5 mg daily, multivitamin daily, calcium supplement tid, vitamin D supplement daily.   **Precautions:** None

Social Supports/Safety Hazards

Patient Living Situation/ Supports/ Hazards: Lives alone

Patient Working Situation/Occupation/ Leisure Activities: High school math teacher full-time. Enjoys travel, taking care of grandchildren

Vital Signs

At rest Temperature: 98.4   BP: 130/76   HR: 72   Resp: 14   O2 sat: 98

Subjective Information

Patient is a female with complaint of pain in the R anterior hip and groin for about 18 months. She c/o pain that is worse after sustained walking and standing after sitting. Recently took grandkids to Disney World and has increased pain since.

Physical Assessment

Orientation: Alert and oriented   **Speech/Vision/Hearing:** Wears glasses   **Skin Integrity:** Intact

ROM: Hip internal rotation 30° R, 40° L. Hip flexion 107° R, 115° L.

Strength: 3+/5 MMT hip abduction B. Otherwise normal.   **Palpation:** No pain on palpation

Muscle Tone: Not tested   **Balance/Coordination:** WNL   **Sensation/Proprioception:** Not tested

Endurance: Not tested   **Posture:** Normal   **Edema:** None

Pain

Pain Rating and Location: At best 0/10   At worst 6/10   **Relieving Factors:** Rest

Aggravating Factors: Walking, standing after sitting   **Irritability:** Pain lasts about 30 minutes after getting up in a.m. With rest, it subsides very quickly.

Functional Assessment

Patient is functionally independent. She continues to work full time. Ambulates with Trendelenburg gait R without devices.

Special Testing

Test Name: Hip scour test   **Result** Positive   **Test Name:**   **Result**

Assessment

Patient has s/s consistent with DJD of the R hip.

Short-Term Treatment Goals

1. Patient will improve in hip abduction strength on R to 4/5.
2. Patient will be independent in HEP.
3. Patient will state a 15% decrease in hip pain.

Long-Term Treatment Goals

1. Patient will improve in hip IR ROM to 35°.
2. Patient will state a 25% decrease in hip pain.

Treatment Plan

Frequency/Duration: 3 times a week for 3 weeks, 2 times a week for 2 weeks

Consisting of: Modalities, therapeutic exercise, neuro re-education, patient education

continued

Patient Case Questions

1. What factors may be contributing to this patient's hip DJD?

2. What data will you collect the first time you see the patient?

3. If the plan of care does not guide you, what modalities might you use with this patient? Why? Are any modalities contraindicated?

4. If the plan of care does not specifically guide you, describe four therapeutic exercises that are indicated for this patient. Justify your choices.

5. What other tests might you use to monitor the patient's progress?

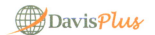 **DavisPlus**   For additional resources, including answers to this case, please visit
http://davisplus.fadavis.com

REFERENCES

1. Cleather, D. J., Goodwin, J. E., & Bull, A. M. J. (2013). Hip and knee joint loading during vertical jumping and push jerking. *Clinical Biomechanics. Bristol, Avon, 28*, 98–103.
2. Daniel, M., Iglic, A., & Kralj-Iglic, V. (2005). The shape of acetabular cartilage optimizes hip contact stress distribution. *Journal of Anatomy, 207*, 85–91.
3. Ferguson, S. J., Bryant, J. T., Ganz, R., & Ito, K. (2003). An in vitro investigation of the acetabular labral seal in hip joint mechanics. *Journal of Biomechanics, 36*, 171–178.
4. Groh, M. M., & Herrera, J. (2009). A comprehensive review of hip labral tears. *Current Reviews in Musculoskeletal Medicine, 2*, 105–117.
5. Rao, J., Zhou, Y. X., & Villar, R. N. (2001). Injury to the ligamentum teres. Mechanism, findings, and results of treatment. *Clinics in Sports Medicine, 20*, 791–799, vii.
6. Byrd, J. W. T., & Jones, K. S. (2004). Traumatic rupture of the ligamentum teres as a source of hip pain. *Arthroscopy, 20*, 385–391.
7. Shbeeb, M. I., & Matteson, E. L. (1996). Trochanteric bursitis (greater trochanter pain syndrome). *Mayo Clinic, Proceedings of the Mayo Clinic. 71*, 565–569.
8. Strauss, E. J., Nho, S. J., & Kelly, B. T. (2010). Greater trochanteric pain syndrome. *Sports Medicine and Arthroscopy Review, 18*, 113–119.
9. Williams, B. S., & Cohen, S. P. (2009). Greater trochanteric pain syndrome: A review of anatomy, diagnosis and treatment. *Anesthesia & Analgesia, 108*, 1662–1670.
10. Tan, V., Seldes, R. M., Katz, M. A., Freedhand, A. M., Klimkiewicz, J. J., & Fitzgerald, R. H. Jr. (2001). Contribution of acetabular labrum to articulating surface area and femoral head coverage in adult hip joints: An anatomic study in cadavera. *American Journal of Orthopedics (Belle Mead, N.J.), 30*, 809–812.
11. Neumann, D. A. (2010). Kinesiology of the hip: A focus on muscular actions. *Journal of Orthopaedic and Sports Physical Therapy, 40*, 82–94.
12. Sajko, S., & Stuber, K. (2009). Psoas Major: A case report and review of its anatomy, biomechanics, and clinical implications. *Journal of the Canadian Chiropractic Association, 53*, 311–318.
13. Kumagai, M., Shiba, N., Higuchi, F., Nishimura, H., & Inoue, A. (1997). Functional evaluation of hip abductor muscles with use of magnetic resonance imaging. *Journal of Orthopaedic Research, Official Publication of the Orthopedic Research Society, 15*, 888–893.

14. Ward, S. R., Winters, T. M., & Blemker, S. S. (2010). The architectural design of the gluteal muscle group: Implications for movement and rehabilitation. *Journal of Orthopaedic and Sports Physical Therapy, 40*, 95–102.
15. Harris-Hayes, M., Czuppon, S., Van Dillen, L. R., Steger-May, K., Sahrmann, S., Schootman, M., Salsich, G. B., et al. (2016). Movement-pattern training to improve function in people with chronic hip joint pain: A feasibility randomized clinical trial. *Journal of Orthopaedic and Sports Physical Therapy, 46*, 452–461.
16. Levangie, P. K., Norkin, C. C. & Levangie, P. K. (2011). *Joint structure and function: A comprehensive analysis.* Philadelphia, PA: F.A. Davis Co.
17. Offierski, C. M., & MacNab, I. (1983). Hip-spine syndrome. *Spine, 8*, 316–321.
18. Ben-Galim, P., Ben-Galim, T., Rand, N., Haim, A., Hipp, J., Dekel, S., & Floman, Y. (2007). Hip-spine syndrome: The effect of total hip replacement surgery on low back pain in severe osteoarthritis of the hip. *Spine, 32*, 2099–2102.
19. Cleland, J., Koppenhaver, S. (2010). *Orthopaedic clinical examination: An evidence based approach.* 2nd edition. Philadelphia, PA: Saunders.
20. Cooper, C., Inskip, H., Croft, P., Campbell, L., Smith, G., McLaren, M., & Coggon, D. (1998). Individual risk factors for hip osteoarthritis: Obesity, hip injury, and physical activity. *American Journal of Epidemiology, 147*, 516–522.
21. Hertling, D., & Kessler, R. M. (2006). *Management of common musculoskeletal disorders: Physical therapy principles and methods.* Philadelphia, PA: Lippincott Williams & Wilkins.
22. Harris-Hayes, M., & Royer, N. K. (2011). Relationship of acetabular dysplasia and femoroacetabular impingement to hip osteoarthritis: A focused review. *PM&R: The Journal of Injury, Function, and Rehabilitation, 3*, 1055–1067.e1.
23. Zebala, L. P., Schoenecker, P. L., & Clohisy, J. C. (2007). Anterior femoroacetabular impingement: A diverse disease with evolving treatment options. *Iowa Orthopaedic Journal, 27*, 71–81.
24. Beck, M., Kalhor, M., Leunig, M., & Ganz, R. (2005). Hip morphology influences the pattern of damage to the acetabular cartilage: Femoroacetabular impingement as a cause of early osteoarthritis of the hip. *Journal of Bone and Joint Surgery, British Volume, 87*, 1012–1018.

25. Tanzer, M., & Noiseux, N. (2004). Osseous abnormalities and early osteoarthritis: The role of hip impingement. *Clinical Orthopaedics and Related Research, 429,* 170–177.

26. McCarthy, J. C., Noble, P. C., Schuck, M. R., Wright, J., & Lee, J. (2001). The Otto E. Aufranc Award: The role of labral lesions to development of early degenerative hip disease. *Clinical Orthopaedics and Related Research, 393,* 25–37.

27. Altman, R., Alarcón, G., Appelrouth, D., Bloch, D., Borenstein, D., Brandt, K., Brown, C., et al. (1991). The American College of Rheumatology criteria for the classification and reporting of osteoarthritis of the hip. *Arthritis & Rheumatism, 34,* 505–514.

28. Stratford, P. W., Kennedy, D. M., & Woodhouse, L. J. (2006). Performance measures provide assessments of pain and function in people with advanced osteoarthritis of the hip or knee. *Physical Therapy, 86,* 1489–1496.

29. Cook, C., & Hegedus, E. J. (2013). *Orthopedic physical examination tests: An evidence-based approach.* New York, NY: Pearson.

30. Wong, M. S. (2009). *Pocket orthopaedics: Evidence-Based survival guide.* Burlington, MA: Jones & Bartlett Learning.

31. Mitchell, B., McCrory, P., Brukner, P., O'Donnell, J., Colson, E., & Howells, R. (2003). Hip joint pathology: Clinical presentation and correlation between magnetic resonance arthrography, ultrasound, and arthroscopic findings in 25 consecutive cases. *Clinical Journal of Sports Medicine, 13,* 152–156.

32. Clohisy, J. C., Knaus, E. R., Hunt, D. M., Lesher, J. M., Harris-Hayes, M., & Prather, H. (2009). Clinical presentation of patients with symptomatic anterior hip impingement. *Clinical Orthopaedics and Related Research, 467,* 638–644.

33. Broadhurst, N. A., & Bond, M. J. (1998). Pain provocation tests for the assessment of sacroiliac joint dysfunction. *Journal of Spinal Disorders, 11,* 341–345.

34. Maitland, G. D. (1975). *The peripheral joints: Examination and recording guide.* Adelaide, Australia: Virgo Press.

35. Cliborne, A. V., Wainner, R. S., Rhon, D. I., Judd, C. D., Fee, T. T., Matekel, R. L., & Whitman, J. M. (2004). Clinical hip tests and a functional squat test in patients with knee osteoarthritis: Reliability, prevalence of positive test findings, and short-term response to hip mobilization. *Journal of Orthopaedic and Sports Physical Therapy, 34,* 676–685.

36. Roddy, E., Zhang, W., Doherty, M., Arden, N. K., Barlow, J., Birrell, F., Carr, A., et al. (2005). Evidence-based recommendations for the role of exercise in the management of osteoarthritis of the hip or knee—The MOVE consensus. *Rheumatology (Oxford, England), 44,* 67–73.

37. Roddy, E., Zhang, W., & Doherty, M. (2005). Home based exercise for osteoarthritis. *Annals of the Rheumatic Diseases, 64,* 170; author reply 170–171.

38. Zhang, W., Moskowitz, R. W., Nuki, G., Abramson, S., Altman, R. D., Arden, N., Bierma-Zeinstra, S., et al. (2008). OARSI recommendations for the management of hip and knee osteoarthritis, Part II: OARSI evidence-based, expert consensus guidelines. *Osteoarthritis and Cartilage, 16,* 137–162.

39. Sutlive, T. G., Lopez, H. P., Schnitker, D. E., Yawn, S. E., Halle, R. J., Mansfield, L. T., Boyles, R. E., et al. (2008). Development of a clinical prediction rule for diagnosing hip osteoarthritis in individuals with unilateral hip pain. *Journal of Orthopaedic and Sports Physical Therapy, 38,* 542–550.

40. Loureiro, A., Mills, P. M., & Barrett, R. S. (2013). Muscle weakness in hip osteoarthritis: A systematic review. *Arthritis Care and Research, 65,* 340–352.

41. Rasch, A., Byström, A. H., Dalen, N., & Berg, H. E. (2007). Reduced muscle radiological density, cross-sectional area, and strength of major hip and knee muscles in 22 patients with hip osteoarthritis. *Acta Orthopaedica, 78,* 505–510.

42. Kisner, C., & Colby, L. A. (2012). *Therapeutic exercise: Foundations and techniques.* Philadelphia, PA: F.A. Davis.

43. MacDonald, C. W., Whitman, J. M., Cleland, J. A., Smith, M., & Hoeksma, H. L. (2006). Clinical outcomes following manual physical therapy and exercise for hip osteoarthritis: A case series. *Journal of Orthopaedic and Sports Physical Therapy, 36,* 588–599.

44. Hinman, R. S., Heywood, S. E., & Day, A. R. (2007). Aquatic physical therapy for hip and knee osteoarthritis: Results of a single-blind randomized controlled trial. *Physical Therapy, 87,* 32–43.

45. Brander, V., & Stulberg, S. D. (2006). Rehabilitation after hip- and knee-joint replacement. An experience- and evidence-based approach to care. *American Journal of Physical Medicine & Rehabilitation, 85,* S98–118.

46. Rooks, D. S., Huang, J., Bierbaum, B. E., Bolus, S. A., Rubano, J., Connolly, C. E., Alpert, S., et al. (2006). Effect of preoperative exercise on measures of functional status in men and women undergoing total hip and knee arthroplasty. *Arthritis and Rheumatism, 55,* 700–708.

47. Wang, A. W., Gilbey, H. J., & Ackland, T. R. (2002). Perioperative exercise programs improve early return of ambulatory function after total hip arthroplasty: A randomized, controlled trial. *American Journal of Physical Medicine & Rehabilitation, 81,* 801–806.

48. Jacobs, C. A., Christensen, C. P., & Berend, M. E. (2009). Sport activity after total hip arthroplasty: Changes in surgical technique, implant design, and rehabilitation. *Journal of Sport Rehabilitation, 18,* 47–59.

49. National Heart, Lung, and Blood Institute, National Institutes of Health. What are the signs and symptoms of deep vein thrombosis? Retrieved from https://www.nhlbi.nih.gov/health/health-topics/topics/dvt/signs (accessed July 30, 2017).

50. Wells, P. S., Anderson, D. R., Rodger, M., Forgie, M., Kearon, C., Dreyer, J., Kovacs, G., et al. (2003). Evaluation of d-dimer in the diagnosis of suspected deep-vein thrombosis. *New England Journal of Medicine, 349,* 1227–1235.

51. Hip Fractures Among Older Adults | Home and Recreational Safety | CDC Injury Center. Retrieved from https://www.cdc.gov/homeandrecreationalsafety/falls/adulthipfx.html (accessed July 30, 2017).

52. Givens-Heiss, D. L., Krebs, D. E., Riley, P. O., Strickland, E. M., Fares, M., Hodge, W. A., & Mann, R. W. (1992). In vivo acetabular contact pressures during rehabilitation, Part II: Postacute phase. *Physical Therapy, 72,* 700–705; discussion 706–710.

53. Fishman, L. M., Dombi, G. W., Michaelsen, C., Ringel, S., Rozbruch, J., Rosner, B., & Weber, C. (2002). Piriformis syndrome: Diagnosis, treatment, and outcome—A 10-year study. *Archives of Physical Medicine and Rehabilitation, 83,* 295–301.

54. Parziale, J. R., Hudgins, T. H., & Fishman, L. M. (1996). The piriformis syndrome. *American Journal of Orthopedics (Belle Mead, N.J.), 25,* 819–823.

55. Papadopoulos, E. C., & Khan, S. N. (2004). Piriformis syndrome and low back pain: A new classification and review of the literature. *Orthopedic Clinics of North America, 35,* 65–71.

56. Smoll, N. R. (2010). Variations of the piriformis and sciatic nerve with clinical consequence: A review. *Clinical Anatomy, 23,* 8–17.

57. Tonley, J. C., Yun, S. M., Kochevar, R. J., Dye, J. A., Farrokhi, S., & Powers, C. M. (2010). Treatment of an individual with piriformis syndrome focusing on hip muscle strengthening and movement reeducation: A case report. *Journal of Orthopaedic and Sports Physical Therapy, 40,* 103–111.

58. Enseki, K., Harris-Hayes, M., White, D. M., Cibulka, M. T., Woehrle, J., Fagerson, T. L., Orthopaedic Section of the American Physical Therapy Association; (Clohisy, J. C., & 2014). Nonarthritic hip joint pain. *Journal of Orthopaedic and Sports Physical Therapy*, 44, A1–32.

59. Carsen, S., Moroz, P. J., Rakhra, K., Ward, L. M., Dunlap, H., Hay, J. A., Willis, R. B., et al. (2014). The Otto Aufranc Award. On the etiology of the cam deformity: A cross-sectional pediatric MRI study. *Clinical Orthopaedics and Related Research*, 472, 430–436.

60. Gerhardt, M. B., Romero, A. A., Silvers, H. J., Harris, D. J., Watanabe, D., & Mandelbaum, B. R. (2012). The prevalence of radiographic hip abnormalities in elite soccer players. *American Journal of Sports Medicine*, 40, 584–588.

61. Kapron, A. L., Anderson, A. E., Aoki, S. K., Phillips, L. G., Petron, D. J., Toth, R., & Peters, C. L. (2011). Radiographic prevalence of femoroacetabular impingement in collegiate football players: AAOS exhibit selection. *Journal of Bone & Joint Surgery, American Volume*, 93, e111 (1–10).

62. Siebenrock, K. A., Ferner, F., Noble, P. C., Santore, R. F., Werlen, S., & Mamisch, T. C. (2011). The cam-type deformity of the proximal femur arises in childhood in response to vigorous sporting activity. *Clinical Orthopaedics and Related Research*, 469, 3229–3240.

63. Silvis, M. L., Mosher, T. J., Smetana, B. S., Chinchilli, V. M., Flemming, D. J., Walker, E. A., & Black, K. P. (2011). High prevalence of pelvic and hip magnetic resonance imaging findings in asymptomatic collegiate and professional hockey players. *American Journal of Sports Medicine*, 39, 715–721.

64. Harris-Hayes, M., Mueller, M. J., Sahrmann, S. A., Bloom, N. J., Steger-May, K., Clohisy, J. C., & Salsich, G. B. (2014). Persons with chronic hip joint pain exhibit reduced hip muscle strength. *Journal of Orthopaedic and Sports Physical Therapy*, 44, 890–898.

65. Casartelli, N. C., Maffiuletti, N. A., Item-Glatthorn, J. F., Staehli, S., Bizzini, M., Impellizzeri, F. M., & Leunig, M. (2011). Hip muscle weakness in patients with symptomatic femoroacetabular impingement. *Osteoarthritis and Cartilage*, 19, 816–821.

66. Austin, A. B., Souza, R. B., Meyer, J. L., & Powers, C. M. (2008). Identification of abnormal hip motion associated with acetabular labral pathology. *Journal of Orthopaedic and Sports Physical Therapy*, 38, 558–565.

67. Kumar, D., Dillon, A., Nardo, L., Link, T. M., Majumdar, S., & Souza, R. B. (2014). Differences in the association of hip cartilage lesions and cam-type femoroacetabular impingement with movement patterns: A preliminary study. *PM&R, the Journal of Injury, Function, and Rehabilitation*, 6, 681–689.

68. Retchford, T. H., Crossley, K. M., Grimaldi, A., Kemp, J. L., & Cowan, S. M. (2013). Can local muscles augment stability in the hip? A narrative literature review. *Journal of Musculoskeletal and Neuronal Interactions*, 13, 1–12.

69. Naal, F. D., Hatzung, G., Müller, A., Impellizzeri, F., & Leunig, M. (2014). Validation of a self-reported Beighton score to assess hypermobility in patients with femoroacetabular impingement. *International Orthopaedics*, 38, 2245–2250.

70. Wahoff, M., & Ryan, M. (2011). Rehabilitation after hip femoroacetabular impingement arthroscopy. *Clinics in Sports Medicine*, 30, 463–482.

71. Reider, B., Davies, G., & Provencher, M. T. (2014). *Orthopaedic rehabilitation of the athlete: Getting back in the game*. New York, NY: Elsevier Health Sciences.

72. Enseki, K. R., Martin, R., & Kelly, B. T. (2010). Rehabilitation after arthroscopic decompression for femoroacetabular impingement. *Clinical Sports Medicine Journal*, 29, 247–255, viii.

73. Kelly, B. T., Weiland, D. E., Schenker, M. L., & Philippon, M. J. (2005). Arthroscopic labral repair in the hip: Surgical technique and review of the literature. *Arthroscopy, The Journal of Arthroscopy and Related Surgery*, 21, 1496–1504.

74. Lewis, C. L., & Sahrmann, S. A. (2006). Acetabular labral tears. *Physical Therapy*, 86, 110–121.

75. Lewis, C. L., Sahrmann, S. A., & Moran, D. W. (2007). Anterior hip joint force increases with hip extension, decreased gluteal force, or decreased iliopsoas force. *Journal of Biomechanics*, 40, 3725–3731.

76. Yazbek, P. M., Ovanessian, V., Martin, R. L., & Fukuda, T. Y. (2011). Nonsurgical treatment of acetabular labrum tears: A case series. *Journal of Orthopaedic and Sports Physical Therapy*, 41, 346–353.

77. Bird, P. A., Oakley, S. P., Shnier, R., & Kirkham, B. W. (2001). Prospective evaluation of magnetic resonance imaging and physical examination findings in patients with greater trochanteric pain syndrome. *Arthritis and Rheumatism*, 44, 2138–2145.

78. Lequesne, M., Mathieu, P., Vuillemin-Bodaghi, V., Bard, H., & Djian, P. (2008). Gluteal tendinopathy in refractory greater trochanter pain syndrome: Diagnostic value of two clinical tests. *Arthritis and Rheumatism*, 59, 241–246.

79. Reese, N. B., & Bandy, W. D. (2003). Use of an inclinometer to measure flexibility of the iliotibial band using the Ober test and the modified Ober test: Differences in magnitude and reliability of measurements. *Journal of Orthopaedic and Sports Physical Therapy*, 33, 326–330.

80. Lewis, C. L. (2010). Extra-articular snapping hip: A literature review. *Sports Health*, 2, 186–190.

81. Cho, K. H., Lee, S. M., Lee, Y. H., Suh, K. J., Kim, S. M., Shin, M. J., & Jang, H. W. (2004). Non-infectious ischiogluteal bursitis: MRI findings. *Korean Journal of Radiology*, 5, 280–286.

82. Magee, D. J. (2013). *Orthopedic physical assessment*. New York, NY: Elsevier Health Sciences.

83. Johnston, C. A., Lindsay, D. M., & Wiley, J. P. (1999). Treatment of iliopsoas syndrome with a hip rotation strengthening program: A retrospective case series. *Journal of Orthopaedic and Sports Physical Therapy*, 29, 218–224.

84. Murphy, C. L., Meaney, J. F., Rana, H., McCarthy, E. M., Howard, D., & Cunnane, G. (2010). Giant iliopsoas bursitis: A complication of chronic arthritis. *Journal of Clinical Rheumatology: Practical Reports of Rheumatic and Musculoskeletal Diseases*, 16, 83–85.

85. Larson, A. N., Sucato, D. J., Herring, J. A., Adolfsen, S. E., Kelly, D. M., Martus, J. E., Lovejoy, J. F., et al. (2012). A prospective multicenter study of Legg-Calvé-Perthes disease: Functional and radiographic outcomes of nonoperative treatment at a mean follow-up of twenty years. *Journal of Bone and Joint Surgery, American Volume*, 94, 584–592.

86. Mose, K. (1980). Methods of measuring in Legg-Calvé-Perthes disease with special regard to the prognosis. *Clinical Orthopaedics and Related Research*, 150, 103–109.

87. Aksoy, M. C., Caglar, O., Yazici, M., & Alpaslan, A. M. (2004). Comparison between braced and non-braced Legg-Calvé-Perthes-disease patients: A radiological outcome study. *Journal of Pediatric Orthopedics, Part B*, 13, 153–157.

88. Brech, G. C., & Guarnieiro, R. (2006). Evaluation of physiotherapy in the treatment of Legg-Calvé-Perthes disease. *Clinics, Sao Paulo Brazil*, 61, 521–528.

89. Kumazaki, T., Ehara, Y., & Sakai, T. (2012). Anatomy and physiology of hamstring injury. *International Journal of Sports Medicine*, 33, 950–954.

90. Agre, J. C. (1985). Hamstring injuries. Proposed aetiological factors, prevention, and treatment. *Sports Medicine, Auckland, NZ*, 2, 21–33.

91. Schache, A. G., Wrigley, T. V., Baker, R., & Pandy, M. G. (2009). Biomechanical response to hamstring muscle strain injury. *Gait & Posture, 29*, 332–338.

92. Bennell, K., Wajswelner, H., Lew, P., Schall-Riaucour, A., Leslie, S., Plant, D., & Cirone, J. (1998). Isokinetic strength testing does not predict hamstring injury in Australian Rules footballers. *British Journal of Sports Medicine, 32*, 309–314.

93. Engebretsen, A. H., Myklebust, G., Holme, I., Engebretsen, L., & Bahr, R. (2010). Intrinsic risk factors for hamstring injuries among male soccer players: A prospective cohort study. *American Journal of Sports Medicine, 38*, 1147–1153.

94. Orchard, J. W. (2001). Intrinsic and extrinsic risk factors for muscle strains in Australian football. *American Journal of Sports Medicine, 29*, 300–303.

95. Verrall, G. M., Slavotinek, J. P., Barnes, P. G., Fon, G. T., & Spriggins, A. J. (2001). Clinical risk factors for hamstring muscle strain injury: A prospective study with correlation of injury by magnetic resonance imaging. *British Journal of Sports Medicine, 35*, 435–439; discussion 440.

96. Woods, C., Hawkins, R. D., Maltby, S., Hulse, M., Thomas, A., Football Association Medical Research Programme. (Hodson, A., 2004). The Football Association Medical Research Programme: An audit of injuries in professional football—Analysis of hamstring injuries. *British Journal of Sports Medicine, 38*, 36–41.

97. Jönhagen, S., Németh, G., & Eriksson, E. (1994). Hamstring injuries in sprinters. The role of concentric and eccentric hamstring muscle strength and flexibility. *American Journal of Sports Medicine, 22*, 262–266.

98. Croisier, J. L., Forthomme, B., Namurois, M. H., Vanderthommen, M., & Crielaard, J. M. (2002). Hamstring muscle strain recurrence and strength performance disorders. *American Journal of Sports Medicine, 30*, 199–203.

99. Opar, D. A., Williams, M. D., Timmins, R. G., Dear, N. M., & Shield, A. J. (2013). Knee flexor strength and bicep femoris electromyographical activity is lower in previously strained hamstrings. *Journal of Electromyography and Kinesiology, Official Journal of the International Society of Electrophysiology and Kinesiology, 23*, 696–703.

100. Orchard, J., Marsden, J., Lord, S., & Garlick, D. (1997). Preseason hamstring muscle weakness associated with hamstring muscle injury in Australian footballers. *American Journal of Sports Medicine, 25*, 81–85.

101. Fousekis, K., Tsepis, E., Poulmedis, P., Athanasopoulos, S., & Vagenas, G. (2011). Intrinsic risk factors of non-contact quadriceps and hamstring strains in soccer: A prospective study of 100 professional players. *British Journal of Sports Medicine, 45*, 709–714.

102. Kannus, P., & Järvinen, M. (1990). Knee flexor/extensor strength ratio in follow-up of acute knee distortion injuries. *Archives of Physical Medicine and Rehabilitation, 71*, 38–41.

103. Knapik, J. J., Bauman, C. L., Jones, B. H., Harris, J. M., & Vaughan, L. (1991). Preseason strength and flexibility imbalances associated with athletic injuries in female collegiate athletes. *American Journal of Sports Medicine, 19*, 76–81.

104. Zeren, B., & Oztekin, H. H. (2006). A new self-diagnostic test for biceps femoris muscle strains. *Clinical Journal of Sport Medicine, Official Journal of the Canadian Academy of Sport Medicine,16*, 166–169.

105. Heiser, T. M., Weber, J., Sullivan, G., Clare, P., & Jacobs, R. R. (1984). Prophylaxis and management of hamstring muscle injuries in intercollegiate football players. *American Journal of Sports Medicine, 12*, 368–370.

106. Reurink, G., Goudswaard, G. J., Tol, J. L., Verhaar, J. A., Weir, A., & Moen, M. H. (2012). Therapeutic interventions for acute hamstring injuries: A systematic review. *British Journal of Sports Medicine, 46*, 103–109.

107. Sherry, M. A., & Best, T. M. (2004). A comparison of 2 rehabilitation programs in the treatment of acute hamstring strains. *Journal of Orthopaedic and Sports Physical Therapy, 34*, 116–125.

108. Petersen, J., & Hölmich, P. (2005). Evidence based prevention of hamstring injuries in sport. *British Journal of Sports Medicine, 39*, 319–323.

109. Schmitt, B., Tim, T., & McHugh, M. (2012). Hamstring injury rehabilitation and prevention of reinjury using lengthened state eccentric training: A new concept. *International Journal of Sports Physical Therapy, 7*, 333–341.

110. Kornberg, C., & McCarthy, T. (1992). The effect of neural stretching technique on sympathetic outflow to the lower limbs. *Journal of Orthopaedic and Sports Physical Therapy, 16*, 269–274.

111. Kujala, U. M., Orava, S., & Järvinen, M. (1997). Hamstring injuries. Current trends in treatment and prevention. *Sports Medicine, Auckland, NZ, 23*, 397–404.

112. Cross, T. M., Gibbs, N., Houang, M. T., & Cameron, M. (2004). Acute quadriceps muscle strains: Magnetic resonance imaging features and prognosis. *American Journal of Sports Medicine, 32*, 710–719.

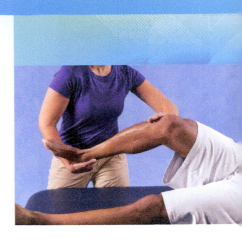

Chapter 11

Orthopedic Interventions for the Knee

Anatomy and Physiology

Common Pathologies

LEARNING OUTCOMES

At the end of this chapter, the student will:

11.1   Describe the anatomy of the knee.

11.2   List normal knee range of motion.

11.3   Describe normal kinematics of the tibiofemoral and patellofemoral joints.

11.4   Describe the mechanics and discuss the purposes of anterior and posterior mobilization techniques of the tibiofemoral joint and glide mobilization techniques of the patellofemoral joint.

11.5   Discuss common knee pathologies and typical presentation.

11.6   Discuss contributing factors to various knee pathologies and, when relevant, preventive measures.

11.7   Describe the clinical tests that the physical therapist may have used to diagnose common knee pathologies and how to administer the tests.

11.8   Discuss common treatment interventions for knee pathologies.

11.9   Describe surgical interventions and post-surgical treatment for the knee, including total knee arthroplasty, anterior cruciate ligament reconstruction, and open reduction, internal fixation for tibial plateau fracture and patellar fracture.

11.10 Compare and contrast related pathologies of the extensor mechanism of the knee, including patellofemoral pain syndrome, patellar tendonitis, patellar tendon rupture, and Osgood-Schlatter disease.

11.11 Discuss the influence of the hip on knee pathologies, including osteoarthritis of the knee, anterior cruciate ligament injury, iliotibial band syndrome, and patellofemoral pain syndrome.

11.12 Describe clinical alerts for select knee pathologies.

KEY WORDS

Allograft	Ligamentization	Patella baja
Arthroscope	Meniscectomy	Patellectomy
Autograft	Necrotization	Q-angle
Bicompartmental	One repetition maximum (1 RM)	Sarcopenia
Clinical prediction rule	Osgood-Schlatter's disease	Sclerosis
Continuous passive motion (CPM)	Osteoarthritis	Screw-home mechanism
Crepitus	Osteophytes	Tricompartmental
Degenerative joint disease (DJD)	Osteotomy	
Effusion	Patella alta	

Anatomy and Physiology

The knee is in the middle of the long, lower extremity kinetic chain. This subjects the knee to high forces and places the knee in a vulnerable position. The bony configuration of the knee, unlike the hip, is not inherently stable. Stability, instead, comes from an abundance of soft tissue structures. Injury and pathology of the knee joint and soft tissues are extremely common because of these factors.

Bone and Joint Anatomy and Physiology

The knee joint complex consists of two joints: the tibiofemoral joint and the patellofemoral joint. As a condyloid joint, the tibiofemoral joint has two degrees of freedom, allowing for flexion and extension as well as rotation. The rounded femoral condyles roll and slide on the flat tibial surface, providing for extensive motion at the knee. The patellofemoral joint is a plane joint that serves an important function in knee biomechanics. Figure 11.1 depicts the bony anatomy.

Tibiofemoral Joint

The normal angle between the tibia and fibula in the frontal plane is a valgus angle of 5° to 10°. An angle of greater than 10° is considered genu valgum (knock knees), and any varus angulation is considered genu varum (bow legs). In the sagittal plane the knee has approximately 140° of flexion and up to 10° of extension.[1] Extension of more than 10° is considered hyperextension, or genu recurvatum. This condition causes overstretching of the posterior capsule of the knee. Figure 11.2 depicts these relationships of the femur and tibia in standing.

In addition to flexion and extension, internal and external rotation also occurs at the tibiofemoral joint.[2–4] This occurs as a component of normal knee flexion and extension. It serves an important role in the knee locking mechanism that increases stability, called the **screw-home mechanism,** which is discussed later in this chapter.

Patellofemoral Joint

The patella sits in the trochlear groove of the anterior femur. It is the site of attachment of the quadriceps muscle and the origin of the patellar tendon, which attaches to the tibial tuberosity. The underside of the patella is covered with articular cartilage. During knee flexion, the contact area on the patella moves progressively more proximally. The compressive forces at this joint are influenced by both degree of joint flexion and whether the movement is performed in closed or open chain.

Table 11-1 summarizes the joints of the knee.

Soft Tissues

Meniscal Cartilage

There are two fibrocartilage menisci in the knee joint: the medial and lateral meniscus. These two menisci help stabilize the femur on the flat tibial plateau by cupping the rounded femoral condyles. This increases joint congruity. Additionally, the menisci help to reduce friction and distribute synovial fluid to the articular cartilage. However, the most important role of the menisci is to absorb

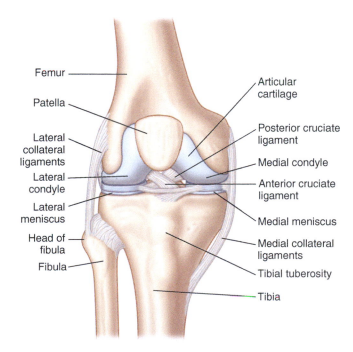

Figure 11.1 The knee contains the tibiofemoral joint and the patellofemoral joint. It is stabilized by the cruciate ligaments and the collateral ligaments.

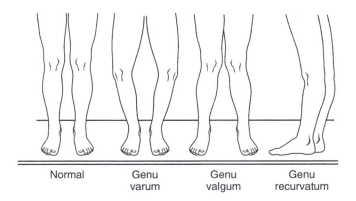

Figure 11.2 The normal relationship between the femur and tibia is slight valgus in the frontal plane and less than 10° hyperextension. Excessive valgus, varus, and recurvatum are all abnormal findings.

Table 11-1   Bone and Joint Anatomy and Physiology
Of the Knee

Joint	Anatomy	Normal ROM and Movements	Landmarks	Clinical Considerations
Tibiofemoral	Condyloid joint with 2 degrees of freedom, allows for flexion and extension and internal and external rotation	Flexion 0°–140°–145°[1] Extension 0°–10°[1] Internal rotation 0°–15°[2] External rotation 0°–20°[2]	Medial and lateral condyles and epicondyles on femur. Intercondylar or trochlear groove between condyles. Tibial plateau is flared surface that articulates with femoral condyles. Tibial tuberosity is attachment site of the patellar tendon.	Common site of pathology of ligaments, menisci, bone, tendons including DJD, ligament tear, patellar tendinopathy, meniscal tear, tibial plateau fracture. Close-packed position: full knee extension with external rotation of tibia. Loose-packed position: about 25° flexion. Capsular pattern: greater limitation in knee flexion than extension.
Patellofemoral	Patella is largest sesamoid bone, imbedded in the quadriceps tendon, rests in the intercondylar groove of the femur.		Inferior pole of patella, tibiofemoral joint line	The patella elevates the quadriceps tendon away from the axis of rotation of the knee and increases strength of the quadriceps by about 25%. Patellofemoral pain syndrome and DJD in patellofemoral joint are common pathologies here.

compressive forces at the knee. The knee is subjected to forces equal to several times body weight. The meniscal cartilages distribute nearly half of the force at the knee.

The medial meniscus is shaped like a C, and the lateral meniscus is shaped like an O. The blood supply to the menisci comes from the joint capsule and synovial membrane and is greatest in the outer third of the rim of cartilage. This area of the meniscus is called the "red zone." The middle one-third ("pink zone") has minimal blood supply, and the inner one-third is described as the "white zone" due to its avascularity (Fig. 11.3). The zones of the meniscus impact the choice made by the surgeon to repair or remove cartilage after a meniscal tear.

While the menisci are loosely attached to the tibia and to each other, they are somewhat moveable. Muscle attachments into the menisci give them a dynamic quality, not an inertness often associated with them.

Capsule and Ligaments

The capsule of the knee encloses both the tibiofemoral and the patellofemoral joints. It is a very large and extensive joint capsule, reinforced on the medial side by the medial collateral ligament (MCL) and on the lateral side by the lateral collateral ligament (LCL). These ligaments are extracapsular, meaning they are outside the joint capsule. The collateral ligaments stabilize the knee in the frontal plane from varus or valgus forces. Specifically, the MCL stabilizes against a valgus force (a force that would tend to cause valgus). The LCL stabilizes against a varus force.

Within the joint capsule (intracapsular) are two ligaments that stabilize the knee in the sagittal plane: the anterior cruciate ligament (ACL) and the posterior cruciate ligament (PCL). The word *cruciate* means cross-shaped, referring to the X-configuration of the ligaments when viewed from the side. The ACL prevents anterior translation of the tibia on the femur and, consequently, posterior translation of the femur on the tibia. The PCL prevents posterior translation of the tibia on the femur and anterior translation of the femur on the tibia. Refer to Figure 11.1 for an illustration of the knee ligaments.

The inner layer of the joint capsule is the synovial membrane. Its purpose is to secrete synovial fluid, which helps to absorb joint forces, reduce friction, and bring nutrients to the joint surfaces. The synovial membrane has folds of tissue that are called plicae, which are remnants of the fetal development of the knee. The plicae in general are not easily palpated, but it is often possible to feel this fold of tissue medial to the patella.

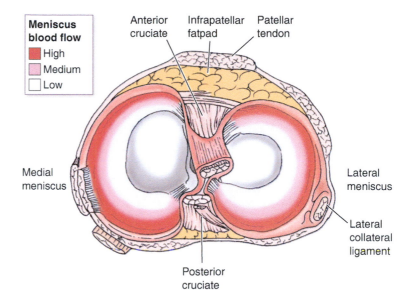

Figure 11.3 The medial and lateral meniscus are loosely attached to the superior tibia. The outer one-third of the meniscus has good blood flow and consequently the ability to heal. The inner two-thirds has poor blood flow. Tears in this area cannot be repaired and usually result in removal of part of the meniscus.

Retinaculum and IT Band

The capsule is further reinforced by retinacula on the medial and lateral side of the patella. These fibrous bands help to stabilize the patella. The medial retinaculum arises from the fascia of vastus medialis. The lateral retinaculum arises from the fascia of vastus lateralis and fibers of the iliotibial (IT) band. Both attach to the patella.

Recall from Chapter 10 that the iliotibial (IT) band originates from the iliac crest and the fascia of gluteus maximus, gluteus medius, and tensor fascia latae. Some of its fibers blend into the lateral retinaculum and attach into the patella, as mentioned. The remainder of the IT band fibers cross over the lateral femoral condyle and attach to the anterolateral tibia, offering lateral support to the knee joint (Fig. 11.4).

Table 11-2 summarizes the soft tissue structures of the knee.

Bursae and Fat Pads

The function of bursae is to cushion soft tissues from bony prominences. As might be expected, there are many bursae in the knee joint; some sources report up to 14. In the anterior knee, there are 4 major bursae, which may contribute to swelling, joint pain, and stiffness. These are the (1) suprapatellar, (2) prepatellar, (3) superficial infrapatellar, and (4) deep infrapatellar bursae. In addition, there is a bursa under the pes anserinus tendons (semitendinosus, sartorius, and gracilis) on the medial aspect of the knee, and under the IT band on the lateral aspect of the knee. The patellar bursae are depicted in Figure 11.5 and summarized in Table 11-3.

Often where there are bursae in the knee they are accompanied by fat pads. Both structures are used to decrease friction. The infrapatellar fat pad lies deep to the patellar tendon and helps distribute synovial fluid to lubricate the knee during flexion and extension. This fat pad is often evident through visual inspection and

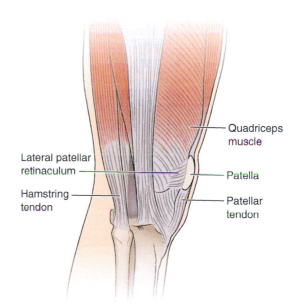

Right leg, lateral view

Figure 11.4 The iliotibial (IT) band originates from the iliac crest and serves as an attachment site for gluteus maximus, gluteus medius, and tensor fascia latae. It courses down the lateral thigh and blends into the lateral retinaculum at the level of the patella. The remainder of the IT band attaches to the proximal tibia.

palpation distal to the patella on either side of the patellar tendon.

Nerves

The sciatic nerve descends through the middle of the posterior thigh. It innervates all the hamstring muscles with the exception of the short head of biceps femoris. Just proximal to the knee, the nerve splits into two branches: the tibial nerve and the common fibular nerve.

Table 11-2   Connective Tissue Anatomy and Physiology
Of the Knee

Structure	Anatomy	Function	Clinical Considerations
Joint capsule	Very large and extensive joint capsule is reinforced on the medial and lateral sides by the collateral ligaments. Lined with synovial membrane. Reinforced by ligaments, medial and lateral retinaculum.	Enclose and stabilize joint.	
Ligaments	Medial collateral ligament (MCL) connects tibia and femur on medial side of knee. Lateral collateral ligament (LCL) connects fibula and femur on lateral knee. Anterior cruciate ligament (ACL) runs from proximal anterior tibia to posterior distal femur. Posterior cruciate ligament (PCL) runs from proximal posterior tibia anterior distal femur.	MCL—stabilizes against a valgus force LCL—stabilizes against a varus force ACL—stabilizes tibia against anterior displacement on femur PCL—stabilizes tibia against posterior displacement on femur	Ligament sprain and tear is common in the knee.
Retinaculum	Medial retinaculum arises from fascia of vastus medialis. Lateral retinaculum arises from fascia of vastus lateralis and part of IT band.	Help stabilize the patella	Tightness of the lateral retinaculum may play a role in patellofemoral pain syndrome.
Meniscal cartilage	Medial and lateral meniscal cartilages attached to the tibia. Blood supply is greatest in outer third and poorest in inner third.	Increase joint congruity, help distribute synovial fluid, reduce friction, and absorb compressive force.	Meniscal cartilage tear is common. Tears in the inner part of the cartilage will not heal due to poor blood supply.
IT Band	Runs from iliac crest down lateral thigh to tibia and patella. Insertion point for gluteus maximus, gluteus medius, and tensor fascia latae.	Provides stability to the lateral knee	May become tight, altering biomechanics of lower extremity Source of pain in IT band friction syndrome

The tibial nerve continues to run through the popliteal space and into the posterior calf. Here it innervates the superficial and deep calf muscles, including gastrocnemius. The common fibular nerve innervates the short head of biceps femoris, then wraps around the lower leg near the head of the fibula and runs down the anterior lower leg, innervating muscles on the anterior and lateral side.

On the anterior thigh, the femoral nerve innervates the pectineus and sartorius muscles and all four heads of the quadriceps femoris. The obturator nerve on the medial anterior thigh innervates the hip adductor group and the gracilis muscle. Figure 11.6 depicts the nerve anatomy around the knee. Table 11-4 summarizes the nerve anatomy.

Muscles

Knee Extensors

The quadriceps femoris group of muscles is the prime mover for knee extension. In open chain, these four muscles extend the tibia on the femur. In closed chain, they extend the femur on the tibia. This group includes rectus femoris (RF), vastus lateralis (VL), vastus intermedius (VI), and vastus medialis (VM). The four heads of quadriceps have a tendinous attachment to the patella (quadriceps tendon) and form an attachment to the tibial tuberosity via the patellar tendon. These muscles are powerful knee extensors. In addition, due to its origin on the AIIS, RF is a hip flexor. VL is the largest and

Table 11-3 Bursae Anatomy and Physiology
Of the Knee

Structure	Anatomy	Function	Clinical Considerations
Suprapatellar bursa	Lies on distal femur, under quadriceps muscle.	Cushions underside of quadriceps muscle from distal femur.	May become inflamed and contribute to knee pain.
Prepatellar bursa	Lies superficial to patella.	Helps skin glide over patella.	May become inflamed and contribute to knee pain (housemaid's knee).
Superficial infrapatellar bursa	Lies between the patellar tendon and the skin.	Helps skin glide over patellar tendon.	May become inflamed and contribute to knee pain associated with patellar tendonitis.
Deep infrapatellar bursa	Lies between proximal tibia and patellar tendon.	Cushions underside of patellar tendon from tibia.	May become inflamed and contribute to knee pain associated with patellar tendonitis.
Anserine bursa	Lies between the medial tibia and the joined tendons of sartorius, gracilis, and semitendinosus.	Cushions pes anserine tendons from medial tibial plateau.	May become inflamed and contribute to medial knee pain.
IT bursa	Lies under the IT band at the lateral femoral condyle.	Cushions the IT band from the femoral condyle.	May become inflamed and contribute to lateral knee pain associated with IT band friction syndrome.

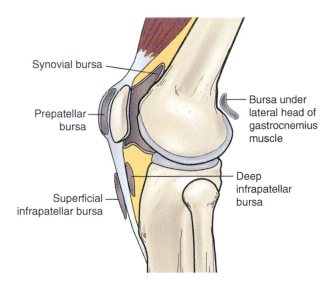

Figure 11.5 Four major bursae in the knee include the suprapatellar, prepatellar, superficial infrapatellar, and deep infrapatellar bursa.

strongest of the quadriceps muscles. VI lies deep to rectus femoris.

Vastus medialis may be divided into two parts: vastus medialis longus (VML) and vastus medialis oblique (VMO). The distal portion of VM where the fiber orientation becomes progressively more horizontal is referred to as VMO. Although the VMO portion of the vastus medialis muscle has not been shown to be anatomically distinct, [5–7] it does have an important functional distinction in its ability to pull the patella medially. This will be discussed further under patellofemoral joint function later in the chapter. All four heads of the quadriceps are capable of contracting with varying timing and to varying degrees, altering the impact on the patella.

Knee Flexors

The hamstring group is the prime mover for knee flexion. The group consists of semimembranosus, semitendinosus, and the short and long heads of biceps femoris. All of these muscles are knee flexors. All except the short head of biceps femoris are also hip extensors. In addition, these three muscles can rotate the tibia.

Gastrocnemius is a weak assister to the hamstrings for knee flexion. This superficial two-joint calf muscle originates from the femoral condyles and inserts on the posterior calcaneus by way of the Achilles tendon. The primary action of gastrocnemius is plantar flexion of the ankle, but secondarily it acts as a knee flexor. The gastrocnemius acts as an antagonist to the ACL at end ranges of extension.[8] Unexpectedly, it also has been shown to act as a knee extensor in closed chain under some circumstances.[9]

Gracilis and sartorius are synergists for the hamstrings in the action of knee flexion. Gracilis is an adductor of the hip but plays a role as a knee flexor and medial knee stabilizer. Sartorius is a long, two-joint strap muscle that has several actions on the hip but at the knee is also a

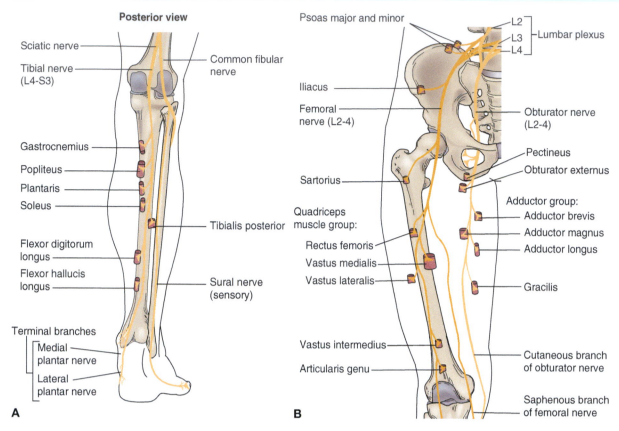

Posterior view

Sciatic nerve

Tibial nerve (L4–S3)

Common fibular nerve

Gastrocnemius

Popliteus

Plantaris

Soleus

Tibialis posterior

Flexor digitorum longus

Flexor hallucis longus

Sural nerve (sensory)

Terminal branches
Medial plantar nerve
Lateral plantar nerve

A

Psoas major and minor

L2
L3   Lumbar plexus
L4

Iliacus

Femoral nerve (L2–4)

Obturator nerve (L2–4)

Sartorius

Pectineus

Obturator externus

Quadriceps muscle group:

Rectus femoris

Vastus medialis

Vastus lateralis

Adductor group:
Adductor brevis
Adductor magnus
Adductor longus

Gracilis

Vastus intermedius

Articularis genu

Cutaneous branch of obturator nerve

Saphenous branch of femoral nerve

B

Figure 11.6 The sciatic nerve splits above the knee into the tibial nerve and the common fibular nerve (A). The tibial nerve innervates the posterior calf muscles, and the common fibular nerve innervates the lateral and anterior lower leg muscles. The obturator and femoral nerves innervate the medial and anterior thigh muscles (B).

Table 11-4   Nerve Anatomy and Physiology

Of the Leg

Structure	Anatomy	Function	Clinical Considerations
Sciatic nerve	Arises from nerve roots of L4–S3.	Innervates most of the hamstring muscles.	May become source of pain in piriformis syndrome.
Tibial nerve	Arises from nerve roots of L4–S3.	Innervates posterior calf muscles.	
Common fibular nerve	Arises from nerve roots of L4–S2.	Innervates anterior lower leg muscles.	Vulnerable to injury as it wraps around the fibular head.
Femoral nerve	Arises from nerve roots of L2–4.	Innervates quadriceps, pectineus, and sartorius.	
Obturator nerve	Arises from nerve roots of L2–4.	Innervates adductor group and gracilis.	

flexor and medial knee stabilizer. On the medial side of the tibia, the sartorius, gracilis, and semitendinosus tendons blend together and have a common insertion. These three tendons are referred to as the pes anserinus tendons, which translates to "goose's foot," named for their resemblance to this structure. The clinical significance of the pes anserinus tendons lies in their role as dynamic medial knee stabilizers, assisting the MCL (Fig. 11.7). Additionally, there is a bursa under these tendons, which may become inflamed, causing medial knee tenderness and pain.

Knee Rotators

The hamstring muscles are rotators of the tibia on the femur. The semimembranosus and semitendinosus attach to the medial side of the tibia and internally rotate the tibia. The biceps femoris attaches to the lateral side of the tibia and the fibula and externally rotates the tibia.

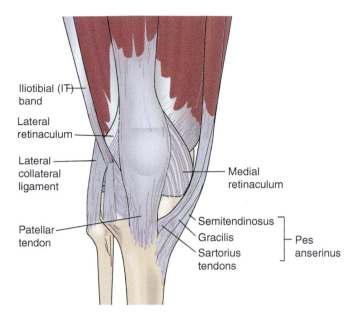

Figure 11.7 The pes anserinus is composed of tendons from semitendinosus, gracilis, and sartorius. It assists the MCL in stabilizing the medial knee.

The function of these muscles in tibial rotation is analogous to directing a horse by pulling on its reins.

In addition to the hamstrings, popliteus plays an important role in rotation of the knee. This small, triangle-shaped muscle on the posterior knee originates on the lateral femoral condyle and inserts on the posterior side of the proximal-medial tibia. Popliteus is an internal rotator of the tibia on the femur in open chain and an external rotator of the femur on the tibia in closed chain. This muscle is the "unlocker" of the screw-home mechanism of the knee (see "Screw-Home Mechanism" later in this chapter).

Table 11-5 summarizes the muscular anatomy of the knee.

Kinematics of the Knee

The normal alignment of the knee is 5° to 10° valgus. Similar to the normal valgus angle of the knee is the quadriceps angle, or **Q-angle.** This angle is an approximate measurement of the line of pull of the quadriceps muscle. It is the angle formed by a line from the ASIS to the center of the patella with a line drawn from the center of the patella through the middle of the tibial tuberosity (Fig. 11.8). In general, the static Q-angle is about 11° to 13° in males and 15° to 17° in females.[10–12]

Patellofemoral Joint

Normal biomechanics of the patellofemoral joint involves tracking of the patella in the trochlear groove of the femur. If the forces acting on the patella are greater laterally than medially, the patella may track abnormally and ride up the lateral side of the groove. This may lead to pathological changes in the patellofemoral joint.

The Q-angle has relevance to understanding the forces acting on the patellofemoral joint. It is helpful to think of the patella imbedded in the quadriceps tendon/patellar tendon as a bead (patella) on a string (muscle/tendon). The force of a quadriceps contraction pulls the patella superiorly but also laterally. The extent of this lateral force on the patella depends largely upon the strength of the quadriceps contraction and the Q-angle. The greater the Q-angle, the more force on the patella to move laterally. In addition, a stronger contraction by VL relative to VMO will increase the tendency of lateral displacement of the patella.

As a counter to the lateral force to which the patella is subjected, there are several soft tissue and bony constraints acting with a goal to keep the patella in the intercondylar groove. These include a higher lateral femoral condyle than medial, the medial retinaculum, and VMO. Table 11-6 summarizes the medial and lateral constraints on the patella.

In addition to the forces acting on the patella to pull it laterally, there are compressive forces between the patella and the femur. These compressive forces are increased in closed chain when performing a squat, progressively increasing with increased knee flexion.[13] In the presence of pathology of the patellofemoral joint, this can cause anterior knee pain. The amount of compression in the patellofemoral joint is a factor of the depth of the squat and the force of the quadriceps contraction. A squat performed with more forward trunk lean will decrease the quadriceps force and increase use of the gluteus maximus. Patients with quadriceps weakness or anterior knee pain may display this movement strategy to decrease the quadriceps force.

Dynamic Valgus and Dynamic Q-angle

Valgus and Q-angle are often considered static, postural references. However, alignment in the frontal plane may change during weight-bearing. In the stance phase of gait, going sit to stand, descending stairs, or landing from a jump, dynamic knee alignment may show an increased valgus due to the momentary forces on the knee. This medial collapse of the knee has been linked to pathologies in the knee. [14–17] It is more common in females.[18–20]

While static Q-angle influences the degree of dynamic Q-angle, the dynamic angle is further increased by internal rotation of the femur, external rotation of the tibia, and pronation of the foot.[15,21–23] Weakness of hip external rotators and abductors are linked with a greater dynamic Q-angle in weight-bearing. Figure 11.9 demonstrates the difference between a static and dynamic Q-angle.

Table 11-5 Muscle Anatomy and Kinesiology
Of the Knee

Muscle	Origin	Insertion	Innervation	Primary Action	Clinical Considerations
Rectus femoris	Anterior inferior iliac spine (AIIS)	Tibial tuberosity	Femoral nerve	Hip flexion and knee extension	Only head of quadriceps muscle that spans hip joint.
Vastus lateralis	Anterior femur	Tibial tuberosity	Femoral nerve	Knee extension	
Vastus medialis	Anterior femur	Tibial tuberosity	Femoral nerve	Knee extension	Distal portion (VMO) exerts medial pull on patella.
Vastus intermedius	Anterior femur	Tibial tuberosity	Femoral nerve	Knee extension	
Semimembranosus	Ischial tuberosity	Medial side of tibia	Sciatic nerve	Hip extension, knee flexion and tibial internal rotation	
Semitendinosus	Ischial tuberosity	Medial side of tibia	Sciatic nerve	Hip extension, knee flexion, and tibial internal rotation	One of three tendons that make up the pes anserine; stabilizes medial knee.
Biceps femoris	Short head: posterior femur Long head: ischial tuberosity	Lateral side of tibia and fibula	Short head: common fibular nerve Long head: sciatic nerve	Hip extension (long head), knee flexion and tibial external rotation	
Gastrocnemius	Femoral condyles	Posterior calcaneus	Tibial nerve	Ankle plantarflexion and knee flexion	
Gracilis	Pubis	Proximal medial tibia	Obturator nerve	Hip adduction. Additionally, it performs weak hip flexion, knee flexion, and is a medial knee stabilizer.	One of three tendons that make up the pes anserine; stabilizes medial knee.
Sartorius	Anterior superior iliac spine (ASIS)	Proximal medial tibia	Femoral nerve	Hip flexion, hip abduction, hip external rotation, and knee flexion	One of three tendons that make up the pes anserine; stabilizes medial knee.
Popliteus	Lateral femoral condyle	Posterior medial tibia	Tibial nerve	Internal rotation of tibia on femur in open chain	Unlocks screw-home mechanism

Dynamic Knee Joint Load

The knee joint is subjected to forces that equal several times body weight. These forces are dampened by the muscles, ligaments, menisci, and other soft tissues around the joint. Especially important in this function is the quadriceps femoris muscle. It has been shown that the quadriceps play a major role in absorbing the compressive forces on the knee,[24] and weakness particularly of the quadriceps muscle is associated with increased risk of pathology in the knee.

Screw-Home Mechanism

As a condyloid joint, the knee allows for rotation. While this movement is not under voluntary control, it is an important accessory movement that locks the tibia into the femur in full extension. There is disagreement regarding the amount of tibial rotation that can occur, but sources agree that the amount of tibial rotation is greatest at 90° of knee flexion and most limited in full extension. Generally, it is thought that the knee allows up to 15°

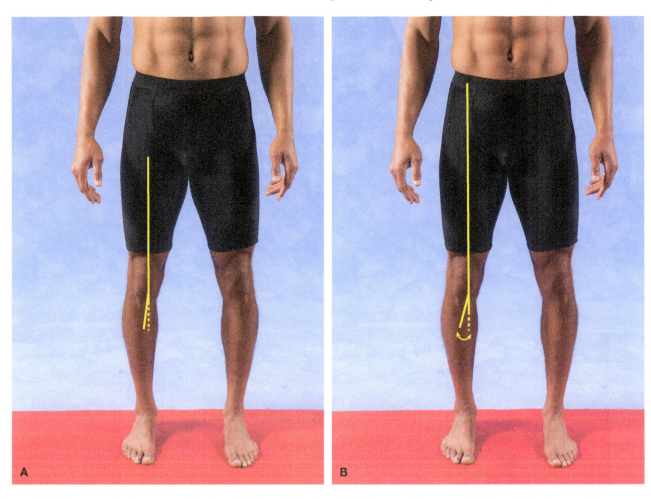

Figure 11.8 The normal alignment of the knee is 5° to 10° valgus (A). The quadriceps angle (Q-angle) is the angle between a line from the ASIS to the midpoint of the patella with a line from the midpoint of the patella through the tibial tuberosity (B). Normal in males is 11° to 13°, and in females it is 15° to 17°.

Table 11-6	Medial/Lateral Constraints on the Patella	
	Medial Constraint	Lateral Constraint
Vastus medialis	✓	
Lateral femoral condyle	✓	
Medial retinaculum tightness	✓	
Vastus lateralis		✓
IT band tightness		✓
Lateral retinaculum tightness		✓

to 20° of internal tibial rotation and 20° to 25° of external tibial rotation.[2]

At the end range of open chain knee extension, the tibia externally rotates on the femur, tightening the ligaments of the knee and bringing the tibia and femur into maximum contact. This phenomenon is known as the screw-home mechanism. In closed chain, the femur is the more moveable bone, and it internally rotates on the tibia as the knee extends. The popliteus plays an active role in unlocking the screw-home mechanism by internally rotating the tibia or externally rotating the femur. As an example, when preparing to sit down from a standing position, the femur must externally rotate on the tibia to unlock the knee. The popliteus is responsible for this motion, allowing the knee to unlock and then flex.

Joint Mobilization

Tibiofemoral Mobilization

To reduce pain or increase range of motion, joint mobilization may be a useful intervention. According to the concave-convex rule, movement of the concave tibia on the convex femoral condyles is accompanied by a slide of the tibia in the same direction as the movement of the tibia. The loose packed position of the knee is slightly flexed, about 25°. Table 11-7 lists the movements of the

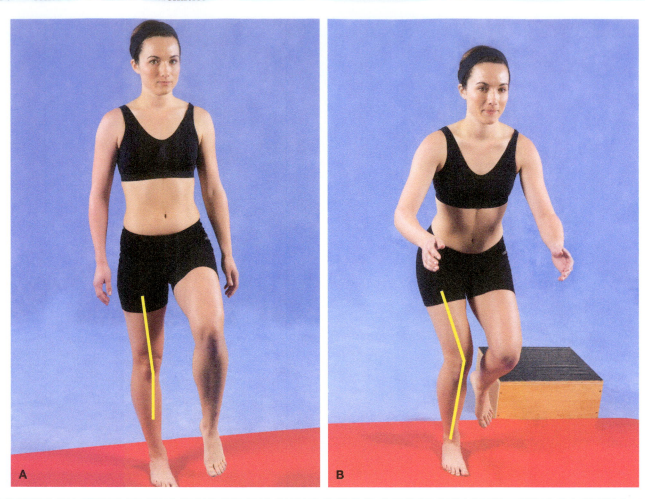

Figure 11.9 Comparison of the static (A) and dynamic (B) valgus angle. Knee valgus and Q-angle are often momentarily increased in gait, going sit-to-stand, and jumping.

knee and the glide mobilizations used to increase range of motion.

Anterior Glide

Anterior tibiofemoral glide is used to increase knee extension. The patient is positioned prone, with the knee flexed and resting on the examiner's shoulder. A towel is placed under the distal femur. The tibia is mobilized with a glide of the tibia anteriorly, as shown in Figure 11.10.

Posterior Glide

Posterior glide is used to increase knee flexion. The patient is positioned supine, with the knee slightly flexed. A towel roll is placed under the distal femur. The tibia is mobilized in a posterior and slightly superior direction, toward the examination table (Fig. 11.11).

Patellofemoral Mobilization

The patellofemoral joint must be mobile to allow for full range of motion. Mobilization of the patella, therefore,

Table 11-7	Direction of Slide Used to Increase Range of Motion
Limited Range	**Direction of Slide in Mobilization**
Flexion	Posterior tibiofemoral glide and inferior patellofemoral glide
Extension	Anterior tibiofemoral glide and superior patellofemoral glide

may be prescribed to increase knee range of motion or to prevent loss of motion. It may also be useful to stretch the soft tissue constraints of the patella to allow for more normal patellar tracking. The most common patellar mobilizations are described as follows.

Superior Glide

Superior glide is used to increase the mobility of the patella to allow full knee extension. It is also used to

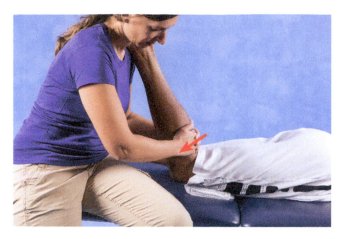

Figure 11.10 Anterior glide of the tibia on the femur increases knee extension.

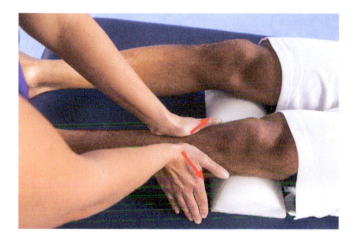

Figure 11.11 Posterior glide of the tibia on the femur increases knee flexion.

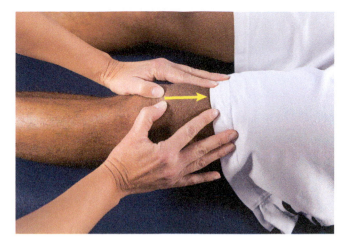

Figure 11.12 Superior glide of the patella on the femur increases knee extension.

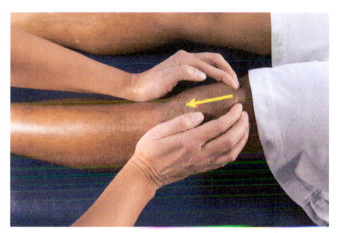

Figure 11.13 Inferior glide of the patella on the femur increases knee flexion.

prevent contracture of the patellar tendon. The patient is placed supine, with the knee extended and the quadriceps relaxed. The examiner grasps the patella with thumb and index finger and slides superiorly (Fig. 11.12).

Inferior Glide

Inferior glide is used to increase the mobility of the patella to allow full knee flexion. The patient is placed in the same position as described above. The examiner grasps the patella with the thumb and index finger and slides it inferiorly (Fig. 11.13).

Medial Glide

Medial glide is used to stretch the lateral structures that tend to displace the patella (IT band, lateral retinaculum). The patient is positioned as described above, and the examiner glides the patella medially (Fig. 11.14).

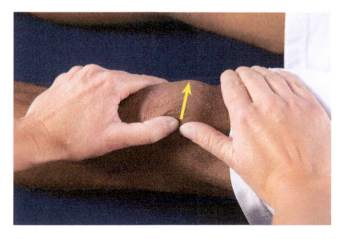

Figure 11.14 Medial glide of the patella on the femur is used to stretch the lateral retinaculum.

Common Pathologies

Osteoarthritis
Anterior Cruciate Ligament Injury
Posterior Cruciate Ligament Injury
Medial Collateral Ligament Injury
Meniscal Tear
Iliotibial Band Syndrome

Patellofemoral Pain Syndrome
Patellar Tendinopathy
Patellar Tendon Rupture
Tibial Plateau Fracture
Patellar Fracture

The knee's location in the middle of two long bones, its lack of bony stability, and its complex soft tissue structure predispose it to injury or pathology. In addition, altered biomechanics in the lower extremity can lead to pain, weakness, inflammation, and damage to the knee joint. In this section, we'll discuss common knee pathologies of the tibiofemoral and patellofemoral joints. Owing to the importance of a basic understanding of surgical treatments, these will be presented when appropriate for osteoarthritis, fracture, meniscal tear, and ligament tear.

Osteoarthritis

Osteoarthritis (OA) is the most common type of arthritis. It is also known as **degenerative joint disease,** or **DJD.** This is a wear-and-tear arthritis, in contrast with rheumatoid arthritis, which is a systemic disease process. As is true in the hip, the manifestations of knee OA include joint pain, stiffness, loss of range of motion, and deformity. Muscle atrophy (**sarcopenia**) may be noticed on physical exam, as well as lax ligaments. A decreased joint space, bone spurs (**osteophytes**), and areas of increased bone density (**sclerosis**) are often disclosed in x-ray findings.

The knee is divided into three compartments: the medial compartment, which includes the medial tibiofemoral joint and medial meniscus; the lateral compartment, which includes the lateral tibiofemoral joint and lateral meniscus; and the patellofemoral compartment, which includes the anterior femur and the patella. OA can affect any or all of these compartments. When OA is found primarily in the medial compartment, the knee develops a varus deformity. With lateral compartment OA, a valgus deformity is seen. If OA affects one side of the tibiofemoral joint and the patellofemoral joint, it is called **bicompartmental** involvement. If it affects both sides of the tibiofemoral joint and the patellofemoral joint, it is considered **tricompartmental** involvement. Figure 11.15 includes a radiograph of a knee with advanced OA.

Causes/Contributing Factors

There are many reported risk factors for OA of the knee. It has been linked to increased stresses on the joint from obesity, previous injury to the meniscus or ACL, occupations that involve kneeling and squatting, overloading through intense exercise, normal aging, and altered biomechanics, especially valgus malalignment and loss of range of motion.[25–37]

Symptoms

The onset of OA is typically slow, with increasing symptoms over several years. Common symptoms include

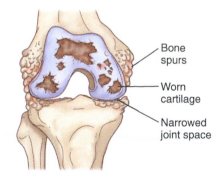

Bone spurs

Worn cartilage

Narrowed joint space

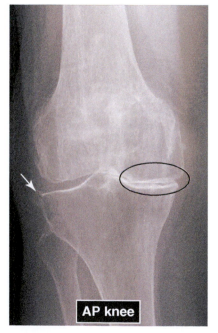

AP knee

Figure 11.15 Illustration of knee osteoarthritis and typical x-ray findings of decreased joint space, osteophytes, and sclerosis.

pain in the knee that is increased with walking and stair climbing, a feeling of stiffness in the joint, visible swelling, knee instability, and **crepitus.** Crepitus is the crackling or popping sound that may accompany joint movement. Morning stiffness lasting less than 1 hour is typical and indicative of OA.[38] If the patellofemoral compartment is particularly involved, the patient may feel anterior knee pain that is increased with ascending or descending stairs or when going from sitting to standing.

Clinical Signs

Many sources of information are used to assign the diagnosis of knee OA, including x-ray findings and patient complaints. The criteria for classification of OA of the knee include age over 50 years, presence of knee crepitus, palpable bony enlargement, bony tenderness to palpation, morning stiffness lasting less than 30 minutes, and absence of palpable warmth of the joint.[39] There are no special tests for knee OA.

Common Interventions

Treatment for OA of the knee will depend upon the severity of symptoms and often includes a combination of physical therapy, pharmacological, and surgical interventions. Patient education regarding the pathology, progression, and contributing factors is important. This should include information regarding weight loss if appropriate.

Therapeutic exercise has been shown to be beneficial in the treatment of OA in terms of pain, strength, and function.[40–49] The plan of care may include manual therapy and therapeutic exercises including joint range-of-motion, strengthening, proprioceptive, aquatic, and aerobic exercises.

Range-of-motion exercises should focus on maintaining knee flexion and extension. Hip range-of-motion exercises may also be included in the plan. Additionally, stretching of the two-joint muscles, hamstrings and rectus femoris, is often included. Rectus femoris stretching is very important if patellofemoral OA is present (Fig. 11.16).

Strengthening exercises are indicated for all the muscles around the knee and the hip, particularly knee extensors (Fig. 11.17).[40,50,51,53] People with knee OA have, on average, 20% less quadriceps strength than their healthy age-matched counterparts.[51] The relationship between quadriceps strength and knee OA is very strong, leading some researchers to question if quadriceps weakness may be a contributor to knee OA, rather than a result.[51,52]

Hip abductors and hip extensors are also key muscles to strengthen to stabilize against varus and valgus forces at the knee.[54–56] By strengthening gluteus maximus and medius, movement into hip adduction, hip internal rotation, and consequently knee valgus is controlled (Fig. 11.18). Additionally, gluteus maximus, gluteus medius,

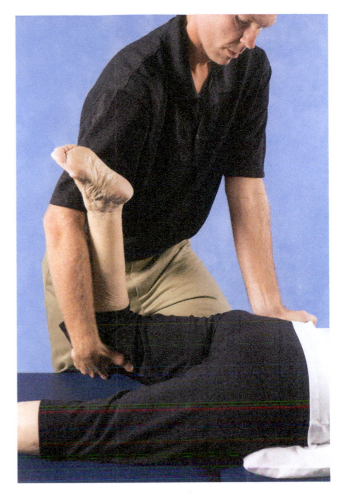

Figure 11.16 Stretching the rectus femoris may be part of the treatment plan for patients with patellofemoral arthritis.

and tensor fascia latae are also capable of providing lateral knee support through their insertion on the iliotibial (IT) band, thus assisting in stabilizing against knee varus.

Patients with OA of the knee often report a feeling of knee instability,[57] and ligament laxity is a common finding. Proprioceptive exercises and balance retraining are beneficial components of the patient's home exercise program.[58–61] Exercises done in a pool to lessen the weight-bearing forces on the knee have also been shown to be beneficial in decreasing pain.[62,63]

Bracing and orthotic devices have been shown to be effective in relieving pain and improving function in patients with knee OA. Lateral wedge insoles may be used to decrease the varus force on the knee.[64,65] Valgus bracing has been shown to help pain and function in patients with a varus deformity.[66] Similar to bracing, taping to reposition the patella may reduce pain and improve function in patients with patellofemoral OA.[67] A description of McConnell taping is found in Box 11-2 later in this chapter.

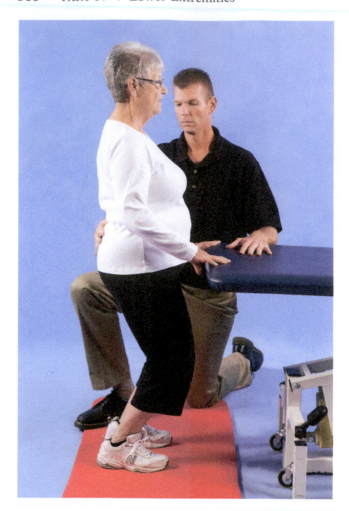

Figure 11.17 Quadriceps strengthening is often included in the POC for tibiofemoral OA.

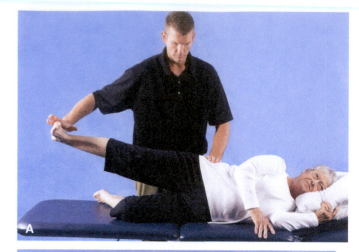

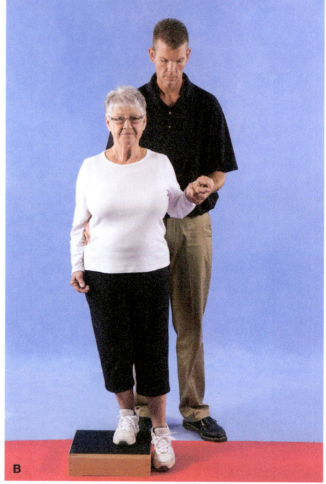

Figure 11.18 Strengthening hip abductors in open chain (A) or closed chain (B) helps increase frontal plane stability.

Gait training with an assistive device to unload the knee is often included in the plan of care. This may decrease pain, slow disease progression, and allow the patient to remain ambulatory. Some studies suggest that modifying the patient's gait to shift the forces within the knee during gait may be helpful. Training the patient to adopt a toe-in gait may help patients with medial compartment OA.[68,69] Likewise, training a patient with lateral compartment OA to toe-out in gait may delay the need for surgery.

If the patient is unsuccessful in controlling knee pain and/or loss of function, surgery may be indicated. The patient may be a candidate for a total knee arthroplasty, a unicompartmental arthroplasty, or a high tibial **osteotomy.** The most common surgical treatment is total knee arthroplasty, in which the distal femur, the proximal tibia, and the underside of the patella are resurfaced. If the patient has advanced OA in only one compartment, a unicompartmental prosthesis may be used. To postpone arthroplasty, an osteotomy may be performed in a younger patient to change the biomechanics of the joint. These three common surgical approaches will be discussed.

What's in the Plan of Care?

Prevention

The risk of OA is decreased by maintaining a high level of physical activity. Encourage patients with early OA to lose weight if appropriate. Avoiding occupations that require kneeling or extreme knee flexion decreases the risk.

The Bottom Line: for patients with knee OA

Description and causes	Deterioration of the knee, which may be due to obesity, abnormal biomechanics, normal aging, injury to the meniscus or ACL, occupations that involve kneeling and squatting, or overloading through intense exercise
Test	No special tests
Stretch	Into knee flexion and extension, focus on stretching rectus femoris and hamstrings
Strengthen	Especially quadriceps, hip extensors and abductors, hamstrings
Train	Proprioception, balance.
Avoid	Occupations that involve excessive kneeling and squatting and sports/exercises that involve extreme overloading

Interventions for the Surgical Patient

Total Knee Arthroplasty

Multiple studies have shown the effectiveness of PT for the OA patient. Preoperative physical therapy increases strength, function, proprioception, aerobic capacity, and range of motion; improves pain; and enhances the likelihood of discharge to home rather than a rehabilitation facility.[42,53,70–72]

Mizner et al. found that the best predictor of postoperative success was preoperative quadriceps strength.[71] An important component of the preoperative phase is strengthening of the quadriceps, hamstrings, and hip flexors. During this time patients are often instructed in gait with a device.

Prior to surgery, the surgeon and patient make several important decisions, including how much of the knee is replaced, what happens to the cruciate ligaments, and if the prosthesis is cemented in place. The decision to replace the whole joint or one compartment depends upon the extent of arthritis. If arthritis is found in only one of the two tibiofemoral compartments, the patient may be a candidate for a partial knee replacement (see "Unicompartmental Knee Arthroplasty" later in this chapter). In surgery, one or both of the cruciate ligaments may be removed or both may be spared. If the cruciates are removed, sagittal plane stability is built into the design of the prosthesis. The prosthesis may have components that require cementing, noncemented components, or a hybrid. Hybrid prostheses usually involve cemented tibial and patellar components with a cementless femoral component. If cementless components are used, the patient will usually be restricted in weight-bearing for a short time; cemented prostheses allow the patient to be weight-bearing as tolerated immediately after surgery.

What's in the Plan of Care?

Surgery

Total knee replacement involves replacing, or more accurately, resurfacing all three compartments of the knee. The surgeon removes the distal part of the femur and cuts it in a shape that allows a metal femoral component to cover the end of the bone. The proximal tibia is removed and a metal tray is attached. A plastic liner is locked onto the tray. Finally, often the underside of the patella is resurfaced with a plastic button that is cemented into place. Figure 11.19 shows the components of a typical total knee prosthesis and a radiograph of an inserted total knee replacement.

Postoperative Phase

The purpose of physical therapy after total knee arthroplasty is to minimize the risk of deep vein thrombosis (DVT), recover range of motion of the knee, increase hip and knee strength, improve function, and decrease pain and swelling.

> ⚑ **CLINICAL ALERT**
>
> During the first few days postoperatively, it is important to teach the patient "ankle pumps" to prevent DVT. The risk of DVT is that the clot will dislodge and become a pulmonary embolism. Signs of a DVT are swelling, pain, or tenderness in the leg that is more noticeable when standing or walking, increased warmth in the area, and red or discolored skin overlying the clot (National Heart, Lung, and Blood Institute, National Institutes of Health, 2011). Wells' criteria offer a **clinical prediction rule** that is often used to assess the likelihood of DVT. See Table 10-3 in Chapter 10 for Wells' criteria.

Many protocols will have the patient performing therapeutic exercises the day after surgery (postoperative day 1, or POD1). These may include quadriceps sets, hamstring sets, and gluteus maximus sets. On POD 1 or 2, knee rehabilitation exercises are initiated, which often include active knee flexion and extension supine (heel slides), hip abduction supine, active knee extension in a shortened arc of motion (short arc quad exercises), straight leg raises, and sitting active-assisted knee flexion stretching. A goal of 90° of AAROM into flexion by the

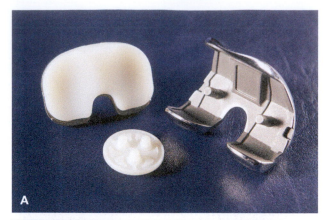

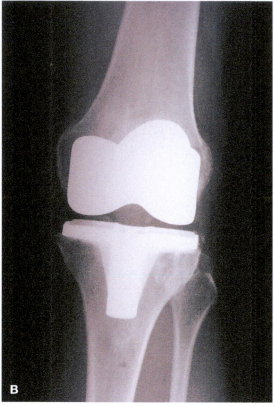

Figure 11.19 The total knee prosthesis consists of femoral, tibial, and patellar components (A). Figure B shows a radiograph after total knee replacement.

time of discharge is typical. During the first few postoperative days, therapy will also work on gait training with an assistive device and functional activities including transfers and bed mobility.

In some instances, the plan of care may include **continuous passive motion (CPM)** after TKA. The patient's lower extremity is placed in the CPM, which mechanically performs range-of-motion of the hip and knee at a selected speed, selected arc of motion, and selected treatment duration. Three meta-analyses have shown that CPM may increase passive and active flexion range of motion, reduce the use of pain medication, decrease the length of hospital stay, and reduce the need for a manipulation of the joint due to limited motion.[73–75] However, the gains in all areas were very minimal. Moreover, several studies have shown no significant benefit to the use of CPM after TKA.[76–80] This decision largely depends upon the philosophy of the surgeon, but the current position of APTA is that the risk of prolonged bedrest while using CPM should be weighed against expected limited benefits.[81]

After discharge, the patient will continue physical therapy in a skilled nursing facility, home health, or outpatient setting. Gradually the patient's therapeutic exercise protocol may be progressed to include passive and active range-of-motion exercises, and open and closed chain strengthening exercises of the quadricep, hamstring, hip extensor, and hip abductor muscles. Recovery of full or near-full range of motion is often the goal. Eccentric exercise and proprioceptive retraining may be included in the plan of care. Gait training may be progressed eventually to include gait without a device and gait on stairs. Cycling, patellar mobilization, tibiofemoral mobilization, and modalities (heat, ice, NMES) may also be utilized.

Recent attention has focused on the persistent weakness of knee extensors and, to a lesser extent, knee flexors after TKA.[81–86] Prior to surgery, quadriceps strength is often decreased on the affected side as compared to the unaffected side. This deficit becomes greater after surgery, until about 6 months postop. At 6 months postop, strength is generally slightly better than at preoperative levels, but declines from that point onward at a faster rate than would be expected due to normal aging. Strength deficits in the quadriceps average 20% as compared to the unaffected side, and between 30% to 48% when compared to healthy age-matched control subjects.

PTAs have an important role in preventing this decline in strength. It is recommended that rehabilitation protocols include more aggressive strengthening of the quadricep and hamstring muscles, including having the patient perform 10 to 15 repetitions at 70% of their **one repetition maximum (1 RM)**.[71,81–83] Eccentric strengthening has the ability to increase strength and cross-sectional area of muscle and will therefore often be included in the plan of care.[82] Proprioceptive retraining, especially if the cruciate ligaments were removed, should be included.[87] See Box 11-1 for information on calculating 70% of 1 RM.

It may be as important to address deficits in power as much as deficits in strength after TKA.[86] It has been shown that after TKA the quadriceps and hamstrings have less capability to generate power. An asymmetry of power in the lower extremities has been associated with an increased risk of falls.[84,88] For this reason, power training may be included in the patient's plan of care.

What's in the Plan of Care?

Box 11-1	How to Calculate 70% of a One Rep Maximum (1 RM)

1 RM is the amount of weight that can be lifted one time, and one time only, for a given exercise. If a patient can lift 10 lb in a biceps curl only one time, then 10 lb is the 1 RM for this exercise for this patient at this time. If you wanted the patient to exercise at 70% of 1 RM, you would instruct the patient to perform biceps curls with 7 lb. The 1 RM increases as the patient improves in strength.

It may be difficult to have patients who are elderly or in discomfort complete an assessment to determine their 1 RM for each exercise. As an alternative, it is commonly accepted that if a patient can perform 10 to 15 repetitions of an exercise, but no more, without signs of muscle fatigue (maintaining good form, no shaking, etc.), then the amount of resistance is equivalent to 70% of their 1 RM.

This technique can be used with elastic resistance as well. Again, if a patient can perform 10 to 15 repetitions of an exercise, but no more than this, the band is providing approximately 70% of 1 RM resistance.

Unicompartmental Knee Arthroplasty

Surgery

If OA is present in only one of the tibiofemoral compartments, the patient may be a candidate for a unicompartmental knee arthroplasty (UKA). While this term may be applied to a patellofemoral replacement, generally it is used to describe a medial or lateral tibiofemoral replacement.

Unicompartmental knee replacement is a shorter, easier surgery than TKA. The prosthesis has femoral and tibial components that resurface half of the knee. The components are smaller, allowing for a smaller incision. Both cruciate ligaments are preserved. This surgery may be done on an outpatient basis or may involve a 1-day stay in the hospital. Recovery is faster than after TKA. Figure 11.20 shows a typical unicompartmental prosthesis and a radiograph of a knee after UKA.

Postoperative Phase

Physical therapy after UKA is similar to that after TKA, except that the recovery time is shorter. Patients usually experience less pain and swelling after UKA. Progression of gait and range of motion is faster.

High Tibial Osteotomy

Surgery

If a young patient has OA, an osteotomy may buy time before a TKA is needed. The purpose of an osteotomy is to change the alignment of the joint to shift the weight-bearing surfaces toward areas that are less damaged. On

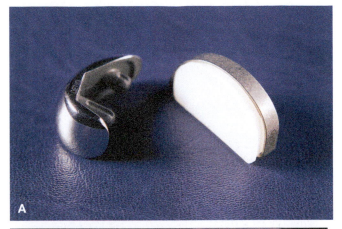

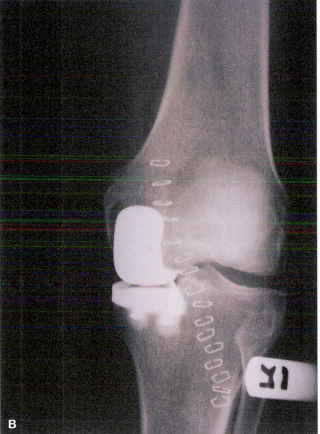

Figure 11.20 The unicompartmental knee prosthesis consists of a femoral and tibial component that resurface half of the tibiofemoral joint (A). Figure B shows a radiograph after unicompartmental knee replacement.

average, the patient will progress to needing a TKA about 10 years after osteotomy.[89]

In the case of medial compartment OA, a wedge of bone can be taken out of the proximal lateral tibia, aligning the knee in decreased varus, which puts more stress on the lateral compartment. In this case, after the wedge of bone is removed, bone surfaces are brought together to realign the joint. This is called a "closing wedge" osteotomy. Alternatively, an "opening wedge" can be created on the medial tibia and spanned by a

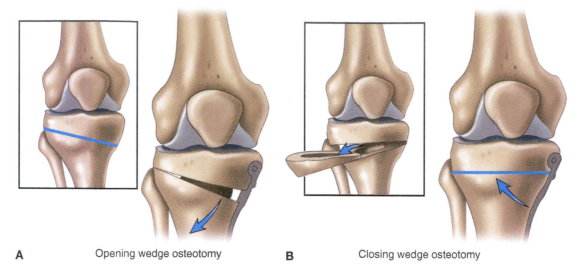

A   Opening wedge osteotomy   **B**   Closing wedge osteotomy

Figure 11.21 Osteotomy may be a temporary solution for younger patients who need a total knee arthroplasty. An opening wedge osteotomy (A) or closing wedge osteotomy (B) will correct a varus deformity as shown here.

plate and screws to achieve the same results. Figure 11.21 depicts an opening wedge and a closing wedge osteotomy for varus deformity.

Postoperative Phase

What's in the Plan of Care? Depending upon whether the osteotomy is opening or closing wedge, and what type of fixation was used, the patient will likely be restricted in weight-bearing for 2 to 8 weeks. The patient may be placed in a hinged knee brace that is locked in extension and removed only for exercises for the first 4 weeks. Eventually the patient will be allowed to ambulate with the brace unlocked. Electrical stimulation and cryotherapy may be included in the early plan of care.

Typical strengthening exercises in the first 4 weeks include heel slides (0° to 90°), quadricep sets, ankle pumps, short arc quadriceps strengthening, resisted ankle dorsiflexion and plantarflexion, and four-plane straight leg raises with the brace locked in full extension (Fig. 11.22). Stretching exercises often include non-weight-bearing gastrocsoleus, hamstring, IT band, and quadricep stretches.

By 4 to 6 weeks, the patient may be allowed to do straight leg raise exercises without the brace if capable of maintaining full knee extension. Use of a stationary bike may be added. Generally, no closed chain exercises are allowed until 6 to 7 weeks postop. By 7 to 8 weeks, open and closed chain quadriceps strengthening in a restricted range may be added.[90,91]

Anterior Cruciate Ligament Injury   CPG

The anterior cruciate ligament (ACL) prevents anterior movement of the tibia on the femur. Injury to the ACL

includes grade I sprain without evidence of joint instability, grade II sprain with some joint instability (anterior cruciate-deficient knee), and grade III rupture or tear of the ACL. Grade I sprain will usually heal without incident. Grade II may require some short-term activity/sport modification, and grade III often requires surgical repair for patients with an active lifestyle.

Causes/Contributing Factors

Most ACL injuries (65% to 95%) are noncontact injuries.[92–95] A common mechanism of injury occurs when the foot is planted on the ground with the knee in a valgus position, combined with femoral internal rotation and tibial external rotation during deceleration (Fig.11.23). Often this occurs after landing on the leg in an attempt to pivot laterally during a sport. Although less likely, it is also possible to tear the ACL in a contact injury, usually when the femur is hit from the front and the knee is hyperextended.[95–97]

Understanding the contributing factors that lead to a torn ACL has been the impetus of research for many years. Anatomical, hormonal, biomechanical, and neuromuscular factors have been identified. These include female gender, decreased intercondylar femoral notch size, shallow tibial plateau, laxity of the knee joint, relative weakness of the hamstrings in relationship to the quadriceps, decreased core and/or extremity proprioception, and poor neuromuscular control of the hip and knee resulting in dynamic knee valgus.[96,98,99] Women are most at risk during the preovulatory phase of the menstrual cycle, days 10 to 14.[96,100–103]

Symptoms

There may be an audible pop or snap at the time of the injury. Immediately after an ACL injury, the patient will often report significant swelling and pain. Knee range

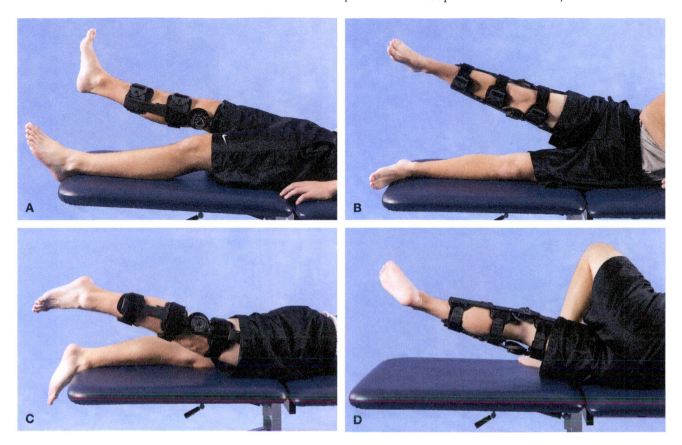

Figure 11.22 After wedge osteotomy, straight leg raises in all four planes with a brace locked in full extension may be indicated.

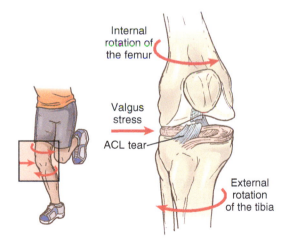

Figure 11.23 The ACL is most often torn without contact when the foot is planted with a valgus knee, internally rotated femur, and externally rotated tibia.

of motion will often be significantly limited, as will quadriceps strength. The knee will feel unstable, as if it will buckle or give away, with a complete ACL tear. It is usually difficult to walk immediately after the injury.

Clinical Signs

The ACL is responsible for preventing anterior translation of the tibia on the femur, so most of the diagnostic tests rely on detecting anterior movement of the tibia with an anteriorly directed force. There are three tests for ACL tear that support the diagnosis. There is dispute about the reliability and validity of the three tests, so often more than one test is used.[104,105]

Lachman Test

The patient is positioned supine with the knee flexed to 30°. The examiner stabilizes the femur with one hand. With the other hand grasping the tibia, and the thumb resting on the tibial tuberosity, the examiner applies an anterior force to the proximal tibia (Fig. 11.24). A positive test is indicated by excessive anterior movement of the tibia as compared to the unaffected side. Some sources suggest that movement of 3 mm in excess of the other side, or a total translation of 10 mm, is indicative of ACL tear.

Anterior Drawer Test

The patient is positioned supine with the knee flexed to 90° and the foot resting on the examination table. The examiner sits on the patient's foot to stabilize the extremity. With thumbs spanning the tibiofemoral joint on the medial and lateral sides, the examiner's fingers grasp the posterior tibia. The patient is instructed to remain relaxed; the examiner palpates the hamstring tendons during the test to ensure relaxation. The examiner simultaneously

The Bottom Line: for patients with ACL tear

Description and causes	Noncontact injury involving a planted foot with valgus knee, internal rotation of the femur, and external rotation of the tibia that tears the ACL
Test	Lachman, anterior drawer, pivot shift
Stretch	To regain knee ROM
Strengthen	Quadriceps and hamstrings, open chain, closed chain extension 0° to 45°
Train	Neuromuscular retraining including proprioception, plyometrics, balance retraining, and feedback on technique.[98,122,123]
Avoid	Collapse into valgus on jump-landing and pivoting

Interventions for the Surgical Patient

If the patient with an ACL-deficient knee is unable to cope with the instability caused by the ligament laxity or tear, it may be necessary to undergo an ACL reconstruction. The graft material used to create a new ACL may be taken from the patient's body (**autograft**) or taken from a cadaver (**allograft**). Most commonly, an autograft from the patellar tendon or the semitendinosus-gracilis muscles is used. Because the graft site impacts the postoperative rehabilitation program, these two surgical techniques and postoperative rehabilitation will be discussed separately.

ACL Reconstruction/Patellar Tendon Graft

Preoperative Phase

Many studies have shown the benefit of preoperative physical therapy for ACL tear. During this phase, education, stretching, strengthening, and neuromuscular training may allow some patients the ability to functionally manage their injury. If the patient elects to have a reconstruction, the outcome will be improved by preoperative exercises. The plan of care often includes exercises that mirror those used for patients who don't require surgical reconstruction.

Preoperative quadriceps muscle strength is a very good indicator of functional outcomes after ACL reconstruction.[111,112,114,124,125] Some researchers suggest that the strength of the quadriceps on the involved side should be at least 90% that of the uninvolved side before surgery. Additionally, it is beneficial to recovery if the patient has full knee extension range of motion, no extension lag during a straight leg raise, and minimal to no **effusion** going into surgery.[114]

Surgery

The middle one-third of the patellar tendon is commonly used for ACL reconstruction. In this surgery, the graft is harvested through an incision down the center of the knee. A piece of bone from the inferior patella and one from the tibial tuberosity are taken as well, creating a bone-patellar tendon-bone (BPTB) graft (Fig. 11.30). The ends of the graft are fixed to the anterior tibia and the posterior femur, mimicking the position of the ACL.

The advantage of the patellar tendon procedure is that the graft is less likely to fail than other graft types. The biggest complication is complaint of anterior knee pain, especially with kneeling. Patients may experience pain in kneeling or knee-walking that persists for many years.

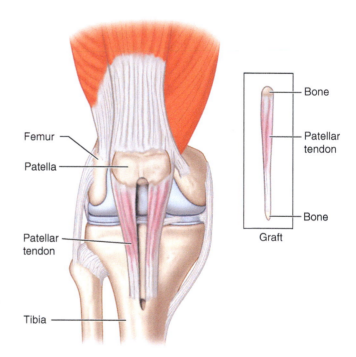

Figure 11.30 The middle third of the patellar tendon may be used for an ACL graft. A piece of the patella and of the tibial tuberosity are used to fix the graft into place.

Because the blood supply to the graft is disrupted when it is removed, the graft will begin to die. This process is called **necrotization** of the graft. Simultaneously, new cells begin to invade the graft and over time come to resemble the collagen of the natural ACL (**ligamentization**). As this process occurs, there is a period of time when the graft is most vulnerable around 6 to 8 weeks postoperatively.[126] The graft will continue to gain in strength over a period of 12 to 24 months.[127,128] It is important that the PTA bear this healing process in mind in the early months of rehabilitation after ACL reconstruction. The graph in Figure 11.31 depicts the process of graft healing.

Postoperative Phase

After an ACL-patellar tendon graft, common components of the plan of care include:

- Patellar mobilizations, focusing on superior glides to prevent **patella baja**, a patella that has been pulled inferiorly
- Pain and effusion control
- Strengthening of the hip (especially the gluteal muscles), quadricep, hamstring, and gastrocsoleus muscles using a combination of isometric, concentric, eccentric, open and closed chain exercises
- Stretching of the hamstrings, gastrocsoleus, and posterior knee with a goal of full extension/hyperextension range of motion and flexion up to 110° by 2 weeks postop[114]
- NMES to the quadriceps
- Cycling
- Perturbation activities such as single-leg standing[129,130]

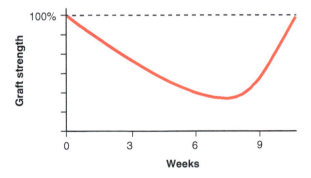

Figure 11.31 The patellar tendon graft is most vulnerable around 6 to 8 weeks postoperatively.

It is usually recommended initially that the patient limit active open chain quadricep strengthening to a range of 90° to 45° to prevent injury to the graft. Closed chain quadricep activities are also done in a limited range, usually from 0° to 60°, to minimize the stress on the graft and on the patellofemoral joint.

The patient will often be placed in a hinged, long-leg brace or an immobilizer to be worn night and day. As the patient's control of knee extension improves, the brace may be unlocked or discontinued. Crutches may be used until the patient is able to ambulate safely without pain.

Recent research indicates that quadriceps weakness is a common problem after ACL injury with or without reconstruction. Studies have shown a persistent deficit in quadriceps strength on the involved side as compared to the uninvolved side up to 2 years after surgery. This deficit averages 20%.[124] More aggressive strengthening of the quadriceps, including the use of neuromuscular training and eccentric exercise, is currently being recommended.[114,131–133] If the patient has concomitant meniscal or articular cartilage injuries that are addressed surgically when the ACL is reconstructed, the plan of care will be more conservative.

What's in the Plan of Care?

ACL Reconstruction/Hamstring Graft

Surgery

The semitendinosus ± gracilis tendons may be used as an autograft for ACL reconstruction. The advantage of this graft type is that anterior knee pain and pain with kneeling is rare. The disadvantage is that the graft is more likely to fail over time. In this procedure, the surgeon harvests the tendon of semitendinosus and possibly gracilis. The tendons are typically doubled and stitched together to create the graft (Fig. 11.32). The graft is inserted in the knee to mimic the position of the ACL.

Postoperative Phase

After ACL-hamstring tendon graft, common components of the plan of care include:

- Pain and effusion control
- Strengthening of the hip (especially the gluteal muscles), quadricep, and gastrocsoleus muscles using a combination of isometric, concentric, eccentric, open and closed chain exercises
- Stretching of the gastrocsoleus and posterior knee with a goal of full extension/hyperextension range of motion and flexion up to 110° by 2 weeks postop[114]
- NMES to the quadriceps
- Cycling
- Perturbation activities such as single-leg standing[129,130]

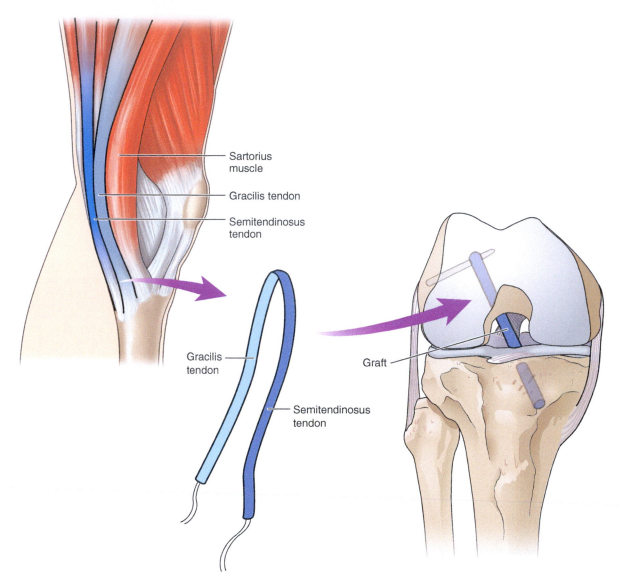

Figure 11.32 The semitendinosus and gracilis tendons may be used as a graft for ACL repair. The tendons are removed, folded, and used to reconstruct an ACL.

Caution must be used in stretching and strengthening the hamstring muscle to avoid injury to the donor site. Generally, gentle hamstring stretching may be performed after 1 week postop but resisted open chain hamstring exercises may not be initiated until 12 weeks postop.

As in the case of ACL repair with a patellar tendon graft, it is usually recommended that the patients with hamstring graft initially limit active open chain quadriceps strengthening to a range of 90° to 45° to prevent injury to the graft. Closed chain quadriceps activities are also done in a limited range, usually from 0° to 60°, to minimize the stress on the graft and on the patellofemoral joint.

The patient will often be placed in a hinged, long-leg brace or an immobilizer to be worn night and day. As the patient's control of knee extension improves, the brace may be unlocked or discontinued. Crutches may be used until the patient is able to ambulate safely without pain.

Some studies indicate that hamstring weakness is more of a problem after ACL reconstruction with a hamstring graft. In the late postoperative phase of rehabilitation, attention should be turned to the strength of the involved side hamstring as compared to the uninvolved side.

What's in the Plan of Care? Again, if the patient has concomitant meniscal or articular cartilage injuries that are addressed surgically when the ACL is reconstructed, the plan of care will be more conservative.

Posterior Cruciate Ligament Injury   CPG

The posterior cruciate ligament (PCL) is stronger, stiffer, and broader than the ACL and thus less prone to injury. The PCL prevents posterior movement of the tibia on the femur. Injury to the PCL includes grade I sprain without evidence of joint instability, grade II sprain with some joint instability (posterior cruciate-deficient knee), and grade III rupture or tear of the PCL. Grade I sprain will usually heal without incident. Grade II may require some short-term activity/sport modification, and grade III may require surgical repair for patients with an active lifestyle.

Causes/Contributing Factors

Injury to the PCL is most frequently caused by a direct blow to the anterior tibia ("dashboard injury"), a fall on a flexed knee with the foot in plantarflexion, or a sudden, violent hyperextension of the knee. Specifically, soccer-related injuries and motorcycle injuries account for the majority of PCL trauma.[92,134]

Symptoms

At the time of injury, common symptoms include pain, swelling, and tenderness in the knee. The patient may complain of a feeling of instability or giving way. Symptoms are likely to be increased during stair climbing or running. Although similar to the symptoms after ACL tear, the symptoms after PCL tear are generally more vague, leading to a frequent failure to diagnose.

Clinical Signs

Making the diagnosis of PCL tear often depends upon a variety of tests. Patient history and complaints, MRI results, and special tests are all useful. The physical therapist is likely to use one of the following special tests in the clinical diagnosis.

Posterior Drawer Test

The patient is positioned supine with the knee flexed to 90° and the foot resting on the examination table. The examiner sits on the patient's foot to stabilize the extremity. With thumbs spanning the tibiofemoral joint on the medial and lateral sides, the examiner pushes on the proximal tibia posteriorly, noting the amount of posterior translation (Fig. 11.33). A positive test is indicated by excessive posterior translation of the tibia as compared to the unaffected side.

Posterior Sag Test

The patient is positioned supine with the hip and knee flexed to 90° and the heel of the leg supported by the examiner. The patient is instructed to relax, and the examiner observes the appearance of the knee joint (Fig.

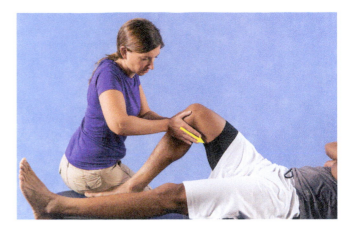

Figure 11.33 Posterior drawer test for PCL tear.

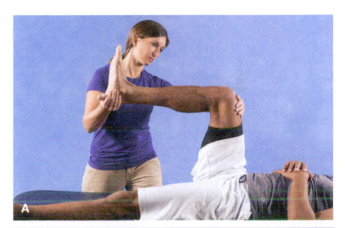

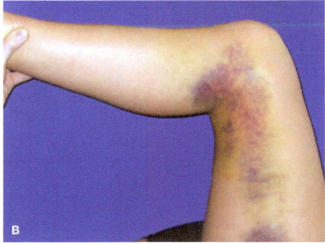

Figure 11.34 Posterior sag test for PCL tear (A). A positive sag test is indicated by posterior translation of the tibia (B).

11.34). If the tibia sags downward as compared to the unaffected side, it is a sign of a PCL tear.

Reverse Pivot Shift Test

The patient is positioned supine with the affected leg in hip flexion and about 70° of knee flexion. The examiner cradles the leg at the heel with one hand, placing the

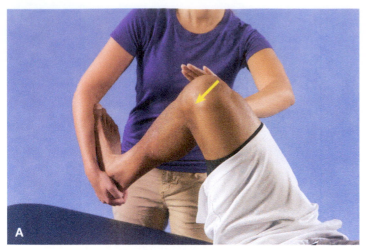

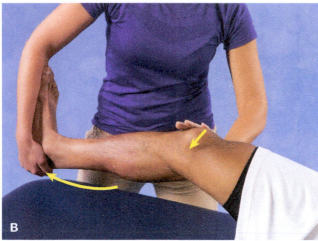

Figure 11.35 Reverse pivot shift test for PCL tear. The examiner applies a valgus force (A) while simultaneously extending the knee (B).

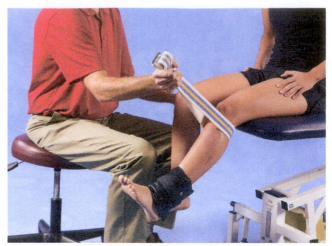

Figure 11.36 A gait belt or pillow case may be used to support the proximal tibia during strengthening exercises to avoid stressing the PCL.

other hand just distal to the knee. The examiner externally rotates the tibia, applies a valgus force, and then extends the knee (Fig. 11.35). If the PCL is lax or torn, the tibia will have been resting in a posterior position on the femur, but as the knee is brought into extension the IT band will reduce the tibia anteriorly and a clunk sound will be detected on the anterior side of the knee.

Common Interventions

Patients are much more likely to recover from PCL injury without the need for surgical intervention than from an ACL injury. Many studies have shown that patients with a grade I or II sprain often return to premorbid sport and activity levels; this may be true even in the case of grade III sprain.[135-139]

In general, rehabilitation after a PCL injury will be slower and more conservative than after an ACL injury.[140] The patient may be in a hinged-knee brace that limits knee flexion. Restoring knee range of motion is a commonly established goal, with or without the use of CPM. Because stress on the PCL increases at end ranges of knee flexion, the PT may limit the amount of knee flexion allowed. Patellar mobilizations may also be included in the plan of care.

Strengthening exercises should focus on the quadriceps, which assist the PCL in preventing posterior movement of the tibia. Closed chain quadriceps exercises in the 0° to 45° range may be preferred to minimize the forces on the patellofemoral joint and on the PCL. Focusing on the eccentric phase has been shown to be effective.[141] Neuromuscular training, core stabilization, and perturbation activities may be included in the plan of care.

> **What's in the Plan of Care?**

> ⚑ **CLINICAL ALERT**
>
> When strengthening patients with PCL tear or repair, care should be taken to support the tibia to prevent it from gliding posteriorly. Figure 11.36 demonstrates the use of a gait belt to support the proximal tibia.

The Bottom Line: for patients with PCL tear

Description and causes	Direct posteriorly directed blow to tibia (dashboard injury) or fall on flexed knee with plantarflexed foot that tears the PCL
Test	Posterior drawer, posterior sag, reverse pivot shift
Stretch	To regain motion, avoiding end range of knee flexion
Strengthen	Knee extensors closed chain 0° to 45°, focus on eccentric
Train	Proprioception
Avoid	End range of knee flexion, posterior sagging of tibia

Interventions for the Surgical Patient

PCL Reconstruction

Prior to surgery, the patient may be seen for therapy with the goals of normalizing range of motion, increasing strength, and optimizing function. The plan of care often includes range-of-motion exercises, quadriceps strengthening, hamstring strengthening in a limited range, patellar mobilizations, straight leg raises in all planes, and perturbation training.[142]

Surgery

Although it is possible to surgically repair the native PCL, reconstruction is the more common approach. Surgical reconstruction often involves use of a graft, similar to ACL reconstruction. Either the middle third of the patellar tendon or semitendinosus tendon is usually used.

Postoperative Phase

The plan of care after PCL reconstruction will generally include stretching, strengthening, gait training, and use of a stationary bike. Knee extension range of motion should be restored to full range as soon as possible. Patellar mobilization is recommended to maintain mobility of this joint.

> ⚑ **CLINICAL ALERT** ────────────
>
> Passive stretching will often be restricted to 90° of knee flexion for at least 2 weeks, with a goal of full knee flexion range of motion by 6 to 12 weeks.

Strengthening in the early postoperative phase often includes isometric quadriceps exercises, straight leg raise into hip flexion/abduction/adduction exercises, and gastrocnemius strengthening against elastic band resistance. Isotonic quadriceps exercises in a restricted range (0° to 60°) are initiated around 2 to 4 weeks *What's in the Plan of Care?* postoperatively. Active and resisted hamstring strengthening are generally not allowed until 18 weeks postop. After PCL reconstruction, the patient will be likely to have restricted weight-bearing for 2 to 4 weeks.

Medial Collateral Ligament Injury   CPG

The most commonly injured ligament in the knee is the medial collateral ligament (MCL). The MCL runs from above the medial epicondyle of the femur to the medial tibial condyle and provides stability to the medial knee to prevent valgus. Injury to this ligament may be of a grade I, II, or III sprain.

Causes/Contributing Factors

MCL sprain is usually the result of a blow to the lateral side of the knee with the foot in contact with the ground. The resulting valgus force stretches or tears the MCL. This is often an athletic injury. Sports in which MCL sprain is common include football, alpine skiing, ice hockey, soccer, rugby, basketball, and baseball.

> **Watch Out For...**
>
> **Watch out for** patients with MCL sprain to have other ligament injury as well. It is rare to have an MCL sprain in isolation, and it often occurs in conjunction with a cruciate ligament injury.

Symptoms

Immediately after MCL injury, knee swelling and complaint of pain are typical. The patient may complain of tenderness on the medial aspect of the knee. The knee may feel as if it's not stable and will give way into valgus.

Clinical Signs

Valgus Stress Test

The patient is positioned supine with the knee flexed to 20°. At 20° of knee flexion, the MCL is the primary restraint to valgus motion. The examiner supports the lower leg while palpating the medial joint line. A valgus force is applied to the knee (Fig. 11.37). Slight gapping is considered normal, but excessive gapping on the medial side of the knee indicates a positive test. The test is then

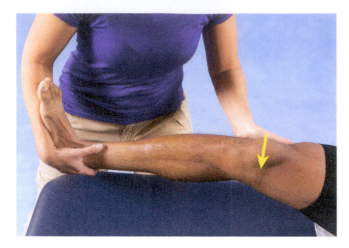

Figure 11.37 Valgus stress test of the knee for MCL injury.

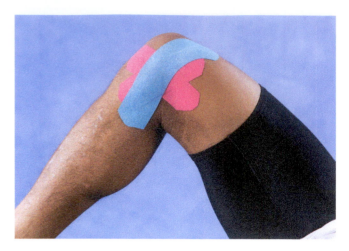

Figure 11.38 Taping of the medial knee may be useful in MCL sprain to provide proprioceptive feedback and increase medial knee stability.

repeated with the knee in full extension. No gapping should be observed in this position.

Common Interventions

The MCL has a greater capacity to heal than the cruciate ligaments.[143,144] Most researchers agree that patients will recover without surgical reconstruction or repair from a grade I or II sprain, and many researchers find that functional outcomes and return to sport are high even with grade III sprain.[145]

Rehabilitation of the patient with an isolated MCL sprain often includes quadriceps strengthening, restoration of normal range of motion, early weight-bearing, and use of a stationary bike. Taping may be used to increase proprioceptive feedback and stability in the medial knee (Fig. 11.38).

> **CLINICAL ALERT**
>
> Valgus stress should be avoided for 3 to 4 weeks to allow the MCL to heal. When the patient demonstrates knee stability with valgus stress testing at 20°, more aggressive side-to-side activities can be added to the therapy program.

The Bottom Line: for patients with MCL tear

Description and causes	Blow to the lateral knee with a planted foot resulting in a tear to the MCL
Test	Valgus stress test
Stretch	To regain normal knee ROM
Strengthen	Quadriceps
Train	Proprioception
Avoid	Valgus stress on knee

Interventions for the Surgical Patient

Repair/Reconstruction of the MCL

If the patient continues to have problems with frontal plane stability, repair or reconstruction of the MCL may be indicated. Repair involves suturing the ends of the ligament back together. In reconstruction, a graft from the semitendinosus tendon is used to re-create the MCL.

Postoperative Phase

In the first 2 weeks after surgery, the plan of care will likely include patellofemoral mobilization, quadriceps and hamstring strengthening in a restricted range (0° to 90°), range-of-motion exercises in this same restricted range, and straight leg raises. Valgus forces and rotation of the tibia should be avoided. The patient may be wearing a hinged knee brace locked in full extension. A non-weight-bearing gait is typical.

After 2 weeks, the patient is allowed to increase flexion range, add hip strengthening exercises, and begin hamstring curls standing. The hinged knee brace may be set to allow some flexion if the patient displays good quadriceps control. Use of a stationary bike may be added to the protocol in this phase. By 6 to 8 weeks, bilateral squats to 70° and proprioception exercises may be added.

Meniscal Tear CPG

The meniscal cartilage in the knee is prone to tear. The ability of a meniscal tear to heal depends upon several factors: where in the meniscus the tear occurs, the cause of the tear, and how large the tear is. This in turn determines treatment options.

Earlier in this chapter we discussed the blood supply to the meniscal cartilage. Blood flow is necessary for healing. If the tear occurs in the outer one-third ("red zone"), it is more likely to heal than a tear in the inner two-thirds of the cartilage. If the tear is due to acute trauma, it is more likely to heal than if associated with degenerative changes. If the tear involves many layers of meniscus with extensive cartilage damage, the likelihood of healing is low. Figure 11.39 depicts common tears seen in the meniscus.

Causes/Contributing Factors

Generally, tears of the meniscal cartilage occur due to acute trauma, chronic degenerative changes, or knee joint laxity. Acute tears are frequently incurred in contact sports and sports that involve cutting and pivoting. Most frequently they occur when pivoting on the leg with the knee in slight flexion. Chronic degenerative tears occur more frequently with age, with increased risk in males over the age of 60 with a history of work-related kneeling, squatting, and/or stair climbing.[146]

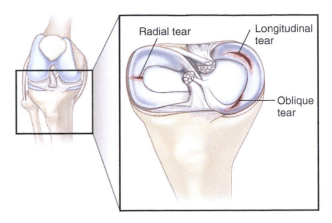

Figure 11.39 Common tears of the meniscus include oblique, radial, and longitudinal tears.

Symptoms

Patients with meniscal tear may have tenderness on palpation of the joint line. Pain and limitation of motion at the end range of flexion as well as limited extension range of motion may be present. The patient may complain of knee locking, clicking, or giving way.

Clinical Signs

There are several tests for meniscal tear. Because the sensitivity and specificity of these tests are questionable, the physical therapist may use a combination of tests to rule a meniscal tear in or out. Although joint line tenderness is not a special test, it is also used as a clinical sign.

McMurray Test

The patient is positioned supine. The examiner supports the patient's leg in hip and full knee flexion. While palpating the medial joint line, the examiner externally rotates the tibia and extends the knee, listening and feeling for a click to assess the medial meniscus. The test is repeated with the tibia in internal rotation, palpating the lateral joint line to test the lateral meniscus (Fig. 11.40). A positive test is indicated by a clicking or reproduction of the patient's symptoms.

Apley Test

The patient is positioned prone with the knee flexed to 90°. The examiner stabilizes the patient's leg by placing one knee on the patient's thigh. The examiner grasps the patient's ankle, pulls upward distracting the knee joint, and then rotates the tibia internally and externally. As evidence of meniscal tear, this part of the test should not reproduce the patient's pain. The examiner then applies a downward force through the tibia, compressing the joint, and then rotates the tibia internally and externally

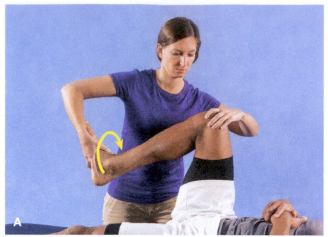

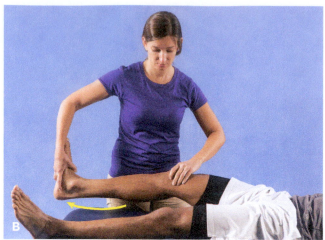

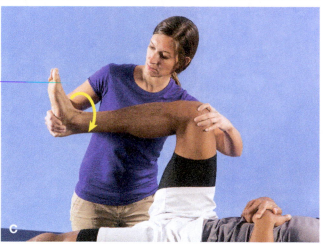

Figure 11.40 McMurray test for medial meniscus tear. The examiner flexes the knee and externally rotates the tibia (A). While extending the knee, the examiner palpates for a click (B) over the medial joint line. The maneuver is repeated with the tibia in internal rotation (C) to test the lateral meniscus.

(Fig. 11.41). A positive test is indicated by reproduction of the patient's pain with this part of the test.

Thessaly Test

The Thessaly test is done at 5° and 20° of knee flexion. The patient is standing on one leg, holding on to the examiner for support. The patient is instructed to flex the knee and then rotate on the leg to the left and to the right in a twisting motion. The motion is repeated three times in each direction (Fig. 11.42). A positive test is indicated by reproduction of the patient's symptoms.[147]

Ege Test

The patient stands with feet 12 to 15 inches apart. The patient squats with both legs in maximal external rotation and then slowly returns to standing. A positive test for medical meniscal tear is indicated if pain or a click is felt by the patient. The patient repeats the test by squatting with both legs in maximal internal rotation and then slowly standing (Fig. 11.43). Pain or a click with this maneuver indicates a lateral meniscal tear.[148]

Common Interventions

The plan of care after a meniscal tear will usually address goals of normalizing range of motion, increasing strength,

and improving neuromuscular control of the knee.[149] Modalities may be included for control of pain or effusion, including NMES.[150]

The strengthening program may include exercises for the quadricep, hamstring, and gastrocnemius muscles. Partial squats, long arc quadriceps, standing toe raises, and hamstring curls may be used. Neuromuscular exercises may include work on dynamic control of knee position and use of an unstable surface (Fig 11.44).

Prevention

Avoiding occupations that involve excessive kneeling, squatting, stair climbing, walking more than 2 hours per day, or carrying heavy objects will decrease the risk of meniscal tear. Patients at risk should be instructed to lose weight if appropriate. If the patient has an ACL deficient knee, they should be advised to talk to their physician about the increased risk of meniscal tear if they elect to postpone surgery.

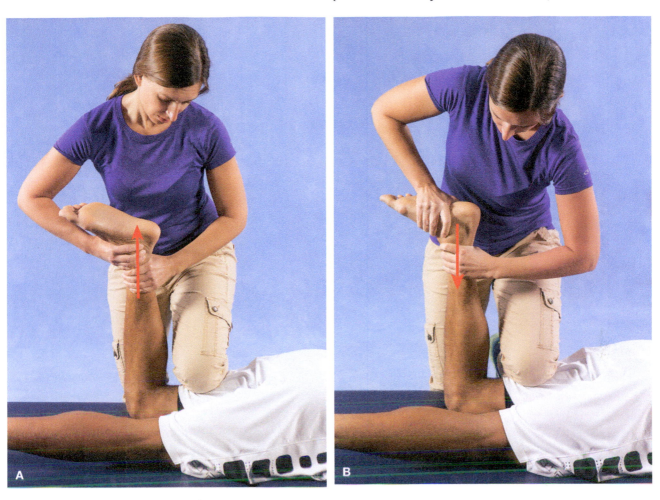

Figure 11.41 Apley distraction (A) and compression (B) test for meniscal tear.

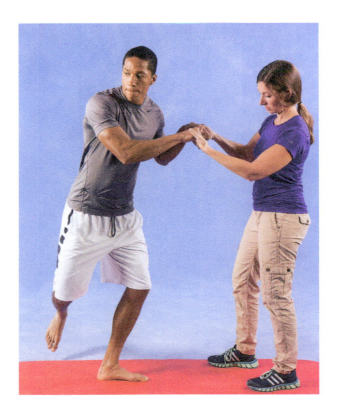

Figure 11.42 Thessaly test for meniscal tear.

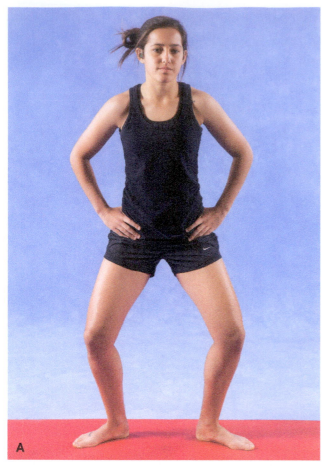

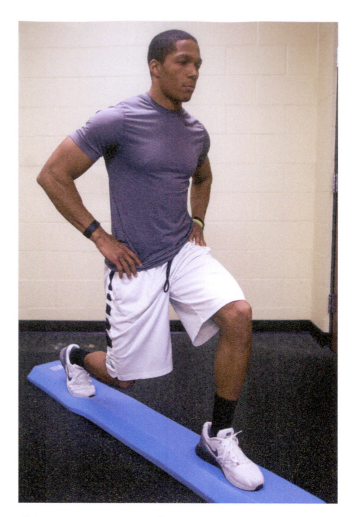

Figure 11.44 Neuromuscular exercises may include use of a foam balance beam to improve knee control.

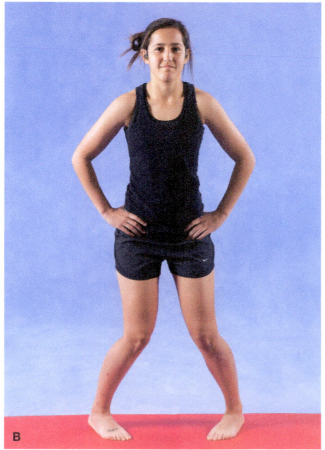

Figure 11.43 The Ege test for meniscal tear. The patient squats with legs in external rotation (A) and then in internal rotation (B).

The Bottom Line: for patients with meniscal tear

Description and causes	Tear of the meniscus as a result of trauma or degenerative changes. Acute trauma often involves pivoting on the leg with the knee in slight flexion.
Test	McMurray, Apley, Thessaly, Ege tests
Stretch	To regain knee ROM
Strengthen	Quadriceps, hamstrings, gastrocsoleus
Train	Proprioception
Avoid	Occupations that involve excessive kneeling, squatting, stair climbing, walking, or carrying heavy objects

Interventions for the Surgical Patient

Surgical treatments for a meniscal tear include repair, removal (**meniscectomy**), or transplantation of the meniscus with cadaver allograft. If the tear is in the outer one-third of the cartilage, a repair is often performed. If the tear is in the inner two-thirds, a partial meniscectomy is common. Meniscal transplantation is a recent surgical advancement. Since rehabilitation after repair and transplantation is the same, these will be presented together.

Meniscectomy

Removal of meniscal tissue is a meniscectomy. Partial meniscectomy is removal of a portion of the tissue near the tear. Complete meniscectomy is removal of the entire meniscus. Partial meniscectomy is preferred over complete meniscectomy, because of the role of the meniscus in distributing forces at the knee. Research has shown accelerated degenerative changes in the knee after removal of the meniscus.[31]

Postoperative Phase

After a meniscectomy, the patient may be seen for physical therapy with goals of controlling swelling and pain, restoring range of motion, improving strength, and normalizing gait. Modalities, including cryotherapy and electrical stimulation, may be used.

The exercise program will generally include strengthening of the hip, quadricep, hamstring, and gastrocnemius muscles.[150] A focus on strengthening of the quadriceps is essential to address quadriceps weakness that commonly persists for 6 months or more after meniscectomy.[151,152] Quadriceps strengthening has the potential to decrease dynamic joint load[24] and improve cartilage health.[153]

Meniscal Repair/Transplantation

In the case of a meniscal tear in the vascular area of the cartilage, a meniscal repair may be performed. This surgical procedure is performed through an **arthroscope**. The surgeon will use sutures or anchors to repair the tear (Fig. 11.45).

If the patient has had a total meniscectomy and is young (less than 50 years old) with pain in the tibio-femoral joint, cartilage transplantation may be beneficial. In this case, a cadaver allograft is inserted into the knee. The allograft consists of the entire meniscal cartilage and a bone bridge that is screwed into the top of the tibia.

Postoperative Phase

The goals for physical therapy after meniscal repair or transplantation will likely address range of motion, strength, gait, and pain. Rehabilitation after transplantation will be less aggressive and proceed more slowly than after a meniscectomy.

> ⚑ CLINICAL ALERT ——————
>
> After surgical repair, range of motion will likely be restricted to 0° to 90° for the first 2 weeks, with full range of motion allowed after 6 weeks. Patients are usually non-weight-bearing for 6 weeks.

The patient may be wearing a hinged, long-leg brace that is initially locked in full extension. The early goal

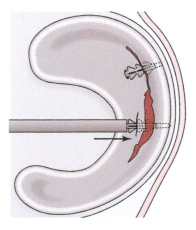

Figure 11.45 Meniscal repair may be performed for tears in the outer third of the meniscus.

is to maintain full knee extension. Patellar mobilizations, stretching into knee flexion to 90°, and into knee extension are typical.

Strengthening exercises initially may include isometric quadriceps sets and straight leg raises. Standing hamstring curls may be added around week 6, as well as limited-arc quadriceps exercises (90° to 30°) and multiple-plane hip exercises into abduction, extension, and flexion. Closed chain quadriceps exercises may be added 6 to 9 weeks after surgery. Early proprioceptive exercises consisting of weight shifting and use of a balance board may be included after 2 to 3 weeks and progressed to more aggressive neuromuscular retraining after 9 to 12 weeks.

Iliotibial (IT) Band Syndrome

Iliotibial band syndrome (ITBS), or iliotibial band friction syndrome, is a disorder characterized by strain or inflammation of the IT band as it crosses the lateral side of the knee (Fig. 11.46). Recall that the IT band is a thickened area of fascia latae that runs down the lateral thigh from the pelvis to the distal femur and lateral tibia. The inflammation occurs in the part of IT band where it crosses over the lateral femoral condyle. ITBS is referred to as "runner's knee."

Causes/Contributing Factors

It has long been believed that ITBS is due to frictional stresses of the IT band rubbing over the lateral femoral condyle with repeated knee flexion and extension.[154] When the knee is extended, the IT band lies anterior to the lateral femoral epicondyle, but with knee flexion of greater than 30°, it appears to move posterior to the epicondyle. Consistent with this is the observation that this disorder occurs most commonly in runners and cyclists, both sports involving repetitive flexion and extension of the knee. Recently, Fairclough et al. proposed that the source of pain with ITBS may be irritation of the fat pad under the IT band as it is compressed at 30° of knee flexion.[155]

Abnormalities in lower extremity kinematics have been linked to ITBS. Runners with ITBS have altered kinematics in the frontal and transverse plane. Specifically, it appears that hip adduction and tibial internal rotation are increased in people who develop ITBS. This position increases the stress on the IT band, which appears to contribute to an inflammation or strain with repeated flexion/extension.[156,157]

Tightness of the IT band and weakness of the hip abductors may increase the likelihood of ITBS. Varus knees may also contribute by increasing the stress on the IT band. Running downhill or on a sidehill increases the risk due to the compensatory altered biomechanics at the knee. Cycling with an in-toeing posture may contribute to ITBS. Leg length discrepancy may also increase risk.

Symptoms

Most commonly the patient will complain of pain on the lateral side of the knee joint that is worse after running or cycling. They may complain of tenderness to palpation about 1 inch proximal to the knee joint line on the lateral side. The hallmark sign is lateral knee pain on weight-bearing at 30° of knee flexion.

Clinical Signs

Clinical signs of ITBS include tenderness over the IT band at the knee and the presence of contributing factors such as a tight IT band. The Noble compression test assesses for tenderness over the area. An Ober test or modified Ober test may have been used by the physical therapist to assess IT band length.

Watch Out For...

Watch out for reassessment using the Ober test. It is important to use the same version of the test (Ober vs. modified Ober) when collecting data; these two tests cannot be used interchangeably.[158]

Ober Test

The patient is positioned in sidelying with the side to be tested upward. The hip and knee on the other side are slightly flexed. The examiner lifts the patient's leg by cradling it in one arm and then stabilizes the pelvis at the iliac crest. With the patient's knee flexed to 90°, the examiner gently guides the leg into hip extension and lets the leg adduct toward the table. According to Ober,

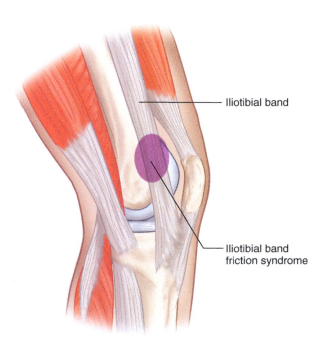

Iliotibial band

Iliotibial band friction syndrome

Figure 11.46 Iliotibial band syndrome causes pain on the lateral knee about an inch proximal to the joint line.

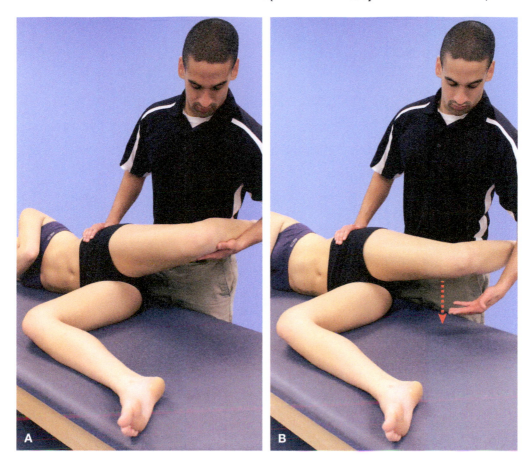

Figure 11.47 Ober test for IT band tightness. The examiner abducts the leg with knee flexion and stabilizes the pelvis (A). The leg is then extended at the hip and allowed to adduct (B).

normal range of motion should allow the leg to drop to the table (Fig. 11.47). A positive test is indicated by a loss of motion or an asymmetry when compared to the uninvolved side.

Modified Ober Test

The modified Ober test is done as previously mentioned with the knee kept in full extension. Again, normal range of motion should allow the leg to drop to the table (Fig. 11.48). A positive test is indicated by a loss of motion or an asymmetry when compared to the uninvolved side.

Noble Compression Test

The patient is positioned supine. The examiner passively flexes the patient's hip and knee to 90°. The examiner then puts pressure on the IT band just proximal to the lateral femoral condyle while passively extending the patient's leg (Fig. 11.49). A positive test is indicated by reproduction of the patient's pain at 30° of knee flexion.

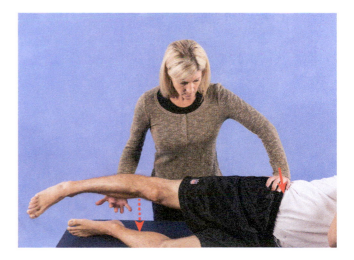

Figure 11.48 Modified Ober test for IT band tightness. In this test the knee is kept extended.

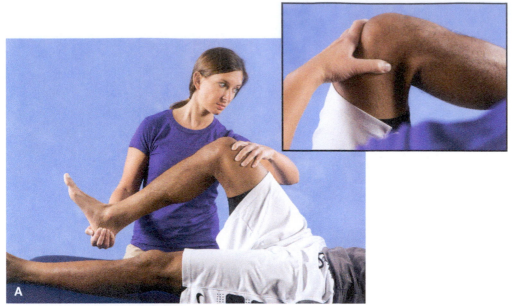

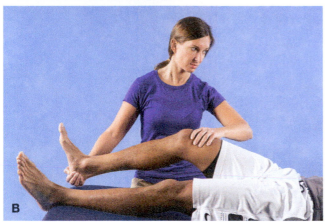

Figure 11.49 Nobel compression test for iliotibial band syndrome. The examiner places the hip and knee in flexion (A) and compresses the IT band (inset) while extending the knee (B).

Common Interventions

The plan of care for ITBS is likely to include modalities, stretching exercises, strengthening exercises, and patient education regarding normal lower extremity kinematics. Cryotherapy, ultrasound, and electrical stimulation may be used initially to decrease inflammation or pain.

IT band stretching is difficult to accomplish.[159] An effective stretch of the IT band is done by having the patient cross the affected leg behind the unaffected leg in a sidelying position, with or without stabilization on the iliac crest (Fig 11.50A–C). The patient may use a foam roller to stretch the IT band by sidelying over the roll and moving the body up and down to get an effect of massage and stretch of the IT band.

Strengthening exercises are a key component in the treatment of ITBS. Hip abduction strength has been shown to be diminished in patients with ITBS as compared to the unaffected side and as compared to a normal control group.[156] Strengthening hip abductor muscles is vital to correcting abnormal kinematics and decreasing the pain of ITBS.[156,157,160–162] Ultimately, running, walking, or cycling kinematics may need to be addressed.[163,164]

Prevention

Several factors have been associated with increased risk of ITBS. Patients at risk of ITBS should avoid overtraining, running on side hills, or downhill running. If a side hill cannot be avoided, alternate the leg that is downhill. Appropriate running shoes provide good support to maintain the foot in neutral alignment. Maintaining strong hip abductors and flexibility in the IT band is important. Cyclists should avoid in-toeing.

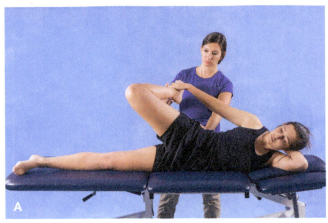

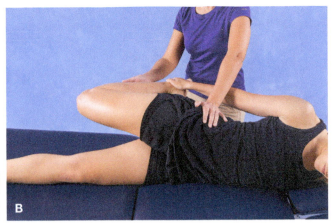

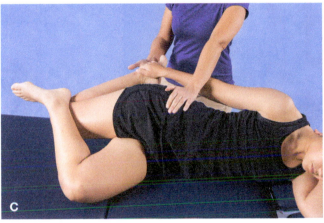

Figure 11.50 Stretching of the IT band can be performed sidelying by abducting the leg with pelvis stabilization (A). The patient then extends the hip (B) and brings the leg into adduction, using the opposite leg to increase the stretch (C).

The Bottom Line:	for patients with IT band syndrome
Description and causes	Inflammation of the IT band as it crosses the lateral femoral condyle associated with a tight IT band and repetitive knee flexion and extension as in running and cycling
Test	Noble compression test, Ober test, modified Ober test
Stretch	IT band
Strengthen	Hip abduction
Train	To avoid medial collapse of the knee
Avoid	Overtraining, running on side hills or downhill, cycling with in-toeing

Patellofemoral Pain Syndrome

Patellofemoral pain syndrome (PFPS) is the most common overuse injury in the lower extremity.[165] This syndrome refers to anterior knee pain that is aggravated by prolonged sitting (moviegoer's sign), squatting, kneeling, and going up or down stairs. It is more common in females, in runners, and in military recruits. People with PFPS are at increased risk to develop patellofemoral OA later in life.[31,165]

We know that the patellofemoral joint is subjected to stresses that exceed body weight. The compressive forces on the patellofemoral joint are estimated to be seven times body weight in squatting and going sit-to-stand. The structures under the patella, including articular cartilage, are assumed to contribute to the pain of PFPS.

Causes/Contributing Factors

This disorder has long been considered to be due to abnormal patellar tracking. We have come to appreciate that the causes or contributors to PFPS are many and involve not just "local" factors in the knee, but biomechanics of the hip and foot/ankle as well. In addition, there appears to be a contribution from central pain pathways.[166] We will discuss the contributors from the hip, knee, and foot/ankle separately.

Table 11-8	Patellofemoral Contributors
Hip	Increased hip adduction
	Increased hip internal rotation
	Weakness in gluteus medius (abduction)
	Weakness in gluteus maximus (extension and external rotation)
Knee	Bony geometry (shallow trochlear groove)
	Large Q-angle
	Relative weakness of VMO vs. VL
	Delayed timing of VMO vs. VL
	Tightness of IT band, lateral retinaculum
Foot/Ankle	Increased pronation/eversion
	Increased supination

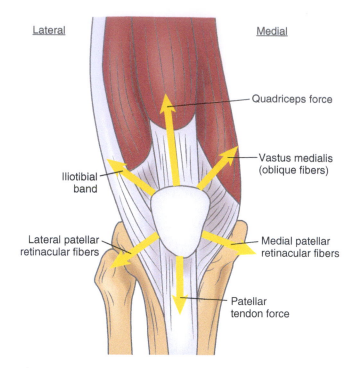

Figure 11.51 Multiple forces act on the patella. In PFPS, the lateral forces may overpower the forces pulling the patella medially.

Hip Contributors

The multiple contributors to PFPS that are proximal to the knee have recently become the subject of much interest. Patients with PFPS are more likely to have altered lower extremity kinematics as compared to normal subjects, especially during tasks such as running, single-leg jumping, and single-leg squatting. Specifically, it appears that subjects with PFPS are more likely to display increased hip adduction and internal rotation. This is especially true in females.

Consistent with these findings is the fact that many people with PFPS also display weakness in hip extensors, abductors, and external rotators. Patients with PFPS repeatedly demonstrate 15% to 25% more weakness in gluteus maximus and gluteus medius as compared to normal subjects.[22,167–173]

Medial collapse of the knee causes the femur to rotate medially under the patella.[15] This increases the contact between the lateral side of the patella and the lateral femoral condyle, contributing to increased wear on the patellofemoral joint. A summary of hip contributors can be found in Table 11-8.

Knee Contributors

Various factors in the knee seem to influence PFPS. These include patellar tracking, Q-angle, strength of the vastus medialis oblique as compared to the vastus lateralis, tightness of lateral structures, and timing of contraction of the medial versus the lateral vasti. Some studies have shown that patients with PFPS demonstrate lateral tracking of the patella. This seems to be related to the geometry of the bone, and extent of lateral tracking increases with increasing static Q-angle. The Q-angle is a measurement that quantifies the tendency of the patella to be pulled laterally.[11,21,165] The Q-angle in females is larger than in males, contributing to the increased tendency for females to experience PFPS.

Dynamic influences on the patella include the vastus medialis oblique (VMO), which has a nearly horizontal line of pull on the medial patella, opposed by the vastus lateralis (VL), which has a lateral attachment to the patella. One factor in PFPS appears to be relative weakness of the VMO versus the VL. Some studies have shown delayed activation of the VMO as compared to the VL, implicating *timing* of contraction rather than *strength*.

Other restraints to movement of the patella in the trochlear groove may pull the patella laterally. Tightness of the IT band, and consequently the lateral retinaculum, may increase lateral displacement. Figure 11.51 illustrates the many forces acting on the patella. A summary of knee contributors to PFPS can be found in Table 11-8.

Foot/Ankle Contributors

There is less consensus about the contribution of the foot to PFPS. Reports in the literature are that patients with PFPS are often pronators and have a low arch.[174] This would tend to increase the valgus force at the knee, thereby increasing the Q-angle. However, Thijs et al. reported that patients with PFPS were more likely to have decreased pronation and weight-bear on the lateral foot compared to normal subjects.[175] The subjects in this study were mostly male, which may explain the conflicting findings. It appears that altered foot biomechanics, either by excessive pronation or supination, can contribute to PFPS. A summary of foot and ankle contributors can be found in Table 11-8.

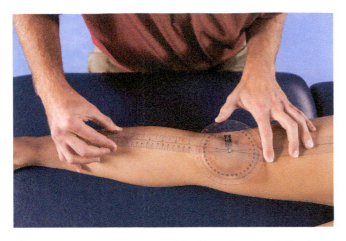

Figure 11.52 Measurement of the Q-angle using ASIS, the center of the patella, and tibial tuberosity as landmarks.

Symptoms

The most common symptoms of PFPS are pain in the anterior knee that is increased with prolonged flexion positioning of the knee and with squatting, stair climbing, running, and kneeling. Patients may have crepitus when squatting or going sit-to-stand. They may complain of stiffness after prolonged knee flexion.

Clinical Signs

Clinical signs of PFPS rely heavily on patient history, findings of tightness or weakness in contributing structures, abnormal tracking of the patella, findings of crepitus, and reproduction of the patient's complaints by compression, squatting, or stair-stepping. The following tests and measures are useful in data collection.

Measurement of Q-angle

Q-angle can be measured in supine or in standing position, with knees flexed or extended, and with the quadriceps muscle relaxed or contracting. The standard Q-angle measurement is performed with the patient supine, knee extended and relaxed. The goniometer is positioned so that the axis of rotation is in the center of the patella. The proximal arm of the goniometer extends to the anterior superior iliac spine (ASIS), and the distal arm bisects the tibial tuberosity (Fig. 11.52). Roughly, this measurement mimics the lines of pull of the quadriceps on the patella and the patellar tendon on the tibia. It provides a relative idea of the force acting on the patella to move it laterally out of the trochlear groove. Normal Q-angle is about 11° to 13° in males and 15° to 17° in females.[10–12]

Ely Test

The Ely test assesses the length of rectus femoris. The patient is positioned prone. The examiner passively flexes the patient's knee, not allowing anterior tilting of the pelvis or extension of the lumbar spine (Fig. 11.53).

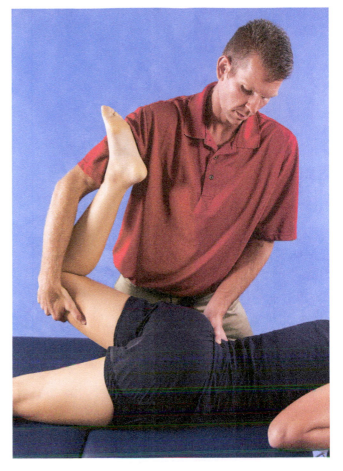

Figure 11.53 Ely test for assessing rectus femoris length.

Normal range of motion is 135°. Less than this indicates tightness in rectus femoris that may be contributing to PFPS.

Functional Activity Tests

The patient performs a variety of functional tests, which include squatting, step ups, step downs, and kneeling. A positive test is indicated by reproduction of the patient's pain. The most common functional activity that reproduces the patient's pain is stepping down or squatting.

Compression Tests

There are several tests that rely on compression of the patella into the trochlear groove. The patient is positioned supine with knee extended. The examiner may either (1) push straight down on the patella, compressing it into the groove, or (2) glide the patella inferiorly and then instruct the patient to perform an isometric quadriceps contraction (Fig. 11.54). A positive sign for both compression tests is reproduction of pain.

Retinaculum Tightness Tests

Tightness of the medial or lateral retinaculum may be assessed as an indicator of PFPS. As an indicator of retinaculum tightness, the patient lies supine with knee

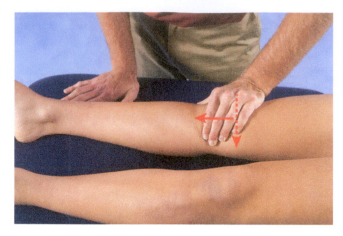

Figure 11.54 Compression test for PFPS. The examiner compresses the patella while gliding it inferiorly and preventing superior glide during a quadriceps set.

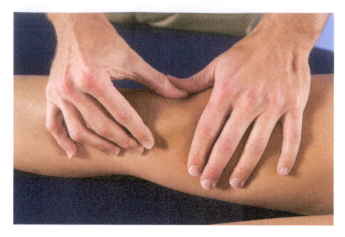

Figure 11.56 Patellar tracking test for PFPS.

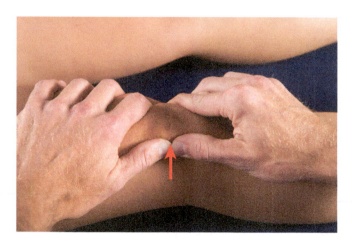

Figure 11.55 Retinaculum tightness test for PFPS.

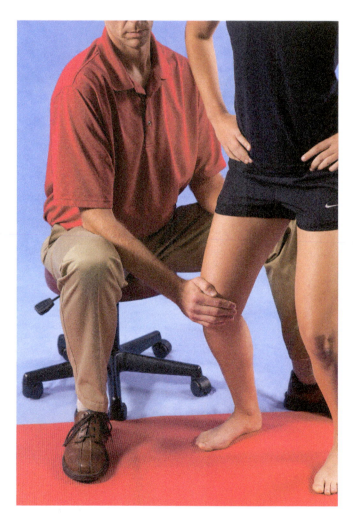

Figure 11.57 Crepitus palpation test for PFPS.

extended and relaxed. The examiner glides the patella medially and laterally. Normal range of patellar motion each way is one-quarter or more of the patellar width.

Alternatively, lateral retinaculum tightness may be assessed by having the patient supine with knee extended and relaxed. The examiner attempts to lift the lateral border of the patella upward (Fig. 11.55). A positive test is indicated by inability to raise the lateral border above the horizontal plane.[176]

Patellar Tracking Test

The patient is positioned supine with knee extended and relaxed. The examiner lightly palpates the patella on each side with enough force to allow observation of the direction the patella moves, but not so much as to prevent or alter movement. The examiner instructs the patient to perform an isometric quadriceps set (Fig. 11.56). Abnormal patellar tracking would be indicated by more lateral movement of the patella than superior movement.

Crepitus Palpation Test

The patient is positioned either supine or standing. The examiner places the heel of the hand on the anterior knee of the patient with light compression. While the patient flexes the knee or performs a squat, the examiner palpates for crepitus (Fig. 11.57). Crepitus is an abnormal finding.

Common Interventions

With an understanding of the many contributors to patellofemoral pain syndrome, it is not surprising that interventions often involve the hip, knee, and ankle. Stretching, strengthening, and neuromuscular re-education exercises are commonly used to improve lower extremity kinematics. Modalities to relieve pain and swelling may be indicated. Use of orthotic devices, tape, and braces may also be included.

Hip Interventions

Contemporary research has highlighted hip weakness or loss of neuromotor control as significant contributors to PFPS. Addressing these deficits is effective in reducing pain for patients with PFPS. Strengthening exercises for hip abductor, extensor, and external rotator muscles are commonly included in the plan of care.[165,177–181] Neuromuscular re-education aimed at normalizing lower extremity kinematics during walking, running, squatting, and jumping may also be included in the plan.

Knee Interventions

Physical therapy for PFPS will often include strengthening of the quadriceps muscle. Because of the ability of the VMO to act as a dynamic restraint to lateral movement, preferred exercises may target this muscle.

> ⚑ **CLINICAL ALERT**
>
> A challenge for the physical therapist assistant is in strengthening the knee extensors but avoiding increased pain due to stress on the patellofemoral joint. In general, PFPS patients tend to tolerate closed chain extension better than open chain. In closed chain, the stress on the patellofemoral joint is lowest in the 0° to 40° range (see Fig.11.58A). In open chain, the stress is lowest in the 60° to 90° range (see Fig. 11.58B).[182]

Initially the patient may perform isometric quadriceps exercises. Quadriceps sets, straight leg raises, and straight leg raises with hip external rotation are all commonly

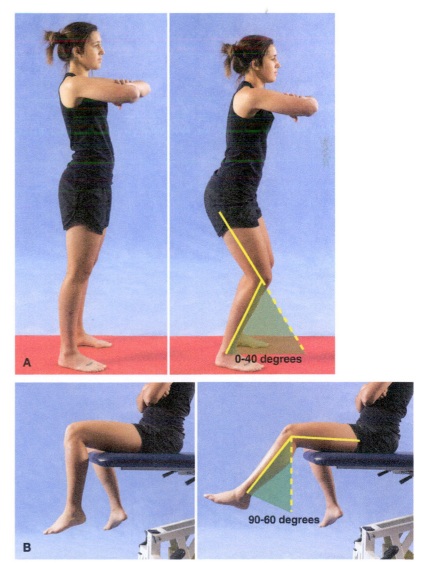

Figure 11.58 Compression on the patellofemoral joint is least in closed chain from 0° to 40° and in open chain from 90° to 60°.

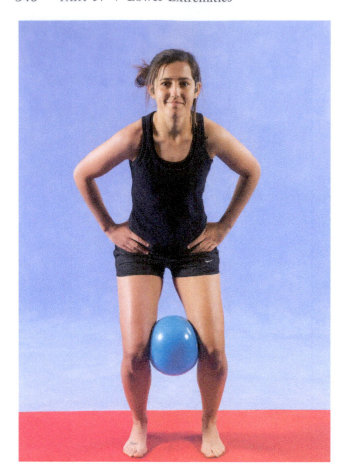

Figure 11.59 Squats with isometric hip adduction can be used to strengthen VMO.

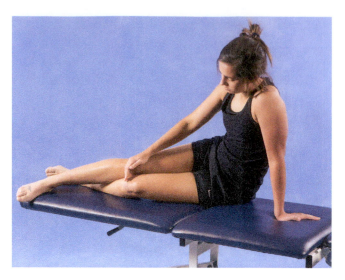

Figure 11.60 Teach the patient to self-stretch the lateral retinaculum by gliding the patella medially.

used.[183,184] As a progression, closed chain exercises (0° to 40°) may be added, such as partial squats, wall squats, and leg press. To facilitate the VMO, the patient may perform squats while simultaneously squeezing a ball (Fig. 11.59). Open chain knee extension exercises (60° to 90° range) may also be used. Timing of the VMO and VL may be addressed by use of biofeedback.[185]

Stretching of tight structures may also be included in the plan of care. This may include stretching the IT band and lateral retinaculum, as well as tensor fascia latae, quadriceps, and hamstring muscles.[176,186] To self-stretch the lateral retinaculum, have the patient perform a medial patellar glide with the knee in extension. This is most effectively done in sidelying position with the affected side up (Fig. 11.60).

Patellar taping using rigid strapping tape or an elastic therapeutic tape may be included in the plan of care. Jenny McConnell[187] first proposed taping the patella to improve alignment and tracking.[190,191] Studies have shown it to be effective in reducing pain. There are many techniques for patellar taping. Box 11-2 details the McConnell technique for PFPS.

Foot/Ankle Interventions

In an attempt to minimize the effect of pronation or supination on the knee, the plan of care may include stretching of the gastrocnemius and soleus muscles. The patient may be fit with orthoses to improve foot control.

Prevention

Risk of PFPS can be reduced by strengthening hip extensors, external rotators, and abductors. Stretching exercises should focus on maintaining flexibility in rectus femoris, hamstring, and gastrocsoleus muscles. The patient may benefit from use of orthoses to correct foot mechanics if appropriate.

Box 11-2   McConnell Taping

Alignment Assessment

The patellar alignment is assessed for glide, medial-lateral tilt, rotation, and superior-inferior tilt. The patient is positioned supine with the knee extended and relaxed.

Glide

The examiner lightly places thumb and index finger on either side of the patella to assess patellar position and palpate, but not interfere with, the movement. The patient is instructed to isometrically contract the quadriceps muscle. The examiner notes if the patella tracks in the trochlear groove or if it tends to track medially or laterally. It is common with patients with PFPS to have lateral tracking.

Medial-Lateral Tilt

The examiner palpates the lateral and medial borders of the patella with thumb and index finger, noting if the patella is level. If one side is lower, the patient has a tilted patella. It is common in patients with PFPS to have a lower lateral side, indicating tightness in the lateral structures.

Superior-Inferior Tilt

The examiner palpates the superior and inferior poles of the patella with thumb and index finger, noting if the patella is level from top to bottom. If one end is lower, the patient has a tilted patella. It is common in patients with PFPS to have a lower inferior pole, which may contribute to irritation of the fat pad distal to the patella.

Rotation

The examiner palpates the superior and inferior poles of the patella, noting if they are in line with the long axis of the femur. If they are not in alignment, the patient has a rotated patella. It is most common in patients with PFPS to have a laterally rotated inferior pole.

Taping Intervention

The glide component is corrected first. The examiner glides the patella medially while applying tape from the lateral patellar border to the medial knee (Fig. A). The patient is then asked to perform the movement that elicits pain to determine the effectiveness of the tape. If the tape is not effective, it is removed.

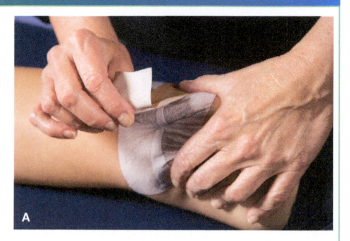

Secondly, the medial tilt component is corrected if an abnormality is detected. If the patient has a high medial patella, a second strip of tape is placed over the first, starting at the vertical midline of the patella (Fig. B). Again, the patient is asked to perform the movement that elicits pain to determine the effectiveness of this piece of tape. If the tape is not effective, it is removed.

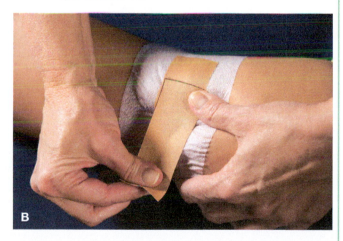

Next, the superior-inferior tilt component is corrected if an abnormality is detected. A strip of tape is placed over the first, starting at the lateral border of the patella. It covers either the superior or inferior half of the patella on the side that is high (Fig. C). Most commonly, patients with PFPS will require tape on the top half to raise the inferior pole out of the fat pad. Again, the patient is asked to perform the movement that elicits pain to determine the effectiveness of this piece of tape. If the tape is not effective, it is removed.

Continued

Box 11-2 McConnell Taping—cont'd

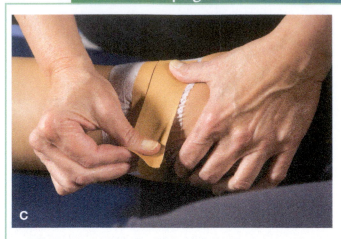

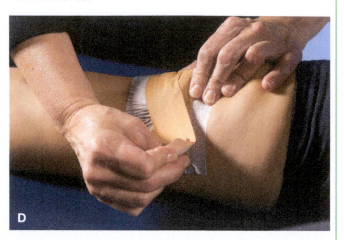

medially while rotating the patella into alignment (Fig. D). As before, if this piece of tape is not effective, it is removed.

Lastly, the rotation component is corrected if an abnormality is detected. If the patient has an inferior pole that is rotated laterally, a piece of tape is applied from the middle of the inferior pole upwards and

The Bottom Line: for patients with patellofemoral pain syndrome

Description and causes	Irritation of the patellofemoral joint that may be due to multiple factors from the hip, knee, and/or ankle and foot
Test	Q-angle measurement, Ely test, functional activity test, compression tests, retinaculum tightness test, patellar tracking test, crepitus palpation test
Stretch	Lateral retinaculum, IT band, rectus femoris, hamstrings, gastrocsoleus
Strengthen	Hip abductors, hip extensors, hip external rotators, VMO
Train	Closed chain 0°–40°, open chain 60°–90°, neuromuscular control, timing of VMO vs. VL
Avoid	Pronation

Interventions for the Surgical Patient

If the instability of the patella is severe and conservative treatment is not successful, the patient may require surgery. Surgical options include release of a tight lateral retinaculum, shortening of an elongated medial retinaculum, reconstruction of the trochlear groove, transfer of the tibial tuberosity to a more medial location, and derotation osteotomy of the tibia or femur.

Patellar Tendinopathy

Patellar tendinopathy refers to a range of conditions from inflammation of the patellar tendon (tendinitis) to chronic degeneration (tendinosus). This pathology is commonly referred to as "jumper's knee." If the tendinopathy becomes chronic, it may predispose the patient to partial or complete rupture. The portion of the tendon that is most commonly affected is the proximal end at the inferior pole of the patella.

In the young, skeletally immature athlete, stresses on the patellar tendon may result in inflammation of the growth plate under the tibial tuberosity referred to as **Osgood-Schlatter's disease.** This is due to repeated trauma caused by overuse of the quadriceps. Shortening of the rectus femoris muscle increases the likelihood of Osgood-Schlatter's disease. It results in increased bone growth at the tibial tuberosity (Fig. 11.61).

Causes/Contributing Factors

Patellar tendinopathy appears to result from eccentric overload/overuse of the patellar tendon. Athletes who participate in sports that involve jumping and running, particularly basketball and volleyball, are at highest risk. The kinematics of jumping and landing may be a factor; patients with patellar tendinopathy display a landing pattern that is more upright with increased stress on the knee extensors as compared to normal controls.[190,191] Figure 11.62 depicts this difference.

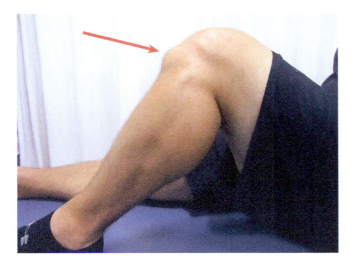

Figure 11.61 Osgood-Schlatter's disease is a result of inflammation of the epiphyseal plate under the tibial tuberosity, resulting in enlargement of the tuberosity.

Limited quadriceps and hamstring length may contribute to patellar tendinopathy.[192] Also shown to be a contributor is limited ankle dorsiflexion range of motion.[193,194] In the presence of limited dorsiflexion, the ankle is unable to effectively absorb the impact from a jump landing, increasing the forces on the knee extensor mechanism.

Symptoms

Patients with patellar tendinopathy will complain of pain over the patellar tendon with jumping, running, and squatting. The onset of symptoms is gradual. The pain may be first noticed after participation in sports but become more constant as inflammation progresses.

Clinical Signs

Clinical signs of patellar tendinopathy are consistent with those of contractile tissue pathology: pain with stretch, contraction, and palpation. Patellar tendinopathy causes tenderness to palpation, usually found at the inferior pole of the patella at the origin of the tendon. To assess for this, palpate the tendon when the patient is supine with the knee extended and quadriceps relaxed. Reproduction of the patient's pain with resisted knee extension is a second clinical sign of patellar tendinopathy. This can be reproduced in open or closed chain. Lastly, in some instances the patient will complain of increased pain with passive knee flexion at end ranges.

In addition, the following tests may be used to diagnose this pathology.[195] Because the inflammation of the patellar tendon is usually in the deeper fibers, tensing of the tendon forms a protective barrier that decreases pain with palpation. These two tests rely on this by comparing tenderness in a relaxed tendon versus a tensed tendon.

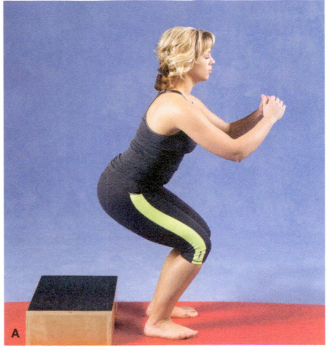

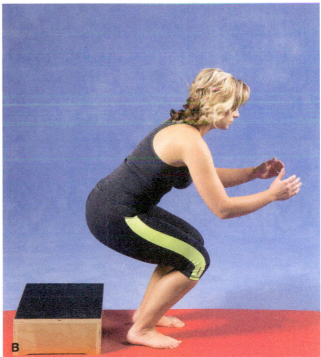

Figure 11.62 Landing pattern associated with jumping athletes at increased risk of patellar tendinopathy. Upright landing (A) increases the stress on the quadriceps and patellar tendon. Squat landing (B) increases use of gluteus maximus.

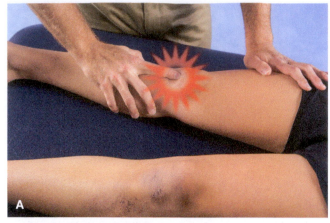

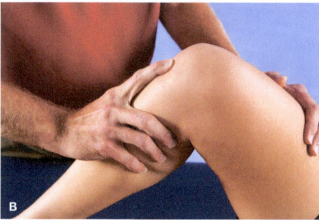

Figure 11.63 Passive flexion-extension test for patellar tendinopathy. With the knee extended and quadriceps relaxed (A), palpation of the tendon is painful. When the knee is flexed and the superficial fibers of the tendon are taut (B), pain on palpation is reduced.

Passive Flexion-Extension Test

The patient is positioned supine with knee extended and quadriceps relaxed. The examiner palpates for the point of maximal tenderness. The patient then flexes the knee to 90°, and pressure is again applied by the examiner (Fig. 11.63). A comparison of the amount of tenderness to palpation in the two positions is made. A positive test is confirmed if the flexed position is less tender.

Standing Active Quadriceps Test

The patient is positioned standing with knee extended and quadriceps relaxed. The examiner palpates for the point of maximal tenderness. The patient is then instructed to stand only on the tested leg and flex the knee to 30°. This point is again palpated, and a comparison of tenderness is made between the two positions (Fig. 11.64). A positive test is confirmed by a reduction in tenderness when the quadriceps muscle is contracted.

Common Interventions

The plan of care for patellar tendinopathy is likely to include modalities, stretching exercises, strengthening exercises, and neuromuscular retraining. Initially, anti-inflammatory modalities including cryotherapy may help control pain and swelling. Stretching exercises to the rectus femoris, hamstring, and gastrocsoleus muscles are effective treatment options.

Strengthening gluteus maximus, quadriceps, and gastrocsoleus muscles is very important. Gluteus maximus is important for sagittal plane control in a jump landing or squat and can ease the stresses on the quadriceps and patellar tendon. Quadriceps strengthening may be done concentrically or eccentrically but is most effective eccentrically.[196–109] Squats performed on a decline board are more effective in treatment of patellar tendinopathy than when performed on level surfaces (Fig. 11.65).[199,200] Strengthening gastrocsoleus in open or closed chain is also an important component in the treatment of patellar tendinopathy.[201]

Prevention

Patients should be encouraged to lose weight if appropriate. Maintaining flexibility of the rectus femoris, hamstring, and gastrocsoleus muscles and strength of the quadriceps and gluteus maximus is beneficial. Encourage the patient to wear orthotic devices for correction of foot mechanics if warranted. Athletes should be instructed to avoid a stiff landing pattern in jump-landing.

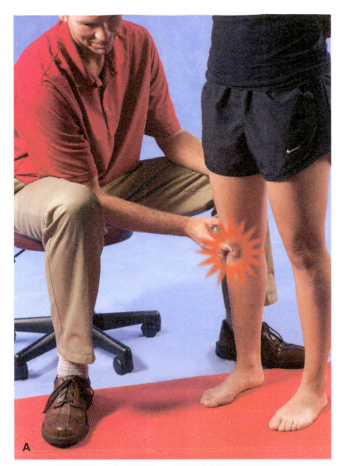

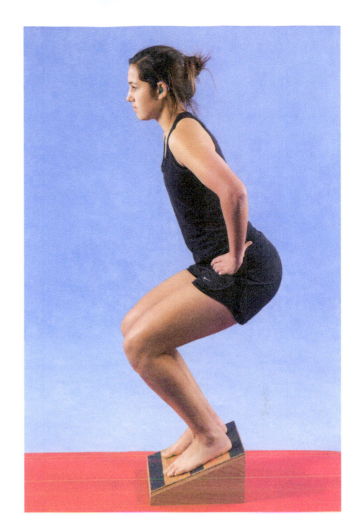

Figure 11.65 Squats performed on a decline board may be included in the plan of care for patellar tendinopathy.

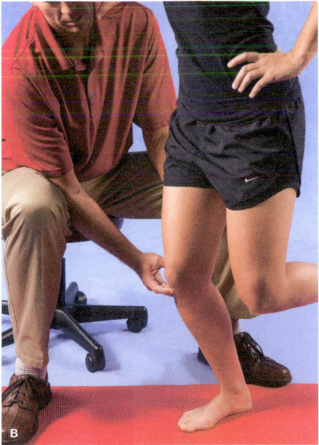

Figure 11.64 Standing active quadriceps test for patellar tendinopathy. Similar to the passive flexion-extension test, with the knee extended and quadriceps relaxed (A), palpation of the tendon is painful. When the knee is flexed and the superficial fibers of the tendon are taut (B), pain on palpation is reduced.

The Bottom Line:	for patients with patellar tendinopathy
Description and causes	Inflammation of the patellar tendon associated with weak gluteus maximus, and tight quadriceps and gastrocsoleus in jumping athletes
Test	Passive flexion-extension test, standing active quadriceps test
Stretch	Quadriceps, hamstrings, gastrocsoleus
Strengthen	Gluteus maximus, quadriceps, gastrocsoleus
Train	Quadriceps eccentrically, landing pattern for jumping athletes
Avoid	Landing from a jump in an upright posture

Patellar Tendon Rupture

Patellar tendon rupture is a rare but very disabling condition that may result from patellar tendinopathy. Rupture of the patellar tendon may be partial or complete. It most often occurs at the patellar tendon's origin on the inferior pole of the patella.

Causes/Contributing Factors

The cause of rupture is often trauma from a jump-landing onto a flexed knee or a fall onto a flexed knee. Rupture is uncommon because the patellar tendon is very thick and strong. When rupture does occur, it is usually in the presence of predisposing factors such as chronic patellar tendinopathy, history of ACL reconstruction using a patellar tendon graft, or steroid injections into the patellar tendon. Other conditions associated with patellar tendon rupture include diabetes mellitus, systemic lupus erythematosus, obesity, chronic renal disease, rheumatoid arthritis, and hyperparathyroidism.

Symptoms

The most indicative symptom of a complete patellar tendon rupture is inability to actively extend the knee. Patients will have pain and difficulty ambulating. They may be unable to ambulate or ambulate by hyperextending the knee in stance phase to compensate. Swelling and bruising may be noticed.

Clinical Signs

The patella will be pulled superiorly because of the lack of distal attachment. This finding is called **patella alta** and may be discovered on x-ray or by palpation. Palpation of the patellar tendon may be impeded by swelling but often will reveal the tendon rupture. There are no special tests for patellar tendon rupture.

Common Interventions

Surgical repair of the tendon will be performed prior to initiating physical therapy.

Interventions for the Surgical Patient

Repair/Reconstruction of the Patellar Tendon

Surgery for patellar tendon rupture may involve suturing the ends of the tendon together, reattaching the end of the tendon to the bone, or use of hamstring autograft or cadaver allograft (often the Achilles tendon) to augment the patellar tendon. Figure 11.66A depicts repair of patellar tendon rupture by suturing, and Figure 11.66B depicts reconstruction using semitendinosus autograft.

Postoperative Phase

Therapy after a patellar tendon repair will depend largely upon the type of repair, as well as on the age and general health of the patient. In general, after an uncomplicated repair, the patient will ambulate with crutches, touch weight-bearing. Often a hinged knee brace is worn locked in full extension.

> **CLINICAL ALERT**
>
> The brace is to be worn at all times unless the patient is performing exercises. Range of motion will likely be restricted from 0° to 30°.

The patient may begin with isometric exercises of the quadriceps, hamstring, and gluteus maximus muscles. Patellar mobilizations may be included. Gentle stretching of hamstring and gastrocnemius muscles may also be included. Use of modalities such as cryotherapy and electrical stimulation are often used to control pain and swelling.

After 3 weeks, the patient may be progressed to allow passive knee flexion to 90°. Active **What's in the Plan of Care?** knee extension will likely remain restricted, as well as passive hyperextension. The patient may begin to perform weight-bearing as tolerated gait, heel slides, and straight leg raises in all planes with the brace locked in extension. By about 7 to 10 weeks postop, the patient will be allowed to actively contract quadriceps and begin some mini-squats in a limited range.

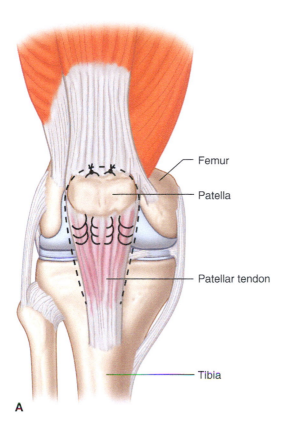

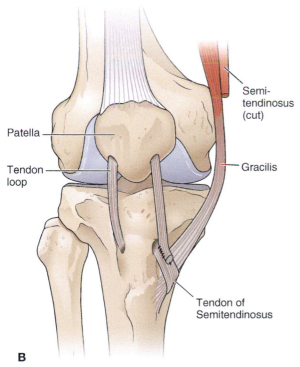

Figure 11.66 Patellar tendon rupture may be surgically repaired by suturing the ends together (A) or by using a graft (B). If the tendon of semitendinosus is used, it is left attached at its insertion and threaded through holes in the patella and tibial tuberosity, as shown.

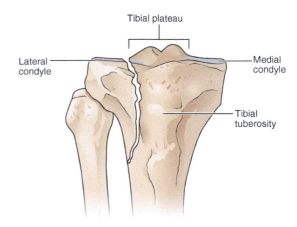

Figure 11.67 Lateral tibial plateau fracture.

Tibial Plateau Fracture

A fracture that involves the proximal tibia and disrupts the tibial weight-bearing surface is called a tibial plateau fracture. These fractures may involve the medial or lateral tibial plateau or the central area. They may be bicondylar, involving both sides of the tibia. In the case of high-impact trauma, the tibia may sustain a transverse fracture, separating the diaphysis from the metaphysis. Figure 11.67 depicts a typical lateral tibial plateau fracture.

Causes/Contributing Factors

Typically, these fractures are caused by a motor vehicle accident, a fall, or a sport injury in which the compression force on the knee is coupled with a varus or valgus force. The lateral tibial plateau is more commonly fractured than the medial side.

Symptoms

The patient will often present with a history of trauma, and complaints of pain and swelling in the knee, with an inability to bear weight. If there is damage to the collateral ligaments or the cruciate ligaments, instability may be a primary complaint.

Clinical Signs

There are no special tests for tibial plateau fracture. Patient symptoms and history will usually lead to x-ray findings.

Common Interventions

If the tibial plateau fracture is nondisplaced, the patient may not need to have a surgical repair. In this case, the patient will usually be placed in a hinged knee brace locked in full extension and will likely be restricted to non-weight-bearing for up to 3 months. Depending upon the type of fracture and other soft tissue damage, the

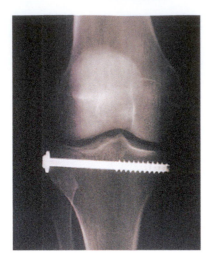

Figure 11.68 ORIF screw fixation of a tibial plateau fracture.

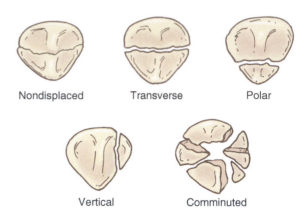

Figure 11.69 Types of fractures of the patella include nondisplaced, transverse, polar, vertical, and comminuted.

patient may be restricted in performing range of motion and/or strengthening exercises for several weeks.

Interventions for the Surgical Patient

ORIF of the Tibial Plateau

If the fracture is displaced, or if there is meniscal or ligamentous injury, the patient will likely undergo surgical repair in the form of an ORIF. This typically involves screw, or plate and screw, fixation (Fig. 11.68).

Postoperative Phase

> ► **CLINICAL ALERT** ——————
>
> After ORIF, the patient will probably be wearing a hinged knee brace locked in full extension for 6 weeks. The brace is removed for therapy only. Gait is usually restricted to non-weight-bearing (NWB) for 12 weeks. AAROM exercises are restricted as healing of the incision allows, but generally 0° to 70° in the acute phase. Commonly, a goal of 90° of flexion by 4 weeks postop is set.

Strengthening initially includes straight leg raises in all planes and quadriceps sets focusing on VMO contraction. Ankle strengthening, strengthening of the unaffected limb, and patellar mobilization are often included in the plan of care. Closed chain strengthening is delayed due to restrictions in the patient's weight-bearing status (6 to 12 weeks). Proprioceptive retraining may also be included in the plan of care when weight-bearing restrictions are lifted.

Patellar Fracture

The patella is susceptible to fracture. The types of fracture that can occur here include transverse, polar (lower or upper pole), vertical, and comminuted, which can be displaced or nondisplaced fractures (Fig. 11.69).

Causes/Contributing Factors

The most common cause of patellar fracture is a direct blow from a fall or motor vehicle accident. They can also occur as an avulsion fracture with forceful contraction of the quadriceps. There are cases of patellar fracture that have occurred after ACL reconstruction using a patellar tendon graft. This is likely due to the fragment of patellar bone that is taken for the graft.

Symptoms

The patient will report pain and swelling in the anterior knee. It will be painful to flex or extend the knee. Walking will usually be painful.

Clinical Signs

There are no special tests for patellar fracture. Patient history and symptoms will usually lead to x-ray findings.

Common Interventions

If the fracture is nondisplaced, it may heal without surgical intervention. In this case, patients will usually be placed in a brace that keeps them in full knee extension and be non-weight-bearing or partial weight-bearing for about 6 weeks. After this period of immobilization, patients will often need physical therapy to restore motion and strength. While patients are immobilized, they can maintain hip function with straight leg raises in all planes and ankle function via stretching and strengthening exercises.

After the period of immobilization, the plan of care will usually include gentle stretching and strengthening. These may not be initiated for several weeks to allow for bone healing. Generally, gentle PROM will begin by 6 weeks after injury, initially avoiding flexion beyond 90°. Gentle active quadriceps contraction is usually begun about 6 to 8 weeks after injury, taking care not to stress the fracture site. By 9 to 12 weeks after injury the patient is usually ready to begin resistive exercises to the quadriceps. The plan of care is likely to have a goal of normalizing range of motion by 12 weeks after injury.

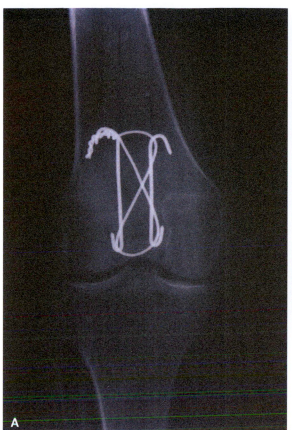

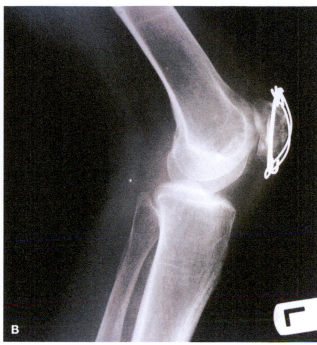

Figure 11.70 ORIF of the patella using tension band wiring for a transverse patellar fracture.

Interventions for the Surgical Patient

ORIF of the Patella

If the fracture is displaced, it is likely that the patient will have an ORIF of the patella. This can be done with pins, wires, and/or screws, depending upon the number of fragments and the location of the fracture. Occasionally it may become necessary to remove small fragments of a comminuted fracture. Rarely is the whole patella removed (**patellectomy**), because this procedure frequently results in long-standing quadriceps weakness due to loss of mechanical leverage. Figure 11.70 depicts tension band wiring of the patella in the case of a displaced transverse fracture.

Postoperative Phase

The rehabilitation plan of care after surgery will depend upon the type of fracture and the fixation used. The patient is likely to be in a hinged knee brace, locked in full or nearly full extension. The patient may be restricted to non- or touch-weight-bearing gait for 6 weeks or may be allowed to be weight-bearing as tolerated (WBAT) initially. Active assisted range-of-motion exercises into flexion and extension may be started within 1 week after surgery.

> **⚑ CLINICAL ALERT**
>
> The patient will often be restricted to 90° of knee flexion until 6 weeks postop, but a common goal is to achieve 90° by week 6.

Strengthening exercises usually will initially include isometric quadriceps and hamstring exercises, hip abduction and adduction sets, and ankle exercises against elastic resistance. At 2 weeks postop, the protocol may include straight leg raises. By 6 to 10 weeks postop, the patient may be using a stationary bicycle, stepper, and low weight resistance.

SUMMARY

The knee joint has little bony stability and relies heavily on ligament and meniscus restraints to handle the forces to which it is subjected. The consequences of altered biomechanics of the knee itself, as well as the hip and foot, are most significant in contributing to knee pathology. In restoring knee function, it is important that the PT-PTA team consider the entire lower extremity kinetic chain.

REVIEW QUESTIONS

1. The patellofemoral joint is least compressed at varying points in the range of motion of the knee. At what point in the range is compression least in open chain? At what point is it least in closed chain? How does this affect your treatment?

2. Patellofemoral pain syndrome is an excellent example of the forces incurred by the knee arising from altered biomechanics of the hip and the foot. Discuss with your lab partner how the hip impacts the knee in patellofemoral pain syndrome. What other pathologies of the knee are impacted by hip biomechanics?

3. Discuss the relevance of the blood supply to the meniscal cartilage.

4. Clinical Practice Guidelines have been created for the pathologies of knee ligament sprain and cartilage lesions. In what way does this impact your patient education or interventions?

5. Compare and contrast related pathologies of the extensor mechanism of the knee, including patellofemoral pain syndrome, patellar tendinopathy, patellar tendon rupture, and Osgood-Schlatter disease.

6. For each of the following special tests, name the pathology that yields a positive test:
   a. Anterior drawer test
   b. Apley test
   c. Crepitus palpation test
   d. Ege test
   e. Ely test
   f. Lachman test
   g. McMurray test
   h. Noble compression test
   i. Ober test
   j. Passive flexion-extension test
   k. Pivot shift test
   l. Posterior drawer test
   m. Posterior sag test
   n. Q-angle measurement
   o. Retinaculum tightness test
   p. Reverse pivot shift test
   q. Standing active quadriceps test
   r. Thessaly test
   s. Valgus stress test

PATIENT CASE: IT Band Syndrome

PT Evaluation

Patient Name: XXXXXX XXXXXXXXX	**Age:** 33	**BMI:** 22.4

Diagnosis/History

Medical Diagnosis: IT band syndrome

PT Diagnosis: Pain in R lateral knee secondary to IT band syndrome

Diagnostic Tests/Results: X-ray - negative

Relevant Medical History: Unremarkable

Prior Level of Function: Very active, runs daily

Patient's Goals: Decrease pain, return to sport

Medications: Ibuprofen 800 mg tid

Precautions: None

Social Supports/Safety Hazards

Patient Living Situation/ Supports/ Hazards: Lives alone

Patient Working Situation/Occupation/ Leisure Activities: Nursing home administrator, runner

Vital Signs

At rest Temperature: 97.8   BP: 126/68   HR: 58   Resp: 12   O2 sat: 99

Subjective Information

Patient is a male with 2-3 month history of pain in his R knee. He states this began for no apparent reason, and is worse especially after running. He runs at least 4 days a week for 45 minutes at a minimum.

Physical Assessment

Orientation: Alert and oriented   **Speech/Vision/Hearing:** Normal   **Skin Integrity:** Intact

ROM: WNL generally in hips B.

Strength: Gluteus medius weakness R 4/5. L 5/5.   **Palpation:** Tender to palpation over lateral knee

Muscle Tone: Not tested   **Balance/Coordination:** not tested   **Sensation/Proprioception:** Not tested

Endurance: Normal   **Posture:** In frontal plane, static alignment of knees 5° varus B.   **Edema:** None

Pain

Pain Rating and Location: **At best** 0/10   **At worst** 7/10   **Relieving Factors:** Rest, ice, ibuprofen

Aggravating Factors: Running, crossing legs   **Irritability:** Patient states after running, his knee hurts for about an hour. He has decreased running distance and frequency.

Functional Assessment

Patient is functionally independent.

Special Testing

Test Name: Modified Ober   **Result** Positive   **Test Name:** Noble compression test   **Result** Positive

Assessment

Patient has s/s consistent with IT band syndrome (runner's knee).

Short-Term Treatment Goals

1. Patient will state a 20% decrease in pain.
2. Patient will have increased strength in gluteus medius as evidenced by tolerance to exercise.
3. Patient will be independent in HEP

Long-Term Treatment Goals

1. Patient will have 5/5 strength in gluteus medius.
2. Patient will state a 50% decrease in pain.
3. Patient will demonstrate awareness of controlling dynamic valgus.

Treatment Plan

Frequency/Duration: 2 times a week for 6 weeks
Consisting of: Modalities, therapeutic exercise, neuro re-education, patient education

continued

Patient Case Questions

1. What factors might be contributing to the patient's IT band syndrome?

2. What would you tell the patient about specific activities to avoid or curtail?

3. What data will you collect the first time you see the patient?

4. If the plan of care does not guide you, what modalities might you use with this patient? Why? Are any modalities contraindicated?

5. If the plan of care does not specifically guide you, describe three therapeutic exercises that are indicated for this patient. Justify your choices.

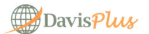

For additional resources, including answers to this case, please visit
http://davisplus.fadavis.com

REFERENCES

1. Reese, N. B., & Bandy, W. D. (2010). *Joint range of motion and muscle length testing.* New York: Elsevier Health Sciences.

2. Almquist, P. O., Arnbjörnsson, A., Zätterström, R., Ryd, L., Ekdahl, C., & Fridén, T. (2002). Evaluation of an external device measuring knee joint rotation: An in vivo study with simultaneous Roentgen stereometric analysis. *Journal of Orthopaedic Research, Official Publication of the Orthopaedic Research Society, 20,* 427–432.

3. Hill, P. F., Vedi, V., Williams, A., Iwaki, H., Pinskerova, V., & Freeman, M. A. (2000). Tibiofemoral movement 2: The loaded and unloaded living knee studied by MRI. *Journal of Bone and Joint Surgery (British volume), 82*–*B,* 1196–1198.

4. Patel, V. V., Hall, K., Ries, M., Lotz, J., Ozhinsky, E., Lindsey, C., Lu, Y., & Majumdar, S. (2004). A three-dimensional MRI analysis of knee kinematics. *Journal of Orthopaedic Research, Official Publication of the Orthopaedic Research Society, 22,* 283–292.

5. Hubbard, J. K., Sampson, H. W., & Elledge, J. R. (1997). Prevalence and morphology of the vastus medialis oblique muscle in human cadavers. *The Anatomical Record, 249,* 135–142.

6. Smith, T. O., Nichols, R., Harle, D., & Donell, S. T. (2009). Do the vastus medialis obliquus and vastus medialis longus really exist? A systematic review. *Clinical Anatomy, 22,* 183–199.

7. Waligora, A. C., Johanson, N. A., & Hirsch, B. E. (2009). Clinical anatomy of the quadriceps femoris and extensor apparatus of the knee. *Clinical Orthopaedics and Related Research, 467,* 3297–3306.

8. Fleming, B. C. Renstrom, P. A., Ohlen, G., Johnson, R. J., Peura, G. D., Beynnon, B. D., & Badger, G. J. (2001). The gastrocnemius muscle is an antagonist of the anterior cruciate ligament. *Journal of Orthopaedic Research, Official Publication of the Orthopaedic Research Society, 19,* 1178–1184.

9. Neptune, R. R., Kautz, S. A., & Zajac, F. E. (2001). Contributions of the individual ankle plantar flexors to support, forward progression and swing initiation during walking. *Journal of Biomechanics, 34,* 1387–1398.

10. Horton, M. G., & Hall, T. L. (1989). Quadriceps femoris muscle angle: Normal values and relationships with gender and selected skeletal measures. *Physical Therapy, 69,* 897–901.

11. Livingston, L. A. (1998). The quadriceps angle: A review of the literature. *Journal of Orthopaedic and Sports Physical Therapy, 28,* 105–109.

12. Woodland, L. H., & Francis, R. S. (1992). Parameters and comparisons of the quadriceps angle of college-aged men and women in the supine and standing positions. *American Journal of Sports Medicine, 20,* 208–211.

13. Escamilla, R. F., Zheng, N., Macleod, T. D., Edwards, W. B., Imamura, R., Hreljac, A., Fleisig, G. S., et al. (2009). Patellofemoral joint force and stress during the wall squat and one-leg squat. *Medicine and Science in Sports and Exercise, 41,* 879–888.

14. Voskanian, N. (2013). ACL Injury prevention in female athletes: Review of the literature and practical considerations in implementing an ACL prevention program. *Current Reviews in Musculoskeletal Medicine, 6,* 158–163.

15. Powers, C. M. (2003). The influence of altered lower-extremity kinematics on patellofemoral joint dysfunction: A theoretical perspective. *Journal of Orthopaedic and Sports Physical Therapy, 33,* 639–646.

16. Powers, C. M. (2010). The influence of abnormal hip mechanics on knee injury: A biomechanical perspective. *Journal of Orthopaedic and Sports Physical Therapy, 40,* 42–51.

17. Ramskov, D., Barton, C., Nielsen, R. O., & Rasmussen, S. (2015). High eccentric hip abduction strength reduces the risk of developing patellofemoral pain among novice runners initiating a self-structured running program: A 1-year observational study. *Journal of Orthopaedic and Sports Physical Therapy, 45,* 153–161.

18. Chappell, J. D., Yu, B., Kirkendall, D. T., & Garrett, W. E. (2002). A comparison of knee kinetics between male and female recreational athletes in stop-jump tasks. *American Journal of Sports Medicine, 30,* 261–267.

19. Malinzak, R. A., Colby, S. M., Kirkendall, D. T., Yu, B., & Garrett, W. E. (2001). A comparison of knee joint motion patterns between men and women in selected athletic tasks. *Clinical Biomechanics (Bristol Avon), 16,* 438–445.

20. Shimokochi, Y., & Shultz, S. J. (2008). Mechanisms of noncontact anterior cruciate ligament injury. *Journal of Athletic Training, 43,* 396–408.

21. Lathinghouse, L. H., & Trimble, M. H. (2000). Effects of isometric quadriceps activation on the Q-angle in women before and after quadriceps exercise. *Journal of Orthopaedic and Sports Physical Therapy, 30,* 211–216.

22. Nakagawa, T. H., Moriya, E. T. U., Maciel, C. D., & Serrão, F. V. (2012). Trunk, pelvis, hip, and knee kinematics, hip strength, and gluteal muscle activation during a single-leg squat in males and females with and without patellofemoral pain syndrome. *Journal of Orthopaedic and Sports Physical Therapy, 42*, 491–501.

23. Souza, R. B., Draper, C. E., Fredericson, M., & Powers, C. M. (2010). Femur rotation and patellofemoral joint kinematics: A weight-bearing magnetic resonance imaging analysis. *Journal of Orthopaedic and Sports Physical Therapy, 40*, 277–285.

24. Mikesky, A. E., Meyer, A., & Thompson, K. L. (2000). Relationship between quadriceps strength and rate of loading during gait in women. *Journal of Orthopaedic Research, Official Publication of the Orthopaedic Research Society, 18*, 171–175.

25. Badlani, J. T., Borrero, C., Golla, S., Harner, C. D., & Irrgang, J. J. (2013). The effects of meniscus injury on the development of knee osteoarthritis: Data from the osteoarthritis initiative. *American Journal of Sports Medicine, 41*, 1238–1244.

26. Egloff, C., Hügle, T., & Valderrabano, V. (2012). Biomechanics and pathomechanisms of osteoarthritis. *Swiss Medical Weekly, 142*, w13583.

27. Felson, D. T., Zhang, Y., Hannan, M. T., Naimark, A., Weissman, B., Aliabadi, P., & Levy, D. (1997). Risk factors for incident radiographic knee osteoarthritis in the elderly: The Framingham Study. *Arthritis & Rheumatism, 40*, 728–733.

28. Felson, D. T., Niu, J., Gross, K. D., Englund, M., Sharma, L., Cooke, T. D., Guermazi, A., et al. (2013). Valgus malalignment is a risk factor for lateral knee osteoarthritis incidence and progression: Findings from the Multicenter Osteoarthritis Study and the Osteoarthritis Initiative. *Arthritis & Rheumatism, 65*, 355–362.

29. Gunardi, A. J., Brennan, S. L., Wang, Y., Cicuttini, F. M., Pasco, J. A., Kotowicz, M. A., Nicholson, G. C., et al. (2013). Associations between measures of adiposity over 10 years and patella cartilage in population-based asymptomatic women. *International Journal of Obesity, 2005, 37*, 1586–1589.

30. Hashikawa, T., Osaki, M., Ye, Z., Tomita, M., Abe, Y., Honda, S., Takamura, N., et al. (2011). Factors associated with radiographic osteoarthritis of the knee among community-dwelling Japanese women: The Hizen-Oshima Study. *Journal of Orthopaedic Science, Official Journal of the Japanese Orthopaedic Association, 16*, 51–55.

31. Kim, Y. M., & Joo, Y. B. (2012). Patellofemoral osteoarthritis. *Knee Surgery & Related Research, 24*, 193–200.

32. Kujala, U. M., Kaprio, J., & Sarna, S. (1994). Osteoarthritis of weight bearing joints of lower limbs in former élite male athletes. *The BMJ, 308*, 231–234.

33. Maetzel, A., Mäkelä, M., Hawker, G., & Bombardier, C. (1997). Osteoarthritis of the hip and knee and mechanical occupational exposure—A systematic overview of the evidence. *Journal of Rheumatology, 24*, 1599–1607.

34. Molloy, M. G., & Molloy, C. B. (2011). Contact sport and osteoarthritis. *British Journal of Sports Medicine, 45*, 275–277.

35. Muthuri, S. G., Hui, M., Doherty, M., & Zhang, W. (2011). What if we prevent obesity? Risk reduction in knee osteoarthritis estimated through a meta-analysis of observational studies. *Arthritis Care & Research, 63*, 982–990.

36. Richmond, S. A., Fukuchi, R. K., Ezzat, A., Schneider, K., Schneider, G., & Emery, C. A. (2013). Are joint injury, sport activity, physical activity, obesity, or occupational activities predictors for osteoarthritis? A systematic review. *Journal of Orthopaedic and Sports Physical Therapy, 43*, 515–524.

37. Shelbourne, K. D., Urch, S. E., Gray, T., & Freeman, H. (2012). Loss of normal knee motion after anterior cruciate ligament reconstruction is associated with radiographic arthritic changes after surgery. *American Journal of Sports Medicine, 40*, 108–113.

38. Stratford, P. W., Kennedy, D. M., & Woodhouse, L. J. (2006). Performance measures provide assessments of pain and function in people with advanced osteoarthritis of the hip or knee. *Physical Therapy, 86*, 1489–1496.

39. Altman, R., Asch, E., Bloch, D., Bole, G., Borenstein, D., Brandt, K., Christy, W., et al. (1986). Development of criteria for the classification and reporting of osteoarthritis. Classification of osteoarthritis of the knee. Diagnostic and Therapeutic Criteria Committee of the American Rheumatism Association. *Arthritis and Rheumatism, 29*, 1039–1049.

40. Alnahdi, A. H., Zeni, J. A., & Snyder-Mackler, L. (2012). Muscle impairments in patients with knee osteoarthritis. *Sports Health, 4*, 284–292.

41. Brakke, R., Singh, J., & Sullivan, W. (2012). Physical therapy in persons with osteoarthritis. *PM&R: The Journal of Injury, Function, and Rehabilitation, 4*, S53–58.

42. Ettinger, W. H., Jr., Burns, R., Messier, S. P., Applegate, W., Rejeski, W. J., Morgan, T., Shumaker, S., et al. (1997). A randomized trial comparing aerobic exercise and resistance exercise with a health education program in older adults with knee osteoarthritis. The Fitness Arthritis and Seniors Trial (FAST). *Journal of the American Medical Association, 277*, 25–31.

43. Felson, D. T., Lawrence, R. C., Hochberg, M. C., McAlindon, T., Dieppe, P. A., Minor, M. A., Blair, S. N., et al. (2000). Osteoarthritis: New insights. Part 2: Treatment approaches. *Annals of Internal Medicine, 133*, 726–737.

44. Iwamoto, J., Sato, Y., Takeda, T., & Matsumoto, H. (2011). Effectiveness of exercise for osteoarthritis of the knee: A review of the literature. *World Journal of Orthopedics, 2*, 37–42.

45. Smith, T. O., King, J. J., & Hing, C. B. (2012). The effectiveness of proprioceptive-based exercise for osteoarthritis of the knee: A systematic review and meta-analysis. *Rheumatology International, 32*, 3339–3351.

46. Tanaka, R., Ozawa, J., Kito, N., & Moriyama, H. (2013). Efficacy of strengthening or aerobic exercise on pain relief in people with knee osteoarthritis: A systematic review and meta-analysis of randomized controlled trials. *Clinical Rehabilitation, 27*, 1059–1071.

47. van Baar, M. E., Assendelft, W. J., Dekker, J., Oostendorp, R. A., & Bijlsma, J. W. (1999). Effectiveness of exercise therapy in patients with osteoarthritis of the hip or knee: A systematic review of randomized clinical trials. *Arthritis and Rheumatism, 42*, 1361–1369.

48. Wang, S. Y., Olson-Kellogg, B., Shamliyan, T. A., Choi, J. Y., Ramakrishnan, R., & Kane, R. L. (2012). Physical therapy interventions for knee pain secondary to osteoarthritis: A systematic review. *Annals of Internal Medicine, 157*, 632–644.

49. Péloquin, L., Bravo, G., Gauthier, P., Lacombe, G., & Billiard, J. S. (1999). Effects of a cross-training exercise program in persons with osteoarthritis of the knee: A randomized controlled trial. *Journal of Clinical Rheumatology: Practical Reports on Rheumatic and Musculoskeletal Diseases, 5*, 126–136.

50. Brandt, K. D., Heilman, D. K., Slemenda, C., Katz, B. P., Mazzuca, S. A., Braunstein, E. M., & Byrd, D. (1999). Quadriceps strength in women with radiographically progressive osteoarthritis of the knee and those with stable radiographic changes. *The Journal of Rheumatology, 26*, 2431–2437.

51. Slemenda, C., Brandt, K. D., Heilman, D. K., Mazzuca, S., Braunstein, E. M., Katz, B. P., & Wolinsky, F. D. (1997).

Quadriceps weakness and osteoarthritis of the knee. *Annals of Internal Medicine, 127,* 97–104.

52. Slemenda, C., Heilman, D. K., Brandt, K. D., Katz, B. P., Mazzuca, S. A., Braunstein, E. M., & Byrd, D. (1998) Reduced quadriceps strength relative to body weight: A risk factor for knee osteoarthritis in women? *Arthritis and Rheumatism, 41,* 1951–1959.

53. Tan, J., Balci, N., Sepici, V., & Gener, F. A. (1995). Isokinetic and isometric strength in osteoarthrosis of the knee. A comparative study with healthy women. *American Journal of Physical Medicine & Rehabilitation, 74,* 364–369.

54. Bennell, K. L., Hunt, M. A., Wrigley, T. V., Hunter, D. J., McManus, F. J., Hodges, P. W., Li, L., & Hinman, R. S. (2010). Hip strengthening reduces symptoms but not knee load in people with medial knee osteoarthritis and varus malalignment: A randomised controlled trial. *Osteoarthritis and Cartilage, 18,* 621–628.

55. Gadikota, H. R., Kikuta, S., Qi, W., Nolan, D., Gill, T. J., & Li, G. (2013). Effect of increased iliotibial band load on tibiofemoral kinematics and force distributions: A direct measurement in cadaveric knees. *Journal of Orthopaedic and Sports Physical Therapy, 43,* 478–485.

56. Sled, E. A., Khoja, L., Deluzio, K. J., Olney, S. J., & Culham, E. G. (2010). Effect of a home program of hip abductor exercises on knee joint loading, strength, function, and pain in people with knee osteoarthritis: A clinical trial. *Physical Therapy, 90,* 895–904.

57. Fitzgerald, G. K., Piva, S. R., & Irrgang, J. J. (2004). Reports of joint instability in knee osteoarthritis: Its prevalence and relationship to physical function. *Arthritis and Rheumatism, 51,* 941–946.

58. Fitzgerald, G. K., Childs, J. D., Ridge, T. M., & Irrgang, J. J. (2002). Agility and perturbation training for a physically active individual with knee osteoarthritis. *Physical Therapy, 82,* 372–382.

59. Lin, D. H., Lin, Y. F., Chai, H. M., Han, Y. C., & Jan, M. H. (2007). Comparison of proprioceptive functions between computerized proprioception facilitation exercise and closed kinetic chain exercise in patients with knee osteoarthritis. *Clinical Rheumatology, 26,* 520–528.

60. Lin, D. H., Lin, C. H. J., Lin, Y. F., & Jan, M. H. (2009). Efficacy of 2 non-weight-bearing interventions, proprioception training versus strength training, for patients with knee osteoarthritis: A randomized clinical trial. *Journal of Orthopaedic and Sports Physical Therapy, 39,* 450–457.

61. Wegener, L., Kisner, C., & Nichols, D. (1997). Static and dynamic balance responses in persons with bilateral knee osteoarthritis. *Journal of Orthopaedic and Sports Physical Therapy, 25,* 13–18.

62. Hinman, R. S., Heywood, S. E., & Day, A. R. (2007). Aquatic physical therapy for hip and knee osteoarthritis: Results of a single-blind randomized controlled trial. *Physical Therapy, 87,* 32–43.

63. Wyatt, F. B., Milam, S., Manske, R. C., & Deere, R. (2001). The effects of aquatic and traditional exercise programs on persons with knee osteoarthritis. *Journal of Strength and Conditioning Research, 15,* 337–340.

64. Keating, E. M., Faris, P. M., Ritter, M. A., & Kane, J. (1993). Use of lateral heel and sole wedges in the treatment of medial osteoarthritis of the knee. *Orthopaedic Review, 22,* 921–924.

65. Sasaki, T., & Yasuda, K. (1987). Clinical evaluation of the treatment of osteoarthritic knees using a newly designed wedged insole. *Clinical Orthopaedics and Related Research, 221,* 181–187.

66. Gaasbeek, R. D. A., Groen, B. E., Hampsink, B., van Heerwaarden, R. J., & Duysens, J. (2007). Valgus bracing in patients with medial compartment osteoarthritis of the knee. A gait analysis study of a new brace. *Gait & Posture, 26,* 3–10.

67. Cushnaghan, J., McCarthy, C., & Dieppe, P. (1994). Taping the patella medially: A new treatment for osteoarthritis of the knee joint? *The BMJ, 308,* 753–755.

68. Shull, P. B., Shultz, R., Silder, A., Dragoo, J. L., Besier, T. F., Cutkosky, M. R., & Delp, S. L. (2013). Toe-in gait reduces the first peak knee adduction moment in patients with medial compartment knee osteoarthritis. *Journal of Biomechanics, 46,* 122–128.

69. Vincent, K. R., Conrad, B. P., Fregly, B. J., & Vincent, H. K. (2012). The pathophysiology of osteoarthritis: A mechanical perspective on the knee joint. *PM&R: The Journal of Injury, Function, and Rehabilitation, 4,* S3–9.

70. Brander, V., & Stulberg, S. D. (2006). Rehabilitation after hip- and knee-joint replacement. An experience- and evidence-based approach to care. *American Journal of Physical Medicine & Rehabilitation, 85,* S98-118; quiz S119-123.

71. Mizner, R. L., Petterson, S. C., Stevens, J. E., Axe, M. J., & Snyder-Mackler, L. (2005). Preoperative quadriceps strength predicts functional ability one year after total knee arthroplasty. *The Journal of Rheumatology, 32,* 1533–1539.

72. Rooks, D. S., Huang, J., Bierbaum, B. E., Bolus, S. A., Rubano, J., Connolly, C. E., Alpert, S., et al. (2006). Effect of preoperative exercise on measures of functional status in men and women undergoing total hip and knee arthroplasty. *Arthritis and Rheumatism, 55,* 700–708.

73. Brosseau, L., Milne, S., Wells, G., Tugwell, P., Robinson, V., Casimiro, L., Pelland, L., et al. (2004). Efficacy of continuous passive motion following total knee arthroplasty: A metaanalysis. *Journal of Rheumatology, 31,* 2251–2264.

74. Harvey, L. A., Brosseau, L., & Herbert, R. D. (2010). Continuous passive motion following total knee arthroplasty in people with arthritis. *Cochrane Database of Systematic Reviews,* CD004260. doi: 10.1002/14651858.CD004260. pub2.

75. Milne, S., Brosseau, L., Robinson, V., Noel, M. J., Davis, J., Drouin, H., Wells, G., et al. (2003). Continuous passive motion following total knee arthroplasty. *Cochrane Database of Systematic Reviews,* CD004260. doi: 10.1002/14651858. CD004260.

76. Beaupré, L. A., Davies, D. M., Jones, C. A., & Cinats, J. G. (2001). Exercise combined with continuous passive motion or slider board therapy compared with exercise only: A randomized controlled trial of patients following total knee arthroplasty. *Physical Therapy, 81,* 1029–1037.

77. Chiarello, C. M., Gundersen, L., & O'Halloran, T. (1997). The effect of continuous passive motion duration and increment on range of motion in total knee arthroplasty patients. *Journal of Orthopaedic and Sports Physical Therapy, 25,* 119–127.

78. Denis, M., Moffet, H., Caron, F., Ouellet, D., Paquet, J., & Nolet, L. (2006). Effectiveness of continuous passive motion and conventional physical therapy after total knee arthroplasty: A randomized clinical trial. *Physical Therapy, 86,* 174–185.

79. MacDonald, S. J., Bourne, R. B., Rorabeck, C. H., McCalden, R. W., Kramer, J., & Vaz, M. (2000). Prospective randomized clinical trial of continuous passive motion after total knee arthroplasty. *Clinical Orthopaedics and Related Research, 30*–35.

80. Maniar, R. N., Baviskar, J. V., Singhi, T., & Rathi, S. S. (2012). To use or not to use continuous passive motion post-total knee arthroplasty: Presenting functional assessment results in early recovery. *Journal of Arthroplasty, 27,* 193–200.e1.

81. Bade, M. J., & Stevens-Lapsley, J. E. (2011). Early high-intensity rehabilitation following total knee arthroplasty improves outcomes. *Journal of Orthopaedic and Sports Physical Therapy, 41,* 932–941.

82. LaStayo, P. C., Meier, W., Marcus, R. L., Mizner, R., Dibble, L., & Peters, C. (2009). Reversing muscle and mobility deficits 1 to 4 years after TKA: A pilot study. *Clinical Orthopaedics and Related Research, 467,* 1493–1500.

83. Meier, W., Mizner, R. L., Marcus, R. L., Dibble, L. E., Peters, C., & LaStayo, P. C. (2008). Total knee arthroplasty: muscle impairments, functional limitations, and recommended rehabilitation approaches. *Journal of Orthopaedic and Sports Physical Therapy, 38,* 246–256.

84. Portegijs, E., Sipilä, S., Pajala, S., Lamb, S. E., Alen, M., Kaprio, J., Kosekenvuo, M., et al. (2006). Asymmetrical lower extremity power deficit as a risk factor for injurious falls in healthy older women. *Journal of the American Geriatrics Society, 54,* 551–553.

85. Silva, M., Shepherd, E. F., Jackson, W. O., Pratt, J. A., McClung, C. D., & Schmalzried, T. P. (2003). Knee strength after total knee arthroplasty. *Journal of Arthroplasty, 18,* 605–611.

86. Valtonen, A., Pöyhönen, T., Heinonen, A., & Sipilä, S. (2009). Muscle deficits persist after unilateral knee replacement and have implications for rehabilitation. *Physical Therapy, 89,* 1072–1079.

87. Fuchs, S., Thorwesten, L., & Niewerth, S. (1999). Proprioceptive function in knees with and without total knee arthroplasty. *American Journal of Physical Medicine & Rehabilitation, 78,* 39–45.

88. Skelton, D. A., Kennedy, J., & Rutherford, O. M. (2002). Explosive power and asymmetry in leg muscle function in frequent fallers and non-fallers aged over 65. *Age and Ageing, 31,* 119–125.

89. Aglietti, P., Buzzi, R., Vena, L. M., Baldini, A., & Mondaini, A. (2003). High tibial valgus osteotomy for medial gonarthrosis: A 10- to 21-year study. *Journal of Knee Surgery, 16,* 21–26.

90. Aalderink, K. J., Shaffer, M., & Amendola, A. (2010). Rehabilitation following high tibial osteotomy. *Clinics in Sports Medicine, 29,* 291–301, ix.

91. Noyes, F. R., Mayfield, W., Barber-Westin, S. D., Albright, J. C., & Heckmann, T. P. (2006). Opening wedge high tibial osteotomy: An operative technique and rehabilitation program to decrease complications and promote early union and function. *American Journal of Sports Medicine, 34,* 1262–1273.

92. Logerstedt, D. S., Scalzitti, D., Risberg, M. A., Engebretsen, L., Webster, K. E., Feller, J., Snyder-Mackler, L., et al. (2017). Knee stability and movement coordination impairments: Knee ligament sprain revision 2017. *Journal of Orthopaedic and Sports Physical Therapy, 47,* A1–A47.

93. Boden, B. P., Breit, I., & Sheehan, F. T. (2009). Tibiofemoral alignment: Contributing factors to noncontact anterior cruciate ligament injury. *The Journal of Bone and Joint Surgery (American), 91,* 2381–2389.

94. Dai, B., Herman, D., Liu, H., Garrett, W. E., & Yu, B. (2012). Prevention of ACL injury, Part I: Injury characteristics, risk factors, and loading mechanism. *Research in Sports Medicine, 20,* 180–197.

95. Krosshaug, T., Nakamae, A., Boden, B. P., Engebretsen, L., Smith, G., Slauterbeck, J. R., Hewett, T. E., et al. (2007). Mechanisms of anterior cruciate ligament injury in basketball: Video analysis of 39 cases. *American Journal of Sports Medicine, 35,* 359–367.

96. Alentorn-Geli, E, Myer, G. D., Silvers, H. J., Samitier, G., Romero, D., Lázaro-Haro, C., & Cugat, R. (2009). Prevention of non-contact anterior cruciate ligament injuries in soccer players. Part 1: Mechanisms of injury and underlying risk factors. *Knee Surgery, Sports Traumatology, Arthroscopy: Official Journal of ESSKA, 17,* 705–729.

97. Koga, H., Nakamae, A., Shima, Y., Iwasa, J., Myklebust, G., Engebretsen, L., Bahr, R., et al. (2010). Mechanisms for noncontact anterior cruciate ligament injuries: Knee joint kinematics in 10 injury situations from female team handball and basketball. *American Journal of Sports Medicine, 38,* 2218–2225.

98. Hewett, T. E., Myer, G. D., Ford, K. R., Paterno, M. V., & Quatman, C. E. (2012). The 2012 ABJS Nicolas Andry Award: The sequence of prevention: A systematic approach to prevent anterior cruciate ligament injury. *Clinical Orthopaedics and Related Research, 470,* 2930–2940.

99. Smith, H. C., Vacek, P., Johnson, R. J., Slauterbeck, J. R., Hashemi, J., Shultz, S., & Beynnon, B. D. (2012). Risk factors for anterior cruciate ligament injury: A review of the literature—Part 1: Neuromuscular and anatomic risk. *Sports Health, 4,* 69–78.

100. Arendt, E. A., Bershadsky, B., & Agel, J. (2002). Periodicity of noncontact anterior cruciate ligament injuries during the menstrual cycle. *Journal of Gender-Specific Medicine, Official Journal of the Partnership in Women's Health at Columbia, 5,* 19–26.

101. Hewett, T. E. (2000). Neuromuscular and hormonal factors associated with knee injuries in female athletes. Strategies for intervention. *Sports Medicine (Auckland, NZ), 29,* 313–327.

102. Hewett, T. E., Zazulak, B. T., & Myer, G. D. (2007). Effects of the menstrual cycle on anterior cruciate ligament injury risk: A systematic review. *American Journal of Sports Medicine, 35,* 659–668.

103. Zazulak, B. T., Paterno, M., Myer, G. D., Romani, W. A., & Hewett, T. E. (2006). The effects of the menstrual cycle on anterior knee laxity: A systematic review. *Sports Medicine (Auckland, NZ), 36,* 847–862.

104. Cooperman, J. M., Riddle, D. L., & Rothstein, J. M. (1990). Reliability and validity of judgments of the integrity of the anterior cruciate ligament of the knee using the Lachman's test. *Physical Therapy, 70,* 225–233.

105. Katz, J. W., & Fingeroth, R. J. (1986). The diagnostic accuracy of ruptures of the anterior cruciate ligament comparing the Lachman test, the anterior drawer sign, and the pivot shift test in acute and chronic knee injuries. *American Journal of Sports Medicine, 14,* 88–91.

106. Buss, D. D., Min, R., Skyhar, M., Galinat, B., Warren, R. F., & Wickiewicz, T. L. (1995). Nonoperative treatment of acute anterior cruciate ligament injuries in a selected group of patients. *American Journal of Sports Medicine, 23,* 160–165.

107. Button, K., van Deursen, R., & Price, P. (2006). Classification of functional recovery of anterior cruciate ligament copers, non-copers, and adapters. *British Journal of Sports Medicine, 40,* 853–859.

108. Ciccotti, M. G., Lombardo, S. J., Nonweiler, B., & Pink, M. (1994). Non-operative treatment of ruptures of the anterior cruciate ligament in middle-aged patients. Results after long-term follow-up. *The Journal of Bone & Joint Surgery (America), 76,* 1315–1321.

109. Fridén, T., Zätterström, R., Lindstrand, A., & Moritz, U. (1991). Anterior-cruciate-insufficient knees treated with physiotherapy. A three-year follow-up study of patients with late diagnosis. *Clinical Orthopaedics and Related Research, 263,* 190–199.

110. Moksnes, H., Snyder-Mackler, L., & Risberg, M. A. (2008). Individuals with an anterior cruciate ligament-deficient knee classified as noncopers may be candidates for nonsurgical rehabilitation. *Journal of Orthopaedic and Sports Physical Therapy, 38,* 586–595.

111. Eitzen, I., Holm, I., & Risberg, M. A. (2009). Preoperative quadriceps strength is a significant predictor of knee function two years after anterior cruciate ligament reconstruction. *British Journal of Sports Medicine, 43,* 371–376.

112. Eitzen, I., Moksnes, H., Snyder-Mackler, L., & Risberg, M. A. (2010). A progressive 5-week exercise therapy program leads to significant improvement in knee function early after anterior cruciate ligament injury. *Journal of Orthopaedic and Sports Physical Therapy, 40,* 705–721.

113. Hartigan, E., Axe, M. J., & Snyder-Mackler, L. (2009). Perturbation training prior to ACL reconstruction improves gait asymmetries in non-copers. *Journal of Orthopaedic Research: Official Publication of the Orthopaedic Research Society, 27*, 724–729.

114. Adams, D., Logerstedt, D. S., Hunter-Giordano, A., Axe, M. J., & Snyder-Mackler, L. (2012). Current concepts for anterior cruciate ligament reconstruction: A criterion-based rehabilitation progression. *Journal of Orthopaedic and Sports Physical Therapy, 42*, 601–614.

115. Mikkelsen, C., Werner, S., & Eriksson, E. (2000). Closed kinetic chain alone compared to combined open and closed kinetic chain exercises for quadriceps strengthening after anterior cruciate ligament reconstruction with respect to return to sports: A prospective matched follow-up study. *Knee Surgery, Sports Traumatology, Arthroscopy: Official Journal of ESSKA, 8*, 337–342.

116. Tagesson, S., Oberg, B., Good, L., & Kvist, J. (2008). A comprehensive rehabilitation program with quadriceps strengthening in closed versus open kinetic chain exercise in patients with anterior cruciate ligament deficiency: A randomized clinical trial evaluating dynamic tibial translation and muscle function. *American Journal of Sports Medicine, 36*, 298–307.

117. Fitzgerald, G. K., Axe, M. J., & Snyder-Mackler, L. (2000). Proposed practice guidelines for nonoperative anterior cruciate ligament rehabilitation of physically active individuals. *Journal of Orthopaedic and Sports Physical Therapy, 30*, 194–203.

118. Kålund, S., Sinkjaer, T., Arendt-Nielsen, L., & Simonsen, O. (1990). Altered timing of hamstring muscle action in anterior cruciate ligament deficient patients. *American Journal of Sports Medicine, 18*, 245–248.

119. Solomonow, M., Baratta, R., Zhou, B. H., Shoji, H., Bose, W., Beck, C., & D'Ambrosia, R. (1987). The synergistic action of the anterior cruciate ligament and thigh muscles in maintaining joint stability. *American Journal of Sports Medicine, 15*, 207–213.

120. Beard, D. J., Dodd, C. A., Trundle, H. R., & Simpson, A. H. (1994). Proprioception enhancement for anterior cruciate ligament deficiency. A prospective randomised trial of two physiotherapy regimes. *The Journal of Bone and Joint Surgery (British), 76*, 654–659.

121. Fitzgerald, G. K., Axe, M. J., & Snyder-Mackler, L. (2000). The efficacy of perturbation training in nonoperative anterior cruciate ligament rehabilitation programs for physically active individuals. *Physical Therapy, 80*, 128–140.

122. Powers, C. M., & Fisher, B. (2010). Mechanisms underlying ACL injury-prevention training: The brain-behavior relationship. *Journal of Athletic Training, 45*, 513–515.

123. Yoo, J. H., Lim, B. O., Ha, M., Lee, S. W., Oh, S. J., Lee, Y. S., & Kim, J. G. (2010). A meta-analysis of the effect of neuromuscular training on the prevention of the anterior cruciate ligament injury in female athletes. *Knee Surgery, Sports Traumatology, Arthroscopy: Official Journal of ESSKA, 18*, 824–830.

124. de Jong, S. N., van Caspel, D. R., van Haeff, M. J., & Saris, D. B. F. (2007). Functional assessment and muscle strength before and after reconstruction of chronic anterior cruciate ligament lesions. *Arthroscopy: The Journal of Arthroscopy & Related Surgery, 23*, 21–28, 28.e1–3.

125. Keays, S. L., Bullock-Saxton, J. E., Newcombe, P., & Keays, A. C. (2003). The relationship between knee strength and functional stability before and after anterior cruciate ligament reconstruction. *Journal of Orthopaedic Research: Official Publication of the Orthopaedic Research Society, 21*, 231–237.

126. Prodromos, C. (2018). *The anterior cruciate ligament: Reconstruction and basic science.* 2nd edition. Philadelphia, PA: Elsevier.

127. Kondo, E., Yasuda, K., Katsura, T., Hayashi, R., Kotani, Y., & Tohyama, H. (2012). Biomechanical and histological evaluations of the doubled semitendinosus tendon autograft after anterior cruciate ligament reconstruction in sheep. *American Journal of Sports Medicine, 40*, 315–324.

128. Marumo, K., Saito, M., Yamagishi, T., & Fujii, K. (2005). The 'ligamentization' process in human anterior cruciate ligament reconstruction with autogenous patellar and hamstring tendons: A biochemical study. *American Journal of Sports Medicine, 33*, 1166–1173.

129. Risberg, M. A., Holm, I., Myklebust, G., & Engebretsen, L. (2007). Neuromuscular training versus strength training during first 6 months after anterior cruciate ligament reconstruction: A randomized clinical trial. *Physical Therapy, 87*, 737–750.

130. White, K., Di Stasi, S. L., Smith, A. H., & Snyder-Mackler, L. (2013). Anterior cruciate ligament-specialized post-operative return-to-sports (ACL-SPORTS) training: A randomized control trial. *BMC Musculoskeletal Disorders, 14*, 108.

131. Gerber, J. P., Marcus, R. L., Leland, E. D., & LaStayo, P. C. (2009). The use of eccentrically biased resistance exercise to mitigate muscle impairments following anterior cruciate ligament reconstruction: A short review. *Sports Health, 1*, 31–38.

132. Gerber, J. P., Marcus, R. L., Dibble, L. E., Greis, P. E., Burks, R. T., & LaStayo, P. C. (2007). Safety, feasibility, and efficacy of negative work exercise via eccentric muscle activity following anterior cruciate ligament reconstruction. *Journal of Orthopaedic and Sports Physical Therapy, 37*, 10–18.

133. Gerber, J. P., Marcus, R. L., Dibble, L. E., Greis, P. E., Burks, R. T., & LaStayo, P. C. (2009). Effects of early progressive eccentric exercise on muscle size and function after anterior cruciate ligament reconstruction: A 1-year follow-up study of a randomized clinical trial. *Physical Therapy, 89*, 51–59.

134. Schulz, M. S., Russe, K., Weiler, A., Eichhorn, H. J., & Strobel, M. J. (2003). Epidemiology of posterior cruciate ligament injuries. *Archives of Orthopaedic and Trauma Surgery, 123*, 186–191.

135. Grassmayr, M. J., Parker, D. A., Coolican, M. R. J., & Vanwanseele, B. (2008). Posterior cruciate ligament deficiency: Biomechanical and biological consequences and the outcomes of conservative treatment. A systematic review. *Journal of Science and Medicine in Sport, 11*, 433–443.

136. Patel, D. V., Allen, A. A., Warren, R. F., Wickiewicz, T. L., & Simonian, P. T. (2007). The nonoperative treatment of acute, isolated (partial or complete) posterior cruciate ligament-deficient knees: An intermediate-term follow-up study. *HSS Journal: The Musculoskeletal Journal of Hospital for Special Surgery, 3*, 137–146.

137. Shelbourne, K. D., Davis, T. J., & Patel, D. V. (1999). The natural history of acute, isolated, nonoperatively treated posterior cruciate ligament injuries. A prospective study. *American Journal of Sports Medicine, 27*, 276–283.

138. Shelbourne, K. D., & Muthukaruppan, Y. (2005). Subjective results of nonoperatively treated, acute, isolated posterior cruciate ligament injuries. *Arthroscopy: The Journal of Arthroscopic & Related Surgery, 21*, 457–461.

139. Toritsuka, Y., Horibe, S., Hiro-Oka, A., Mitsuoka, T., & Nakamura, N. (2004). Conservative treatment for rugby football players with an acute isolated posterior cruciate ligament injury. *Knee Surgery, Sports Traumatology, Arthroscopy: Official Journal of ESSKA, 12*, 110–114.

140. Lee, B. K., & Nam, S. W. (2011). Rupture of posterior cruciate ligament: Diagnosis and treatment principles. *Knee Surgery & Related Research, 23*, 135–141.

141. MacLean, C. L., Taunton, J. E., Clement, D. B., Regan, W. D., & Stanish, W. D. (1999). Eccentric kinetic chain exercise as a conservative means of functionally rehabilitating chronic isolated insufficiency of the posterior cruciate ligament.

Clinical Journal of Sports Medicine: Official Journal of the Canadian Academy of Sport Medicine, 9, 142–150.

142. Beecher, M., Garrison, J. C., & Wyland, D. (2010). Rehabilitation following a minimally invasive procedure for the repair of a combined anterior cruciate and posterior cruciate ligament partial rupture in a 15-year-old athlete. *Journal of Orthopaedic and Sports Physical Therapy, 40,* 297–309.

143. Indelicato, P. A. (1995). Isolated medial collateral ligament injuries in the knee. *Journal of the American Academy of Orthopaedic Surgeons, 3,* 9–14.

144. Woo, S. L., Vogrin, T. M., & Abramowitch, S. D. (2000). Healing and repair of ligament injuries in the knee. *Journal of the American Academy of Orthopaedic Surgeons, 8,* 364–372.

145. Laprade, R. F., & Wijdicks, C. A. (2012). The management of injuries to the medial side of the knee. *Journal of Orthopaedic and Sports Physical Therapy, 42,* 221–233.

146. Snoeker, B. A. M., Bakker, E. W. P., Kegel, C. A. T., & Lucas, C. (2013). Risk factors for meniscal tears: A systematic review including meta-analysis. *Journal of Orthopaedic and Sports Physical Therapy, 43,* 352–367.

147. Karachalios, T., Hantes, M., Zibis, A. H., Zachos, V., Karantanas, A. H., & Malizos, K. N. (2005). Diagnostic accuracy of a new clinical test (the Thessaly test) for early detection of meniscal tears. *Journal of Bone & Joint Surgery (American), 87,* 955–962.

148. Akseki, D., Ozcan, O., Boya, H., & Pinar, H. (2004). A new weight-bearing meniscal test and a comparison with McMurray's test and joint line tenderness. *Arthroscopy: The Journal of Arthroscopic and Related Surgery, 20,* 951–958.

149. Stensrud, S., Roos, E. M., & Risberg, M. A. (2012). A 12-week exercise therapy program in middle-aged patients with degenerative meniscus tears: A case series with 1 year follow up. *Journal of Orthopaedic and Sports Physical Therapy, 42,* 919–931.

150. Logerstedt, D. S., Scalzitti, D. A., Bennell, K. L., Hinman, R. S., Silvers-Granelli, H., Ebert, J., Hambly, K., et al. (2018). Knee pain and mobility impairments: Meniscal and articular cartilage lesions revision 2018. *Journal of Orthopaedic and Sports Physical Therapy, 48,* A1–A50.

151. Glatthorn, J. F., Berendts, A. M., Bizzini, M., Munzinger, U., & Maffiuletti, N. A. (2010). Neuromuscular function after arthroscopic partial meniscectomy. *Clinical Orthopaedics and Related Research, 468,* 1336–1343.

152. McLeod, M. M., Gribble, P., Pfile, K. R., & Pietrosimone, B. G. (2012). Effects of arthroscopic partial meniscectomy on quadriceps strength: A systematic review. *Journal of Sport Rehabilitation, 21,* 285–295.

153. Roos, E. M., & Dahlberg, L. (2005). Positive effects of moderate exercise on glycosaminoglycan content in knee cartilage: A four-month, randomized, controlled trial in patients at risk of osteoarthritis. *Arthritis and Rheumatism, 52,* 3507–3514.

154. Jelsing, E. J., Finnoff, J. T., Cheville, A. L., Levy, B. A., & Smith, J. (2013). Sonographic evaluation of the iliotibial band at the lateral femoral epicondyle: Does the iliotibial band move? *Journal of Ultrasound in Medicine: Official Journal of the American Institute of Ultrasound in Medicine, 32,* 1199–1206.

155. Fairclough, J., Hayashi, K., Toumi, H., Lyons, K., Bydder, G., Phillips, N., Best, T. M., et al. (2006). The functional anatomy of the iliotibial band during flexion and extension of the knee: Implications for understanding iliotibial band syndrome. *Journal of Anatomy, 208,* 309–316.

156. Fredericson, M., Cookingham, C. L., Chaudhari, A. M., Dowdell, B. C., Oestreicher, N., & Sahrmann, S. A. (2000). Hip abductor weakness in distance runners with iliotibial band syndrome. *Clinical Journal of Sport Medicine: Official Journal of the Canadian Academy of Sport Medicine, 10,* 169–175.

157. Noehren, B., Davis, I., & Hamill, J. (2007). ASB clinical biomechanics award winner 2006 prospective study of the biomechanical factors associated with iliotibial band syndrome. *Clinical Biomechanics (Bristol Avon), 22,* 951–956.

158. Reese, N. B., & Bandy, W. D. (2003). Use of an inclinometer to measure flexibility of the iliotibial band using the Ober test and the modified Ober test: Differences in magnitude and reliability of measurements. *Journal of Orthopaedic and Sports Physical Therapy, 33,* 326–330.

159. Falvey, E. C., Clark, R. A., Franklyn-Miller, A., Bryant, A. L., Briggs, C., & McCrory, P. R. (2010). Iliotibial band syndrome: An examination of the evidence behind a number of treatment options. *Scandinavian Journal of Medicine & Science in Sports, 20,* 580–587.

160. Baker, R. L., Souza, R. B., & Fredericson, M. (2011). Iliotibial band syndrome: Soft tissue and biomechanical factors in evaluation and treatment. *PM&R: The Journal of Injury, Function, and Rehabilitation, 3,* 550–561.

161. Beers, A., Ryan, M., Kasubuchi, Z., Fraser, S., & Taunton, J. E. (2008). Effects of multi-modal physiotherapy, including hip abductor strengthening, in patients with iliotibial band friction syndrome. *Physiotherapy Canada, 60,* 180–188.

162. Fredericson, M., & Wolf, C. (2005). Iliotibial band syndrome in runners: Innovations in treatment. *Sports Medicine (Auckland, NZ), 35,* 451–459.

163. Ferber, R., Noehren, B., Hamill, J., & Davis, I. S. (2010). Competitive female runners with a history of iliotibial band syndrome demonstrate atypical hip and knee kinematics. *Journal of Orthopaedic and Sports Physical Therapy, 40,* 52–58.

164. van der Worp, M. P., van der Horst, N., de Wijer, A., Backx, F. J. G., & Nijhuis-van der Sanden, M. W. G. (2012). Iliotibial band syndrome in runners: A systematic review. *Sports Medicine (Auckland, NZ), 42,* 969–992.

165. Davis, I. S., & Powers, C. M (2010). Patellofemoral pain syndrome: proximal, distal, and local factors. An International Retreat, April 30–May 2, 2009, Fells Point, Baltimore, MD. *Journal of Orthopaedic and Sports Physical Therapy, 40,* A1-16.

166. Rathleff, M. S., Roos, E. M., Olesen, J. L., Rasmussen, S., & Arendt-Nielsen, L. (2013). Lower mechanical pressure pain thresholds in female adolescents with patellofemoral pain syndrome. *Journal of Orthopaedic and Sports Physical Therapy, 43,* 414–421.

167. Bolgla, L. A., Malone, T. R., Umberger, B. R., & Uhl, T. L. (2008). Hip strength and hip and knee kinematics during stair descent in females with and without patellofemoral pain syndrome. *Journal of Orthopaedic and Sports Physical Therapy, 38,* 12–18.

168. Cichanowski, H. R., Schmitt, J. S., Johnson, R. J., & Niemuth, P. E. (2007). Hip strength in collegiate female athletes with patellofemoral pain. *Medicine and Science in Sports and Exercise, 39,* 1227–1232.

169. Ireland, M. L., Willson, J. D., Ballantyne, B. T., & Davis, I. M. (2003). Hip strength in females with and without patellofemoral pain. *Journal of Orthopaedic and Sports Physical Therapy, 33,* 671–676.

170. Prins, M. R., & van der Wurff, P. (2009). Females with patellofemoral pain syndrome have weak hip muscles: A systematic review. *Australian Journal of Physiotherapy, 55,* 9–15.

171. Robinson, R. L., & Nee, R. J. (2007). Analysis of hip strength in females seeking physical therapy treatment for unilateral patellofemoral pain syndrome. *Journal of Orthopaedic and Sports Physical Therapy, 37,* 232–238.

172. Souza, R. B., & Powers, C. M. (2009). Differences in hip kinematics, muscle strength, and muscle activation between

subjects with and without patellofemoral pain. *Journal of Orthopaedic and Sports Physical Therapy, 39,* 12–19.

173. Willson, J. D., & Davis, I. S. (2009). Lower extremity strength and mechanics during jumping in women with patellofemoral pain. *Journal of Sport Rehabilitation, 18,* 76–90.

174. Barton, C. J., Bonanno, D., Levinger, P., & Menz, H. B. (2010). Foot and ankle characteristics in patellofemoral pain syndrome: A case-control and reliability study. *Journal of Orthopaedic and Sports Physical Therapy, 40,* 286-96.

175. Thijs, Y., Van Tiggelen, D., Roosen, P., De Clercq, D., & Witvrouw, E. (2007). A prospective study on gait-related intrinsic risk factors for patellofemoral pain. *Clinical Journal of Sport Medicine: Official Journal of the Canadian Academy of Sport Medicine, 17,* 437–445.

176. Piva, S. R., Fitzgerald, K., Irrgang, J. J., Jones, S., Hando, B. R., Browder, D. A., & Childs, J. D. (2006). Reliability of measures of impairments associated with patellofemoral pain syndrome. *BMC: Musculoskeletal Disorders, 7,* 33.

177. Boling, M., Padua, D., Marshall, S., Guskiewicz, K., Pyne, S., & Beutler, A. (2010). Gender differences in the incidence and prevalence of patellofemoral pain syndrome. *Scandinavian Journal of Medicine & Science in Sports, 20,* 725–730.

178. Dolak, K. L., Silkman, C., Medina McKeon, J., Hosey, R. G., Lattermann, C., & Uhl, T. L. (2011). Hip strengthening prior to functional exercises reduces pain sooner than quadriceps strengthening in females with patellofemoral pain syndrome: A randomized clinical trial. *Journal of Orthopaedic and Sports Physical Therapy, 41,* 560–570.

179. Fukuda, T. Y., Melo, W. P., Zaffalon, B. M., Rossetto, F. M., Magalhães, E., Bryk, F. F., & Martin, R. L. (2012). Hip posterolateral musculature strengthening in sedentary women with patellofemoral pain syndrome: A randomized controlled clinical trial with 1-year follow-up. *Journal of Orthopaedic and Sports Physical Therapy, 42,* 823–830.

180. Mascal, C. L., Landel, R., & Powers, C. (2003). Management of patellofemoral pain targeting hip, pelvis, and trunk muscle function: 2 case reports. *Journal of Orthopaedic and Sports Physical Therapy, 33,* 647–660.

181. Nakagawa, T. H., Muniz, T. B., Baldon Rde, M., Dias Maciel, C., de Menezes Reiff, R. B., & Serrão, F. V. (2008). The effect of additional strengthening of hip abductor and lateral rotator muscles in patellofemoral pain syndrome: A randomized controlled pilot study. *Clinical Rehabilitation, 22,* 1051–1060.

182. Steinkamp, L. A., Dillingham, M. F., Markel, M. D., Hill, J. A., & Kaufman, K. R. (1993). Biomechanical considerations in patellofemoral joint rehabilitation. *American Journal of Sports Medicine, 21,* 438–444.

183. Kaya, D., Doral, M. N., & Callaghan, M. (2012). How can we strengthen the quadriceps femoris in patients with patellofemoral pain syndrome? *Muscles, Ligaments and Tendons Journal, 2,* 25–32.

184. Roush, M. B., Sevier, T. L., Wilson, J. K., Jenkinson, D. M., Helfst, R. H., Gehlsen, G. M., & Basey, A. L. (2000). Anterior knee pain: a clinical comparison of rehabilitation methods. *Clinical Journal of Sport Medicine: Official Journal of the Canadian Academy of Sport Medicine, 10,* 22–28.

185. Ng, G. Y. F., Zhang, A. Q., & Li, C. K. (2008). Biofeedback exercise improved the EMG activity ratio of the medial and lateral vasti muscles in subjects with patellofemoral pain syndrome. *Journal of Electromyography and Kinesiology: Official Journal of the International Society of Electrophysiology and Kinesiology, 18,* 128–133.

186. Puniello, M. S. (1993). Iliotibial band tightness and medial patellar glide in patients with patellofemoral dysfunction. *Journal of Orthopaedic and Sports Physical Therapy, 17,* 144–148.

187. McConnell, J. (1986). The management of chondromalacia patellae: A long term solution. *Australian Journal of Physiotherapy, 32,* 215–223.

188. Warden, S. J., Hinman, R. S., Watson, M. A., Jr, Avin, K. G., Bialocerkowski, A. E., & Crossley, K. M. (2008). Patellar taping and bracing for the treatment of chronic knee pain: A systematic review and meta-analysis. *Arthritis and Rheumatism, 59,* 73–83.

189. Whittingham, M., Palmer, S., & Macmillan, F. (2004). Effects of taping on pain and function in patellofemoral pain syndrome: A randomized controlled trial. *Journal of Orthopaedic and Sports Physical Therapy, 34,* 504–510.

190. Bisseling, R. W., Hof, A. L., Bredeweg, S. W., Zwerver, J., & Mulder, T. (2008). Are the take-off and landing phase dynamics of the volleyball spike jump related to patellar tendinopathy? *British Journal of Sports Medicine, 42,* 483–489.

191. Bisseling, R. W., Hof, A. L., Bredeweg, S. W., Zwerver, J., & Mulder, T. (2007). Relationship between landing strategy and patellar tendinopathy in volleyball. *British Journal of Sports Medicine, 41,* e8.

192. Witvrouw, E., Bellemans, J., Lysens, R., Danneels, L., & Cambier, D. (2001). Intrinsic risk factors for the development of patellar tendinitis in an athletic population. A two-year prospective study. *American Journal of Sports Medicine, 29,* 190–195.

193. Backman, L. J., & Danielson, P. (2011). Low range of ankle dorsiflexion predisposes for patellar tendinopathy in junior elite basketball players: A 1-year prospective study. *American Journal of Sports Medicine, 39,* 2626–2633.

194. Malliaras, P., Cook, J. L., & Kent, P. (2006). Reduced ankle dorsiflexion range may increase the risk of patellar tendon injury among volleyball players. *Journal of Science and Medicine in Sport, 9,* 304–309.

195. Rath, E., Schwarzkopf, R., & Richmond, J. C. (2010). Clinical signs and anatomical correlation of patellar tendinitis. *Indian Journal of Orthopaedics, 44,* 435–437.

196. Jonsson, P., & Alfredson, H. (2005). Superior results with eccentric compared to concentric quadriceps training in patients with jumper's knee: A prospective randomised study. *British Journal of Sports Medicine, 39,* 847–850.

197. Larsson, M. E. H., Käll, I., & Nilsson-Helander, K. (2012). Treatment of patellar tendinopathy—A systematic review of randomized controlled trials. *Knee Surgery, Sports Traumatology, Arthroscopy: Official Journal of ESSKA, 20,* 1632–1646.

198. Saithna, A., Gogna, R., Baraza, N., Modi, C., & Spencer, S. (2012). Eccentric exercise protocols for patella tendinopathy: Should we really be withdrawing athletes from sport? A systematic review. *Open Orthopaedics Journal, 6,* 553–557.

199. Purdam, C. R., Jonsson, P., Alfredson, H., Lorentzon, R., Cook, J. L., & Khan, K. M. (2004). A pilot study of the eccentric decline squat in the management of painful chronic patellar tendinopathy. *British Journal of Sports Medicine, 38,* 395–397.

200. Young, M. A., Cook, J. L., Purdam, C. R., Kiss, Z. S., & Alfredson, H. (2005). Eccentric decline squat protocol offers superior results at 12 months compared with traditional eccentric protocol for patellar tendinopathy in volleyball players. *British Journal of Sports Medicine, 39,* 102–105.

201. Janssen, I., Steele, J. R., Munro, B. J., & Brown, N. A. (2013). Predicting the patellar tendon force generated when landing from a jump. *Medicine and Science in Sports and Exercise, 45,* 927–934.

Chapter 12

Orthopedic Interventions for the Ankle and Foot

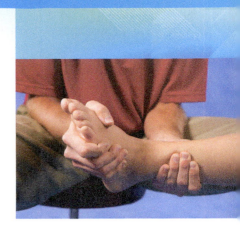

Anatomy and Physiology

Common Pathologies

LEARNING OUTCOMES

At the end of this chapter, the student will:

12.1   Describe the anatomy of the ankle and foot.

12.2   List normal ankle and foot range of motion.

12.3   Describe normal kinematics of the ankle and foot joints, including how the foot changes from being a flexible accommodator to a rigid propulsor in gait.

12.4   Describe the "top-down" versus the "bottom-up" philosophies of lower extremity control.

12.5   Describe the mechanics, and discuss the purposes, of anterior, posterior, medial, lateral, and distraction mobilization techniques of select ankle and foot joints.

12.6   Describe common ankle and foot pathologies and typical presentations.

12.7   Discuss contributing factors to various ankle and foot pathologies and, when relevant, preventive measures.

12.8   Describe the clinical tests that are used to diagnose common ankle and foot pathologies and how to administer the tests.

12.9   Discuss common treatment interventions for ankle and foot pathologies.

12.10 Describe surgical interventions and postsurgical considerations for the ankle and foot including ankle ORIF and Achilles tendon repair.

12.11 Explain the impact of excessive or prolonged pronation on plantar fasciitis, posterior tibialis tendon dysfunction, medial tibial stress syndrome, and tarsal tunnel syndrome.

12.12 Describe clinical alerts for select ankle and foot pathologies.

KEY WORDS

Bimalleolar fracture	Periostitis	Syndesmosis
Diastasis	Ray	Tarsal tunnel
Fasciotomy	Rearfoot	Trimalleolar fracture
Forefoot	Rectus	Windlass mechanism
Midfoot	Stress fracture	
Mortise	Subtalar joint neutral	

Anatomy and Physiology

As the most distal component in the lower extremity kinetic chain, the ankle and foot are subject to extreme rotational and weight-bearing stresses. When the foot contacts the ground, it must be flexible enough to absorb and dissipate forces at initial contact and to accommodate to uneven terrain. But it must be stable enough to provide a base of support for the body and to transmit forces at push-off in the gait cycle. Moreover, the foot must be able to change from a flexible to a rigid structure in fractions of a second. These somewhat conflicting functions are largely accomplished by the anatomical structure of the foot and will be discussed in this chapter.

Bone and Joint Anatomy and Physiology

Like the intricate nature of the hand, the ankle and foot are structurally and functionally very complex. This area contains 28 bones and 30 joints. They include the distal tibia and fibula, the tarsals (talus, calcaneus, navicular, cuboid, and three cuneiforms), the metatarsals, and the phalanges.

The joints in the foot and ankle include the distal tibiofibular joint, the ankle joint between the lower leg bones and the talus, the subtalar joint between the talus and calcaneus, the talonavicular and calcaneocuboid joints between the **rearfoot** and **midfoot,** and joints within and between the bones of the midfoot and **forefoot.**

When viewed from the medial and lateral side, the foot has an arch shape from the heel to the heads of the metatarsals. These are the medial and lateral longitudinal arches. The foot also has a transverse arch from medial to lateral.

The bones of the foot and ankle are depicted in Figure 12.1 and summarized in Table 12-1. Regions of the foot are summarized in Box 12-1. Because terminology is variably used and often confusing, a clarification of the movements of the foot is essential to understanding the joints of this region. See Box 12-2 for review of the terminology of movement and position.

Distal Tibiofibular Joint

The distal tibiofibular joint forms the proximal part of the ankle joint. The joint is stabilized by tibiofibular ligaments. This joint is not a synovial joint, but a **syndesmosis.**

The bones are held in close approximation by multiple ligaments. Limited movement occurs here, and stability of this joint is important to preserve the function of the ankle joint. The two bones separate minimally in ankle dorsiflexion as the anterior talus acts as a wedge.

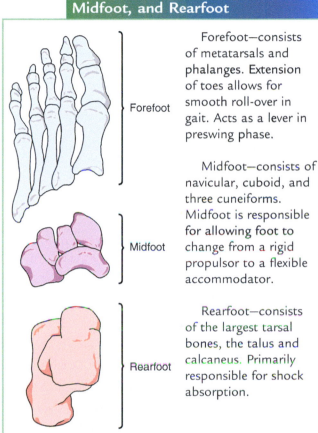

Box 12-1 | **The Foot Is Functionally Divided into Three Regions: The Forefoot, Midfoot, and Rearfoot**

Forefoot—consists of metatarsals and phalanges. Extension of toes allows for smooth roll-over in gait. Acts as a lever in preswing phase.

Midfoot—consists of navicular, cuboid, and three cuneiforms. Midfoot is responsible for allowing foot to change from a rigid propulsor to a flexible accommodator.

Rearfoot—consists of the largest tarsal bones, the talus and calcaneus. Primarily responsible for shock absorption.

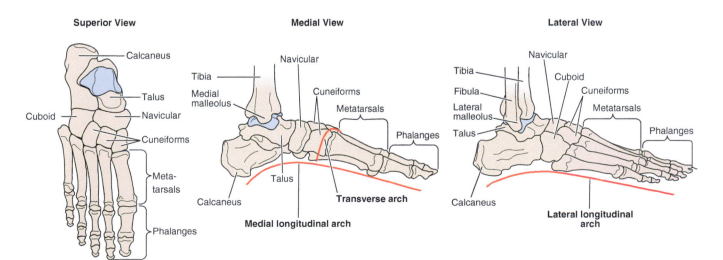

Figure 12.1 The ankle and foot area include the distal tibia and fibula and the twenty-six bones of the foot.

Table 12-1 Bone and Joint Anatomy and Physiology

Of the Ankle and Foot

Joint	Anatomy	Normal ROM and Movements	Landmarks	Clinical Considerations
Distal tibiofibular	Syndesmosis between the two lower leg bones, stabilized by the joint capsule, the anterior and posterior tibiofibular ligaments, and the interosseous ligament.	Very little movement occurs here. Dorsiflexion widens the distance between the two bones.		A high ankle sprain involves this joint.
Tibiotalar (Talocrural)	Hinge joint between tibia, fibula, and dome of the talus. Stabilized laterally by several small ligaments, and medially by the strong deltoid ligament.	Dorsiflexion 20° Plantarflexion 50°		Limited ankle dorsiflexion contributes to plantar fasciitis, toe deformities, Achilles tendinopathy, and gait deviations. Loose packed position 10° of plantarflexion and neutral inversion/ eversion.
Subtalar	Joint between talus and calcaneus with several articulating surfaces. Talocalcaneal ligaments stabilize.	Supination (off-weight: inversion, plantarflexion, and adduction of calcaneus). Pronation (off-weight: eversion, dorsiflexion, and abduction of calcaneus).		Movement of talus on calcaneus occurs through gait cycle. Subtalar joint is supinated at initial contact, pronates during mid stance, and supinates in late stance.
Transverse tarsal joint	This joint consists of: • talonavicular joint • calcaneocuboid joint			Two axes of motion in this joint that make the foot rigid with supination and flexible with pronation.
Tarsometatarsal joints (TMT)	Plane joints that allow minimal gliding movements		The base of the fifth metatarsal is palpated on the lateral side of the foot. This is just distal to the fifth TMT joint.	
Metatarsophalangeal joints (MTP)	Condyloid joints with two degrees of freedom stabilized by collateral ligaments	Flexion and extension. Abduction and adduction.		Limited great big toe extension can contribute to plantar fasciitis and hallux valgus deformity.
Interphalangeal joints	Hinge joints with one degree of freedom	Flexion and extension		

Box 12-2 Review of Terminology of Ankle and Foot Movements and Positions

Dorsiflexion/Plantarflexion

Dorsiflexion and plantarflexion occur mostly at the tibiotalar joint in a sagittal plane around a frontal (medial-lateral) axis. Dorsiflexion and plantarflexion are shown in the following figure.

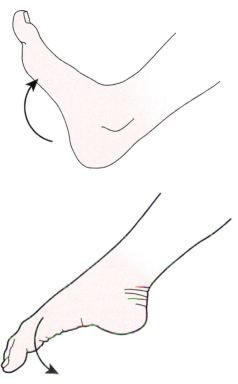

Inversion/Eversion

Inversion and eversion refer to movements that occur at the subtalar and midfoot joints in a frontal plane around a sagittal (anterior-posterior) axis. Foot inversion brings the bottom of the foot medially. Eversion brings it laterally. These movements usually occur in combination with other movements.

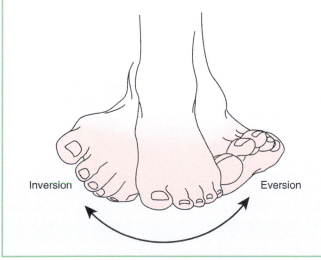

Inversion   Eversion

Inversion and eversion may also refer to the position of the calcaneus. An inverted calcaneus is also called an adducted calcaneus. An everted calcaneus is abducted.

Abduction/Adduction

The terms *abduction* and *adduction* may be used to refer to movement or position of the big toe, forefoot, talus, or calcaneus. Abduction/adduction of the big toe occurs at the first metatarsophalangeal joint. Abduction/adduction of the forefoot occur at the tarsometatarsal joints and at all joints distal to this. The following figure depicts abduction and adduction of the big toe and forefoot.

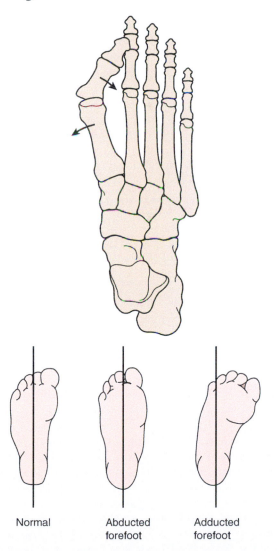

Normal   Abducted   Adducted
                forefoot   forefoot

In addition to forefoot abduction and adduction, the calcaneus can abduct or adduct on the talus. These terms are most consistently used when discussing open chain movement. Abduction of the calcaneus

Continued

Box 12-2   Review of Terminology of Ankle and Foot Movements and Positions—cont'd

accompanies calcaneal eversion. When discussing closed chain movement at the subtalar joint, the talus rather than the calcaneus is considered the moving bone. In closed chain pronation, the talus adducts on the calcaneus; in closed chain supination the talus abducts on the calcaneus. This is discussed under "Subtalar Joint" mechanics.

Varus/Valgus

Varus and *valgus* are terms that describe the position of two segments separated by a joint. Varus denotes a distal segment that is aligned toward the midline relative to the proximal segment. Valgus denotes a distal segment that is aligned away from the midline relative to the proximal segment. In the foot, these terms are commonly used to describe the calcaneus relative to the talus and lower leg, and to describe the forefoot relative to the rearfoot. This figure illustrates varus and valgus of these two areas.

Pronation/Supination

Pronation and *supination* are combination movements that occur at the subtalar and transverse tarsal joints. Off-weight pronation is a position of calcaneal dorsiflexion, eversion, and abduction. On-weight pronation describes this same type of alignment, with a flat foot and everted calcaneus. The talus is adducted on the calcaneus.

Off-weight supination includes components of calcaneal plantarflexion, inversion, and adduction. On-weight supination refers to this same type of alignment, with a high medial arch and inverted calcaneus. The talus is abducted on the calcaneus. This figure depicts pronation and supination in off- and on-weight positions.

Posterior view, right foot

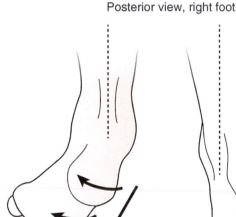
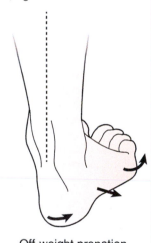

Off-weight supination   Off-weight pronation

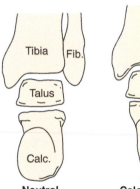
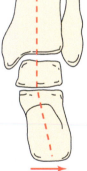

Tibia   Fib.
Talus
Calc.

Neutral   Calcaneal valgus   Calcaneal varus

Posterior View

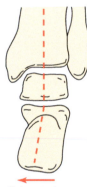

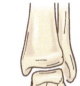

Forefoot varus   Neutral   Forefoot valgus

Right leg, posterior view

Posterior view, right foot

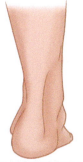
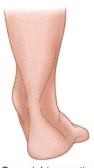

On-weight supination   On-weight pronation

High ankle sprain disrupts this joint. We will discuss this pathology later. Figure 12.2 illustrates this joint.

Tibiotalar (Talocrural) Joint

The joint between the talus and the distal tibia and fibula is called the tibiotalar (talocrural) joint or ankle joint. This joint forms the distal part of the ankle joint and is a hinge joint that allows for movement primarily in the sagittal plane. Most of the dorsiflexion and plantarflexion of the ankle-foot complex occurs here. The tibiotalar joint is often referred to as a **mortise** joint. A mortise is a structure with a groove or slot that accepts an interlocking piece. The distal tibia and fibula form the mortise that fits over the superior talus, as shown in Figure 12.2. This interconnecting joint increases the stability of the ankle-foot complex.

Subtalar Joint

The joint between the talus and calcaneus is referred to as the talocalcaneal or subtalar joint. This articulation is

the first of three key joints in the foot. The talus doesn't sit directly on top of the calcaneus, but toward the medial side. During pronation the talus slides down and in on the calcaneus, and the calcaneus tilts into valgus. During supination, the talus slides up and out on the calcaneus, and the calcaneus tilts into varus. This movement allows the subtalar joint to dampen the rotational forces from the leg during weight acceptance. Internal rotation of the lower leg causes the talus to slide medially and the foot to pronate. With external rotation of the lower leg, the foot supinates. Figure 12.3 depicts the movement of the talus on the calcaneus during pronation and supination.

Talonavicular Joint

The talonavicular articulation is the second of three key joints in the foot. With internal rotation of the lower leg and sliding of the talus down and in, the navicular follows the talus and is pulled down, flattening the medial longitudinal arch of the foot. With external rotation of the lower leg, the navicular follows the talus and is pulled up, elevating the medial longitudinal arch. Figure 12.4 depicts the effect of pronation and supination on the navicular. This relationship can be seen in the *navicular drop test* as described later in the chapter.

Transverse Tarsal Joint

The third of three key joints in the foot, the transverse tarsal joint is the S-shaped articulation between the talus and calcaneus proximally and the navicular and cuboid distally. This joint has two axes of movement, a longitudinal and oblique axis, as shown in Figure 12.5. The axes are crossed during supination and are uncrossed in pronation.[1] When the axes are crossed, the tarsals in the midfoot lock up and the foot becomes rigid. When the axes are uncrossed, the foot is flexible. This joint allows the foot to accomplish the conflicting functions of being rigid for stability and for push-off in gait, yet flexible for dampening rotational forces and accommodating to uneven surfaces. We will discuss this further under "Kinematics."

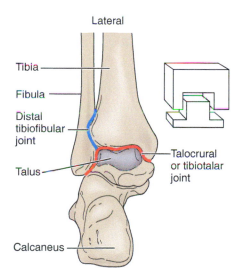

Figure 12.2 The distal tibiofibular and tibiotalar joints are the two joints of the ankle. The tibiotalar joint is also called the ankle mortise.

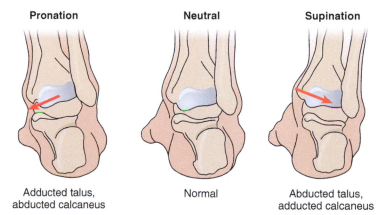

Figure 12.3 The subtalar joint is one of three key joints in the foot. When the foot is pronated, the talus slides down and in on the calcaneus and the calcaneus everts. In supination, the talus slides up and out on the calcaneus and the calcaneus inverts.

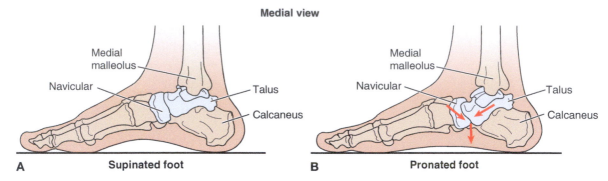

Medial view

A **Supinated foot**

B **Pronated foot**

Figure 12.4 The talonavicular joint is one of three key joints in the foot. When the foot is supinated, the talus sits high on the calcaneus and the navicular follows. This elevates the medial longitudinal arch (A). In pronation, the talus slides down and the navicular follows. It may become a point of weight-bearing in a pronated foot (B).

Soft Tissues

Ligaments

The ligaments of the distal tibiofibular joint include the anterior tibiofibular and posterior tibiofibular ligaments. Additionally, the interosseous membrane continues into this area as the interosseous ligament. During ankle dorsiflexion, slight widening of the ankle mortise is necessary to accommodate the wider part of the talus. The ligaments of the tibiofibular joints allow this slight movement to occur while maintaining joint stability.

The ankle joint is stabilized by a strong ligament system on the medial side and three smaller ligaments on the lateral side. The ligament complex on the medial side is called the deltoid ligament or medial collateral ligament. This fan-shaped ligament has both a superficial and deep region with bands that connect the medial malleolus of the tibia to the navicular, talus, and calcaneus. The deltoid ligament provides significant stability to the medial ankle against eversion or valgus forces.

The three ligaments on the lateral side comprise the lateral collateral ligament. They are the anterior talofibular ligament, posterior talofibular ligament, and calcaneofibular ligament. These three ligaments are not as strong as the deltoid ligament on the medial side but help to control inversion or varus forces.

Numerous ligaments on the plantar surface of the foot help to support the longitudinal arches. The two most important of these ligaments are the spring ligament (plantar calcaneonavicular ligament) and the long plantar ligament. The spring ligament supports the medial longitudinal arch. The long plantar ligament provides arch support to the lateral side of the foot. They are reinforced by the plantar fascia. Figure 12.7 illustrates the ligaments of the ankle and foot.

Plantar Fascia

Also called the plantar aponeurosis, the plantar fascia is a thick band of connective tissue that runs from the inferior calcaneus to the proximal phalanges (Fig. 12.8).

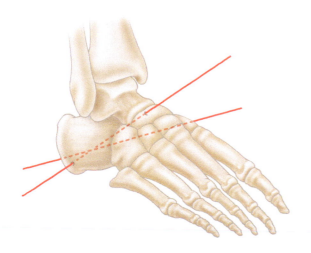

Figure 12.5 The transverse tarsal joint of the midfoot has two axes of motion. When the foot is pronated the axes are nearly parallel, making the foot flexible. But in supination the axes cross, causing the foot to transform into a rigid structure.

Tarsometatarsal Joints

Tarsometatarsal (TMT) joints are the articulations between the metatarsals distally and the corresponding tarsal proximally. The term *ray* is used to describe the combined tarsal and first through fifth metatarsal. For example, first ray is used to indicate the first cuneiform and first metatarsal. Fifth ray refers to the cuboid and fifth metatarsal. The tarsometatarsal joints allow for movement in all three planes. Figure 12.6 depicts the TMT joints, and the first and fifth rays.

Metatarsophalangeal Joints

The convex distal ends of the metatarsals articulate with the concave proximal phalanx on each digit at the metatarsal (MTP) joints. These joints allow two degrees of freedom. Unlike the hand, the MTP joints of the foot have more extension than flexion. This extension permits heel rise while maintaining toe contact with the floor in late-stance phase of gait.

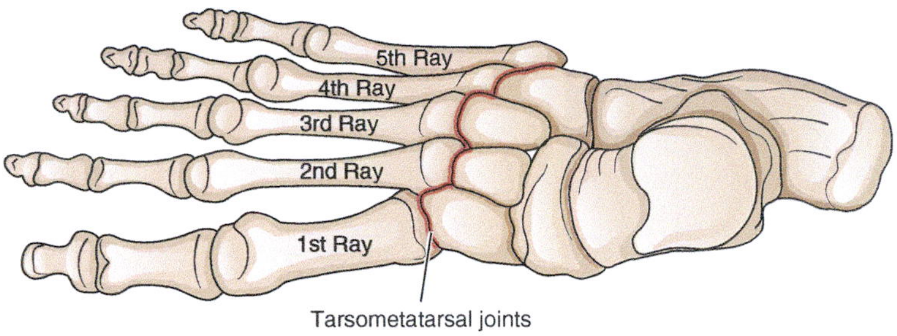

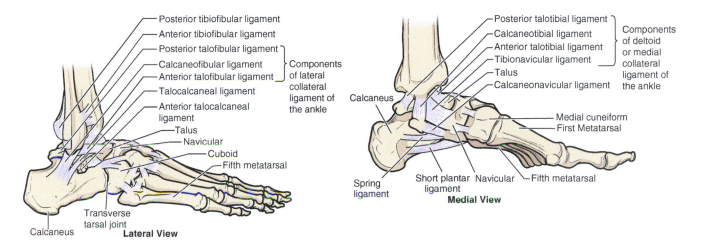

Figure 12.6 The tarsometatarsal joint is shown by the red line. The tarsals and metatarsals with which they articulate are called rays. The first ray is formed by the cuneiform and the first metatarsal, ' the fifth ray by the cuboid and fifth metatarsal.

Figure 12.7 The ligaments of the medial and lateral ankle.

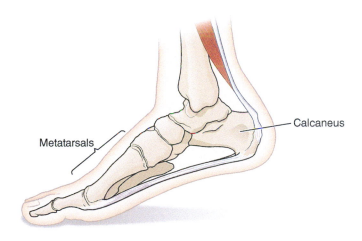

Figure 12.8 The plantar fascia is important in the biomechanics of the foot and bears up to 14% of the load on the foot.

This aponeurosis provides up to 14% of the load-bearing capacity of the ankle-foot complex.[2] The plantar fascia acts as a superficial ligament to stabilize the longitudinal arches. This structure will be discussed further under the pathology *Plantar Fasciitis*.

Flexor Retinaculum

A wide band of connective tissue, the flexor retinaculum runs from the medial malleolus to the medial side of the calcaneus. This retinaculum holds the tendons of the

posterior extrinsic muscles of the foot in place. It forms the roof of the tarsal tunnel.

Table 12-2 summarizes the ligaments of the foot and ankle.

Tarsal Tunnel

The **tarsal tunnel** is a structure that is formed by the flexor retinaculum running superficially over the medial ankle, forming the roof of the tunnel. The floor of the tunnel is comprised of the medial malleolus of the tibia,

Table 12-2 Connective Tissue Anatomy and Physiology
Of the Ankle and Foot

Structure	Anatomy	Function	Clinical Considerations
Joint capsule	Spans the tibiotalar joint. Reinforced by thickened areas anteriorly and posteriorly. Medially and laterally there are strong ligaments to reinforce.		Anterior capsule may be injured in a plantarflexion injury.
Distal tibiofibular ligaments	Three ligaments stabilize the distal tibiofibular joint: • anterior tibiofibular ligament • posterior tibiofibular ligament • interosseous tibiofibular ligament.	Stabilizes the distal tibiofibular joint. Allow the ankle mortise to widen with dorsiflexion and narrow with plantarflexion.	Stabilizes the tibiotalar joint in plantar- and dorsiflexion. May be injured in a high ankle sprain.
Medial (deltoid) ankle ligaments	Triangular system of layered ankle ligaments. Ligaments run from medial malleolus to talus, calcaneus, and navicular.	Support the tibiotalar joint on the medial side.	May be referred to as the medial collateral ligament of the ankle. Stabilizes the ankle against eversion. Very broad, thick ligament structure that is infrequently injured.
Lateral ankle ligaments	Three ligaments on the lateral side: • anterior talofibular • posterior talofibular • calcaneofibular.	Support the tibiotalar joint on the lateral side.	May be referred to as the lateral collateral ligament of the ankle. Stabilizes the ankle against inversion. Anterior talofibular is the most frequently sprained ligament in the ankle.[3].
Plantar calcaneonavicular (spring) ligament	On the plantar surface of the foot, runs from calcaneus to navicular.	Supports the medial longitudinal arch and the head of the talus.	Ligament rupture leads to flatfoot deformity.
Long plantar ligament	On the lateral plantar surface of the foot, runs from the middle of the calcaneus to the cuboid and metatarsals 3–5.	Supports the lateral longitudinal arch.	
Plantar fascia	On the plantar surface of the foot, runs from the calcaneus to the MTP joint and proximal phalanx.[4,5]	Supports the longitudinal arch of the foot. Promotes increased arch height with big toe extension through the windlass mechanism.	Plantar fasciitis is a common pathology.
Flexor retinaculum	Runs from the medial malleolus to the medial side of the calcaneus.	Holds the tendons of the posterior extrinsic muscles of the foot in place.	Forms the roof of the tarsal tunnel. Swelling in the area may lead to tarsal tunnel syndrome.

the talus, and the calcaneus. Through this tunnel run the tendons of posterior tibialis, flexor digitorum longus, flexor hallucis longus, and the tibial artery and nerve (Fig. 12.9). The bony floor and ligamentous roof of the tarsal tunnel make the size of the tunnel relatively fixed, which can lead to compression of the nerve in the tunnel.

Bursae

There are two bursae on the posterior calcaneus: a large subcutaneous calcaneal bursa and the retrocalcaneal bursa. The subcutaneous calcaneal bursa lies superficial to the Achilles tendon. The retrocalcaneal bursa lies between the Achilles tendon and the calcaneus, proximal to the insertion of the tendon. These bursae may become

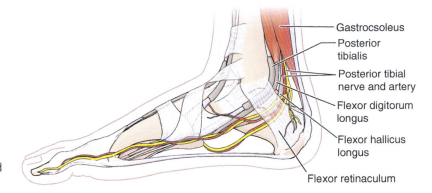

Figure 12.9 The tarsal tunnel is formed by the flexor retinaculum, which runs from medial malleolus to calcaneus. The tibial nerve runs through the tunnel and may become compressed here.

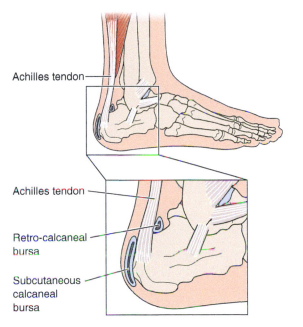

Figure 12.10 Two calcaneal bursae, a subcutaneous calcaneal bursa and a retrocalcaneal bursa, may be a source of posterior heel pain.

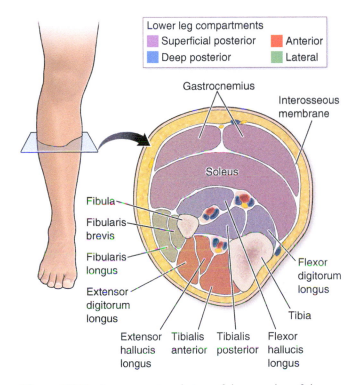

Figure 12.11 A cross-sectional view of the muscles of the lower leg. The muscles are grouped into four groups of three muscles, which are separated by a thick fascia. Fibularis tertius is not showing in this cross-sectional view, as it originates below the cut.

inflamed and cause posterior heel pain. Figure 12.10 depicts the bursae.

Ankle and Foot Muscles

Ankle and extrinsic foot muscles are found in the lower leg. There are 12 of these muscles, and they can best be understood by studying them in four groups. A group of three is found on the anterior lower leg. On the posterior lower leg there is a superficial group and a deep group, each with three muscles. The deep posterior group mirrors the anterior group, with opposing actions. The last group of three is found on the lateral lower leg. Each of these four groups is separated from each other by a fascia. Figure 12.11 depicts a cross section of the lower leg illustrating these groupings.

The muscles of the ankle and foot are frequently named for their action, insertion, or location. As in the wrist and hand, a muscle name that includes "flexor" or

"extensor" will foretell its action. Muscles with the name "digiti" or "digitorum" are toe muscles, and "hallucis" are big toe muscles. Muscles that have tibialis in the name will run on the medial leg and foot, and muscles that have fibularis in the name will run on the lateral leg and foot.

The muscles, origin, insertion, innervation, and action are summarized in Table 12-3.

Anterior Lower Leg Muscles

The mnemonic of "Tom, Dick, and Harry" can be used to remember these muscles: anterior **t**ibialis, extensor **d**igitorum longus, and extensor **h**allucis longus. All three of these muscles can dorsiflex the ankle because they cross the ankle anterior to the malleoli. In addition, anterior tibialis inverts the foot. Extensor digitorum longus extends toes 2 to 5, and extensor hallucis longus extends the big toe.

Lateral Lower Leg Muscles

The three fibularis muscles are the ankle evertors: fibularis longus, fibularis brevis, and fibularis tertius. In addition to ankle eversion, by passing anterior or posterior to the lateral malleolus, they can assist in ankle dorsiflexion or plantarflexion. respectively.

Posterior Lower Leg Muscles—Superficial Group

The posterior muscles—gastrocnemius, soleus, and plantaris—are the ankle plantarflexors. They are the muscles that give the calf its definition and shape. Frequently, gastrocnemius and soleus are referred to as gastrocsoleus due to their common tendinous insertion.

Table 12-3 Muscle Anatomy and Kinesiology
Of the Ankle and Foot

Muscle	Origin	Insertion	Innervation	Primary Action	Clinical Considerations
Anterior tibialis	Proximal tibia	First metatarsal and second cuneiform	Common fibular nerve	Dorsiflexion and inversion of the ankle	
Extensor digitorum longus	Proximal tibia, fibula, and interosseous membrane	Middle and distal phalanx of toes 2–5	Common fibular nerve	Extension of toes 2–5, weak assister of ankle dorsiflexion	
Extensor hallucis longus	Middle third of the fibula and the interosseous membrane	Distal phalanx of the big toe	Common fibular nerve	Big toe extension, weak assister of ankle dorsiflexion and inversion	
Fibularis longus	Proximal half of the fibula	Base of the first metatarsal and first cuneiform.	Common fibular nerve	Ankle eversion and plantarflexion; in addition, it functions as a dynamic supporter of the transverse arch.	
Fibularis brevis	Distal half of the fibula	Base of the fifth metatarsal	Common fibular nerve	Ankle eversion and plantarflexion	
Fibularis tertius	Anterior aspect of the fibula	Base of the fifth metatarsal	Common fibular nerve	Ankle eversion and dorsiflexion	
Gastrocnemius	Femoral condyles	Posterior calcaneus	Tibial nerve	Ankle plantarflexion, knee flexion	Joins with soleus and plantaris to form the Achilles tendon. Tendinopathy of this tendon is common.
Soleus	Posterior tibia and fibula	Posterior calcaneus	Tibial nerve	Ankle plantarflexion	To stretch soleus without gastrocnemius becoming the limiting factor, bend the knee.

Table 12-3   Muscle Anatomy and Kinesiology—cont'd

Of the Ankle and Foot

Muscle	Origin	Insertion	Innervation	Primary Action	Clinical Considerations
Plantaris	Lateral epicondyle of the femur	Posterior calcaneus	Tibial nerve	Weak plantarflexor and knee flexor.[6] Its role appears to be primarily one of proprioception.[7]	Similar to the palmaris longus in the upper extremity, this muscle is missing in 7% to 20% of the population.[8] The tendon may be harvested for a tendon graft without compromise of ankle plantarflexion strength.
Posterior tibialis	Posterior aspect of the proximal tibia	Dividing into three bands, the insertion is broad: the navicular, middle and lateral cuneiform, cuboid, and the base of metatarsals 2–4.	Tibial nerve	Plantarflexion and inversion of ankle	Key stabilizer of the medial ankle and foot. Tendon dysfunction affects medial arch.
Flexor digitorum longus	Posterior aspect of the tibia	Distal phalanx of toes 2–5	Tibial nerve	Flexion of toes 2–5 and ankle plantarflexion, weak ankle inversion	
Flexor hallucis longus	Posterior surface of the fibula	Distal phalanx of the big toe	Tibial nerve	Big toe flexion and ankle plantarflexion, weak ankle inversion	
Lumbricals	Tendon of flexor digitorum longus	Extensor expansion of the toes	Tibial nerve	Flexion of the MTP joints, and extension of the PIP and DIP joints.	
Plantar and dorsal interossei	Between the metatarsals	Dorsal: base of proximal phalanges 2–4 Plantar: base of proximal phalanges 3–5.	Tibial nerve	Abduction and adduction of toes; support the longitudinal arches of the foot[9].	
Quadratus plantae	Plantar surface of calcaneus	Tendon of flexor digitorum longus	Tibial nerve	Assists toe flexion by straightening the pull of FDL.	

Posterior Lower Leg Muscles—Deep Group

The deep posterior muscles are a reflection the anterior muscles of the lower leg. Again, the mnemonic of "Tom, Dick, and Harry" can be used to remember these muscles: posterior tibialis, flexor digitorum longus, and flexor hallucis longus. All three muscles are capable of plantarflexing and inverting the ankle because they enter the foot posterior to the medial malleolus. Additionally, flexor digitorum longus flexes toes 2 to 5 and flexor hallucis longus flexes the big toe.

Intrinsic Muscles of the Foot

Muscles that originate and insert in the foot are called intrinsic muscles. These include the lumbricals, dorsal interossei, plantar interossei, and quadratus plantae.

Nerves

Branches of the sciatic nerve provide the innervation to the muscles distal to the knee. Recall that just proximal to the knee on the posterior leg, the sciatic nerve splits into two nerves: the tibial nerve and the common fibular nerve.

The tibial nerve continues into the posterior calf and innervates all the posterior leg muscles: the gastrocnemius, soleus, plantaris, posterior tibialis, flexor digitorum longus, and flexor hallucis longus. It enters the plantar surface of the foot through the tarsal tunnel and innervates the intrinsic muscles of the foot including the lumbricals and interossei. Figure 12.12A depicts the tibial nerve.

The common fibular nerve wraps around the head of the fibula and runs down the anterior lower leg. It

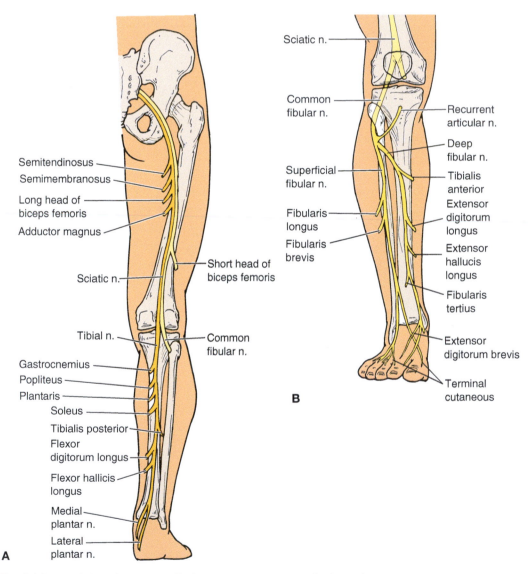

Figure 12.12 The tibial nerve (A) and common fibular nerve (B) innervate the lower leg and foot muscles.

Table 12-4　Nerve Anatomy and Physiology

Of the Lower Leg

Structure	Anatomy	Function	Clinical Considerations
Tibial nerve	Branch of sciatic nerve that runs down posterior calf and into the bottom of the foot.	Innervates the posterior calf muscles and foot intrinsic muscles.	Tarsal tunnel syndrome is impingement of this nerve at the medial ankle.
Common fibular nerve	Branch of the sciatic nerve that crosses fibular head and runs down anterior lower leg.	Innervates anterior and lateral muscle groups.	

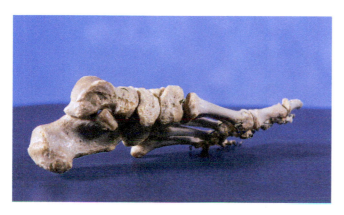

Figure 12.13 Foot alignment displays a forefoot varus. The calcaneus is perpendicular to the floor. Notice the inversion of the forefoot.

innervates the anterior tibialis, extensor digitorum longus, and extensor hallucis longus, as well as all three fibularis muscles: fibularis longus, fibularis brevis, and fibularis tertius. Figure 12.12B depicts the common fibular nerve. Nerve anatomy is summarized in Table 12-4.

Kinematics of the Ankle and Foot

Static Alignment

Static foot alignment refers to the position of the calcaneus and the forefoot when the foot is in a neutral subtalar joint position, referred to as **subtalar joint neutral** (STJN). In this position, normal alignment would indicate the calcaneus to be in line with the lower leg. It shouldn't be inverted or everted. This position is called calcaneal **rectus**. Normal available range of motion from this neutral position is 20° of calcaneal inversion and 10° of calcaneal eversion. The forefoot and rearfoot should not be rotated relative to each other. If the forefoot is turned in relative to the rearfoot, it is called a forefoot varus. If it is turned out, the forefoot is in valgus. Figure 12.13 demonstrates the skeleton of a foot with forefoot varus.

Dynamic Alignment

Static alignment impacts dynamic alignment in gait. When off-weight, if the patient displays a static alignment of calcaneal varus and/or forefoot varus, on-weight the patient will often compensate by excessive pronation. Conversely, if the patient has a static alignment of calcaneal valgus and/or forefoot valgus off-weight, the on-weight compensation is usually supination. An off-weight foot that appears to be supinated will become a pronated foot on-weight, and vice versa.

> ## Watch Out For...
>
> **Watch out for** the effect of weight-bearing on foot pronation and supination. A foot that appears very inverted and supinated off-weight will cause a compensation of pronation to get the first ray to the floor.

In addition to dynamic alignment being affected by static alignment, muscle strength and timing of contraction also play a role in dynamic alignment. Three important muscles in maintaining the dynamic alignment of the foot are the posterior tibialis, fibularis longus, and gastrocsoleus.

- Posterior tibialis is the strongest ankle invertor. When the heel hits the ground on initial contact, the foot pronates as it accepts weight. Posterior tibialis slows down foot pronation by eccentrically contracting, controlling the collapse of the medial arch. By midstance, posterior tibialis is contracting concentrically to help pull the foot back up into a supinated position for terminal stance and preswing. In this way, posterior tibialis plays a primary role in controlling pronation and supination in gait.
- Fibularis longus provides dynamic transverse arch support as it crosses from lateral to medial on the underside of the foot. Because of its attachment on the first metatarsal and first cuneiform, it is capable of everting the foot to assist in transferring weight-bearing to the medial side of the foot and the big toe at preswing.[10] Illustration of the fibularis longus and posterior tibialis muscles and how they impact foot dynamic alignment is found in Figure 12.14.

- Normal gait requires about 10° of dorsiflexion with knee extension in terminal stance. Gastrocsoleus must be long enough to allow this range of motion. If gastrocsoleus limits dorsiflexion, patients may gain the necessary range by flattening the midfoot and longitudinal arch (Fig. 12.15). This can lead to excessive pronation in gait and to pathologies of the foot and ankle.

Normal Biomechanics of the Foot in Gait

Pronation of the foot in the gait cycle from initial contact through midstance accomplishes two important functions of the foot. It allows the foot to dissipate the internal

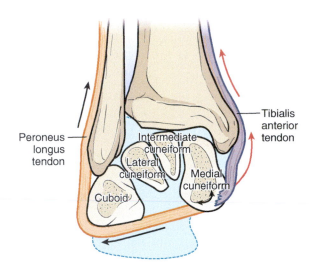

Figure 12.14 Posterior tibialis and fibularis longus are crucial stabilizers of the medial longitudinal arch and the transverse arch of the foot. Together they form a sling under the arch of the foot.

rotation force from the lower leg, and it transforms the foot from rigid to flexible.

While the axis of motion of the ankle joint lies mostly in the frontal plane, it is obliquely oriented in a posterior and inferior direction from medial to lateral. Basically, the foot is externally rotated on the lower leg. This creates an internal rotation force at the foot on initial contact. This rotational force is absorbed largely by the sliding of the talus down and in on the calcaneus, resulting in foot pronation.

In addition to absorbing the rotation of the lower leg on initial contact, pronation of the foot also unlocks the transverse tarsal joint by uncrossing the axes of motion. This joint unlocking allows the foot to be momentarily flexible and accommodate to uneven surfaces.

From midstance through preswing, the foot must begin to supinate. This converts the foot into a rigid lever to allow the force from the plantarflexors to propel the body forward. If the foot remained loose and flexible, the function of the gastrocsoleus would be reduced. Figure 12.16 illustrates the changes in foot pronation and supination during the stance phase of gait.

Windlass Mechanism of the Plantar Fascia

One mechanism that assists the foot in supinating late in stance is called the **windlass mechanism.** Recall that the plantar fascia extends from the calcaneus to the proximal phalanges. The windlass effect refers to the elevation of the longitudinal arch of the foot caused by lengthening the plantar fascia over the big toe (Fig. 12.17).

In preswing, the pivot point becomes the MTP joint of the big toe. From terminal stance to preswing, extension quickly increases at the MTP joint, up to about 80°. This extension lengthens the fascia over the MTP joint, causing it to shorten between the calcaneus and the metatarsal heads, elevating the longitudinal arch. The elevation of the arch supinates the foot and increases its rigidity for push-off.

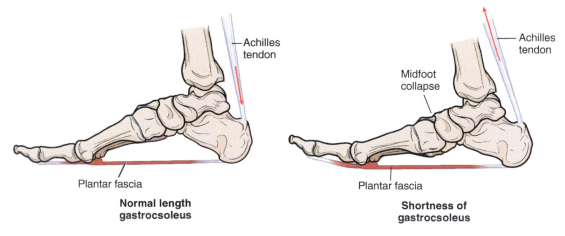

Figure 12.15 Normal gastrocsoleus length allows for 10° dorsiflexion with knee extension necessary during gait. If gastrocsoleus is short, a compensation is to collapse the midfoot and flatten the medial longitudinal arch.

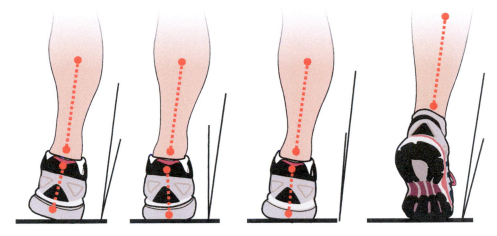

Figure 12.16 The foot pronates from initial contact through midstance, and then begins to supinate. Pronation absorbs rotational forces and supination converts the foot into a rigid lever.

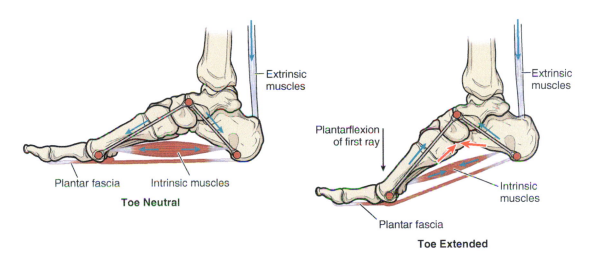

Figure 12.17 Lengthening of the plantar fascia over the first MTP joint shortens it between the calcaneus and metatarsal heads and elevates the longitudinal arch.

Effect of Excessive Pronation or Supination in Gait

Commonly, we observe abnormalities in gait that are related to excessive pronation or supination. Patients that excessively pronate will have difficulty getting into a position of supination before push-off. The force generated by gastrocsoleus will not be as effective when propelling the body off a soft foot. The patient may roll off the medial side of the foot as opposed to pushing off the big toe.

Patients that excessively supinate will have difficulty accommodating to uneven terrain and to the rotational force of the tibia. Forces will be spread throughout the foot, which may lead to degenerative changes. These patients are at high risk to suffer ankle sprain due to the relative inflexibility of the foot.

Top-down or Bottom-up Approach

Static alignment of the ankle and foot complex may affect or be affected by the alignment of the segments above, including the pelvis, hip, and knee. It has long been believed that the foot controls the position of the knee and hip in a "bottom-up" control of the limb. Researchers have studied the foot as a contributor to knee and hip problems and found evidence to support this belief.[11]

But recently researchers have begun to appreciate the influence of proximal segments on foot position; a "top-down" type of control. As an example, patients with weakness in hip external rotators and abductors have difficulty controlling the knee. Dynamic knee valgus may be increased in these patients during running and jumping. This increased valgus may contribute to excessive pronation of the foot on-weight.

Because the current evidence supports both approaches, when rehabilitating a patient consider the foot to be both influenced by, and an influence on, proximal joints. Bear in mind a top-down *and* bottom-up approach.

Joint Mobilization

Joint mobilization in the ankle and foot may be used to increase range of motion or to decrease pain. The loose packed position of the ankle is 10° of plantarflexion and neutral inversion/eversion. Table 12-5 lists the major movements of the ankle and foot with the associated direction of a glide mobilization of the distal segment to increase range of motion.

Distal Tibiofibular Joint

Anterior/Posterior Glide

Anterior or posterior glide of the fibula on the tibia is used to increase range of motion into ankle dorsiflexion, since this joint must separate slightly during dorsiflexion. The patient is lying supine. The examiner stabilizes on the top of the foot with one hand. With the other hand an anterior or posterior force is applied to the fibula (Fig. 12.18).

Tibiotalar Joint

Anterior Glide

Anterior glide of the convex talus on the concave tibia and fibula is used to increase range of motion into ankle plantarflexion. The patient is supine with a towel roll under the lower leg. The examiner stabilizes the lower leg with one hand. With the other hand the examiner cups the calcaneus and applies an upward force to glide the talus anteriorly (Fig. 12.19).

Posterior Glide

Posterior glide of the talus on the tibia and fibula is used to increase range of motion into ankle dorsiflexion. The patient is supine with a towel roll under the lower leg. The examiner palpates the joint line with one hand anterior to the joint. With the web space of the other hand the examiner applies a posterior force across the talus (Fig. 12.20).

Distraction

Distraction of the talus away from the tibia and fibula is used for general joint restrictions. The patient may be sitting or supine. The examiner stabilizes the distal tibia with one hand. With the other hand the examiner grasps across the talus and pulls distally (Fig. 12.21). Alternatively, the examiner may clasp both hands over the talus and pull distally.

Table 12-5 Direction of Slide Used to Increase Range of Motion	
Limited Range	Direction of Slide in Mobilization
Ankle dorsiflexion	Anterior/posterior glide of tibiofibular joint Posterior glide of tibiotalar joint
Ankle plantarflexion	Anterior glide of tibiotalar joint
Calcaneal inversion	Lateral glide of subtalar joint
Calcaneal eversion	Medial glide of subtalar joint
General ankle motion	Distraction of tibiotalar joint

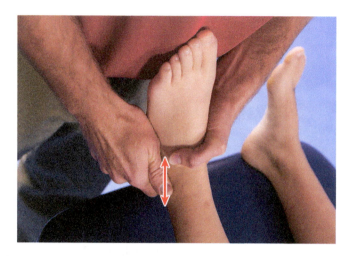

Figure 12.18 Anterior/posterior glide of the tibiofibular joint to increase ankle dorsiflexion.

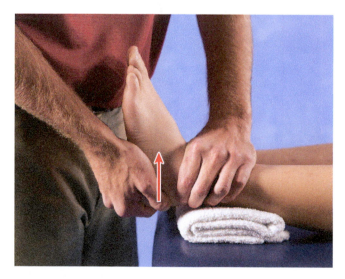

Figure 12.19 Anterior glide of the tibiotalar joint for ankle plantarflexion.

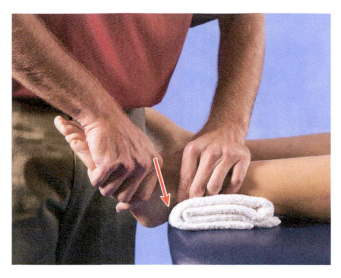

Figure 12.20 Posterior glide of the tibiotalar joint for ankle dorsiflexion.

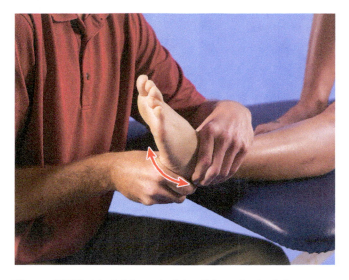

Figure 12.22 Medial/lateral glide of the subtalar joint to increase eversion/inversion.

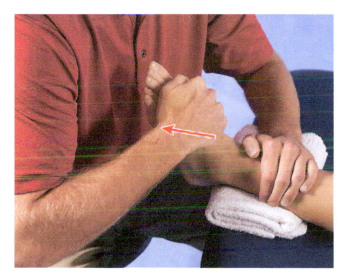

Figure 12.21 Distraction of the tibiotalar joint for general joint restrictions.

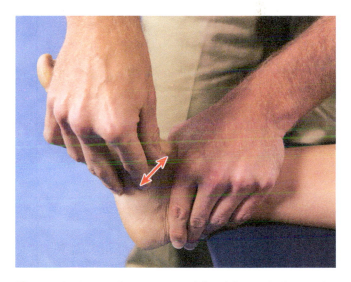

Figure 12.23 Anterior/posterior glide of the navicular on the talus for midfoot restriction.

Subtalar Joint

Medial/Lateral Glide

The calcaneus may be mobilized on the talus to increase inversion and eversion. The patient may be positioned sitting or supine with the foot off the end of the table. The examiner stabilizes the talus with one hand and grasps the calcaneus with the other hand. A slight distraction force is accompanied by a medial or lateral glide (Fig. 12.22). A medial glide will increase eversion and a lateral glide will increase inversion.

Tarsal Joints

Intertarsal joints may be mobilized using an anterior-posterior glide. The examiner uses the thumb and index finger of one hand to stabilize a tarsal bone, and with the thumb and index finger of the other hand applies an anterior and posterior glide to an adjacent tarsal bone. Tarsometatarsal joints may also be mobilized with anterior-posterior glides. These mobilizations are used to address restrictions in the midfoot. Figure 12.23 shows a mobilization of the navicular on the talus.

Metatarsophalangeal and Interphalangeal Joints

MTP and IP joints may be mobilized using the concave-convex rule. The proximal segment of these joints is convex and the distal segment is concave.

Common Pathologies

Lateral Ankle Sprain
Syndesmotic Sprain (High Ankle Sprain)
Plantar Fasciitis
Achilles Tendinopathy
Posterior Tibialis Tendon Dysfunction
Medial Tibial Stress Syndrome

Compartment Syndrome
Tarsal Tunnel Syndrome
Ankle and Calcaneal Fractures
Stress Fracture
Toe Deformities

We have discussed the need for the foot to be flexible early in stance phase and yet rigid late in stance phase. The mechanism by which this is accomplished is through pronation and supination at the transverse tarsal joint. Normal gait involves the ankle and foot pronating and supinating with every step, thousands of times a day. In addition, the foot must absorb both internal rotational forces and compressive forces often equal to several times body weight. It is easy to understand that pathologies due to abnormal biomechanics, overuse, or injury are common given these circumstances. In this section, we will discuss the common pathologies of the ankle and foot that are treated with physical therapy.

Lateral Ankle Sprain   CPG

Stability of the lateral ankle primarily comes from bony joint congruity, the fibularis muscles, and three ligaments. The ligaments that stabilize the lateral ankle are the anterior talofibular, the calcaneofibular, and the posterior talofibular ligaments. In lateral ankle sprain, one or more of these ligaments are injured or torn. Almost 75% of lateral ankle sprains involve isolated injury to the anterior talofibular ligament.[3] Figure 12.24 depicts lateral ankle sprain.

Ankle sprain is graded based on severity. Grade I ankle sprain is the result of stretching of the ankle ligaments, grade II is the result of partial tearing, and grade III is the result of a complete tear of one or more of the ligaments.

Causes/Contributing Factors

Inversion with plantarflexion is the most common mechanism of injury, such as occurs in landing on the side of the foot after a jump or stepping into a hole. Nearly half of these injuries are sports-related. The highest risk involves running and jumping sports, especially basketball, football, and soccer.

Symptoms

After lateral ankle sprain, the patient will usually complain of pain on the lateral aspect of the ankle, just distal to the lateral malleolus. Pain is increased with weight-bearing. Swelling and bruising is often noted in the area. The patient may have a feeling of instability in the ankle.

Clinical Signs

Tenderness, swelling, and pain are key elements of patient assessment after ankle sprain. In addition, ligament laxity

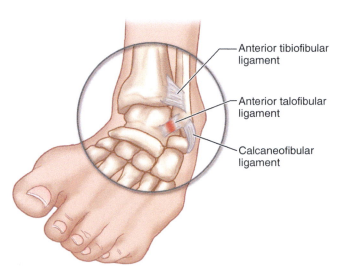

Anterior tibiofibular ligament

Anterior talofibular ligament

Calcaneofibular ligament

Figure 12.24 Lateral ankle sprain most commonly affects the anterior talofibular ligament and occurs with a plantarflexion and inversion injury.

or pain reproduction on the following tests may be an indicator of the degree of injury and recovery.

Anterior Drawer Test

This test is used to assess the integrity of the anterior talofibular ligament. The patient is positioned sitting with the foot off the floor. The examiner stabilizes the lower leg with one hand on the anterior surface above the ankle. With the patient's foot in slight plantarflexion, the examiner grasps around the calcaneus with the other hand and distracts the joint. Maintaining distraction of the calcaneus, the examiner applies an anteriorly directed force on the calcaneus and talus (Fig. 12.25). A positive test is indicated by a reproduction of the patient's symptoms over the anterior talofibular ligament or displacement of the foot of greater than 5 mm.

Watch Out For...

Watch out for use of the descriptor anterior drawer test in your documentation. The anterior drawer test can be performed on many joints, including the shoulder, knee, and ankle. Documentation should include the joint to which you are administering the test. For example, document "anterior drawer test of the ankle."

Medial Talar Tilt Stress Test

This test is used to assess the integrity of each of the lateral ankle ligaments. The patient is positioned sitting with the foot off the floor. The examiner stabilizes on the medial surface of the lower leg above the ankle with one hand. With the patient's foot in full plantarflexion, the examiner grasps around the calcaneus with the other hand and distracts the joint. Maintaining distraction of the calcaneus, the examiner applies a medially directed force on the calcaneus and talus, inverting the foot. This

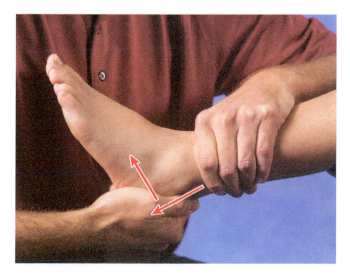

Figure 12.25 Anterior drawer test for anterior instability of the ankle. This test may be positive in lateral ankle sprain.

maneuver assesses the anterior talofibular ligament. The test is repeated with the patient's foot in neutral to assess the calcaneofibular ligament, and in dorsiflexion to assess the posterior talofibular ligament (Fig. 12.26). A positive test is indicated by a reproduction of the patient's symptoms over the lateral ankle ligaments.

Common Interventions

Protected Phase

Immediately after injury, the patient's ankle will be protected during the acute phase of tissue healing. During this time, the patient will likely be wearing a splint or cast. Progressive weight-bearing through this phase has been shown to be beneficial. Modalities including cryotherapy, diathermy, or electrical stimulation may be used to control swelling, pain, and inflammation.

During the protected phase, studies have shown benefit from manual therapy, including lymph drainage, soft tissue mobilization, and grade I and II joint mobilizations within the limits of pain. Joint mobilizations that have been found to be beneficial include anterior-posterior glides of the talus and of the distal tibiofibular joint. The patient may begin active range-of-motion into plantar- and dorsiflexion. Gentle resistive exercises, including exercise to foot intrinsic muscles, may be initiated during this time.[12]

> **CLINICAL ALERT**
> End ranges of plantarflexion and of inversion should be avoided during this time due to the stress on the healing lateral ligaments.

Training Phase

In phase two, the goals include decreasing pain and normalizing range of motion, strength, proprioception, and coordination. Manual therapy may include long axis distraction, talar glides, and mobilization with movement.[12] Mobilization with movement (MWM) for lateral ankle sprain involves a posterior glide of the talus. This is done by providing a posteriorly directed force to the talus in closed chain while the patient moves the ankle into dorsiflexion. The force may be provided by a resistance band or manually (Fig. 12.27).

Range-of-motion exercises may be done passively and actively. A balance board may be used in a seated position to promote normal range, as shown in Figure 12.28. Strengthening ankle plantarflexion, dorsiflexion, inversion, and eversion with resistive bands or weights may be added. Emphasis should be placed on ankle inversion and eversion.

It is crucial as this phase progresses to incorporate proprioceptive retraining to minimize the likelihood of recurrence.[13–16] The risk of reinjury is very high; research suggests up to 73% for some sports. Indeed, previous injury is the most agreed-upon risk factor for ankle sprain.

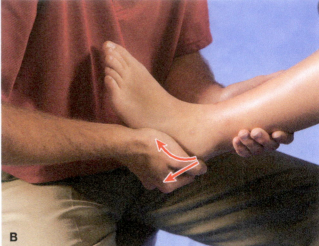

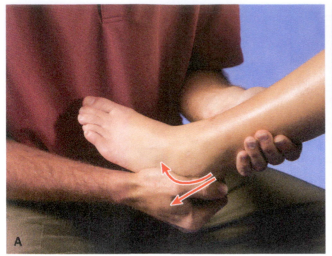

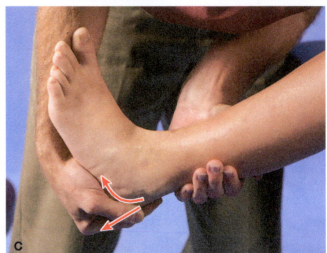

Figure 12.26 Medial talar tilt stress test for lateral ankle instability after sprain. The ankle is positioned in plantarflexion (A) to test the anterior talofibular ligament, neutral (B) to test the calcaneofibular ligament, and dorsiflexion (C) to test the posterior talofibular ligament. In each position the ankle is distracted and a medial force is applied.

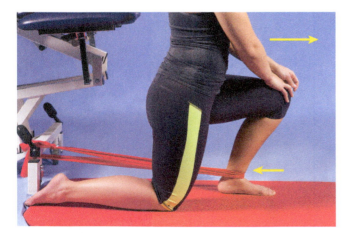

Figure 12.27 Posterior mobilization of the talus with movement of the ankle into dorsiflexion.

The PTA can lower the risk of recurrence through interventions that include proprioceptive retraining. Weight-bearing functional exercises such as stepping up and down, heel and toe raises, standing on an unstable surface, and standing perturbation activities, as shown in Figure 12.29, may be used. Encouraging patients to use a brace or tape to enhance stability also decreases reinjury risk.

Prevention

Because the risk of recurrent ankle sprain is so high, prevention is important. In high-risk sports, patients can decrease risk by wearing a lace-up brace or taping the ankles.[17–19] Including proprioceptive exercises in the training regimen and participating in warm-up exercises before play will result in lower risk.[20,21]

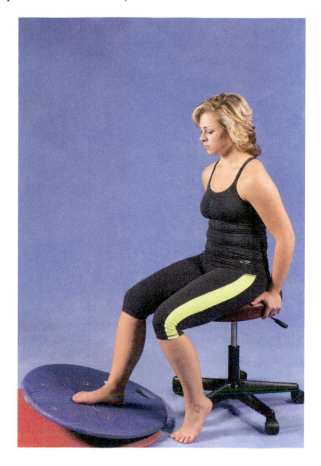

Figure 12.28 A balance board may be used with the patient seated in the early phases of ankle rehabilitation to promote ankle range of motion.

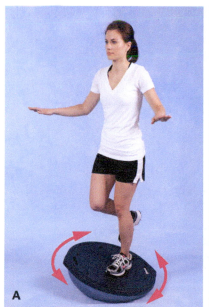

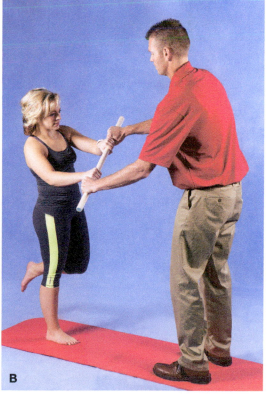

Figure 12.29 Standing perturbation exercises for proprioceptive retraining are an important component in the plan of care for ankle sprain to decrease the risk of recurrence. The patient may be challenged on an unstable surface (A) or with the application of external forces (B).

The Bottom Line: for patients with lateral ankle sprain

Description and causes	Injury to the lateral ankle ligaments, most often the anterior talofibular ligament, due to inversion of the ankle
Test	Anterior drawer test, medial talar tilt stress test
Stretch	In pain-free range.
Strengthen	All ankle movements, with focus on inversion and eversion
Train	Proprioception
Avoid	Plantarflexion and inversion initially

Syndesmotic Sprain (High Ankle Sprain)

Syndesmotic sprain of the ankle is also referred to as high ankle sprain. Rather than a sprain of the ligaments on the outside of the foot, this injury involves the ligaments of the distal tibiofibular joint (Fig. 12.30). The stability of the ankle mortise may be compromised depending upon the severity of the sprain.

The distal tibiofibular joint is a fibrous syndesmosis. The two bones are normally held in very close approximation so they can lock onto the talus like a wrench on a bolt. Disruption of the ligaments of this joint may lead to widening of the ankle mortise, called **diastasis.** When this occurs, the ankle joint stability is lost. Syndesmotic injury results in more pain than lateral ankle sprain and takes about twice as long to recover.[22]

This type of ankle sprain is less common than lateral ankle sprain. Literature reports between 1% and 18% of ankle sprains are syndesmotic injuries.[23] However, it is somewhat more difficult to diagnose, and mild injury to the syndesmosis may go undetected.

Causes/Contributing Factors

As opposed to the inversion mechanism of lateral ankle sprain, high ankle sprain is most commonly due to external rotation of the foot on the tibia. It may also be due to extreme dorsiflexion or sudden eversion of the talus within the ankle mortise. Any of these mechanisms tend to separate the distal tibia and fibula, spraining the ligaments that stabilize the joint. Syndesmosis injuries are commonly associated with turf sports such as football and soccer and with sports that immobilize the foot in a boot such as skiing and hockey.

Symptoms

Patients with high ankle sprain most commonly complain of pain and tenderness over the anterior aspect of the distal tibiofibular joint. They may have increased pain with foot external rotation or ankle dorsiflexion. Pain may extend up the lower leg. If a patient diagnosed with

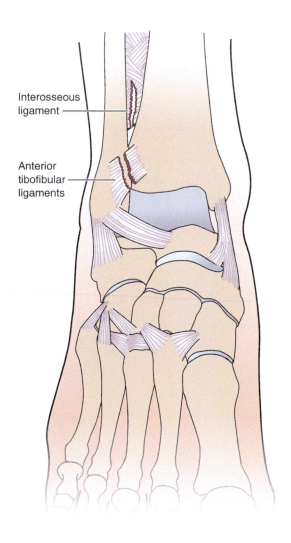

Interosseous ligament

Anterior tibiofibular ligaments

Figure 12.30 Syndesmotic ankle sprain, or high ankle sprain, involves the distal tibiofibular joint and usually the interosseous membrane.

lateral ankle sprain has symptoms that persist, high ankle sprain should be considered.

Clinical Signs

Anterior ankle pain with dorsiflexion or foot external rotation are strong indicators of high ankle sprain. In

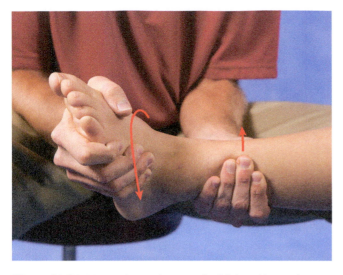

Figure 12.31 External rotation test for high ankle sprain.

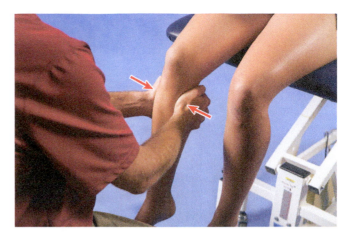

Figure 12.32 Squeeze test for high ankle sprain.

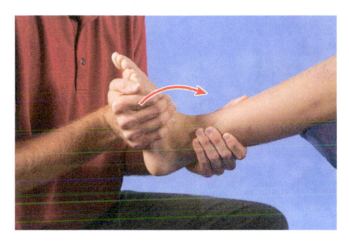

Figure 12.33 Dorsiflexion maneuver for high ankle sprain.

addition, pain reproduction on the following tests may be used to diagnose this pathology.

External Rotation Test

The external rotation test is done with the patient sitting or supine. The examiner flexes the patient's knee to 90°, and the ankle is held in a neutral position. The foot is passively externally rotated on the tibia (Fig. 12.31). A positive test is indicated by pain over the area of the syndesmotic ligaments.

Squeeze Test

The squeeze test is done with the patient sitting or supine. The examiner compresses the fibula to the tibia above the midpoint of the calf (Fig. 12.32). This causes separation of the two bones at the distal joint. A positive test is indicated by pain over the area of the syndesmotic ligaments. Patients with a positive squeeze test have been shown to have a much longer recovery time and slower return to sport.[22,24]

Dorsiflexion Maneuver

The dorsiflexion maneuver is done with the patient sitting. The examiner stabilizes the patient's leg with one hand and passively dorsiflexes the patient's ankle with the other hand (Fig. 12.33). A positive test is indicated by pain over the area of the syndesmotic ligaments.

Dorsiflexion Compression Test

This test is a variation of the dorsiflexion maneuver. The patient is standing and flexes both knees to bring the ankles into dorsiflexion. The patient reports the level of pain in dorsiflexion and the examiner notes the amount of dorsiflexion range available. The test is then repeated with the examiner providing manual compression around the malleoli to maintain the ankle mortise (Fig. 12.34).

A positive test is indicated by an improvement with compression. The patient may report decreased pain and/or an increase in range of motion with compression.

Common Interventions

Protected Phase

Initially, the patient will be in a protected phase with no weight-bearing to prevent further damage to the ligaments. Cryotherapy or electrical stimulation may be used to control swelling, pain, and inflammation. The patient may be immobilized in a cast or splint depending upon the extent of the injury.

CLINICAL ALERT

Care should be taken to avoid tightening a splint around the upper calf as it may separate the two bones distally. Active range of motion in the pain-free range may be included in the plan of care, being cautious about end-range ankle dorsiflexion.

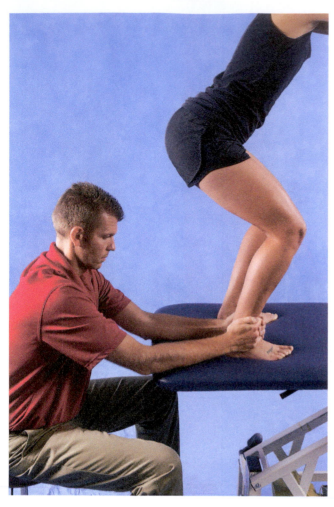

Figure 12.34 Dorsiflexion compression test for high ankle sprain.

Training Phase

What's in the Plan of Care? As pain and swelling subside, the patient may begin a partial weight-bearing gait. A heel lift may be used to prevent excessive dorsiflexion during ambulation. Low-level balance retraining on two legs, and gentle strengthening of the ankle muscles may be initiated. The focus should be on the fibularis muscle group and gastrocsoleus.[25] Cycling and aquatic exercise may be included in this phase.

As the patient tolerates more weight-bearing, the plan of care may include more aggressive exercises, including single-leg weight-bearing strengthening, double- and single-leg heel raises, and single-leg balance retraining. Before return to sport, interventions may include sport-specific drills, including running, jumping, and cutting.

The Bottom Line: for patients with high ankle sprain

Description and Causes	Injury to the distal tibiofibular joint that results in loss of stability of the ankle mortise, often due to external rotation, eversion, or extreme dorsiflexion on a planted foot
Test	External rotation test, squeeze test, dorsiflexion maneuver, dorsiflexion compression test
Stretch	To regain ankle ROM, in pain-free range.
Strengthen	Fibularis muscles, gastrocsoleus
Train	Proprioception
Avoid	End-range dorsiflexion

Interventions for the Surgical Patient

If conservative measures are not successful due to separation of the ankle mortise, surgical fixation may be necessary. Often patients that require surgery have some disruption to the deltoid ligament or a fibular fracture in addition to the syndesmotic sprain.

Screw Fixation (ORIF)

One or two screws are placed through the fibula and into the tibia to hold the bones together until the ligaments heal. These screws are left in place for 9 to 16 weeks while healing occurs. The surgeon may arthroscopically debride the distal tibiofibular joint prior to the ORIF.

The deltoid ligament may be repaired or reconstructed during the surgical procedure as well.

Postoperative Phase

After surgery, the patient is kept non-weight-bearing or touch weight-bearing for 6 to 8 weeks or more. Some surgeons recommend keeping the patient non-weight-bearing until the screws are removed.

After the screws are removed, the patient may be in a cast boot with limited weight-bearing until the screw holes fill in. Initial goals are to decrease swelling and pain. The plan of care will usually include active range of motion of the ankle in the pain-free range beginning about 2 to 4 weeks after surgery. Cycling and aquatic exercise may be included in the plan of care.

At about 6 to 8 weeks, gentle strengthening may be initiated. Proprioceptive retraining with double-leg standing may be started. Progression to running and jumping may be included in the plan of care about 12 to 16 weeks postoperatively.

Plantar Fasciitis   CPG

The superficial plantar fascia runs from the calcaneus to the proximal phalanges on the underside of the foot. Plantar fasciitis is a condition characterized by inflammation and degeneration at the origin of the fascia that leads to heel pain (Fig. 12.35).[26] This condition may also be called plantar fasciopathy. The plantar fascia often becomes thickened and tight. The inflammation, and ultimately the degeneration, of the fascia is thought to be due to abnormal stresses placed on it, which lead to microtearing and scarring.

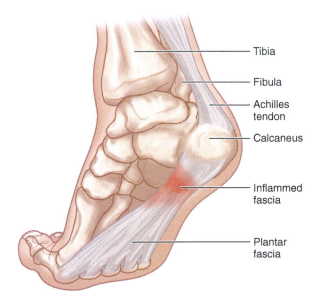

Tibia

Fibula

Achilles tendon

Calcaneus

Inflammed fascia

Plantar fascia

Figure 12.35 Plantar fasciitis, inflammation of the plantar fascia, causes pain in the plantar aspect of the heel.

Causes/Contributing Factors

The causes of plantar fasciitis are still not completely understood, but it is linked to abnormal foot biomechanics[27], obesity, limited dorsiflexion range of motion[28], and limited big toe extension. In general, plantar fasciitis occurs in people with excessive foot pronation[27,29,30] or supination[31]. Among athletes there is a link to running sports, especially in runners with increased supination. People whose occupation involves standing and walking on hard surfaces are more susceptible to plantar fasciitis.[32]

The literature supports a relationship between plantar fasciitis and limited range of motion of ankle dorsiflexion or big toe extension. There is also evidence that overpronation and oversupination may lead to fasciitis. Let's explore each cause in more detail.

Limitation of Ankle Dorsiflexion

A contributor to plantar fasciitis is limited range of motion into dorsiflexion. In the gait cycle, immediately before the heel rises, the tibia has advanced over the talus, causing dorsiflexion of the ankle. Ten degrees of ankle dorsiflexion with knee extension is necessary for normal gait. If the gastrocsoleus is short and doesn't allow for this range, the motion may be gained by dropping the talus down and flattening the medial longitudinal arch, as shown in Figure 12.15 (page 382). The flattening of the arch stretches the plantar fascia, leading to inflammation.

Limitation of Big Toe Extension

Another contributor is limited range of motion of big toe extension. During terminal stance, the MTP joint of the big toe becomes the pivot point as the body advances past the foot. As the big toe extends, it becomes a winch to shorten the plantar fascia between the calcaneus and the metatarsal heads. This activates the windlass mechanism that raises the longitudinal arch. If the MTP joint of the big toe is limited, due to hallux rigidus or osteoarthritis for example, the pivot point of the foot shifts back toward the midfoot, stretching the plantar fascia (Fig. 12.36).

Overpronation and Oversupination

Limited range of motion in ankle dorsiflexion or big toe extension leads to overpronation and stress on the fascia as described above. But regardless of the cause, overpronation lengthens the fascia, leading to stress, inflammation, and degeneration. Excessive supination also stresses the fascia. In a supinated position, the body weight forces that are normally dissipated by foot pronation are instead transmitted throughout the foot structure. The fascia is one structure that absorbs this excess force. In addition, in both abnormal pronation and supination the fascia is not running in a straight plane from rearfoot to forefoot but is slightly twisted, like a dish rag when it is wrung.

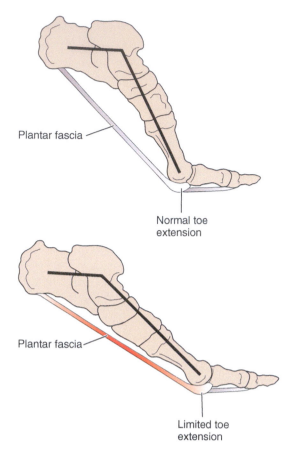

Figure 12.36 Normal extension motion of the big toe helps raise the arch and supinate the foot in late stance. If big toe extension is limited, it contributes to inflammation of the plantar fascia.

Symptoms

Patients with plantar fasciitis will complain of pain in the plantar aspect of the medial heel. This area may be tender to palpation. Pain is worse when weight-bearing after prolonged inactivity. A classic complaint is of pain when first getting out of bed in the morning. Pain also may increase with prolonged weight-bearing, for example, standing on the feet all day.

Clinical Signs

Diagnosis is largely based on patient symptoms and clinical signs. Palpation over the origin of the fascia on the medial plantar calcaneus may elicit tenderness. The fascia may be thickened and tight. Range of motion into ankle dorsiflexion may be limited. The patient may display a bone spur on x-ray growing into the fascia, as shown in Figure 12.37.

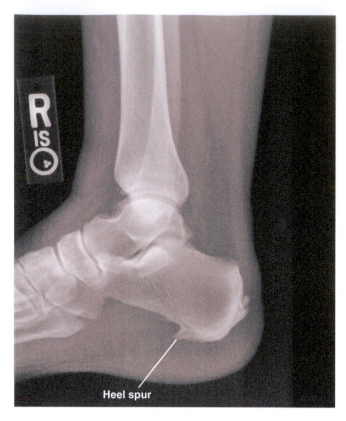

Figure 12.37 Sagittal view x-ray of the foot. The calcaneus has a heel spur that is growing into the plantar fascia, indicative of plantar fasciitis.

Windlass Test

The patient can be standing or sitting for this test, but the test has been shown to be more sensitive when weight-bearing.[33] The patient stands on a stool with the metatarsal heads supported and the toes off the edge. Instruct the patient to stand with equal weight on both feet. Allowing the IP joint of the big toe to flex, the examiner passively extends the MTP joint of the big toe. A positive test is indicated by reproduction of the patient's pain. To objectify the results of this test, the range-of-motion of big toe extension at the point of pain may be assessed (Fig. 12.38).

Navicular Drop Test

This test is not used to diagnose plantar fasciitis, but rather to provide information on pronation as a contributing factor. The patient is standing. The examiner positions the patient in a subtalar neutral position (STJN). The navicular tuberosity is palpated on the medial aspect of the foot. The distance from the tuberosity to the floor is measured. The patient is then instructed to assume a relaxed standing posture, and the measurement is again taken (Fig. 12.39). In patients with excessive pronation, the navicular tuberosity will drop toward the floor. There is disagreement about the amount of drop that should be considered a positive test, but in general more than 10 mm has been considered positive.[34]

Common Interventions

Most patients will recover with conservative measures, including activity modification, shoe wear modification, physical therapy, and weight loss. Initially, the physical

therapy plan of care may include manual therapy, stretching and strengthening exercises, taping, the use of orthoses and/or night splints, and education.

Manual therapy, consisting of joint and soft tissue mobilization, is effective in addressing symptoms of plantar fasciitis.[35-37] Specifically, soft tissue mobilization of the gastrocsoleus may be used to increase calf mobility. Range of motion of the lower extremity may be normalized using joint mobilization.

Exercise to stretch gastrocsoleus and the plantar fascia is also effective.[38-40] When stretching gastrocsoleus, keeping the foot rigid ensures that the calf muscles are getting the maximum stretch without allowing the midfoot to flatten. This can be done by placing a medial arch support under the patient's foot while performing a weight-bearing stretch (Fig. 12.40).[41]

Stretching the plantar fascia is done by extending the big toe until a stretch sensation is felt. This may be accompanied by massage of the fascia up into the arch to provide a further stretch. A common technique that is employed to stretch the fascia is to roll the foot over a dowel rod. Figure 12.41 shows plantar fascia stretching techniques.

Strengthening exercises may also be included in the plan of care. The focus of strengthening exercises is commonly the foot intrinsic muscles and the posterior tibialis. Towel scrunches, single-leg standing, and ankle inversion against resistance may be employed to address the plan of care. Figure 12.42 depicts foot intrinsic exercises.

Taping,[39,42,43] orthoses,[44-48] and night splints[49-51] may be used to control the position of the foot. There is

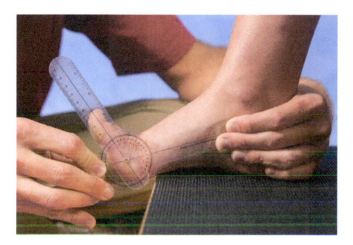
Figure 12.38 Windlass test for plantar fasciitis.

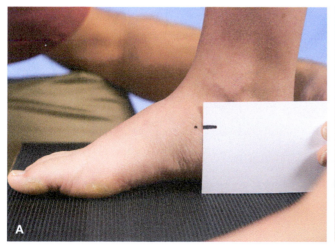 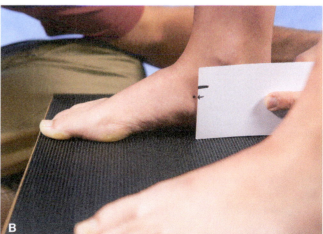

Figure 12.39 Navicular drop test for assessment of foot pronation. The distance from the navicular tuberosity to the floor is measured in a STJN position (A) and in a relaxed standing position (B). A drop of more than 10 mm indicates excessive pronation.

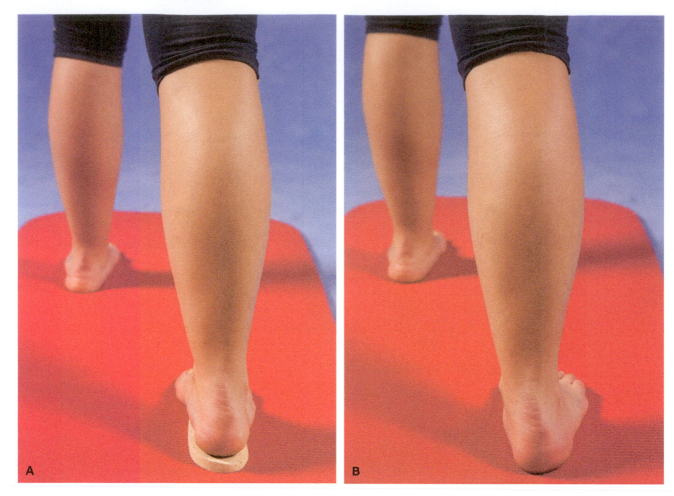

Figure 12.40 Gastrocsoleus stretch with a medial arch support supinates the foot, locking the midfoot (A). This maximizes the stretch of the calf muscles and prevents midfoot collapse (B).

evidence that all are effective. Taping to control pronation, called low-Dye or high-Dye, may be included in the plan of care. These techniques are named after the podiatrist who first described the technique, Dr. Ralph Dye. Using the low-Dye taping technique, the examiner applies tape below the ankle; the high-Dye technique involves taping into the lower third of the leg. Both techniques control pronation, but high-Dye taping has been shown to better control the rearfoot if that is desired.[52] Box 12-3 depicts the low-Dye technique.

Modalities may be included in the plan of care, including cryotherapy, iontophoresis, or phonophoresis.

While evidence is weak regarding the effectiveness of these modalities, some research has shown improvement through their use.

Education regarding heel spur is often beneficial. Patients will assume the spur is the source of their pain and that until it is removed the pain will not subside. An understanding that the spur is a symptom of the fasciitis, and not the cause, is important. As the fascia becomes thickened and tight, it pulls on the calcaneus, causing bone to grow into the fascia. The pain that the patient is experiencing is from the fasciitis itself, not the spur. Furthermore, as the fascia is treated, and symptoms resolve, the spur will be reabsorbed and go away.

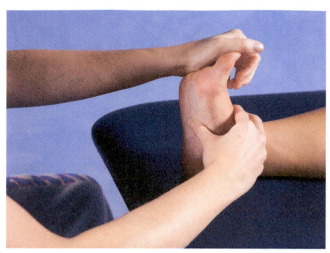

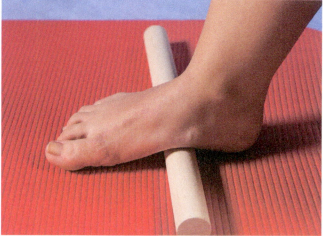

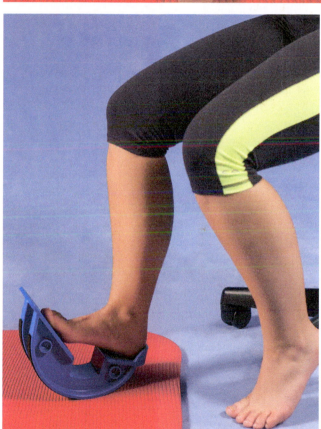

Figure 12.41 Three methods to stretch the plantar fascia. The fascia is stretched by extending the big toe with pressure into the arch of the foot.

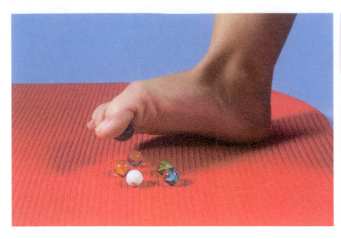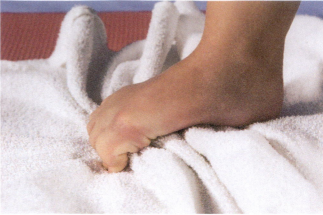

Figure 12.42 Toe intrinsic strengthening exercises are often included in the plan of care for plantar fasciitis to help stabilize the fascia. Common methods are using the toes to pick up marbles or to scrunch a towel.

Box 12-3 Low-Dye Taping for Plantar Fasciitis.

There are many methods of taping for fasciitis. If the tape stays below the malleoli, it is commonly referred to as low-Dye taping. The following depicts one method.

General Instructions:
1. Use rigid strapping tape or athletic tape, about 1-1/2 inches wide.
2. Skin should be clean and dry.
3. Start with the foot in a neutral position.
4. As you apply the tape, smooth any wrinkles.
5. Instruct the patient to remove the tape if any numbness, pain, or bluing of the nails occurs.

Step 1. Apply a strip of tape from just below the 5th metatarsal, around the heel, and up to the base of the first metatarsal (Fig. A).

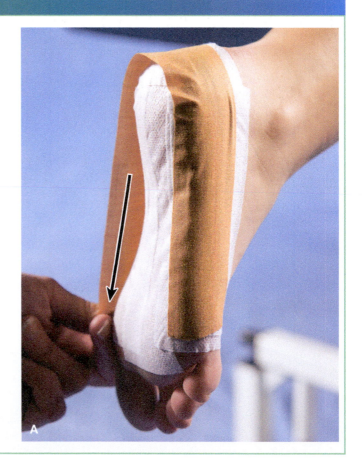

Box 12-3 Low-Dye Taping for Plantar Fasciitis.—cont'd

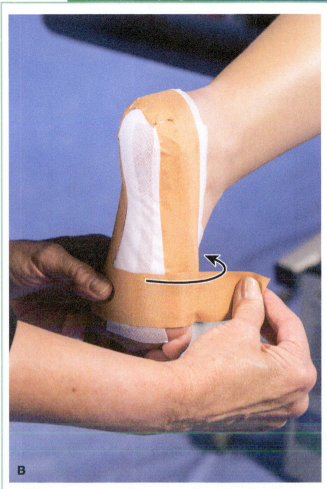

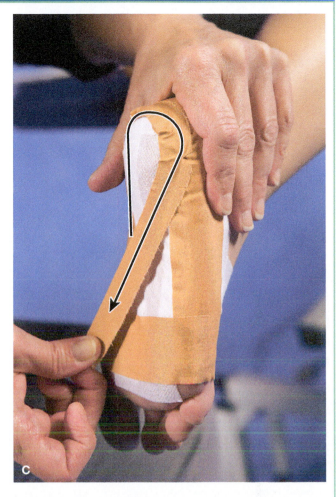

Step 2. Wrap a strip of tape around the foot and across the metatarsal heads. The ends of the tape should be on the top of the foot (Fig. B).

Step 3. Tear a long strip of tape in half lengthwise, so the tape is ¾" wide. Starting at the first metatarsal head, tape across the foot, around the calcaneus, and back to the starting point (Fig. C).

Continued

Box 12-3   Low-Dye Taping for Plantar Fasciitis.—cont'd

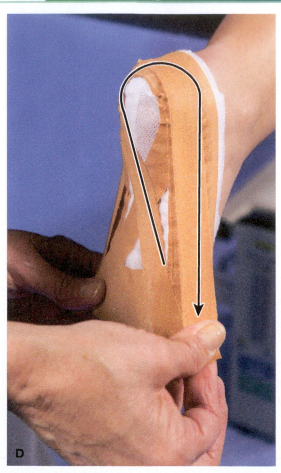

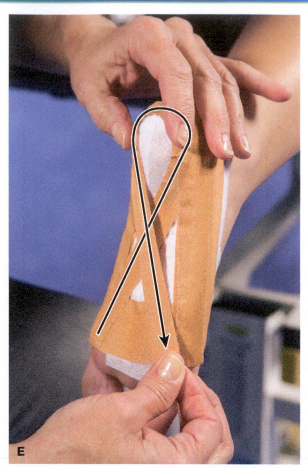

Step 4. Using the narrow width as above, tape from the fifth metatarsal head, across the foot, around the calcaneus, and back to the starting point. The tape now forms an "X" shape across the bottom of the foot (Fig. D).

Step 5. Using the narrow width as above, tape from the first metatarsal head, across the foot, around the calcaneus, across the foot again, ending at the fifth metatarsal head (Fig. E).

Box 12-3 **Low-Dye Taping for Plantar Fasciitis.—cont'd**

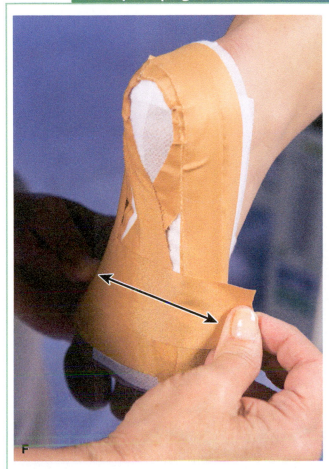

Step 6. Using the full width of the tape, apply a strip across the foot about ½" proximal to piece #2, starting and ending on the sides of the foot on piece #1 (Fig. F).

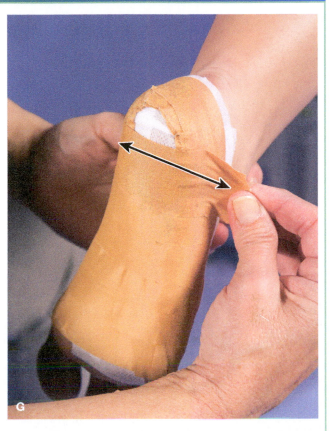

Step 7. Continue to apply strips across the foot with 50% overlap, closing in the plantar surface of the foot. Leave the calcaneus open as shown (Fig. G).

Continued

Box 12-3 Low-Dye Taping for Plantar Fasciitis.—cont'd

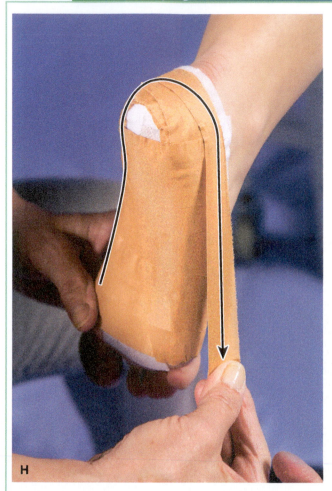

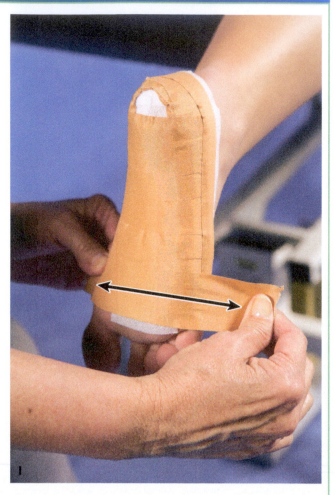

Step 8. Apply a full-width strip around the foot as in step #1, covering the ends of the closing-in strips (Fig. H).

Step 9. Apply a full-width strip across the metatarsal heads, as in step #2 (Fig. I).

Step 10. Having the patient stand with weight-bearing on the foot, rewrap the strips that cross the top of the foot to ensure they are not too tight.

Prevention

Plantar fasciitis has been linked to limited ankle dorsiflexion, obesity, and occupations that involve prolonged standing or walking. Prevention efforts include weight loss, stretching exercises, and foot wear to provide shock absorption. Rocker bottom shoes, as shown in Figure 12.43, may be worn to decrease the stress on the fascia.[53]

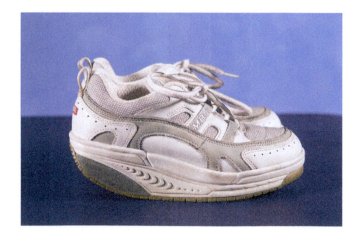

Figure 12.43 Rocker bottom shoes decrease the stress on the plantar fascia.

The Bottom Line:	for patients with plantar fasciitis
Description and Causes	Inflammation of the plantar fascia linked to abnormal foot biomechanics, obesity, and limited ROM into dorsiflexion or big toe extension
Test	Windlass test, navicular drop test
Stretch	Gastrocsoleus, plantar fascia
Strengthen	Foot intrinsic muscles, posterior tibialis
Train	NA
Avoid	Allowing the patient to worry about the heel spur

Achilles Tendinopathy   CPG

The Achilles tendon is the largest and strongest tendon in the body. This common tendon from gastrocnemius and soleus inserts on the posterior calcaneus. Achilles tendinopathy includes acute inflammation (tendonitis) and chronic degenerative change (tendinosis) of the Achilles tendon.

Acutely, Achilles tendonitis is thought to result from overuse. It is found most commonly in athletes involved in running sports, but other athletes and nonathletes may experience it. As a degenerative tendinopathy, it is thought to be the result of structural changes that occur in the tendon with age and a history of overuse. Figure 12.44 depicts Achilles tendinopathy.

Causes/Contributing Factors

There are multiple contributors to developing Achilles tendinopathy. For example, it has been attributed to a decreased dorsiflexion range of motion, abnormal subtalar joint motion, weakness in gastrocsoleus, overpronation, poor footwear, an increase in running volume or pace, and obesity.

People with limited ankle dorsiflexion range of motion, with less than about 12° when measured with the knee extended, are at greater risk.[55] Abnormal subtalar joint range of motion, either excessive inversion[55] or less than 25° of total motion,[56] leads to increased risk. Weakness in plantarflexion strength or endurance also increases the likelihood of developing Achilles tendinopathy.[57,58] People who overpronate in gait have an increased risk.[56,58] There is an association between developing Achilles tendinopathy in runners with sudden increase in pace or mileage, or with an increase in hill training.

As evidence that this pathology is frequently due to chronic degeneration of the tendon and not inflammation, abnormal tendon structure may precede symptoms and contribute to Achilles tendinopathy.[59,60] Medical risk factors that are associated with Achilles tendinopathy include obesity, hypertension, hyperlipidemia, and diabetes mellitus.

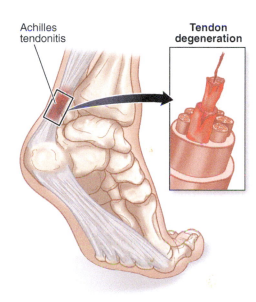

Figure 12.44 Achilles tendinopathy is a deterioration and/or inflammation of the gastrocsoleus tendon.

Symptoms

Patients with this disorder will often complain of pain and stiffness around the Achilles tendon. The most common complaints arise from the middle third of the tendon to its insertion on the calcaneus. The symptoms are increased when weight-bearing after a period of inactivity, especially when getting up in the morning. Some activity will often lead to a decrease in symptoms, so patients may report feeling best in the late morning. However, prolonged standing, walking, or running will cause increased pain.

Clinical Signs

Clinical signs of Achilles tendinopathy include pain with stretch, contraction, and palpation. Pain and limited range of motion into dorsiflexion are common. Patients will usually display weakness, decreased endurance, and pain in single-leg heel raises. Palpation over the tendon may cause pain. A localized area of swelling may be palpated.

Three special tests may be useful to assess the patient with Achilles tendinopathy. The first two are palpation tests that are more powerful when used in combination.[61] The last test may be useful to determine if the Achilles tendon has ruptured.

Arc Sign

The patient is positioned prone with the ankles hanging relaxed over the edge of the table. The examiner palpates the Achilles tendon for an area of localized swelling. Lightly continuing to palpate this area, the patient is instructed to actively plantarflex and dorsiflex the ankle (Fig. 12.45). A positive test is indicated by movement of the area of swelling during plantarflexion and dorsiflexion.

Royal London Hospital Test

The patient is positioned prone with the ankles hanging relaxed over the end of the table. The examiner palpates the Achilles tendon for an area of maximal tenderness. The patient is instructed to actively dorsiflex the ankle. The examiner again palpates this area while the ankle is in maximal dorsiflexion (Fig. 12.46). A positive test is indicated by tenderness that decreases or disappears when the tendon is stretched during full dorsiflexion.

Thompson Test

The patient is positioned prone with the knee flexed to 90°. The examiner stabilizes the leg by grasping around the ankle with one hand. With the other hand, the examiner squeezes the patient's calf (Fig. 12.47). A normal finding is plantarflexion of the foot when the calf is squeezed. A positive test is indicated by a lack of a response in the foot, indicating that the Achilles tendon is ruptured.

Common Interventions

Physical therapy is very effective in the treatment of Achilles tendinopathy. The plan of care is likely to involve some rest and anti-inflammatory modalities initially and progress to stretching and strengthening exercises. Use of orthoses, heel lift, or antipronation taping may be indicated.

Acute Phase

Rest for the tendon may involve use of an assistive device. A heel lift may be beneficial to relieve the stress on the tendon. Patient education to avoid walking up hills and walking barefoot may be helpful to minimize tendon stress. Anti-inflammatory modalities may include cryotherapy, iontophoresis, or low-level laser. Stretching exercises are beneficial to restore dorsiflexion and subtalar joint range of motion. Soft tissue and joint mobilization may also be indicated.

Subacute Phase

As the patient progresses, strengthening exercises that focus on eccentric loading of the tendon are beneficial.[62–65] Eccentric strengthening is most effective in patients with pain in the middle third of the Achilles tendon and less effective in patients with pain at the insertion.

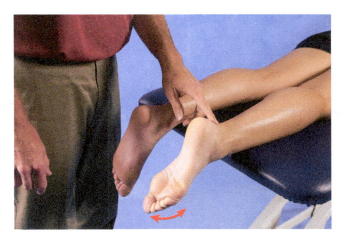

Figure 12.45 Arc sign for Achilles tendinopathy.

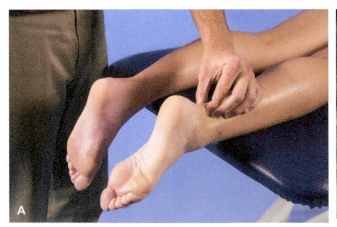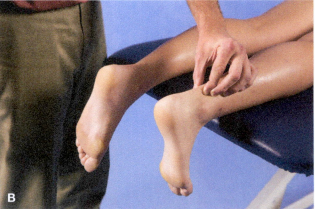

Figure 12.46 Royal London Hospital test for Achilles tendinopathy. The examiner palpates the tendon with the ankle relaxed (A). The tenderness elicited is compared to that in the position of ankle dorsiflexion (B).

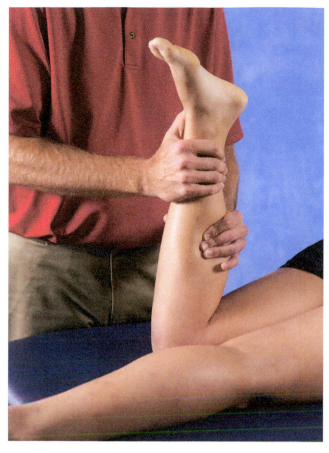

Figure 12.47 Thompson test for Achilles tendon rupture. If the foot doesn't plantarflex when the calf is squeezed, it indicates a rupture.

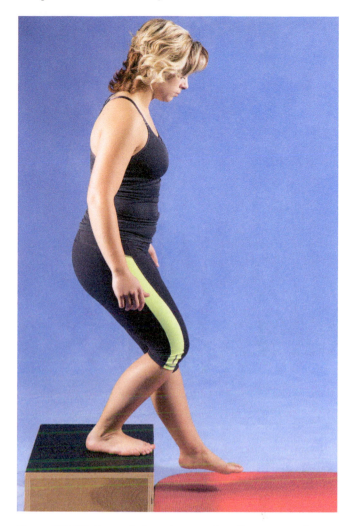

Figure 12.48 Eccentric lowering exercises for gastrocsoleus. The patient may be progressed by increasing the step height.

To strengthen the gastrocnemius and soleus eccentrically, patients may perform controlled-descent lowering exercises off the edge of a step (Fig. 12.48).[66] Eccentric strengthening of gastrocsoleus may also be performed off-weight using a resistance band.

If conservative treatment is not successful, the patient may become a candidate for surgical debridement of the tendon. However, the more common reason that a patient with Achilles tendinopathy would require surgery is for tendon rupture. Tendinopathy leads to degeneration of the tendon, which can lead to tendon failure. This will be discussed under surgical interventions below.

Prevention

Because Achilles tendinopathy is most common in running athletes, education regarding use of caution when increasing running pace or volume, adding in hill training, and returning to sport after a layoff is important in prevention. Wearing proper shoes may prevent Achilles tendinopathy.

The Bottom Line: for patients with Achilles tendinopathy

Description and causes	Inflammation or deterioration of the gastrocsoleus tendon linked to decreased ankle dorsiflexion ROM, abnormal biomechanics, gastrocsoleus weakness, poor footwear, running volume, and obesity
Test	Arc sign, Royal London Hospital test, Thompson test
Stretch	Gastrocsoleus, subtalar joint
Strengthen	Gastrocsoleus
Train	Eccentrically
Avoid	Increasing running pace or volume quickly

Interventions for the Surgical Patient

Repair of Achilles Tendon Rupture

Surgical repair may be done through an open incision or percutaneously through several small incisions. The two ends of the Achilles tendon are approximated and sewn together. The patient may be immobilized for a short period in a cast or splint. If the surgeon has difficulty approximating the tendon ends, the patient may be immobilized in a position of plantarflexion for the first few weeks.

Postoperative Phase

Initially, the patient is likely to be non-weight-bearing on the affected side. After 2 to 3 weeks, the patient is usually permitted to weight-bear as tolerated. Progressively more range of motion into dorsiflexion is allowed. By about 6 weeks, the plan of care often includes progressing range of motion of the ankle into plantarflexion and dorsiflexion, strengthening exercises with resistance bands, and bilateral heel raises. The entire course of rehabilitation may take 6 to 12 months.

Posterior Tibialis Tendon Dysfunction

Posterior tibialis is one of the deep posterior muscles, lying under gastrocsoleus. It runs behind the medial malleolus and has a broad insertion on the medial and plantar surfaces of the foot. In normal foot biomechanics, posterior tibialis is the primary dynamic stabilizer of the medial longitudinal arch. When posterior tibialis contracts, the foot plantarflexes and inverts, raising the medial longitudinal arch. In this supinated position, the midtarsal joint is locked and the foot is rigid. The mechanism of allowing the foot to change from flexible to rigid relies heavily on a normal posterior tibialis.

In posterior tibialis tendon dysfunction (PTTD), these crucial biomechanics are altered due to an insufficient posterior tibialis. The disorder is staged from I to IV. In stage I, the tendon is intact and functioning but is beginning the process of inflammation or degeneration

(Fig. 12.49). Patients may begin to show changes in gait related to excessive pronation in stage I.[67]

As the degeneration progresses, the tendon elongates and becomes dysfunctional. The foot takes on a very flat appearance by stage III. Eventually, the tibiotalar joint also becomes involved (Fig. 12.50). Box 12-4 summarizes the stages of PTTD.

Box 12-4	Stages of PTTD

Stage I: inflamed or degenerative tendon with some discomfort on palpation. Medial longitudinal arch is maintained. Excessive pronation in gait may be observed.

Stage II: posterior tibialis tendon is elongated and dysfunctional. The medial longitudinal arch has flattened. The patient will be diagnosed with an acquired flatfoot deformity. The deformity can be passively corrected.

Stage III: the flatfoot deformity is rigid. Subtalar joint degeneration is visible on x-ray.

Stage IV: the changes of stage III remain, with degenerative changes seen in the tibiotalar joint on x-ray.

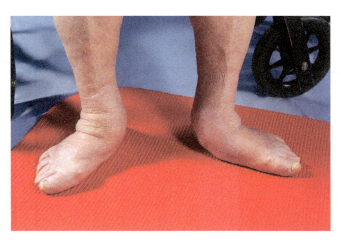

Figure 12.50 Acquired flat foot appearance associated with posterior tibialis tendon dysfunction after stage II.

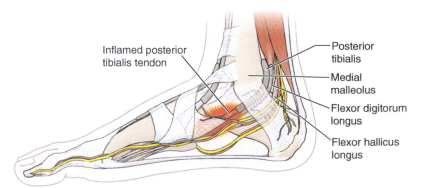

Inflamed posterior tibialis tendon

Posterior tibialis

Medial malleolus

Flexor digitorum longus

Flexor hallicus longus

Figure 12.49 Posterior tibialis tendon dysfunction begins with an inflammation or degeneration of the tendon.

Causes/Contributing Factors

The causes of PTTD are not completely understood, but it seems to be related to abnormal arch structure, weakness in foot inversion, and altered biomechanics in gait. PTTD is most common in middle-aged women, although stage I of the disorder is observed in younger runners. It occurs more commonly in people who excessively pronate.[68,69] It is also more common in people with hypertension, diabetes mellitus, and a history of steroid injections near the tendon.

There are consistent findings related to PTTD that may be causative or an effect of the arch collapse. For example, people with PTTD have been found to have decreased inversion strength.[70,71] There are changes evident in the spring ligament in people with PTTD by stage II.[72] Women who have PTTD have weakness in hip extensors and abductors as compared to women without PTTD.[73]

Symptoms

The early symptoms of PTTD are pain and/or swelling posterior to the medial malleolus and along the medial longitudinal arch. The patient may notice a flattening of the arch of the foot. These two signs are very indicative of PTTD. In addition, the patient may complain of a decrease in walking ability or balance.

Clinical Signs

The diagnosis of PTTD is based largely on patient history and symptoms. The following two tests may have been performed on the initial evaluation.

Unilateral Single Heel Raise Test

The patient is standing unsupported. The examiner instructs the patient to do a single heel raise on the unaffected and then on the affected side. The examiner notes the ability to perform a heel raise. In addition, the examiner observes from the medial or posterior side for *quality* of the heel raise (Fig. 12.51). A positive test is indicated by an inability to perform a single heel raise unsupported, as an indication of stages II to IV PTTD. Early in the progression of the tendinopathy, the patient may be able to perform a heel raise, but the movement pattern is altered as shown in Figure 12.52.[71,74]

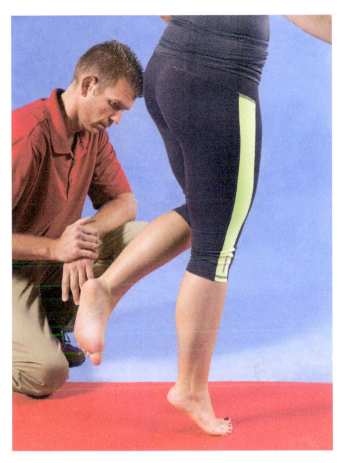

Figure 12.51 Unilateral single heel raise test for posterior tibialis tendon dysfunction.

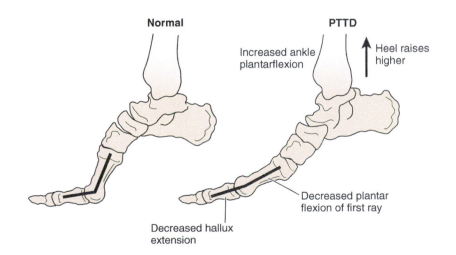

Figure 12.52 Patients with PTTD show an altered movement pattern in heel raise that includes less plantarflexion of the metatarsals and decreased extension of the great big toe. Compensation occurs by increasing ankle plantarflexion.

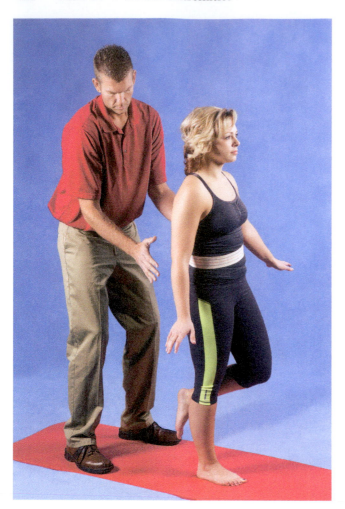

Figure 12.53 Unipedal standing balance test for posterior tibialis tendon dysfunction. This test may be used as an alternate for the heel raise test.

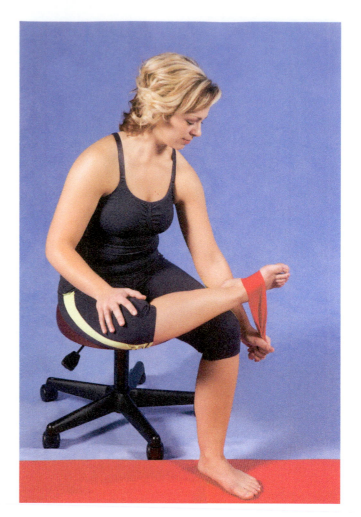

Figure 12.54 Patients can use elastic resistance to strengthen posterior tibialis by adducting the foot in a plantarflexed position. Emphasizing the eccentric phase is important for PTTD.

Unipedal Standing Balance Test

This test may be used as a substitute if the patient is unable to perform a single heel raise.[75] The patient is standing. The examiner instructs the patient to stand on one leg. The examiner assists if needed (Fig. 12.53). A positive test is indicated by the inability to stand on the affected leg without hand support for 10 seconds.

Common Interventions

Recognizing PTTD in stage I is necessary for effective treatment. By stage II, the arch collapse has occurred. Exercise in patients with stage I of the disorder has been effective in decreasing pain and increasing function.[70,76,77] Orthoses to support the medial longitudinal arch are beneficial.[76]

Exercises that have been effective include gastrocnemius and soleus stretching, and strengthening of posterior tibialis, anterior tibialis, gastrocsoleus, and fibularis muscles.[70,77] Foot adduction in a plantarflexed position has been the most effective exercise to activate posterior tibialis.[78] In a study by Kulig, eccentric tendon loading and orthoses were more effective than concentric exercise with orthoses in decreasing pain and improving function.[76] In Figure 12.54, a patient is performing posterior tibialis tendon exercises, concentrating on the eccentric phase.

In addition to stretching and strengthening the muscles of the ankle and foot, the plan of care may include strengthening of the hip extensors, abductors, and external rotators. Core strength and control of the pelvis and hip may be beneficial in treatment of PTTD.[73]

The Bottom Line:	for patients with posterior tibialis tendon dysfunction
Description and causes	Inflammation and deterioration of the tibialis posterior tendon related to overpronation, weakness in foot invertors, hip abductors, and hip extensors.
Test	Unilateral single heel raise test, unipedal standing balance test
Stretch	Gastrocnemius, soleus stretching
Strengthen	Posterior tibialis, anterior tibialis, gastrocsoleus, fibularis muscles, hip abductors, hip extensors, and hip external rotators
Train	Posterior tibialis eccentrically
Avoid	Medial collapse of the knee

Medial Tibial Stress Syndrome

Medial tibial stress syndrome (MTSS) is an overuse injury to the tibia or the origins of posterior tibialis and soleus. It is commonly referred to as "shin splints." This disorder was originally thought to be caused by inflammation of the periosteum (**periostitis**) at the origin of posterior tibialis or soleus. But new evidence indicates that the pain may be related to bone resorption along the tibia, bone stress, or tendinopathy at the muscle origins.[79,80]

Causes/Contributing Factors

Several factors are related to increased risk of developing MTSS. It is largely a disorder of runners and more common in females.[81,82] Runners with excessive pronation are more likely to experience MTSS.[81,83–85] MTSS is more common in people who overtrain by running long distances every day and running on hills or uneven terrain.[86] It also appears related to high body mass index (BMI).[82,87,88]

Tightness or imbalance in lower extremity muscles may also contribute to MTSS. Particularly, tightness in gastrocnemius and soleus with limited dorsiflexion is a contributing factor.[89–91]

Symptoms

The chief complaint of patients with MTSS is pain on the lower leg just medial to the tibia. The pain is worse immediately after running and typically gets better with rest. The patient may notice tenderness along the medial tibia. Swelling may be present.

Clinical Signs

The diagnosis of MTSS is based on clinical signs and symptoms of exercise-induced pain that is accompanied by tenderness along the distal third of the tibia (Fig. 12.55). The physical therapist will rule out other disorders, including tibial **stress fracture** and compartment syndrome, when making this diagnosis. There are no special tests used to confirm MTSS.

Common Interventions

Protected Phase

Rest, ice, and elevation are commonly used initially to alleviate the symptoms of MTSS. It is very important that the runner cut back or stop running until symptoms subside. Iontophoresis, phonophoresis, and ultrasound may be effective.[92]

The plan of care is likely to include lower extremity stretching and strengthening exercises. Stretching gastrocnemius and soleus has been effective.[89–91,93,94] Use of cycling or aquatic therapy during this stage may be used to maintain fitness. Strengthening of hip extensors, abductors, and external rotators may be included in the plan of care to address abnormal biomechanics of running.

Subacute Phase

As the symptoms subside, the patient may begin strengthening anterior tibialis, posterior tibialis, and gastrocsoleus. Focusing on eccentric control of these muscles may be effective in treatment.[95] Before the runner returns to the sport, footwear should be addressed. Shock-absorbing

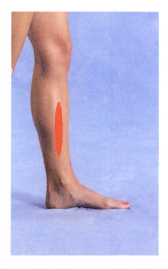

Figure 12.55 Area of tenderness and pain in medial tibial stress syndrome.

insoles[96] or orthoses to control pronation[94] may be useful in treatment.

Prevention

Runners should be instructed to vary the distance they run, alternating long and short distance running every other day. They should avoid running predominantly on hills or rough terrain.[86] Instruct runners to slowly progress their weekly distance, with a recommendation of less than 30% increase per week.[34] Orthoses should be recommended for people who excessively pronate.

The Bottom Line:	for patients with medial tibial stress syndrome
Description and Causes	Stress on tibia or at the origin of posterior tibialis and soleus common in runners who overpronate
Test	None
Stretch	Gastrocsoleus
Strengthen	Gastrocsoleus, anterior tibialis, posterior tibialis, hip abductors, hip extensors, and hip external rotators
Train	Eccentrically anterior tibialis, posterior tibialis, and gastrocsoleus
Avoid	Medial collapse of the knee, overtraining

Compartment Syndrome

As discussed earlier in this chapter, the lower leg muscles are grouped into three anterior muscles, three lateral muscles, and two groups of three posterior muscles. Each of these groups is enclosed by a thick layer of fascial tissue. The fascia has little elasticity and doesn't expand. Compartment syndrome is an extremely painful condition in which the pressure within a compartment increases, causing a decrease in blood flow to the muscles and nerves in the compartment. It most frequently occurs in the leg or arm.

The two main types of compartment syndrome are acute and chronic. Acute compartment syndrome is an emergency condition that can lead to permanent tissue injury. Lack of blood flow to the muscles and nerves can cause paralysis. Chronic compartment syndrome is related to repetitive activities that temporarily increase the pressure within a compartment. This usually resolves with cessation of the activity.

Causes/Contributing Factors

Acute compartment syndrome is caused by trauma that results in bleeding and swelling in the tissues. It is often associated with fracture, crush injuries, or a cast that is too tight. Chronic compartment syndrome is typically related to exercise or activity. It is common in sports that involve repetitive movements, such as cycling and running.

Symptoms

In acute compartment syndrome, the symptoms begin usually within hours of the injury. Deep aching pain is the main symptom. The patient may report a sensation of pins and needles and a feeling of tightness in the extremity. Swelling and bruising is typical (Fig. 12.56).

The symptoms of chronic compartment syndrome, or exertional compartment syndrome, are the same. It is different, however, in the link to exercise and to the decline of symptoms with rest.

Clinical Signs

The symptoms of compartment syndrome are usually sufficient to lead the patient to seek medical attention. If compartment syndrome is suspected, clinical signs are increased pain with muscle contraction or muscle stretch. The patient will display a prolonged capillary refill time.

Capillary Refill Test

The patient is positioned supine. The examiner holds the body part above the heart and applies pressure to the end of a toe to cause blanching. When the pressure is stopped, the examiner notes how long it takes for the area to turn pink (Fig. 12.57). A positive test is indicated by capillary refill time of more than 2 seconds.

Common Interventions

In acute compartment syndrome, the patient must get medical assistance. Surgical opening of the compartment, called **fasciotomy,** may be necessary. Patients with symptoms of chronic compartment syndrome may first report the symptoms to their PT or PTA. Recognition of the symptoms may lead to appropriate treatment. Physical therapy intervention for these patients may include soft tissue mobilization, stretching, and patient education regarding exercise modification.

> ⚑ CLINICAL ALERT ————
>
> It is important for the PTA to recognize early signs of acute compartment syndrome in patients who are casted or wearing elastic bandages.

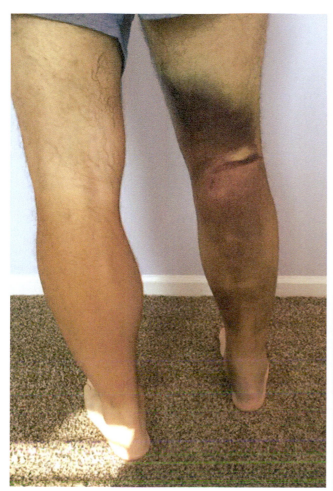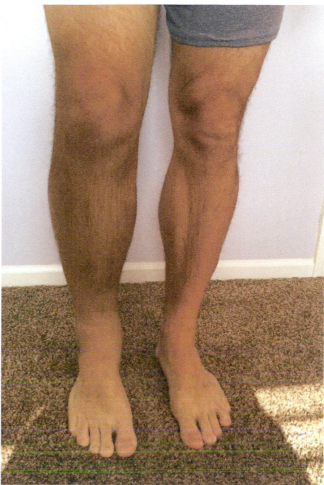

Figure 12.56 Acute compartment syndrome after trauma often occurs with swelling and bruising.

Tarsal Tunnel Syndrome

The tarsal tunnel on the medial ankle and foot contains the tendons of the deep posterior muscles and the tibial nerve. Tarsal tunnel syndrome is a neuropathy that results from compression or entrapment of the tibial nerve or its plantar branches under the flexor retinaculum.

After the tibial nerve passes through the tarsal tunnel, it divides into three branches: a branch to the calcaneus, the medial plantar nerve, and the lateral plantar nerve (Fig. 12.58). The neuropathy may involve any or all of these nerves.

Causes/Contributing Factors

Tarsal tunnel syndrome can be caused by anything that produces compression on the tibial nerve. It is most typically found in people who have increased pronation. As the talus slides down and in, and the calcaneus everts, the tibial nerve and tendons that run through the tunnel may be stretched or compressed between the retinaculum and the tarsal bones. It may also occur in people who develop an abnormal structure in this area that takes up space, such as a tumor, varicose vein, arthritic spur, or

cyst. If the structures that pass through the tarsal tunnel swell due to inflammation or injury, tarsal tunnel syndrome may occur.

Symptoms

Patients may complain of pain, numbness, tingling, burning, or a cramping sensation in the sole of the foot. This may be limited to the medial aspect of the plantar surface or be felt across the whole sole. Pain is usually increased with standing and walking and relieved by being off-weight. Patients may also note weakness in the foot muscles.

Clinical Signs

Tarsal tunnel syndrome may cause weakness of the foot intrinsic muscles. The patient may be tender along the tibial nerve. Sensory loss on the plantar foot may be detected using monofilament testing.

Tinel's Sign

Tinel's sign is a test used to detect nerve irritation in multiple sites by tapping on the nerve. For this pathology, Tinel's sign is performed by tapping over the tibial nerve

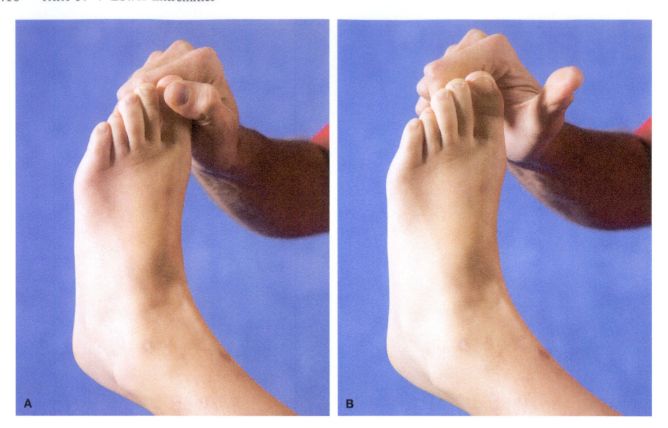

Figure 12.57 Capillary refill test for compartment syndrome. The examiner applies pressure to the end of a toe (A). When pressure is released (B), the examiner times how long it takes for the toe to turn pink, indicating a return of blood flow. Less than 2 seconds is normal refill time.

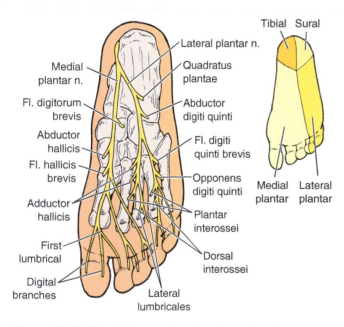

Figure 12.58 The tibial nerve has three branches that provide sensation to the sole of the foot as shown. In tarsal tunnel syndrome, the patient may complain of burning or numbness on the medial plantar aspect or entire sole of the foot.

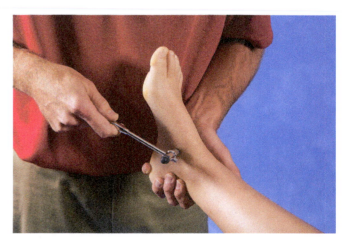

Figure 12.59 Tinel's sign for tarsal tunnel syndrome. The tibial nerve is tapped on the medial side of the ankle.

at the medial ankle using a finger or reflex hammer (Fig. 12.59). A positive test is indicated by a pins and needles sensation into the sole of the foot in a tibial nerve distribution.

Common Interventions

Relieving the cause of pressure on the tibial nerve through stretching, strengthening, and splinting is commonly included in the plan of care. Gastrocsoleus tightness may contribute to this pathology by causing midfoot flattening to gain the motion necessary in gait. Strengthening posterior tibialis also helps to improve control of pronation and minimize the stress on the tarsal tunnel. Strengthening of the foot intrinsic muscles is also important, as weakness is common. The patient may be fitted with orthoses to control pronation. Alternatively, antipronation taping may be beneficial.

The Bottom Line:	for patients with tarsal tunnel syndrome
Description and causes	Compression of the tibial nerve in the tarsal tunnel associated with overpronation, weakness of posterior tibialis, and limited dorsiflexion ROM
Test	Tinel's sign at the medial ankle
Stretch	Gastrocsoleus
Strengthen	Posterior tibialis, foot intrinsic muscles
Train	NA
Avoid	Overpronation

Ankle and Calcaneal Fractures

Fractures of the ankle and foot are very common. Fractures can occur in any of the bones in the lower leg, ankle, and foot, but common complete fractures involve the tibia, fibula, and calcaneus.

A fracture of the ankle usually involves the distal tibia and/or fibula. This frequently occurs as a result of a fall or motor vehicle accident. If the distal end of the tibia and fibula are both fractured, it is referred to as a **bimalleolar fracture.** If the posterior malleolus of the tibia is also fractured, **trimalleolar fracture** is the classification. Figure 12.60 is an x-ray that depicts a trimalleolar fracture.

A common site of fracture in the foot is the calcaneus. This occurs in a fall from a height, often from a ladder or roof. Calcaneal fractures frequently occur bilaterally or in conjunction with fractures of the hip or pelvis. These fractures are associated with a high rate of disability, protracted pain, and eventual osteoarthritis.

Causes/Contributing Factors

Fractures of the ankle and foot are frequently caused by a fall, motor vehicle accident, or sports-related injury.

Symptoms

Pain is the most frequent indicator of a fracture. The patient will also complain of limited motion, difficulty walking, and possibly a deformity. Swelling is likely to be present.

Clinical Signs

With a history of trauma and complaint of pain with movement, limited movement, deformity, and difficulty walking, fracture will be suspected. X-rays are used to confirm the diagnosis of fracture.

Common Interventions

In general, after fracture the patient will be immobilized by splint, casting, internal fixation, or external fixation.

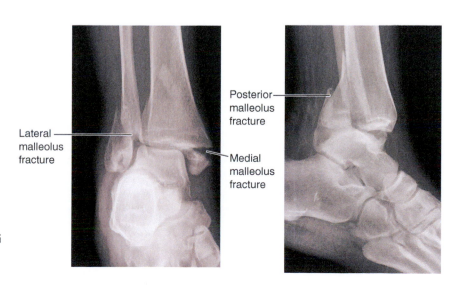

Figure 12.60 Trimalleolar fracture of the ankle involves the medial and lateral malleoli as well as the posterior malleolus on the back of the tibia.

The patient should be instructed to elevate the extremity to minimize swelling. Ice may be used for the first several days. It is important to maintain mobility of the nearby unaffected joints without compromising the fracture site.

Distal Tibia and/or Fibula Fracture

If a distal tibia or fibula fracture is stable and in good alignment, the patient may simply be casted. For unstable, bimalleolar, or trimalleolar fractures, the patient may undergo open reduction, internal fixation (ORIF) (Fig. 12.61).

The initial plan of care is variable in the postoperative stage, from cast immobilization to early mobilization in restricted planes. Early mobilization decreases risk of deep vein thrombosis but may carry an increased risk of surgical site infection and fixation failure.[97] Motion and strength should be maintained in uninvolved joints.

The cast or brace is usually removed about 6 to 8 weeks postoperatively. At this time the patient may be placed in a walking boot or air splint. Active and active-assisted range-of-motion exercises are usually initiated at this time, beginning with dorsiflexion and plantarflexion, and progressing to inversion and eversion. A stationary bike may be used. Weight-bearing is usually increased to weight-bearing-as-tolerated by 8 weeks.

What's in the Plan of Care?

Strengthening of ankle plantarflexion, dorsiflexion, inversion, and eversion is usually included in the plan of care about 2 months after injury. In addition, the patient may benefit from general lower body strengthening and proprioceptive retraining.

Calcaneus Fracture

Rehabilitation after calcaneal fracture is slower. Initially, whether nonoperative or postoperative ORIF, the patient will be immobilized in a cast. No weight-bearing is allowed in this phase. The patient may be seen for exercises to maintain motion and strength in uninvolved joints and to maintain cardiovascular capacity using an arm ergometer.

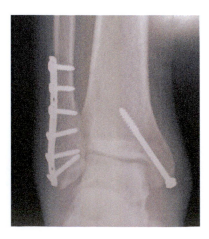

Figure 12.61 ORIF for bimalleolar fracture of the ankle.

By 6 to 8 weeks after surgery or injury, the patient is often allowed to begin to weight-bear on the affected extremity. Range of motion to the ankle and foot joints may be included in the plan of care at this time. Exercises to the unaffected joints and cardiovascular exercises are continued.

By 9 to 12 weeks after surgery or injury, weight-bearing is progressed to full if tolerated. Joint mobilization to tibiotalar and subtalar joints may be included in the plan of care. Soft tissue mobilization to gastrocsoleus and plantar fascia may be beneficial. Progressive isometric to isotonic strengthening of the ankle including gastrocsoleus may be initiated.

Stress Fracture

Stress fractures are small cracks in the bone and are most common in the leg and foot, particularly in the tibia, navicular, and metatarsals.

Causes/Contributing Factors

When the bone is subjected to repeated stresses without sufficient time to heal, stress fracture occurs. Stress fractures of the lower leg and foot are most common as an overuse injury in runners. Development of stress fracture has been linked to static alignment, muscle strength and endurance, bone mass, and training.

Stress fractures are more common in people with high arches,[98] increased external rotation of the hip,[99] leg-length discrepancy,[99,100] and flat feet.[101] It has been linked to overpronation in gait and running.[102-104]

Normal muscle strength, timing, and endurance are important to prevent stress fracture. Muscles help to dissipate the forces of impact. When muscles are weakened, easily fatigued, or have abnormal timing, they are less able to attenuate shock. Fatigue also may lead to altered biomechanics in running, further increasing the risk of stress fracture. Stress fractures are related to muscle strength and size; smaller muscle mass leads to increased risk of stress fractures.[89,100,105,106]

Bone strength is also important. Stress fractures occur in bone that has less mass and less density. This may be one reason that they are more common in women. Osteoporosis increases the risk.

Studies have looked at the training surface as a contributor to stress fracture. The firmness of the surface is not as much a contributor as a change in the surface. If the runner has been training on a firm surface, changing to a softer surface (grass, sand) increases risk of stress fracture. Changing from a soft to a firm surface also increases risk.

Symptoms

Stress fractures present as a gradual onset of pain that is worse after running. Swelling and tenderness may also be present.

Clinical Signs

Stress fracture is initially suspected by patient history. X-rays may not be helpful in diagnosis of acute stress fracture; a bone scan or MRI may be more informative.

Common Interventions

After diagnosis of stress fracture, it is important that the area be rested. This involves modifying running, use of crutches, and splints or cushioned footwear to protect the site. Aquatic therapy may be useful to maintain fitness while minimizing weight-bearing forces.

As pain subsides, progressive weight-bearing is encouraged. The patient is allowed to walk without a device, walking faster and longer distances as pain allows. As an example, one program restricts the runner from return to sport until being pain-free for a week. At this point, the patient is allowed to run every other day for 2 weeks but at half the usual pace and distance.[107] For patients with stress fracture, it is helpful if the PT or PTA provides a specific protocol for return to sport, with criteria for advancement.

Prevention

Stress fracture has been linked to increasing the distance run too quickly, poor footwear, and obesity. Female runners with low muscle mass should be informed of the risk prior to initiating a running program.

The Bottom Line:	for patients with stress fractures
Description and causes	Small cracks in the bone related to high arches, increased external rotation ROM of the hip, leg-length discrepancy, decreased bone mass, and flat feet
Test	NA
Stretch	Leg and foot muscles that are shortened
Strengthen	Leg and foot muscles that are weak
Train	Using a return to running protocol that gradually increases volume
Avoid	Changing running surface, running fatigue

Toe Deformities

Hallux Valgus

Hallux valgus is a foot deformity that is commonly referred to as bunion. In this deformity, the big toe abducts, leading to a prominent first MTP joint (Fig. 12.62). The condition is painful and makes it difficult to wear shoes comfortably.

The factors that lead to hallux valgus are not completely known, but it can be a result of flat feet or ligament laxity. Shoes with a narrow toe box seem to increase the deformity. As the deformity progresses, the second toe may cross over or under the big toe. Generally, this deformity does not require surgical correction, but if the pain and limitation caused by the bunion warrant, osteotomy may be performed to remove excess bone and realign the big toe.

Claw Toe and Hammer Toe

A claw toe deformity is characterized by extension of the MTP joint and flexion of the PIP and DIP joints of the toes. It may occur in toes 2 to 5; often it occurs in the second toe in the presence of a bunion in the big toe. This deformity may be attributed to rheumatoid arthritis.

Hammer toe is similar to claw toe in the extension of the MTP and flexion of the PIP. But in hammer toe, the DIP joint does not flex but is extended to be flat on the floor. Hammer toe also may occur in toes 2 to 5. Figure 12.63 depicts claw toe and hammer toe deformities.

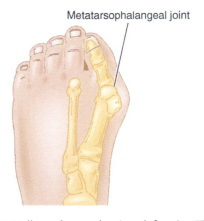

Metatarsophalangeal joint

Figure 12.62 Hallux valgus or bunion deformity. The big toe is abducted and the first MTP joint is prominent, swollen, and painful.

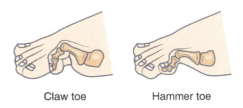

Claw toe   Hammer toe

Figure 12.63 Claw toe and hammer toe deformities.

SUMMARY

Altered biomechanics in the lower extremity kinetic chain can impact the ankle and foot, leading to pathology. Conversely, altered biomechanics of the ankle may affect the lower extremity chain. An understanding of lower limb biomechanics as well as the anatomy and pathologies of the ankle and foot are necessary to effectively treat and prevent problems in this area.

REVIEW QUESTIONS

1. It is important that the foot be able to change from flexible to rigid. How is this accomplished in the foot? At what point in the gait cycle does the foot need to be flexible? When does it need to be rigid?

2. Many pathologies of the foot have over-pronation as a contributor. List four of these pathologies. Taking a top-down approach, how might the plan of care address this? What about a bottom-up approach?

3. Compare and contrast the pathologies of PTTD and MTSS.

4. Many pathologies have gastrocsoleus tightness as a contributor. List four pathologies. With your lab partner, explain the implications of limited dorsiflexion range-of-motion on the midfoot that leads to pathology.

5. Clinical Practice Guidelines have been created for the pathologies of Achilles tendinopathy, ankle sprain, and plantar fasciitis. In what way does this impact your patient education or interventions?

6. For each of the following special tests, name the pathology that yields a positive test:
   a. Anterior drawer test
   b. Arc sign
   c. Capillary refill test
   d. Dorsiflexion maneuver
   e. External rotation test
   f. Medial talar tilt stress test
   g. Navicular drop test
   h. Royal London Hospital test
   i. Squeeze test
   j. Thompson test
   k. Tinel's sign
   l. Unilateral single heel raise test
   m. Windlass test

PATIENT CASE: Plantar Fasciitis

PT Evaluation			

Patient Name: XXXXXXX XXXXXXXXXXXX	**Age:** 48	**BMI:** 29.4

Diagnosis/History

Medical Diagnosis: Plantar fasciitis

PT Diagnosis: Pain in L heel secondary to plantar fasciitis

Diagnostic Tests/Results: X-ray – heel spur

Relevant Medical History: Dyslipidemia, COPD, OA, lymphedema

Prior Level of Function: Minimally active

Patient's Goals: Decrease pain, work without pain

Medications: Crestor 20 mg daily, ibuprofen 800 mg tid

Precautions: None

Social Supports/Safety Hazards

Patient Living Situation/ Supports/ Hazards: Lives alone
Patient Working Situation/Occupation/ Leisure Activities: Employed full-time as a cashier. Enjoys watching TV, visiting friends, cooking

Vital Signs

At rest Temperature: 98.4   BP: 140/88   HR: 82   Resp: 14   O2 sat: 95

Subjective Information

Patient is a female with 2-3 month history of pain in her L heel. She states this began for no apparent reason. Her complaint is of pain that is very bad when she gets up in the morning, and when she goes back to the cash register after her lunch break. She states that she can hardly walk at these times for several minutes.

Physical Assessment

Orientation: Alert and oriented   **Speech/Vision/Hearing:** Normal   **Skin Integrity:** Intact
ROM: Ankle dorsiflexion limited to 10° with knee extension, B. Big toe extension 40° B due to OA.
Strength: Grossly 4/5 in all LE muscles   **Palpation:** No tenderness elicited   **Muscle Tone:** Not tested
Balance/Coordination: not tested   **Sensation/Proprioception:** Not tested   **Posture:** Increased thoracic kyphosis.
Endurance: Patient is short of air after walking 30 feet.   **Edema:** B LE lymphedema, feet to knees. 2+ pitting.

Pain

Pain Rating and Location: At best 0/10   **At worst** 9/10   **Relieving Factors:** rest, ibuprofen
Aggravating Factors: Getting up after sitting or sleeping   **Irritability:** Patient states after walking for a few minutes, her pain goes away.

Functional Assessment

Patient is functionally independent.

Special Testing

Test Name: Navicular drop test   **Result** positive (10 mm B)   **Test Name:**   **Result**

Assessment

Patient has s/s consistent with plantar fasciitis L

Short-Term Treatment Goals

1. Patient will state a 15% decrease in pain.
2. Patient will have increased ROM into dorsiflexion to at least 15° with knee extension B.
3. Patient will be independent in a HEP.

Long-Term Treatment Goals

1. Patient will have 20° dorsiflexion with knee extension B.
2. Patient will state a 35% decrease in pain.
3. Patient will demonstrate awareness of stretching before getting out of bed.

Treatment Plan

Frequency/Duration: 3 times a week for 2 week, 1 time a week for 4 weeks
Consisting of: Modalities, therapeutic exercise, neuro re-education, patient education

continued

Patient Case Questions

1. What factors might be contributing to the patient's plantar fasciitis?

2. What would you tell the patient about specific activities to avoid or curtail?

3. What data will you collect the first time you see the patient?

4. If the plan of care does not guide you, what modalities might you use with this patient? Why? Are any modalities contraindicated?

5. If the plan of care does not specifically guide you, describe three therapeutic exercises that are indicated for this patient. Justify your choices.

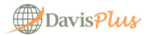 For additional resources, including answers to this case, please visit
http://davisplus.fadavis.com

REFERENCES

1. Martin, R. L., Davenport, T. E., Reischl, S. F., McPoil, T. G., Matheson, J. W., Wukich, D. K., & McDonough, C. M. (2014). Heel pain—Plantar fasciitis: Revision 2014. *Journal of Orthopaedic and Sports Physical Therapy, 44*, A1–A33.

2. Kim, W. & Voloshin, A. S. (1995). Role of plantar fascia in the load bearing capacity of the human foot. *Journal of Biomechanics, 28*, 1025–1033.

3. Golanó, P., Vega, J., de Leeuw, P. A., Malagelada, F., Manzanares, M. C., Götzens, V., & van Dijk, C. N. (2010). Anatomy of the ankle ligaments: A pictorial essay. *Knee Surgery, Sports Traumatology, Arthroscopy, 18*, 557–569.

4. Chen, D., Li, B., Aubeeluck, A., Yang, Y. F., Huang, Y. G., Zhou, J. Q., & Yu, G. R. (2014). Anatomy and biomechanical properties of the plantar aponeurosis: A cadaveric study. *PLoS ONE, 9*.

5. Hicks, J. H. (1954). The mechanics of the foot. II. The plantar aponeurosis and the arch. *Journal of Anatomy, 88*, 25–30.

6. Spina, A. A. (2007). The plantaris muscle: Anatomy, injury, imaging, and treatment. *Journal of the Canadian Chiropractic Association, 51*, 158–165.

7. Moore, K. L. (2013). *Clinically oriented anatomy.* Philadelphia, PA: Lippincott Williams & Wilkins.

8. Simpson, S. L., Hertzog, M. S., & Barja, R. H. (1991). The plantaris tendon graft: An ultrasound study. *Journal of Hand Surgery, 16*, 708–711.

9. Palastanga, N. (1994). *Anatomy and human movement: Structure and function.* Woburn, MA: Butterworth-Heinemann.

10. Andrews, J. R., Harrelson, G. L., & Wilk, K. E. (2012). *Physical rehabilitation of the injured athlete.* Amsterdam, The Netherlands: Elsevier Health Sciences.

11. Levinger, P., & Gilleard, W. (2004). An evaluation of the rearfoot posture in individuals with patellofemoral pain syndrome. *Journal of Sports Science and Medicine, 3*, 8–14.

12. Martin, R. L., Davenport, T. E., Paulseth, S., Wukich, D. K.,Orthopaedic Section American Physical Therapy Association. (Godges, J. J., & 2013). Ankle stability and movement coordination impairments: Ankle ligament sprains. *Journal of Orthopaedic and Sports Physical Therapy, 43*, A1–40.

13. Ben Moussa Zouita, A., Majdoub, O., Ferchichi, H., Grandy, K., Dziri, C., & Ben Salah, F. Z. (2013). The effect of 8-weeks proprioceptive exercise program in postural sway and isokinetic strength of ankle sprains of Tunisian athletes. *Annals of Physical and Rehabilitation Medicine, 56*, 634–643.

14. Postle, K., Pak, D. & Smith, T. O. (2012). Effectiveness of proprioceptive exercises for ankle ligament injury in adults: A systematic literature and meta-analysis. *Manual Therapy, 17*, 285–291.

15. Schiftan, G. S., Ross, L. A., & Hahne, A. J. (2014). The effectiveness of proprioceptive training in preventing ankle sprains in sporting populations: A systematic review and meta-analysis. *Journal of Science and Medicine in Sport, Sports Medicine Australia, 18*, 238–244.

16. Webster, K. A., & Gribble, P. A. (2010). Functional rehabilitation interventions for chronic ankle instability: A systematic review. *Journal of Sport Rehabilitation, 19*, 98–114.

17. Aaltonen, S., Karjalainen, H., Heinonen, A., Parkkari, J., & Kujala, U. M. (2007). Prevention of sports injuries: Systematic review of randomized controlled trials. *Archives of Internal Medicine, 167*, 1585–1592.

18. Bahr, R., & Bahr, I. A. (1997). Incidence of acute volleyball injuries: A prospective cohort study of injury mechanisms and risk factors. *Scandinavian Journal of Medicine & Science in Sports, 7*, 166–171.

19. Dizon, J. M. R., & Reyes, J. J. B. (2010). A systematic review on the effectiveness of external ankle supports in the prevention of inversion ankle sprains among elite and recreational players. *Journal of Science and Medicine in Sport, Sports Medicine Australia, 13*, 309–317.

20. LaBella, C. R., Huxford, M. R., Grissom, J., Kim, K. Y., Peng, J., & Christoffel, K. K. (2011). Effect of neuromuscular warm-up on injuries in female soccer and basketball athletes in urban public high schools: Cluster randomized controlled trial. *Archives of Pediatric and Adolescent Medicine, 165*, 1033–1040.

21. Wedderkopp, N., Kaltoft, M., Lundgaard, B., Rosendahl, M., & Froberg, K. (1999). Prevention of injuries in young female players in European team handball. A prospective intervention study. *Scandinavian Journal of Medicine & Science in Sports, 9*, 41–47.

22. Hopkinson, W. J., St Pierre, P., Ryan, J. B., & Wheeler, J. H. (1990). Syndesmosis sprains of the ankle. *Foot and Ankle, 10*, 325–330.

23. Lin, C.-F., Gross, M. L., & Weinhold, P. (2006). Ankle syndesmosis injuries: Anatomy, biomechanics, mechanism of injury, and clinical guidelines for diagnosis and intervention. *Journal of Orthopaedic and Sports Physical Therapy, 36*, 372–384.

24. Nussbaum, E. D., Hosea, T. M., Sieler, S. D., Incremona, B. R., & Kessler, D. E. (2001). Prospective evaluation of syndesmotic ankle sprains without diastasis. *American Journal of Sports Medicine, 29,* 31–35.

25. Williams, G. N., & Allen, E. J. (2010). Rehabilitation of syndesmotic (high) ankle sprains. *Sports Health, 2,* 460–470.

26. Lemont, H., Ammirati, K. M., & Usen, N. (2003). Plantar fasciitis: A degenerative process (fasciosis) without inflammation. *Journal of the American Podiatric Medical Association, 93,* 234–237.

27. Pohl, M. B., Hamill, J., & Davis, I. S. (2009). Biomechanical and anatomic factors associated with a history of plantar fasciitis in female runners. *Clinical Journal of Sport Medicine, Official Journal of the Canadian Academy of Sport Medicine, 19,* 372–376.

28. Patel, A., & DiGiovanni, B. (2011). Association between plantar fasciitis and isolated contracture of the gastrocnemius. *Foot & Ankle International, 32,* 5–8.

29. Irving, D. B., Cook, J. L., Young, M. A., & Menz, H. B. (2007). Obesity and pronated foot type may increase the risk of chronic plantar heel pain: A matched case-control study. *BMC Musculoskeletal Disorders, 8,* 41.

30. Wearing, S. C., Smeathers, J. E., Urry, S. R., Hennig, E. M., & Hills, A. P. (2006). The pathomechanics of plantar fasciitis. *Sports Medicine (Auckland, NZ), 36,* 585–611.

31. Ribeiro, A. P., Trombini-Souza, F., Tessutti, V., Rodrigues Lima, F., Sacco Ide, C., & João, S. M. (2011). Rearfoot alignment and medial longitudinal arch configurations of runners with symptoms and histories of plantar fasciitis. *Clinics (São Paulo, Brazil), 66,* 1027–1033.

32. Werner, R. A., Gell, N., Hartigan, A., Wiggerman, N., & Keyserling, W. M. (2010). Risk factors for plantar fasciitis among assembly plant workers. *PM&R: The Journal of Injury, Function, and Rehabilitation, 2,* 110–116.

33. De Garceau, D., Dean, D., Requejo, S. M., & Thordarson, D. B. (2003). The association between diagnosis of plantar fasciitis and Windlass test results. *Foot & Ankle International, 24,* 251–255.

34. Nielsen, R. G., Rathleff, M. S., Simonsen, O. H., & Langberg, H. (2009). Determination of normal values for navicular drop during walking: A new model correcting for foot length and gender. *Journal of Foot and Ankle Research, 2,* 12.

35. Brantingham, J. W., Bonnefin, D., Perle, S. M., Cassa, T. K., Globe, G., Pribicevic, M., Hicks, M., et al. (2012). Manipulative therapy for lower extremity conditions: Update of a literature review. *Journal of Manipulative and Physiological Therapeutics, 35,* 127–166.

36. Cleland, J. A., Abbott, J. H., Kidd, M. O., Stockwell, S., Cheney, S., Gerrard, D. F., & Flynn, T. W. (2009). Manual physical therapy and exercise versus electrophysical agents and exercise in the management of plantar heel pain: A multicenter randomized clinical trial. *Journal of Orthopaedic and Sports Physical Therapy, 39,* 573–585.

37. Renan-Ordine, R., Alburquerque-Sendín, F., de Souza, D. P. R., Cleland, J. A., & Fernández-de-Las-Peñas, C. (2011). Effectiveness of myofascial trigger point manual therapy combined with a self-stretching protocol for the management of plantar heel pain: A randomized controlled trial. *Journal of Orthopaedic and Sports Physical Therapy, 41,* 43–50.

38. Garrett, T. R., & Neibert, P. J. (2013). The effectiveness of a gastrocnemius-soleus stretching program as a therapeutic treatment of plantar fasciitis. *Journal of Sport Rehabilitation, 22,* 308–312.

39. Landorf, K. B., & Menz, H. B. (2008). Plantar heel pain and fasciitis. *BMJ Clinical Evidence, 02,* 1111.

40. Sweeting, D., Parish, B., Hooper, L., & Chester, R. (2011). The effectiveness of manual stretching in the treatment of plantar heel pain: A systematic review. *Journal of Foot and Ankle Research, 4,* 19.

41. Jung, D. Y., Koh, E. K., Kwon, O. Y., Yi, C. H., Oh, J. S., & Weon, J. H. (2009). Effect of medial arch support on displacement of the myotendinous junction of the gastrocnemius during standing wall stretching. *Journal of Orthopaedic and Sports Physical Therapy, 39,* 867–874.

42. Franettovich, M., Chapman, A., Blanch, P., & Vicenzino, B. (2008). A physiological and psychological basis for anti-pronation taping from a critical review of the literature. *Sports Medicine (Auckland, NZ), 38,* 617–631.

43. van de Water, A. T. M., & Speksnijder, C. M. (2010). Efficacy of taping for the treatment of plantar fasciosis: A systematic review of controlled trials. *Journal of the American Podiatric Medical Association, 100,* 41–51.

44. Al-Bluwi, M. T., Sadat-Ali, M., Al-Habdan, I. M., & Azam, M. Q. (2011). Efficacy of EZStep in the management of plantar fasciitis: A prospective, randomized study. *Foot and Ankle Specialist, 4,* 218–221.

45. Drake, M., Bittenbender, C., & Boyles, R. E. (2011). The short-term effects of treating plantar fasciitis with a temporary custom foot orthosis and stretching. *Journal of Orthopaedic and Sports Physical Therapy, 41,* 221–231.

46. Hume, P., Hopkins, W., Rome, K., Maulder, P., Coyle, G., & Nigg, B. (2008). Effectiveness of foot orthoses for treatment and prevention of lower limb injuries: A review. *Sports Medicine (Auckland, NZ), 38,* 759–779.

47. Lee, S. Y., McKeon, P., & Hertel, J. (2009). Does the use of orthoses improve self-reported pain and function measures in patients with plantar fasciitis? A meta-analysis. *Physical Therapy in Sport: Official Journal of the Association of Chartered Physiotherapists in Sports Medicine, 10,* 12–18.

48. Uden, H., Boesch, E., & Kumar, S. (2011). Plantar fasciitis—To jab or to support? A systematic review of the current best evidence. *Journal of Multidisciplinary Healthcare, 4,* 155–164.

49. Beyzadeoğlu, T., Gökçe, A., & Bekler, H. (2007). The effectiveness of dorsiflexion night splint added to conservative treatment for plantar fasciitis. *Acta Orthopaedica et Traumatologica Turcica, 41,* 220–224.

50. Lee, W. C. C., Wong, W. Y., Kung, E., & Leung, A. K. L. (2012). Effectiveness of adjustable dorsiflexion night splint in combination with accommodative foot orthosis on plantar fasciitis. *Journal of Rehabilitation Research and Development, 49,* 1557–1564.

51. Sheridan, L., Lopez, A., Perez, A., John, M. M., Willis, F. B., & Shanmugam, R. (2010). Plantar fasciopathy treated with dynamic splinting: A randomized controlled trial. *Journal of the American Podiatric Medical Association, 100,* 161–165.

52. Keenan, A. M., & Tanner, C. M. (2001). The effect of high-Dye and low-Dye taping on rearfoot motion. *Journal of the American Podiatric Medical Association, 91,* 255–261.

53. Fong, D. T. P., Pang, K. Y., Chung, M. M. L., Hung, A. S. L., & Chan, K. M. (2012). Evaluation of combined prescription of rocker sole shoes and custom-made foot orthoses for the treatment of plantar fasciitis. *Clinical Biomechanics (Bristol Avon), 27,* 1072–1077.

54. Carcia, C. R., Martin, R. L., Houck, J., Orthopaedic Section of the American Physical Therapy Association. (Wukich, D. K., & 2010). Achilles pain, stiffness, and muscle power deficits: Achilles tendinitis. *Journal of Orthopaedic and Sports Physical Therapy, 40,* A1–26.

55. Kaufman, K. R., Brodine, S. K., Shaffer, R. A., Johnson, C. W., & Cullison, T. R. (1999). The effect of foot structure and range of motion on musculoskeletal overuse injuries. *American Journal of Sports Medicine, 27,* 585–593.

56. Kvist, M. (1994). Achilles tendon injuries in athletes. *Sports Medicine (Auckland, NZ), 18,* 173–201.

57. Mahieu, N. N., Witvrouw, E., Stevens, V., Van Tiggelen, D., & Roget, P. (2006). Intrinsic risk factors for the development of achilles tendon overuse injury: A prospective study. *American Journal of Sports Medicine, 34*, 226–235.

58. McCrory, J. L., Martin, D. F., Lowery, R. B., Cannon, D. W., Curl, W. W., Read, H. M. Jr, Hunter, D. M., et al. (1999). Etiologic factors associated with Achilles tendinitis in runners. *Medicine and Science in Sports and Exercise, 31*, 1374–1381.

59. Fredberg, U., Bolvig, L., Pfeiffer-Jensen, M., Clemmensen, D., Jakobsen, B. W., & Stengaard-Pedersen, K. (2004). Ultrasonography as a tool for diagnosis, guidance of local steroid injection and, together with pressure algometry, monitoring of the treatment of athletes with chronic jumper's knee and Achilles tendinitis: A randomized, double-blind, placebo-controlled study. *Scandinavian Journal of Rheumatology, 33*, 94–101.

60. Fredberg, U., Bolvig, L., Lauridsen, A., & Stengaard-Pedersen, K. (2007). Influence of acute physical activity immediately before ultrasonographic measurement of Achilles tendon thickness. *Scandinavian Journal of Rheumatology, 36*, 488–489.

61. Maffulli, N., Kenward, M. G., Testa, V., Capasso, G., Regine, R., & King, J. B. (2003). Clinical diagnosis of Achilles tendinopathy with tendinosis. *Clinical Journal of Sport Medicine: Official Journal of the Canadian Academy of Sport Medicine, 13*, 11–15.

62. Ohberg, L., Lorentzon, R., Alfredson, H., & Maffulli, N. (2004). Eccentric training in patients with chronic Achilles tendinosis: Normalised tendon structure and decreased thickness at follow up. *British Journal of Sports Medicine, 38*, 8–11.

63. Rompe, J. D., Furia, J., & Maffulli, N. (2009). Eccentric loading versus eccentric loading plus shock-wave treatment for midportion achilles tendinopathy: A randomized controlled trial. *American Journal of Sports Medicine, 37*, 463–470.

64. Rompe, J. D., Nafe, B., Furia, J. P., & Maffulli, N. (2007). Eccentric loading, shock-wave treatment, or a wait-and-see policy for tendinopathy of the main body of tendo Achillis: A randomized controlled trial. *American Journal of Sports Medicine, 35*, 374–383.

65. Silbernagel, K. G., Thomeé, R., Eriksson, B. I., & Karlsson, J. (2007). Full symptomatic recovery does not ensure full recovery of muscle-tendon function in patients with Achilles tendinopathy. *British Journal of Sports Medicine, 41*, 276–280; discussion 280.

66. Alfredson, H., Pietilä, T., Jonsson, P., & Lorentzon, R. (1998). Heavy-load eccentric calf muscle training for the treatment of chronic Achilles tendinosis. *American Journal of Sports Medicine, 26*, 360–366.

67. Rabbito, M., Pohl, M. B., Humble, N., & Ferber, R. (2011). Biomechanical and clinical factors related to stage I posterior tibial tendon dysfunction. *Journal of Orthopaedic and Sports Physical Therapy, 41*, 776–784.

68. Dyal, C. M., Feder, J., Deland, J. T., & Thompson, F. M. (1997). Pes planus in patients with posterior tibial tendon insufficiency: Asymptomatic versus symptomatic foot. *Foot & Ankle International, 18*, 85–88.

69. Williams, D. S., McClay, I. S., & Hamill, J. (2001). Arch structure and injury patterns in runners. *Clinical Biomechanics (Bristol Avon), 16*, 341–347.

70. Alvarez, R. G., Marini, A., Schmitt, C., & Saltzman, C. L. (2006). Stage I and II posterior tibial tendon dysfunction treated by a structured nonoperative management protocol: An orthosis and exercise program. *Foot & Ankle International, 27*, 2–8.

71. Houck, J. R., Neville, C., Tome, J., & Flemister, A. S. (2009). Foot kinematics during a bilateral heel rise test in participants with stage II posterior tibial tendon dysfunction. *Journal of Orthopaedic and Sports Physical Therapy, 39*, 593–603.

72. Shibuya, N., Ramanujam, C. L., & Garcia, G. M. (2008). Association of tibialis posterior tendon pathology with other radiographic findings in the foot: A case-control study. *Journal of Foot and Ankle Surgery: Official Publication of the American College of Foot and Ankle Surgeons, 47*, 546–553.

73. Kulig, K., Popovich, J. M., Noceti-Dewit, L. M., Reischl, S. F., & Kim, D. (2011). Women with posterior tibial tendon dysfunction have diminished ankle and hip muscle performance. *Journal of Orthopaedic and Sports Physical Therapy, 41*, 687–694.

74. Kohls-Gatzoulis, J., Angel, J. C., Singh, D., Haddad, F., Livingstone, J., & Berry, G. (2004). Tibialis posterior dysfunction: A common and treatable cause of adult acquired flatfoot. *BMJ, 329*, 1328–1333.

75. Kulig, K., Lee, S. P., Reischl, S. F., & Noceti-DeWit, L. (2014). Effect of tibialis posterior tendon dysfunction on unipedal standing balance test. *Foot & Ankle International, 36*, 83–89.

76. Kulig, K., Reischl, S. F., Pomrantz, A. B., Burnfield, J. M., Mais-Requejo, S., Thordarson, D. B., & Smith, R. W. (2009). Nonsurgical management of posterior tibial tendon dysfunction with orthoses and resistive exercise: A randomized controlled trial. *Physical Therapy, 89*, 26–37.

77. Kulig, K., Lederhaus, E. S., Reischl, S., Arya, S., & Bashford, G. (2009). Effect of eccentric exercise program for early tibialis posterior tendinopathy. *Foot & Ankle International, 30*, 877–885.

78. Kulig, K., Burnfield, J. M., Requejo, S. M., Sperry, M., & Terk, M. (2004). Selective activation of tibialis posterior: Evaluation by magnetic resonance imaging. *Medicine and Science in Sports and Exercise, 36*, 862–867.

79. Galbraith, R. M., & Lavallee, M. E. (2009). Medial tibial stress syndrome: Conservative treatment options. *Current Reviews in Musculoskeletal Medicine, 2*, 127–133.

80. Moen, M. H., Tol, J. L., Weir, A., Steunebrink, M., & De Winter, T. C. (2009). Medial tibial stress syndrome: A critical review. *Sports Medicine (Auckland, NZ), 39*, 523–546.

81. Bennett, J. E., Reinking, M. F., Pluemer, B., Pentel, A., Seaton, M., & Killian, C. (2001). Factors contributing to the development of medial tibial stress syndrome in high school runners. *Journal of Orthopaedic and Sports Physical Therapy, 31*, 504–510.

82. Plisky, M. S., Rauh, M. J., Heiderscheit, B., Underwood, F. B., & Tank, R. T. (2007). Medial tibial stress syndrome in high school cross-country runners: Incidence and risk factors. *Journal of Orthopaedic and Sports Physical Therapy, 37*, 40–47.

83. Messier, S. P., & Pittala, K. A. (1988). Etiologic factors associated with selected running injuries. *Medicine and Science in Sports and Exercise, 20*, 501–505.

84. Sommer, H. M., & Vallentyne, S. W. (1995). Effect of foot posture on the incidence of medial tibial stress syndrome. *Medicine and Science in Sports and Exercise, 27*, 800–804.

85. Viitasalo, J. T., & Kvist, M. (1983). Some biomechanical aspects of the foot and ankle in athletes with and without shin splints. *American Journal of Sports Medicine, 11*, 125–130.

86. Rauh, M. J. (2014). Summer training factors and risk of musculoskeletal injury among high school cross-country runners. *Journal of Orthopaedic and Sports Physical Therapy, 44*, 793–804.

87. Hamstra-Wright, K. L., Huxel Bliven, K. C., & Bay, C. (2015). Risk factors for medial tibial stress syndrome in physically active individuals such as runners and military personnel: A systematic review and meta-analysis. *British Journal of Sports Medicine, 49*, 362–369.

88. Yagi, S., Muneta, T., & Sekiya, I. (2013). Incidence and risk factors for medial tibial stress syndrome and tibial stress

fracture in high school runners. *Knee Surgery, Sports Traumatology, Arthroscopy: Official Journal of ESSKA, 21,* 556–563.

89. Beck, B. R. (1998). Tibial stress injuries. An aetiological review for the purposes of guiding management. *Sports Medicine (Auckland, NZ), 26,* 265–279.

90. Fredericson, M. (1996). Common injuries in runners. Diagnosis, rehabilitation and prevention. *Sports Medicine (Auckland, NZ), 21,* 49–72.

91. Wilder, R. P., & Sethi, S. (2004). Overuse injuries: Tendinopathies, stress fractures, compartment syndrome, and shin splints. *Clinical Sports Medicine, 23,* 55–81, vi.

92. Winters, M., Eskes, M., Weir, A., Moen, M. H., Backx, F. J., & Bakker, E. W. (2013). Treatment of medial tibial stress syndrome: A systematic review. *Sports Medicine (Auckland, NZ), 43,* 1315–1333.

93. Dugan, S. A., & Weber, K. M. (2007). Stress fractures and rehabilitation. *Physical Medicine and Rehabilitation Clinics of North America, 18,* 401–416, viii.

94. Loudon, J. K., & Dolphino, M. R. (2010). Use of foot orthoses and calf stretching for individuals with medial tibial stress syndrome. *Foot & Ankle Specialist, 3,* 15–20.

95. Herring, K. M. (2006). A plyometric training model used to augment rehabilitation from tibial fasciitis. *Current Sports Medicine Reports, 5,* 147–154.

96. Thacker, S. B., Gilchrist, J., Stroup, D. F., & Kimsey, C. D. (2002). The prevention of shin splints in sports: A systematic review of literature. *Medicine and Science in Sports and Exercise, 34,* 32–40.

97. Keene, D. J., Williamson, E., Bruce, J., Willett, K., & Lamb, S. E. (2014). Early ankle movement versus immobilization in the postoperative management of ankle fracture in adults: A systematic review and meta-analysis. *Journal of Orthopaedic and Sports Physical Therapy, 44,* 690–701.

98. Simkin, A., Leichter, I., Giladi, M., Stein, M., & Milgrom, C. (1989). Combined effect of foot arch structure and an orthotic device on stress fractures. *Foot & Ankle, 10,* 25–29.

99. Finestone, A., Shlamkovitch, N., Eldad, A., Wosk, J., Laor, A., Danon, Y. L., Milgrom, C. (1991). Risk factors for stress fractures among Israeli infantry recruits. *Military Medicine, 156,* 528–530.

100. Bennell, K. L., Malcolm, S. A., Thomas, S. A., Reid, S. J., Brukner, P. D., Ebeling, P. R., & Wark, J. D. (1996). Risk factors for stress fractures in track and field athletes. A twelve-month prospective study. *American Journal of Sports Medicine, 24,* 810–818.

101. Sullivan, D., Warren, R. F., Pavlov, H., & Kelman, G. (1984). Stress fractures in 51 runners. *Clinical Orthopaedics and Related Research, 187,* 188–192.

102. Dixon, S. J., Creaby, M. W., & Allsopp, A. J. (2006). Comparison of static and dynamic biomechanical measures in military recruits with and without a history of third metatarsal stress fracture. *Clinical Biomechanics (Bristol Avon), 21,* 412–419.

103. Milner, C. E., Hamill, J., & Davis, I. S. (2010). Distinct hip and rearfoot kinematics in female runners with a history of tibial stress fracture. *Journal of Orthopaedic and Sports Physical Therapy, 40,* 59–66.

104. Pohl, M. B., Mullineaux, D. R., Milner, C. E., Hamill, J., & Davis, I. S. (2008). Biomechanical predictors of retrospective tibial stress fractures in runners. *Journal of Biomechanics, 41,* 1160–1165.

105. Armstrong, D. W., Rue, J.-P. H., Wilckens, J. H., & Frassica, F. J. (2004). Stress fracture injury in young military men and women. *Bone, 35,* 806–816.

106. Hoffman, J. R., Chapnik, L., Shamis, A., Givon, U., & Davidson, B. (1999). The effect of leg strength on the incidence of lower extremity overuse injuries during military training. *Military Medicine, 164,* 153–156.

107. Miller, M. D., DeLee, J., & Thompson, S. R. (2014). *DeLee & Drez's orthopaedic sports medicine: Principles and practice.* Philadelphia, PA: Elsevier/Saunders.

Appendix

Special Test Cross-Reference		
Name	Region	Pathology
Acromioclavicular resisted extension test	Shoulder	AC strain/separation[1]
Active compression test (O'Brien)	Shoulder	SLAP lesion, AC strain/separation[2,3]
Adam's forward flexion test	Thoracic/Lumbar spine	Scoliosis[4]
Adson's test	Shoulder	Thoracic outlet syndrome[5-7]
Anterior drawer test	Ankle	Lateral ankle sprain[8]
Anterior drawer test	Knee	ACL tear[9]
Anterior drawer test	Shoulder	Anterior instability[10]
Apley compression and distraction test	Knee	Meniscal tear[11,12]
Apprehension test	Shoulder	Instability[2,10]
Arc sign	Ankle	Achilles tendinopathy[13,14]
Cervical distraction test	Cervical spine	Cervical radiculopathy[15]
Cervical flexion-rotation test	Cervical spine	Cervicogenic headache[16,17]
Compression tests	Knee	Patellofemoral pain syndrome[18]
Costoclavicular test (military bracing test)	Shoulder/UE	Thoracic outlet syndrome[5-7]
Craniocervical flexion test	Cervical spine	Whiplash, cervicogenic headache[19]
Crepitus palpation test	Knee	Patellofemoral pain syndrome, patellofemoral OA[20]
Cross-body adduction stress test	Shoulder	AC strain/separation[1,21]
Crossed straight leg raise test	Lumbar spine	Lumbar radiculopathy[22]
Deep neck flexor endurance test	Cervical spine	Whiplash, cervicogenic headache[23]
Dorsiflexion compression test	Ankle	High ankle sprain[24]
Dorsiflexion maneuver	Ankle	High ankle sprain[24]
Drop arm test	Shoulder	Rotator cuff tear[3,25]
ECU synergy test	Wrist/Hand	Extensor carpi ulnaris tendinopathy[26]
Ege tests	Knee	Meniscal tear[12]
Eichhoff test	Wrist/Hand	de Quervain's tenosynovitis[27]
Elbow flexion test	Elbow	Cubital tunnel syndrome[28]
Ely test	Hip/Knee	Rectus femoris strain, patellofemoral pain syndrome[29]
Empty can test	Shoulder	Impingement syndrome, supraspinatus tear.[2,30,31]
Extension-rotation test	Lumbar spine	Facet DJD[32]
External rotation lag test	Shoulder	Infraspinatus or teres minor tear[25,31]
External rotation test	Ankle	High ankle sprain[33]
FABER test	Hip	OA of hip, SI pathology, FAI, labral tear, GTPS[34,35]
FADIR test	Hip	Piriformis syndrome, FAI, labral tear[36]

Continued

Special Test Cross-Reference—cont'd

Name	Region	Pathology
FAIR test	Hip	Piriformis syndrome, FAI[37]
Finkelstein test	Wrist/Hand	de Quervain's tenosynovitis[38]
Full can test	Shoulder	Impingement syndrome, supraspinatus tear[2,30,31]
Functional activity test	Knee	Patellofemoral pain syndrome[29]
Hawkins test	Shoulder	SAIS[2,3]
Hyperabduction test	Shoulder/UE	Thoracic outlet syndrome[5,6]
Infraspinatus test	Shoulder	Infraspinatus tendonitis/tear[39]
Internal rotation lag test	Shoulder	Rotator cuff tear, esp. subscapularis[25,31,40]
Kim test	Shoulder	Posteroinferior instability or posteroinferior labral tear[3,41]
Kyphosis index using flexicurve ruler	Thoracic spine	Hyperkyphosis[42]
Lachman test	Knee	ACL tear[9]
Lasegue's test	Lumbar spine	Lumbar radiculopathy[22]
McMurray test	Knee	Meniscal tear[11,12,43]
Medial talar tilt stress test	Ankle	Lateral ankle sprain[44,45]
Moving valgus stress test	Elbow	Medial collateral ligament strain[46]
Navicular drop test	Ankle/Foot	Plantar fasciitis, measure of degree of pronation[47]
Neer test	Shoulder	SAIS[2,3]
Noble compression test	Knee	IT band syndrome[48]
Ober and Modified Ober tests	Hip/Knee	GTPS, IT band syndrome[49]
Occiput-to-wall distance	Thoracic spine	Compression fractures, hyperkyphosis[50,51]
Pain-free grip test	Elbow	Medial and lateral epicondylalgia
Painful arc test	Shoulder	SAIS[2]
Passive flexion-extension test	Knee	Patellar tendinopathy[52]
Passive lumbar extension test	Lumbar spine	spondylosis/spondylolisthesis[53]
Patellar tracking test	Knee	Patellofemoral pain syndrome[54]
Phalen's test	Wrist/Hand	Carpal tunnel syndrome[55]
Pivot shift test	Knee	ACL tear[9]
Posterior drawer test	Knee	PCL tear[56]
Posterior drawer test	Shoulder	Posterior shoulder instability[10]
Posterior impingement test	Hip	Labral tear[57]
Posterior sag test	Knee	PCL tear[56]
Q-angle measurement	Knee	Patellofemoral pain syndrome[58,59]
Range of motion, resisted movement, and palpation tests	Temporomandibular joint	TMJ dysfunction
Resisted SLR test (Stinchfield)	Hip	FAI, hip labral tear[35]
Retinaculum tightness test	Knee	Patellofemoral pain syndrome
Reverse pivot shift test	Knee	PCL tear[56]
Rib-to-pelvis distance	Thoracic spine	Compression fracture, hyperkyphosis[60]
Roos test	Shoulder/UE	Thoracic outlet syndrome[5-7]

Special Test Cross-Reference—cont'd

Name	Region	Pathology
Rowe's test	Shoulder	Multidirectional instability[10]
Royal London Hospital test	Ankle	Achilles tendinopathy[14]
Scouring/quadrant test	Hip	OA of hip, labral tears[34,35,61]
Sign of the buttock test	Hip	Ischiogluteal bursitis[62]
Single leg standing test	Hip	GTPS[63]
Slump sit test	Lumbar spine	Lumbar radiculopathy[22]
Speed's test	Shoulder	Bicipital tendonitis, SLAP lesion[64]
Spurling's test	Cervical spine	Cervical radiculopathy[65]
Squeeze test	Ankle	High ankle sprain[33,66]
Standing active quadriceps test	Knee	Patellar tendinopathy[67]
Straight leg raise test	Lumbar spine	Lumbar radiculopathy[22]
Sulcus sign	Shoulder	Inferior instability[10]
Surprise test	Shoulder	Anterior instability[2,10]
Taking off the shoe test	Knee	Hamstring strain[73,74]
Thessaly test	Knee	Meniscal tear[12,43,68,69]
Thomas test	Hip	Hip flexor tightness, iliopsoas syndrome[70]
Thompson test	Ankle	Achilles tendinopathy[13]
Tinel's sign	Ankle	Tarsal tunnel syndrome[71]
Tinel's sign	Elbow	Cubital tunnel syndrome[72]
Tinel's sign	Wrist/Hand	Carpal tunnel syndrome[55]
Trendelenburg sign	Hip	GTPS[75]
Two-stage bicycle test	Lumbar spine	Lumbar stenosis[76]
Two-stage treadmill test	Lumbar spine	Lumbar stenosis[77,78]
Unilateral single heel raise test	Ankle/Foot	Posterior tibialis tendon dysfunction[79]
Unipedal standing balance test	Ankle/Foot	Posterior tibialis tendon dysfunction[80]
Upper cut test	Shoulder	Bicipital tendonitis, SLAP lesion[64]
Upper limb tension test	Cervical spine	Cervical radiculopathy[65]
Valgus stress test	Elbow	Medial collateral ligament strain[46]
Valgus stress test	Knee	Medial collateral ligament strain[81]
Windlass test	Foot	Plantar fasciitis[82]
Wright test	Shoulder/UE	Thoracic outlet syndrome[5-7]

REFERENCES

1. Chronopoulos, E., Kim, T. K., Park, H. B., Ashenbrenner, D., & McFarland, E. G. (2004). Diagnostic value of physical tests for isolated chronic acromioclavicular lesions. *American Journal of Sports Medicine, 32,* 655–661.
2. Hegedus, E. J., Goode, A. P., Cook, C. E., Michener, L., Myer, C. A., Myer, D. M., & Wright, A. A. (2012). Which physical examination tests provide clinicians with the most value when examining the shoulder? Update of a systematic review with meta-analysis of individual tests. *British Journal of Sports Medicine, 46,* 964–978.
3. Cadogan, A., Laslett, M., Hing, W., McNair, P., & Williams, M. (2011). Interexaminer reliability of orthopaedic special tests used in the assessment of shoulder pain. *Manual Therapy, 16,* 131–135.
4. Reamy, B. V., & Slakey, J. B. (2001). Adolescent idiopathic scoliosis: Review and current concepts. *American Family Physician, 64,* 111–116.
5. Nord, K. M., Kapoor, P., Fisher, J., Thomas, G., Sundaram, A., Scott, K., & Kothari, M. J. (2008). False positive rate of thoracic outlet syndrome diagnostic maneuvers. *Electromyography and Clinical Neurophysiology, 48,* 67–74.
6. Novak, C. B., Mackinnon, S. E., & Patterson, G. A. (1993). Evaluation of patients with thoracic outlet syndrome. *Journal of Hand Surgery, 18,* 292–299.

7. Gillard, J., Pérez-Cousin, M., Hachulla, E., Remy, J., Hurtevent, J. F., Vinckier, L., Thévenon, A., et al. (2001). Diagnosing thoracic outlet syndrome: Contribution of provocative tests, ultrasonography, electrophysiology, and helical computed tomography in 48 patients. *Joint Bone Spine, 68,* 416–424.

8. Croy, T., Koppenhaver, S., Saliba, S., & Hertel, J. (2013). Anterior talocrural joint laxity: Diagnostic accuracy of the anterior drawer test of the ankle. *Journal of Orthopaedic and Sports Physical Therapy, 43,* 911–919.

9. Benjaminse, A., Gokeler, A., & van der Schans, C. P. (2006). Clinical diagnosis of an anterior cruciate ligament rupture: A meta-analysis. *Journal of Orthopaedic and Sports Physical Therapy, 36,* 267–288.

10. Eshoj, H., Ingwersen, K. G., Larsen, C. M., Kjaer, B. H., & Juul-Kristensen, B. (2018). Intertester reliability of clinical shoulder instability and laxity tests in subjects with and without self-reported shoulder problems. *BMJ Open, 8,* e018472.

11. Hegedus, E. J., Cook, C., Hasselblad, V., Goode, A., & McCrory, D. C. (2007). Physical examination tests for assessing a torn meniscus in the knee: A systematic review with meta-analysis. *Journal of Orthopaedic and Sports Physical Therapy, 37,* 541–550.

12. Ockert, B., Haasters, F., Polzer, H., Grote, S., Kessler, M. A., Mutschler, W., & Kanz, K. G. (2010). Value of the clinical examination in suspected meniscal injuries. A meta-analysis. *Der Unfallchirurg, 113,* 293–299.

13. Maffulli, N. (1998). The clinical diagnosis of subcutaneous tear of the Achilles tendon. A prospective study in 174 patients. *American Journal of Sports Medicine, 26,* 266–270.

14. Reiman, M., Burgi, C., Strube, E., Prue, K., Ray, K., Elliott, A., & Goode, A. (2014). The utility of clinical measures for the diagnosis of achilles tendon injuries: A systematic review with meta-analysis. *Journal of Athletic Training, 49,* 820–829.

15. Rubinstein, S. M., Pool, J. J. M., van Tulder, M. W., Riphagen, I. I., & de Vet, H. C. W. (2007). A systematic review of the diagnostic accuracy of provocative tests of the neck for diagnosing cervical radiculopathy. *European Spine Journal, 16,* 307–319.

16. Hall, T., Briffa, K., Hopper, D., & Robinson, K. L. (2010). Long-term stability and minimal detectable change of the cervical flexion-rotation test. *Journal of Orthopaedic and Sports Physical Therapy, 40,* 225–229.

17. Ogince, M., Hall, T., Robinson, K., & Blackmore, A. M. (2007). The diagnostic validity of the cervical flexion-rotation test in C1/2-related cervicogenic headache. *Manual Therapy, 12,* 256–262.

18. Cook, C., Mabry, L., Reiman, M. P., & Hegedus, E. J. (2012). Best tests/clinical findings for screening and diagnosis of patellofemoral pain syndrome: A systematic review. *Physiotherapy, 98,* 93–100.

19. Jull, G., & Falla, D. (2016). Does increased superficial neck flexor activity in the craniocervical flexion test reflect reduced deep flexor activity in people with neck pain? *Manual Therapy, 25,* 43–47.

20. Crossley, K. M., Stefanik, J. J., Selfe, J., Collins, N. J., Davis, I. S., Powers, C. M., McConnell, J., et al. (2016). 2016 Patellofemoral pain consensus statement from the 4th International Patellofemoral Pain Research Retreat, Manchester. Part 1: Terminology, definitions, clinical examination, natural history, patellofemoral osteoarthritis and patient-reported outcome measures. *British Journal of Sports Medicine, 50,* 839–843.

21. Krill, M. K., Rosas, S., Kwon, K., Dakkak, A., Nwachukwu, B. U., & McCormick, F. (2018). A concise evidence-based physical examination for diagnosis of acromioclavicular joint pathology: A systematic review. *The Physician and Sportsmedicine, 46,* 98–104.

22. van der Windt, D. A., Simons, E., Riphagen, I. I., Ammendolia, C., Verhagen, A. P., Laslett, M., Devillé, W., et al. (2010). Physical examination for lumbar radiculopathy due to disc herniation in patients with low-back pain. *Cochrane Database of Systematic Reviews, 17,* CD007431.

23. Domenech, M. A., Sizer, P. S., Dedrick, G. S., McGalliard, M. K., & Brismee, J. M. (2011). The deep neck flexor endurance test: Normative data scores in healthy adults. *PM & R: The Journal of Injury, Function, and Rehabilitation, 3,* 105–110.

24. Alonso, A., Khoury, L., & Adams, R. (1998). Clinical tests for ankle syndesmosis injury: Reliability and prediction of return to function. *Journal of Orthopaedic and Sports Physical Therapy, 27,* 276–284.

25. Miller, C. A., Forrester, G. A., & Lewis, J. S. (2008). The validity of the lag signs in diagnosing full-thickness tears of the rotator cuff: A preliminary investigation. *Archives of Physical Medicine and Rehabilitation, 89,* 1162–1168.

26. Ruland, R. T., & Hogan, C. J. (2008). The ECU synergy test: An aid to diagnose ECU tendonitis. *Journal of Hand Surgery [American], 33,* 1777–1782.

27. Elliott, B. G. (1992). Finkelstein's test: A descriptive error that can produce a false positive. *Journal of Hand Surgery [British], 17,* 481–482.

28. Buehler, M. J., & Thayer, D. T. (1988). The elbow flexion test. A clinical test for the cubital tunnel syndrome. *Clinical Orthopaedics and Related Research, 233,* 213–216.

29. Cook, C., Hegedus, E., Hawkins, R., Scovell, F., & Wyland, D. (2010). Diagnostic accuracy and association to disability of clinical test findings associated with patellofemoral pain syndrome. *Physiotherapy Canada, 62,* 17–24.

30. Boettcher, C. E., Ginn, K. A., & Cathers, I. (2009). The 'empty can' and 'full can' tests do not selectively activate supraspinatus. *Journal of Science and Medicine in Sport, 12,* 435–439.

31. Jain, N. B., Luz, J., Higgins, L. D., Dong, Y., Warner, J. J., Matzkin, E., & Katz, J. N. (2017). The diagnostic accuracy of special tests for rotator cuff tear: The ROW cohort study. *American Journal of Physical Medicine and Rehabilitation, 96,* 176–183.

32. Stuber, K., Lerede, C., Kristmanson, K., Sajko, S., & Bruno, P. (2014). The diagnostic accuracy of the Kemp's test: A systematic review. *Journal of the Canadian Chiropractic Association, 58,* 258–267.

33. Sman, A. D., Hiller, C. E., & Refshauge, K. M. (2013). Diagnostic accuracy of clinical tests for diagnosis of ankle syndesmosis injury: A systematic review. *British Journal of Sports Medicine, 47,* 620–628.

34. Sutlive, T. G., Lopez, H. P., Schnitker, D. E., Yawn, S. E., Halle, R. J., Mansfield, L. T., Boyles, R. E., et al. (2008). Development of a clinical prediction rule for diagnosing hip osteoarthritis in individuals with unilateral hip pain. *Journal of Orthopaedic and Sports Physical Therapy, 38,* 542–550.

35. Pacheco-Carrillo, A., & Medina-Porqueres, I. (2016). Physical examination tests for the diagnosis of femoroacetabular impingement. A systematic review. *Physical Therapy in Sport, 21,* 87–93.

36. Reiman, M. P., Goode, A. P., Cook, C. E., Hölmich, P., & Thorborg, K. (2015). Diagnostic accuracy of clinical tests for the diagnosis of hip femoroacetabular impingement/labral tear: A systematic review with meta-analysis. *British Journal of Sports Medicine, 49,* 811.

37. Kean Chen, C., & Nizar, A. J. (2013). Prevalence of piriformis syndrome in chronic low back pain patients. A clinical diagnosis with modified FAIR test. *Pain Practice, 13,* 276–281.

38. Dawson, C., & Mudgal, C. S. (2010). Staged description of the Finkelstein test. *Journal of Hand Surgery [American], 35,* 1513–1515.

39. Boettcher, C. E., Ginn, K. A., & Cathers, I. (2009). Which is the optimal exercise to strengthen supraspinatus? *Medicine and Science in Sports and Exercise, 41,* 1979–1983.

40. Pennock, A. T., Pennington, W. W., Torry, M. R., Decker, M. J., Vaishnav, S. B., Provencher, M. T., Millett, P. J., et al. (2011). The influence of arm and shoulder position on the bear-hug, belly-press, and lift-off tests: An electromyographic study. *American Journal of Sports Medicine, 39,* 2338–2346.

41. Kim, S. H., Park, J. S., Jeong, W. K., & Shin, S. K. (2005). The Kim test: A novel test for posteroinferior labral lesion of the shoulder—a comparison to the jerk test. *American Journal of Sports Medicine, 33,* 1188–1192.

42. Siminoski, K., Warshawski, R. S., Jen, H., & Lee, K. C. (2011). The accuracy of clinical kyphosis examination for detection of thoracic vertebral fractures: Comparison of direct and indirect kyphosis measures. *Journal of Musculoskeletal & Neuronal Interactions, 11,* 249–256.

43. Smith, B. E., Thacker, D., Crewesmith, A., & Hall, M. (2015). Special tests for assessing meniscal tears within the knee: A systematic review and meta-analysis. *Evidence-Based Medicine, 20,* 88–97.

44. Rosen, A. B., Ko, J., & Brown, C. N. (2015). Diagnostic accuracy of instrumented and manual talar tilt tests in chronic ankle instability populations. *Scandinavian Journal of Medicine & Science in Sports, 25,* e214–221.

45. Hertel, J., Denegar, C. R., Monroe, M. M., & Stokes, W. L. (1999). Talocrural and subtalar joint instability after lateral ankle sprain. *Medicine and Science in Sports and Exercise, 31,* 1501–1508.

46. O'Driscoll, S. W. M., Lawton, R. L., & Smith, A. M. (2005). The 'moving valgus stress test' for medial collateral ligament tears of the elbow. *American Journal of Sports Medicine, 33,* 231–239.

47. Picciano, A. M., Rowlands, M. S., & Worrell, T. (1993). Reliability of open and closed kinetic chain subtalar joint neutral positions and navicular drop test. *Journal of Orthopaedic and Sports Physical Therapy, 18,* 553–558.

48. Noble, C. A. (1979). The treatment of iliotibial band friction syndrome. *British Journal of Sports Medicine, 13,* 51–54.

49. Willett, G. M., Keim, S. A., Shostrom, V. K., & Lomneth, C. S. (2016). An anatomic investigation of the Ober test. *American Journal of Sports Medicine, 44,* 696–701.

50. Nair, P., Bohannon, R. W., Devaney, L., Maloney, C., & Romano, A. (2017). Reliability and validity of nonradiologic measures of forward flexed posture in Parkinson disease. *Archives of Physical Medicine and Rehabilitation, 98,* 508–516.

51. Heuft-Dorenbosch, L., Vosse, D., Landewé, R., Spoorenberg, A., Dougados, M., Mielants, H., van der Tempel, H., et al. (2004). Measurement of spinal mobility in ankylosing spondylitis: Comparison of occiput-to-wall and tragus-to-wall distance. *Journal of Rheumatology, 31,* 1779–1784.

52. Calmbach, W. L., & Hutchens, M. (2003). Evaluation of patients presenting with knee pain: Part II. Differential diagnosis. *American Family Physician, 68,* 917–922.

53. Kasai, Y., Morishita, K., Kawakita, E., Kondo, T., & Uchida, A. (2006). A new evaluation method for lumbar spinal instability: Passive lumbar extension test. *Physical Therapy, 86,* 1661–1667.

54. Fredericson, M., & Yoon, K. (2006). Physical examination and patellofemoral pain syndrome. *American Journal of Physical Medicine & Rehabilitation, 85,* 234–243.

55. Valdes, K., & LaStayo, P. (2013). The value of provocative tests for the wrist and elbow: A literature review. *Journal of Hand Therapy, 26,* 32–42; quiz 43.

56. Rubinstein, R. A., Jr, Shelbourne, K. D., McCarroll, J. R., VanMeter, C. D., & Rettig, A. C. (1994). The accuracy of the clinical examination in the setting of posterior cruciate ligament injuries. *American Journal of Sports Medicine, 22,* 550–557.

57. Gómez-Hoyos, J., Martin, R. L., Schröder, R., Palmer, I. J., & Martin, H. D. (2016). Accuracy of 2 clinical tests for ischiofemoral impingement in patients with posterior hip pain and endoscopically confirmed diagnosis. *Arthroscopy, 32,* 1279–1284.

58. Almeida, G. P., Silva, A. P., França, F. J., Magalhães, M. O., Burke, T. N., & Marques, A. P. (2016). Q-angle in patellofemoral pain: Relationship with dynamic knee valgus, hip abductor torque, pain and function. *Revista Brasileira de Ortopedia, 51,* 181–186.

59. Silva Dde, O., Briani, R. V., Pazzinatto, M. F., Gonçalves, A. V., Ferrari, D., Aragão, F. A., & de Azevedo, F. M. (2015). Q-angle static or dynamic measurements, which is the best choice for patellofemoral pain? *Clinical Biomechanics (Bristol, Avon), 30,* 1083–1087.

60. Siminoski, K., Warshawski, R. S., Jen, H., & Lee, K. C. (2003). Accuracy of physical examination using the rib-pelvis distance for detection of lumbar vertebral fractures. *The American Journal of Medicine, 115,* 233–236.

61. Narvani, A. A., Tsiridis, E., Kendall, S., Chaudhuri, R., & Thomas, P. (2003). A preliminary report on prevalence of acetabular labrum tears in sports patients with groin pain. *Knee Surgery, Sports Traumatology, Arthroscopy, 11,* 403–408.

62. Magee, D. J. (2013). *Orthopedic physical assessment.* Philadelphia, PA: Elsevier Health Sciences.

63. Fearon, A., Neeman, T., Smith, P., Scarvell, J., & Cook, J. (2017). Pain, not structural impairments may explain activity limitations in people with gluteal tendinopathy or hip osteoarthritis: A cross sectional study. *Gait & Posture, 52,* 237–243.

64. Ben Kibler, W., Sciascia, A. D., Hester, P., Dome, D., & Jacobs, C. (2009). Clinical utility of traditional and new tests in the diagnosis of biceps tendon injuries and superior labrum anterior and posterior lesions in the shoulder. *American Journal of Sports Medicine, 37,* 1840–1847.

65. Wainner, R. S., Fritz, J. M., Irrgang, J. J., Boninger, M. L., Delitto, A., & Allison, S. (2003). Reliability and diagnostic accuracy of the clinical examination and patient self-report measures for cervical radiculopathy. *Spine, 28,* 52–62.

66. de César, P. C., Avila, E. M., & de Abreu, M. R. (2011). Comparison of magnetic resonance imaging to physical examination for syndesmotic injury after lateral ankle sprain. *Foot & Ankle International, 32,* 1110–1114.

67. Rath, E., Schwarzkopf, R., & Richmond, J. C. (2010). Clinical signs and anatomical correlation of patellar tendinitis. *Indian Journal of Orthopaedics, 44,* 435–437.

68. Goossens, P., Keijsers, E., van Geenen, R. J., Zijta, A., van den Broek, M., Verhagen, A. P., Scholten-Peeters, G. G. (2015). Validity of the Thessaly test in evaluating meniscal tears compared with arthroscopy: A diagnostic accuracy study. *Journal of Orthopaedic and Sports Physical Therapy, 45,* 18–24, B1.

69. Karachalios, T., Hantes, M., Zibis, A. H., Zachos, V., Karantanas, A. H., & Malizos, K. N. (2005). Diagnostic accuracy of a new clinical test (the Thessaly test) for early detection of meniscal tears. *Journal of Bone and Joint Surgery [American], 87,* 955–962.

70. McCarthy, J. C., & Busconi, B. (1995). The role of hip arthroscopy in the diagnosis and treatment of hip disease. *Orthopedics, 18,* 753–756.

71. Oloff, L. M., & Schulhofer, S. D. (1998). Flexor hallucis longus dysfunction. *Journal of Foot and Ankle Surgery, 37,* 101–109.

72. Beekman, R., Schreuder, A. H. C. M. L., Rozeman, C. A. M., Koehler, P. J., & Uitdehaag, B. M. J. (2009). The diagnostic value of provocative clinical tests in ulnar neuropathy at the elbow is marginal. *Journal of Neurology, Neurosurgery, and Psychiatry, 80,* 1369–1374.

73. Zeren, B., & Oztekin, H. H. (2006). A new self-diagnostic test for biceps femoris muscle strains. *Clinical Journal of Sports Medicine, 16,* 166–169.

74. Reiman, M. P., Loudon, J. K., & Goode, A. P. (2013). Diagnostic accuracy of clinical tests for assessment of hamstring injury: A systematic review. *Journal of Orthopaedic and Sports Physical Therapy, 43,* 223–231.

75. Youdas, J. W., Madson, T. J., & Hollman, J. H. (2010). Usefulness of the Trendelenburg test for identification of patients with hip joint osteoarthritis. *Physiotherapy: Theory and Practice, 26,* 184–194.

76. Zanoli, G., Jönsson, B., & Strömqvist, B. (2006). SF-36 scores in degenerative lumbar spine disorders: Analysis of prospective data from 451 patients. *Acta Orthopaedica, 77,* 298–306.

77. Fritz, J. M., Erhard, R. E., Delitto, A., Welch, W. C., & Nowakowski, P. E. (1997). Preliminary results of the use of a two-stage treadmill test as a clinical diagnostic tool in the differential diagnosis of lumbar spinal stenosis. *Journal of Spinal Disorders, 10,* 410–416.

78. Barz, T., Melloh, M., Staub, L., Roeder, C., Lange, J., Smiszek, F. G., Theis, J. C., et al. (2008). The diagnostic value of a treadmill test in predicting lumbar spinal stenosis. *European Spine Journal, 17,* 686–690.

79. Kulig, K., Popovich, J. M., Noceti-Dewit, L. M., Reischl, S. F., & Kim, D. (2011). Women with posterior tibial tendon dysfunction have diminished ankle and hip muscle performance. *Journal of Orthopaedic and Sports Physical Therapy, 41,* 687–694.

80. Kulig, K., Lee, S. P., Reischl, S. F., & Noceti-DeWit, L. (2015). Effect of tibialis posterior tendon dysfunction on unipedal standing balance test. *Foot & Ankle International, 36,* 83–89.

81. Harilainen, A. (1987). Evaluation of knee instability in acute ligamentous injuries. *Annales Chirurgaie Gynaecologiae, 76,* 269–273.

82. De Garceau, D., Dean, D., Requejo, S. M., & Thordarson, D. B. (2003). The association between diagnosis of plantar fasciitis and Windlass test results. *Foot & Ankle International, 24,* 251–255.

Glossary

Abstract: The first paragraph of a research article that provides a brief summary of the study purpose, methods, and findings

Accessory movement: Nonvoluntary movement that occurs between the joint surfaces including rolling, spinning, and sliding. Occurs with physiological movement of the joint

Acromioplasty: Surgical procedure used to decompress the structures underlying the coracoacromial arch that involves removing part of the acromion process

Ala: Projection on either side of the base of the sacrum

Allograft: Tissue graft in which the donor is of the same species but is not the recipient or an identical twin

AMBRI: Acronym to describe shoulder instability that is **A**traumatic, **M**ultidirectional, frequently **B**ilateral, responding to **R**ehabilitation, and, if therapy is not successful, requiring a surgical correction called an **I**nferior capsular shift

Anatomical snuff box: Depression on the posterior hand formed by the scaphoid and trapezium as the base, the tendons of the abductor pollicis longus and extensor pollicis brevis on the lateral side, and the tendon of extensor pollicis longus on the medial side. Tenderness on the floor of the snuff box indicates possible scaphoid fracture. De Quervain's tenosynovitis involves the tendons on the lateral border of the snuff box

Angle of inclination: The angle of the femoral neck with the shaft in the frontal plane. Normal angle of inclination is 120° to 135°

Angle of torsion: The angle of rotation of the femoral head and neck with the femoral shaft in the transverse plane. Normal angle of torsion is 12° to 15°. Abnormal angle of torsion may result in retroversion or anteversion of the hip

Anteversion: A position of increased rotation of the femoral head and neck on the shaft of the femur to more than 25° resulting in increased internal rotation of the lower extremity and in-toeing

Ape hand: Resting appearance of the hand after a median nerve injury in which the thenar eminence is atrophied, the thumb is pulled into the plane of the fingers, and opposition is weakened. The second and third fingers may be pulled into hyperextension at the MCP, and flexion of the IP joints, due to weakness of the lateral two lumbricals

Arthrogenic: Arising from the joint

Arthroplasty: Surgical replacement or reconstruction of a joint

Arthroscope: Surgical instrument through which joint surgery is performed. Several small incisions are used to access the joint

Autograft: Tissue graft in which the donor is the recipient. Often ACL surgery is performed using an autograft of the patient's patellar tendon or hamstring tendon

Avascular necrosis: Death of the bone due to loss of blood flow. Avascular necrosis commonly occurs in the hip as a result of subcapital fracture or dislocation

Avulsion fracture: A fracture of bone that results from ligament or tendon that attaches to the bone pulling off a piece of the bone. This type of fracture is most common at the elbow, hip, and ankle

Axonotmesis: A more severe form of nerve damage than neurapraxia, with injury to some axons. The endoneurium may be intact or partially disrupted. The perineurium and epineurium remain intact, and recovery is possible

Bankart lesion: A detachment of the anterior labrum of the shoulder and the inferior GH ligament that typically results from an anterior shoulder dislocation

Benediction hand: Appearance of the hand after a median nerve injury on attempts to make a fist. Only fourth and fifth digits flex fully, leaving the thumb, second, and third digits extended. Also called Bishop's hand

Bicompartmental: Involving two of the compartments of the knee, often one of the tibiofemoral compartments (medial or lateral) and the patellofemoral compartment

Bimalleolar fracture: A common ankle fracture involving the distal malleolus of the tibia (medial malleolus) and the distal fibular malleolus (lateral malleolus). This is an unstable fracture and requires surgical fixation

Black flags: Policies or rules involving the employee's return to work that impact recovery

Blind: A method used in research that prevents subjects from knowing the group to which they are assigned in order to reduce bias

Blue flags: Perceived work-related factors that impact recovery

Bone mineral density (BMD): Measurement of the density of calcium in bone. Low BMD is called osteopenia or osteoporosis and is associated with risk of fracture

Boxer's fracture: Fracture of the neck of the metacarpal that results when hitting an object with a closed fist. This most commonly involves the fifth metacarpal

Bruxism: Grinding or clenching the teeth, which can lead to TMJ joint dysfunction. This may occur during the day or at night

Capsular pattern: A pattern of joint limitation caused by capsular restriction. Capsular patterns are unique to each joint

Carpal tunnel: Anatomical structure formed by the carpal bones and the transverse carpal ligament. Flexor tendons to the thumb and fingers and the median nerve run through the tunnel into the hand

Carrying angle: The valgus angle formed between the humerus and the ulna, which is generally 5° to 15°

Case series study: A study design in which a group of similar subjects are studied to determine the effects of an intervention. Case series studies have no control group

Case study: A study design that provides an in-depth discussion of one subject's findings

Case-control study: A study design in which subjects with a condition (case subjects) are compared to subjects that appear similar except for the absence of the condition (control subjects) in an attempt to identify contributing factors to the condition

Central sensitization: An amplification of neural signaling within the CNS that elicits pain hypersensitivity

Centralization: Change in location of symptoms of radiculopathy toward the spine that is considered to reflect an improvement in symptoms

Cervical myelopathy: Spinal cord compression in the neck that often results in pain, weakness, and numbness in the arms. The legs may become affected as well

Cervicogenic: Arising from the cervical spine. Cervicogenic headaches, for example, are caused by a pathology of the cervical spine

Clinical practice guidelines: Statements that provide recommendations for best practice that are developed by a systematic review of the literature. CPGs are in the highest tier of evidence

Clinical prediction rule: Criteria that are given weight to mathematically determine likelihood of a condition. Wells criteria for DVT is an example of a clinical prediction rule. Clinical prediction rules help clinical decision making

Closed reduction: Procedure to align bone ends after a fracture that does not require surgery. Closed reduction may be done under a local or general anesthetic

Cluster of tests: A group of special tests that have greater sensitivity or specificity when performed together

Coaptation: Surgically connecting the ends of separated tissue, as in a severed nerve

Cohort study: A longitudinal study design in which subjects that have similar characteristics (for example, medical condition, gender, age) are studied prospectively to determine how differences in the group lead to different outcomes

Collagen fibers: Protein fibers produced by fibroblasts, which are a major component of soft tissue. Collagen fibers provide tensile strength to tissue

Colles' fracture: Fracture of the distal radius with or without the ulna. A Colles' fracture frequently results in a wrist malalignment called a dinner fork deformity

Comminuted fracture: A fracture of bone that involves more than two fragments

Compound fracture: A fracture that involves damage to surrounding tissue as the bone end pierces the skin. Also called an open fracture

Conclusion: The section of a research report in which the author summarizes the study findings

Congenital hypermobility syndrome: A benign, congenital syndrome characterized by increased laxity of ligaments, joint capsules, and intervertebral discs, resulting in increased range of motion and increased risk of joint instability and dislocation

Continuous passive motion (CPM): Intervention in which a limb is positioned in a machine that passively moves the joint through a determined range of motion in one plane. CPM may be used after knee surgery

Control group: The subjects in a research study who receive no intervention. These subjects are used as a comparison group to determine the results of the intervention under study

Coracoacromial arch: Anatomical structure in the shoulder, formed by the coracoid, coracoacromial ligament, and acromion process

Coracoacromial ligament resection: Surgical procedure to decompress the structures underlying the coracoacromial arch by removal of the coracoacromial ligament. This is often accompanied by an acromioplasty

Counternutation: The position of extension of the sacrum in which the base (top) of the sacrum tilts posteriorly

Coxa valga: Abnormal position of the hip that is caused by the angle of inclination between the femoral neck and shaft being greater than 135°. This finding is a component of developmental dysplasia of the hip

Coxa vara: Abnormal position of the hip that is caused by the angle of inclination between the femoral neck and shaft being less than 120°

Crepitus: Crackling or popping sound that may accompany joint movement. This may be an early sign of degenerative changes in a joint

Cubital tunnel: A confined space with the elbow joint capsule as its floor and a ligament as its roof. The ulnar nerve runs through the cubital tunnel

Deep vein thrombosis (DVT): A clot in the deep venous system, which may dislodge and become a pulmonary embolism. Signs of a DVT include pain, swelling, warmth, and redness in the area, but the DVT may be asymptomatic. Wells criteria is a screening tool used for DVT, with a score of 2 or greater indicating DVT is probable

Degenerative joint disease (DJD): Osteoarthritis or wear-and-tear arthritis. DJD most commonly affects weight-bearing joints (hips, knees, and spine) and finger DIP joints. This is the most common type of arthritis

Denervated: The condition of lacking a nerve supply. In the case of a denervated muscle, the loss of the nerve renders the muscle unable to contract intentionally and leads to muscle atrophy

Dermatome: The area of skin that is given its sensation from a single spinal nerve root. Dermatomes are fairly consistent from person to person and thereby provide information on the health of the corresponding nerve root level

Diastasis: Abnormal separation of two parts of the body. Diastasis recti is a condition of separation of the two straps of the rectus abdominis muscle

Directional preference: Finding in patients with neck or back pain that is characterized by decreased symptoms or centralization of symptoms with movement in one direction

Discectomy: Surgical removal of part or all of the intervertebral disc

Discussion: The section of a research report in which the author discusses the findings in the context of the hypothesis

Dislocation: Abnormal position of a joint in which the joint surfaces have lost all contact as one bone has slipped off the other

Distal clavicle excision: Surgical procedure used to decompress the structures underlying the coracoacromial arch in which the distal end of the clavicle is removed leaving the coracoclavicular ligaments intact. May be done in conjunction with acromioplasty and coracoacromial ligament resection

Double-blind: A method used in research that prevents the subject and the investigator from knowing the group to which the subject is assigned in order to reduce bias

Dynamic stability: Stability of a joint or structure that comes from muscle contraction, normal muscle timing, and muscles acting together as force couples

Dyskinesia: Abnormal movement

Dysplasia: Abnormal growth of a tissue. For example, a shallow acetabulum and coxa valgus are found in degenerative hip dysplasia

Effusion: Joint swelling that is an indication of pathology or trauma

Elastic response: Tissue response to stretch that results in a return to the previous length of the tissue. This is the response to a low level of tissue stress

Elastin fibers: Protein fiber that gives soft tissue flexibility. Elastin fibers provide the ability to stretch and return to their original length

Electromyography/nerve conduction velocity (EMG/NCV): A diagnostic test in which needle electrodes are inserted into muscle to hear electrical activity of the muscle (EMG) and inserted into nerves to assess the speed of impulse conduction of a nerve (NCV). This test is used to determine the function of the neuromuscular system

Endoprosthesis: Device that is placed in the body to replace a body part. *Endoprosthesis* is the term for the device used in joint replacement

Epicondylalgia: Pain in the area of an epicondyle of the humerus. This term is used interchangeably with epicondylitis and epicondylosis. It is the most general of the three terms, since it does not presume the presence of tissue degeneration or inflammation

Epicondylitis: Painful inflammation of tendons that attach to an epicondyle of the humerus. This term is used interchangeably with epicondylosis and epicondylalgia

Epicondylosis: Degeneration without inflammation in tendons that attach to an epicondyle of the humerus. This term is used interchangeably with epicondylitis and epicondylalgia

Epidural steroid injection: Medical outpatient procedure in which a steroid is injected into the epidural space near an inflamed nerve root to provide relief of symptoms

Evidence-based practice (EBP): An explicit and formal problem-solving strategy that considers current research in making decisions about patients

Excision: Removal of tissue, often done surgically

Experimental group: The subjects in a research study who receive the intervention. This group is also called the treatment group

Extension bias: Selection of spinal exercises used for patients with a directional preference of extension. These include McKenzie exercises

Extensor expansion: Aponeurosis on the dorsum of the fingers that provides an insertion for the finger extensors, lumbricals, and interossei. Also known as the dorsal hood

External fixation: Surgical method of stabilizing a fracture that involves hardware outside of the body

Extraarticular ligaments: Ligaments that are outside the joint and often are part of the joint capsule. In the knee, the collateral ligaments are extraarticular

Extruded disc: A progression of herniation of a protruded intervertebral disc in which the displacement of the nucleus is greater and the annular rings are likely completely torn through. The disc material remains connected to the disc of origin

Fasciectomy: Partial or complete surgical removal of an area of fascia. Used in treatment of Dupuytren's contracture

Fasciotomy: Cutting of the fascia without removal. Used in treatment of Dupuytren's contracture and compartment syndrome

Flexion bias: Selection of spinal exercises used for patients with a directional preference of flexion

FOOSH: Acronym for fall on an outstretched hand. FOOSH injuries tend to have predictable consequences, which makes this acronym useful

Foraminotomy: Surgical decompression of the spinal nerve root in the neural (intervertebral) foramen

Force couple: Two or more muscles acting in different directions to cause rotation of a joint. For example, in the shoulder, the deltoids and rotator cuff are a force couple to create arm elevation

Forefoot: Part of the bony anatomy of the foot consisting of the metatarsals and phalanges

Forward head posture: Abnormal postural alignment characterized by anterior displacement of the head. Forward head posture positions the lower cervical spine in increased flexion and the upper cervical spine in increased extension

Fracture hematoma: A blood clot that forms at the site of a fracture. Fracture hematoma precedes the formation of a soft callus

Gate theory of pain control: A theory proposed by Melzack and Wall for modulation of pain by stimulation of non-noxious nerve fibers that close a gate on the pain at the spinal cord level

Golgi tendon organ (GTO): Sensory receptor in the proximal tendon that senses tension in the muscle-tendon unit. Stimulation of the GTO is caused by increased tension and results in inhibition of the muscle

Ground substance: Gelatinous matrix that provides nutrition to collagen, elastin, and reticulin fibers in soft tissue

Guyon's canal: An anatomical structure on the anterior aspect of the medial wrist, superior to the transverse carpal ligament, that contains the ulnar nerve. Compression of the ulnar nerve may occur in this space-restricted structure

Hard callus: Bump of bone bridging the area of a fracture that is the result of osteoblasts converting a soft callus to bone

Hemiarthroplasty: Surgical procedure that involves inserting an endoprosthesis on one side of a joint. Hemiarthroplasty is often used to treat subcapital fracture of the hip

Hypothesis: A testable assumption that describes the relationship between two variables

Idiopathic: Having no known cause

In-parallel addition: Addition of sarcomeres primarily as a result of strengthening, in which the muscle fiber becomes thicker

In-series addition: Addition of sarcomeres primarily as a result of stretching, in which the muscle fiber becomes longer

Instability: Tendency to sublux or dislocate, as in the shoulder

Intertrochanteric fracture: Fracture of the hip involving the greater or lesser trochanter. This fracture is usually stabilized by an ORIF

Intraarticular ligaments: Ligaments that are inside the joint. In the knee, the cruciate ligaments are intraarticular

Introduction: The section of a research report in which the author introduces the problem being studied, provides a review of the literature, and states a purpose or hypothesis of the study

Irritability: Degree of sensitivity of the tissues to intervention, measured by the amount of pain after intervention. Reflects the level of inflammation

Kyphoplasty: Medical procedure for compression fracture that includes inflating a balloon in the vertebral body to restore vertebral body height and filling the space with bone cement. Similar to vertebroplasty

Laminectomy: A spinal surgical procedure in which the lamina of one or more vertebrae is removed to provide access to the neural structures

Lateral shift: Postural deviation seen in patients with lumbar HNP in which the patient's shoulders are not directly over the patient's hips. This posture decreases nerve root compression

Ligamentization: The conversion of a tendinous graft used in ACL repair to assume the microscopic properties of a ligament

Literature review: The section of a research report in which the author presents the pertinent literature on the topic being studied. It is part of the introduction and often illuminates the reason for the study

Longitudinal study: A study design that involves repeated observations over a long period of time

Lumbopelvic rhythm: The normal kinematic interplay of motion occurring throughout the lumbar spine and at the hip during forward bending. Normal lumbopelvic rhythm includes movement at the spine and at the hip

Manipulation under anaesthetic (MUA): Movement of a joint through the full range of motion performed while the patient is under a general anaesthetic. This procedure is most often used in the case of frozen shoulder and knee contracture

Meniscectomy: Surgical removal of the meniscal cartilage in a joint. This is a common surgical procedure in the knee

Meta-analysis: A synthesis of research findings that quantitatively integrates the results of multiple studies

Method: The section of a research report in which the author describes the study design, the selection of subjects, the intervention, and the method of data collection

Microfracture: Surgical technique that involves making small holes in the chondral surface of a joint to stimulate healing. This is used most commonly in the knee for articular cartilage defects

Microtearing: Small tears in soft tissue, visible at a microscopic level. The tissue integrity is not compromised

Midfoot: Part of the bony anatomy of the foot consisting of the smaller tarsal bones: the navicular, cuboid, and three cuneiform bones

Minimal clinically important difference (MCID): Statistical analysis that determines the smallest treatment outcome that a patient would perceive as beneficial or important

Mortise: Structure with a groove or slot that accepts an interlocking piece. The ankle joint is a mortise-type joint

Multidirectional instability: Instability in two or, uncommonly, three directions. For example, multidirectional instability of the shoulder often occurs in an anterior and inferior direction

Multiple angle isometrics: A form of isometric exercise in which the patient performs a contraction without moving at various angles throughout the range of motion, generally at intervals of 20° or less. This method of establishing multiple stop points is used to accomplish strengthening throughout the entire available range of motion

Muscle spindle: Sensory receptor in the muscle that senses amount and velocity of changing muscle length. Stimulation of the muscle spindle results in contraction of the muscle, as is seen in reflex testing

Myogenic: Arising from the muscle

Myotome: A group of muscles that are innervated by a single spinal nerve root. Myotomes are fairly consistent from person to person and thereby may be used to provide information on the health of the corresponding nerve root level

Necrotization: The process of death or tissue destruction, as in a ligament graft

Neurapraxia: The least severe form of nerve injury in which the endoneurium remains intact. Full recovery is expected. This may be due to a nerve stretch or compression

Neuritis: Inflammation of a nerve

Neuromatrix: Network of nerves in the brain that generate pain

Neuromatrix theory of pain control: Theory of pain modulation based on the assumption that pain is a decision the brain makes when it determines the person is in danger

Neuropathic pain: Pain that is the result of disease or a lesion of the nervous system

Neuroplasticity: The ability of the nervous system to change in structure or function

Neurotag: The pathways and locations in the brain that are consistently activated by a given sensory input

Neurotmesis: Injury to a nerve in which everything is disrupted except possibly the epineurium. In the most severe cases, the nerve is completely severed. Recovery is not possible without surgical repair

Nocioceptive pain: Pain that is a result of actual or threatened damage to non-nervous tissue

Nociplastic pain: Pain in which changes (plasticity) in central nervous system sensitization appear to be contributing to the chronicity of the symptoms

Nutation: The position of flexion of the sacrum in which the base (top) of the sacrum tilts anteriorly

Occult fracture: Fracture that does not initially show up on x-ray. Signs of fracture, including pain, swelling, and limited ROM are present

One repetition maximum (1 RM): The maximal amount of weight a person can lift one time in a given exercise. On the second attempt to lift the load, fatigue or weakness makes it impossible to lift and maintain a steady contraction with good form. Resistance may be calculated by a percentage of the patient's 1 RM

Open reduction, internal fixation (ORIF): Surgical treatment of a fracture that involves an incision (open) and approximation of bone ends (reduction), followed by stabilization of the fracture with plates, screws, nails, etc. (internal fixation)

Orange flags: Findings of psychiatric illness during patient examination

Orthostatic hypotension: Decrease in blood pressure related to a change to a more upright position. Generally considered a decrease in systolic blood pressure greater than 20 mm Hg within 3 minutes of standing from a sitting or supine position

Osgood-Schlatter's disease: Inflammation of the growth plate at the tibial tuberosity; most common in adolescent athletes due to overuse

Osteoarthritis (OA): Degenerative joint disease or wear-and-tear arthritis. OA most commonly affects weight-bearing joints (hips, knees, and spine) and finger DIP joints. This is the most common type of arthritis

Osteoblast: Cell that creates bone

Osteochondrosis: Orthopedic disease characterized by interrupted blood supply to the bone, followed by necrosis and eventual bone rebuilding. Legg-Calvé-Perthes disease is a type of osteochondrosis

Osteoclast: Cell that absorbs or destroys bone

Osteopenia: Abnormal condition of bone characterized by decreased bone density but to a lesser degree than osteoporosis

Osteophyte: Bone spur associated with degenerative joint disease

Osteoplasty: Surgical reshaping of bone, as in reshaping the femoral neck in femoroacetabular impingement

Osteoporosis: Abnormal condition of bone characterized by decreased bone density that leads to increased risk of fracture

Osteotomy: Surgical removal or reshaping of bone

Paresthesia: Tingling, tickling, pricking, itching, or burning sensation of nerve origin

Paratenon: Outer covering of a tendon that is a loose connective sheath within which the tendon moves freely

Patella alta: Abnormal position of the patella in which it lies higher than normal. May be caused by patellar tendon rupture

Patella baja: Abnormal position of the patella in which it lies lower than normal. Often associated with restricted range of motion, pain, and crepitus. May be a complication after ACL reconstruction with patellar tendon graft

Patellectomy: Surgical removal of part or all of the patella

Periostitis: Inflammation of the periosteum

Peripheralization: Change in location of symptoms of radiculopathy away from the spine and toward the distal extremity that is considered to reflect a decline in status

Perturbation: Effort to disrupt balance; for example, having patient sway to limits of base of support

Physiological movement: Voluntary movement of one bone on another. Occurs with accessory movement within the joint

Plan of care: A result of the physical therapist's examination and evaluation in which the treatment interventions, goals, and precautions are detailed

Plane of the scapula: The plane in which the scapula rests, that is about 30° to 45° forward from the frontal plane toward the sagittal plane

Plastic response: Tissue response to stretch that results in a permanent change in length of the tissue. This is the response to a high level of tissue stress that causes microtearing of the tissues

Posterior elements: Part of the spine excluding the vertebral bodies. The posterior elements include the pedicles, laminae, transverse processes, facet joints, and spinous processes

Power: The ability of the analysis to detect a true effect of an intervention. Power may be increased by the study design or by increasing the number of participants in the study. Meta-analysis increases power by combining multiple studies

Premorbid: Existing prior to a disease or disorder

PRICE approach to treatment: Protection, Rest, Ice, Compression, Elevation. These interventions have been found to be effective in the early stages of tissue healing. Protection may take the form of bracing or splinting and use of assistive devices

Prospective study: A method of study that examines individuals in a group and follows the subjects going forward in time to determine the relationship between an intervention (or cause) and an effect. This type of study is also called a cohort study

Protruded disc: An intervertebral disc that is minimally displaced outside the boundaries of the end plates. The annular rings are likely still intact

Purpose: A statement in the introduction of a research report that provides the reason for conducting the study

p-value: A statistically generated value that provides the likelihood of committing a type I error. If *p* is less than 0.05, there is less than a 5% chance of committing a type I error. There is an inverse relationship between the *p*-value and the statistical strength of the results

Q-angle (quadriceps angle): The angle formed between a line from ASIS to the midpoint of the patella and a line from the midpoint of the patella to the tibial tuberosity. This angle roughly inscribes the path of the quadriceps and is an indicator of the extent of lateral displacing force on the patella. Normal Q-angle is generally considered to be 11° to 13° in males and 15° to 17° in females

Radiculopathy: Pathology of a nerve root often due to compression, which may result in pain, weakness, loss of sensation, tingling, or diminished reflexes in the arm or leg

Randomization: A method of distributing subjects to groups that statistically decreases the differences between the groups

Randomized control trial (RCT): A study design in which subjects are assigned to one of two or more groups. One group is designated as a control group

Ray: Term used in the hand to refer to the metacarpal and phalanges and in the foot to refer to the tarsal, metatarsal, and phalanges. Rays are numbered 1 to 5, with bones of the thumb and great toe numbered as first rays

Rearfoot: Part of the bony anatomy of the foot consisting of the talus and calcaneus. May also be called the hindfoot

Rectus: A Latin word for "straight." This term is used in muscle names (rectus abdominis) and may be applied to a position of a bone or segment, as in calcaneal rectus

Red flags: Signs of a serious pathology that indicate the need to refer the patient to another medical professional

Reflex arc: A nerve pathway that is assessed by eliciting a muscular contraction by a quick stretch of a muscle. Testing of the presence and relative briskness of a reflex may provide information on the health of the corresponding nerve root level

Reliability: The degree to which a test or measure produces the same or similar results under consistent circumstances

Results: The section of a research report in which the author presents the raw data and statistical analysis of the results without a subjective interpretation

Reticulin fibers: A thin collagen fiber found in connective tissue that adds bulk and support

Retrospective study: A method of study of an individual or group in terms of an outcome and that examines, by looking back in time, a likely cause or causes

Retroversion: A position of decreased rotation of the femoral head and neck on the shaft of the femur to less than 8° resulting in increased external rotation of the lower extremity and out-toeing

Rib hump: A physical finding in patients with rotoscoliosis in which the ribs are more prominent on the convex side of the curve. This becomes more apparent with forward bending

Rotoscoliosis: An abnormal curvature of the spine that occurs primarily in the frontal plane, but with a significant degree of vertebral rotation and finding of a rib hump

Sacral promontory: Anterior aspect of the body of the first sacral vertebra

Sarcomere: The contractile unit of a muscle from Z-band to adjacent Z-band

Scaption: Elevation of the arm at the shoulder in the scapular plane. This plane lies 30° to 40° into horizontal adduction from the frontal plane

Scapular stabilizers: The group of muscles that includes upper trapezius, middle trapezius, lower trapezius, serratus anterior, rhomboids, and levator scapulae

Scapulohumeral rhythm: Kinematic relationship seen in shoulder elevation that includes movement of the scapula on the thorax and movement of the humerus on the glenoid. Normal scapulohumeral rhythm is 2° of glenohumeral motion for every 1° of scapulothoracic motion for a total of 120° of motion at the glenohumeral joint and 60° of motion at the scapulothoracic joint

Sclerosis: Hardening of a tissue. In bone, sclerosis is detected on x-ray by increased whiteness and is a finding in arthritis

Scoliosis: An abnormal curvature of the spine that occurs primarily in the frontal plane. Scoliosis has a component of vertebral rotation as well

Screw-home mechanism: Biomechanical occurrence in the knee in which the tibia laterally rotates on the femur at the end range of knee extension, increasing joint congruity

Sensitivity: A measurement of the ability of a test to correctly detect a case

Sequestered disc: A progression of herniation of an extruded intervertebral disc in which a fragment of disc material breaks away and is not attached to the disc of origin. This free-floating mass of disc material can migrate away from the original location

Shoulder abduction relief sign: Finding of decreased radicular arm pain with the arm in full abduction due to decreased stretch on the nerve root

Simple fracture: A fracture that does not break through the skin. Also called a closed fracture

Sliders: A type of nerve exercise that involves sliding or flossing the nerve with little overall change in nerve length

Soft callus: A soft bump bridging the area of a fracture consisting of fibrocartilage produced by fibroblasts and chondrocytes

Special tests: Maneuvers used in physical therapy assessment with results indicative of various pathologies

Specificity: A measurement of the ability of a test to correctly rule out a non-case

Spica: A type of cast that is used to immobilize a joint that involves one very large and one smaller body part. Spica casts may be used to immobilize the hip by spanning the trunk and one or both legs. A thumb spica immobilizes the MCP joint of the thumb

Stabilization exercises: Selection of exercises that increase the stability of a structure. For example, spinal stabilization exercises focus on core strength

Static stability: Stability of a joint or structure that comes from static structures, including bone shape, ligaments, and capsules

Stenosing tenosynovitis: Inflammation and progressive narrowing of the synovial sheath of a tendon

Stenosis: Narrowing or constriction of a passage

Strain: Tissue elongation or deformation due to stress

Stress: An applied load to a tissue

Stress fracture: A type of fracture characterized by small cracks in the bone due to repetitive stress

Subcapital fracture: Fracture of the neck of the femur. This fracture is associated with a high likelihood of avascular necrosis

Subluxation: Abnormal position of a joint in which the joint surfaces have partially lost contact as one bone has slid on the other

Subtalar joint neutral: Reference position of the foot in which the talus is positioned in neither pronation nor supination but is equally palpated on medial and lateral sides. In this position, with the application of slight dorsiflexion, the calcaneus is positioned directly under the talus

Subtrochanteric fracture: Fracture of the femur that occurs below the lesser trochanter

Syndesmosis: Fibrous joint that allows for very little motion. The distal tibiofibular joint is an example of a syndesmosis

Synovial sheath: Outer lining of a tendon that produces synovial fluid to allow the tendon to move freely. Synovial sheaths are found in places where the tendons cross multiple joints, such as in the hand

Systematic review: A synthesis of research findings from multiple studies using a formal protocol

Tarsal tunnel: Structure on the medial side of the ankle formed by the tarsal bones and the flexor retinaculum. Tendons of flexor hallucis longus, flexor digitorum longus, tibialis posterior, and the posterior tibial nerve run through this tunnel. This becomes a site of compression of the posterior tibial nerve

Tendinopathy: An inclusive term used to describe pathologies of the tendon with or without inflammation

Tendinosis: Degenerative changes in the tendon without signs of inflammation

Tendonitis: Inflammation of the tendon, which may lead to degeneration

Tenosynopathy: An inclusive term used to describe pathologies of the tendon and its synovial sheath

Tenosynovitis: Inflammation of the tendon and its synovial sheath

Tensile strength: The ability of a tissue to withstand tension or stress along its length

Tensioners: A type of nerve exercise that involves gently stretching the nerve over the joints resulting in a lengthening of the nerve over the joints and increased neural tension

Therapeutic neuroscience education: Body of education provided to patients that explains pain. This includes the concepts of the neuromatrix theory of pain control and neuroplasticity

Tissue necking: Thinning of tissue due to stress that precedes rupture

Total hip arthroplasty: Surgical replacement of both the acetabular and the femoral portions of the hip joint with an endoprosthesis

Trendelenburg sign/gait, compensated: Trunk lean toward the affected side in stance phase on the affected side caused by pain or by weakness in the hip lateral tilt force couple of either gluteus medius, quadratus lumborum, or both

Trendelenburg sign/gait, uncompensated: Lateral pelvis drop on the unaffected side in swing phase on the unaffected side caused by weakness in the hip lateral tilt force couple of either gluteus medius, quadratus lumborum, or both

Triangular fibrocartilage complex (TFCC): Anatomical structure at the distal end of the ulna consisting of a meniscal cartilage, radioulnar ligaments, and ulnar collateral ligaments. Cushions and stabilizes the distal radioulnar and ulnocarpal joints

Tricompartmental: Involving all three of the compartments of the knee: the medial tibiofemoral compartment, the lateral tibiofemoral compartment, and the patellofemoral compartment

Trimalleolar fracture: A common ankle fracture involving the distal malleolus of the tibia (medial malleolus), the distal fibular malleolus (lateral malleolus), and the posterior tibial malleolus. This is an unstable fracture and requires surgical fixation

TUBS: Acronym to describe shoulder instability that is Traumatic, Unidirectional, causing a Bankart lesion, and usually requiring Surgery to correct

Type I error: An error in which we incorrectly conclude that a relationship exists; a false positive is accepted as true

Type II error: An error in which we incorrectly conclude that no relationship exists; a false negative is accepted as true

Ulnar claw: Resting appearance of the hand after ulnar nerve injury in which the fourth and fifth digits are held in MCP hyperextension, PIP and DIP flexion due to weakness of the medial two lumbricals. This appearance is accentuated on attempts to extend the fingers

Validity: The degree to which the test or instrument is measuring what it is supposed to measure

Vertebroplasty: Medical procedure for compression fracture that includes injecting the vertebral body with bone cement. Similar to kyphoplasty

Volkmann's ischemic contracture: Flexion contracture of the wrist and hand caused by a lack of blood flow to the muscles of the forearm. Supracondylar fracture may lead to a Volkmann's ischemic contracture

Wallerian degeneration: Deterioration of axons that are disconnected from the cell body after a nerve injury. This occurs in the nerve axons distal to the injury

Windlass mechanism: Biomechanical effect of elevation of the medial longitudinal arch of the foot that occurs with extension of the big toe as a result of tension in the plantar fascia

Wrist drop: Weakness in the wrist and finger extensor muscles resulting from a radial nerve lesion. The wrist assumes a flexed position

Yellow flags: Psychosocial factors that impact patient care, including beliefs the patient has about his or her physical problems

Index

Note: Page numbers with f indicate figures; those with t indicate tables; those with b indicate boxes.